QUICK REFERENCE TO

VETERINARY

MEDICINE

SECOND EDITION

QUICK REFERENCE TO

VETERINARY MEDICINE

S E C O N D E D I T I O N

William R. Fenner, D.V. M.

Diplomate, American College of Veterinary Internal Medicine
Associate Professor, Department of Veterinary Clinical Sciences
College of Veterinary Medicine
The Ohio State University
Columbus, Ohio

With 27 Additional Contributors

J.B. Lippincott Company **Philadelphia**
New York London Hagerstown

I dedicate this book to three people:
to my parents for the example that helped me achieve my
  goals,
to Terry for the support, encouragement, and understanding
  that have sustained me.

Acquisitions Editor: Nancy Mullins
Production Manager: Janet Greenwood
Production: P. M. Gordon Associates
Compositor: Bi-Comp, Incorporated
Printer/Binder: R. R. Donnelley & Sons Company

Second Edition

Library of Congress Cataloging-in-Publication Data

Quick reference to veterinary medicine / [edited by] William R. Fenner;
    with 27 additional contributors.—2nd ed.
        p.   cm.
    Includes bibliographical references and index.
    ISBN 0-397-50895-6
    1. Veterinary medicine—Diagnosis—Handbooks, manuals, etc.
2. Veterinary medicine—Handbooks, manuals, etc.   I. Fenner,
William R.   II. Title: Veterinary medicine.
    [DNLM: 1. Animal Diseases—diagnosis—handbooks.   SF 771 Q65]
SF771.Q53   1991
636.089'6075—dc20
DNLM/DLC   90–13699
for Library of Congress   CIP

6 5 4 3 2 1

The authors and publisher have exerted every effort to ensure that drug selection and dosage set forth in this text are in accord with current recommendations and practice at the time of publication. However, in view of ongoing research, changes in government regulations, and the constant flow of information relating to drug therapy and drug reactions, the reader is urged to check the package insert for each drug for any change in indications and dosage and for added warnings and precautions. This is particularly important when the recommended agent is a new or infrequently employed drug.

CONTRIBUTORS

Larry Berkwitt, D.V.M.
Diplomate American College of Veterinary
  Internal Medicine
Staff Internist
Darien Animal Hospital
Darien, Connecticut

John D. Bonagura, D.V.M.
Diplomate American College of Veterinary
  Internal Medicine (Cardiology and Internal
  Medicine)
Department of Veterinary Clinical Sciences
College of Veterinary Medicine
The Ohio State University
The Ohio State University Veterinary Teaching
  Hospital
Columbus, Ohio

Marcia Carothers, D.V.M.
Associate
Internal Medical Referral Practice of Cleveland
Cleveland, Ohio

John S. Cave, D.V.M.
Diplomate American College of Veterinary
  Internal Medicine
Private Practice
Henderson, Kentucky

Dennis J. Chew, D.V.M.
Diplomate American College of Veterinary
  Internal Medicine
Professor
College of Veterinary Medicine
The Ohio State University
The Ohio State University Veterinary Teaching
  Hospital
Columbus, Ohio

C. Guillermo Couto, D.V.M.
Diplomate American College of Veterinary
  Internal Medicine
Department of Veterinary Clinical Sciences
College of Veterinary Medicine
The Ohio State University
Chief, Clinical Oncology Service
The Ohio State University Veterinary Teaching
  Hospital
Columbus, Ohio

Deborah J. Davenport, D.V.M., M.S.
Diplomate American College of Veterinary
  Internal Medicine
Associate in Clinical Nutrition
Mark Morris Associates
Topeka, Kansas

Stephen P. DiBartola, D.V.M.
Diplomate American College of Veterinary
  Internal Medicine
Associate Professor
Department of Veterinary Clinical Sciences
College of Veterinary Medicine
The Ohio State University
Columbus, Ohio

Donna S. Dimski, D.V.M., M.S.
Assistant Professor
Department of Veterinary Clinical Sciences
Louisiana State University
Veterinary Clinician
Veterinary Teaching Hospital and Clinics
Baton Rouge, Louisiana

Roy Fenner, D.V.M.
Private Practice
Port Lavaca, Texas

William R. Fenner, D.V.M.
Diplomate American College of Veterinary
  Internal Medicine (Neurology)
Associate Professor
College of Veterinary Medicine
The Ohio State University
Staff Neurologist
The Ohio State University Veterinary Teaching
  Hospital
Columbus, Ohio

James M. Fingeroth, D.V.M.
Diplomate American College of Veterinary
  Surgeons
Animal Hospital Pittsford
Rochester, New York

Diane F. Gerken, D.V.M., Ph.D.
Diplomate A.B.V.T., A.B.R.
Associate Professor
College of Veterinary Medicine
The Ohio State University
Columbus, Ohio

Alan S. Hammer, D.V.M.
Assistant Professor
Department of Veterinary Clinical Sciences
College of Veterinary Medicine
The Ohio State University
Columbus, Ohio

Bernard Hansen, D.V.M.
Visiting Instructor
North Carolina State University College of
  Veterinary Medicine
Director of Intensive Care
North Carolina State University Veterinary
  Teaching Hospital
Raleigh, North Carolina

Kirk H. Haupt, D.V.M.
Diplomate American College of Veterinary
  Internal Medicine
Cats Exclusive Veterinary Hospital
Edmonds, Washington

Catherine W. Kohn, V.M.D.
Diplomate American College of Veterinary
  Internal Medicine
Associate Professor
Department of Veterinary Clinical Sciences
College of Veterinary Medicine
The Ohio State University
Columbus, Ohio

Kenneth W. Kwochka, D.V.M.
Diplomate American College of Veterinary
  Dermatology
Assistant Professor of Dermatology
Department of Veterinary Clinical Sciences
College of Veterinary Medicine
The Ohio State University
Chief of Dermatology Service
The Ohio State University Veterinary Teaching
  Hospital
Columbus, Ohio

Ronald Lyman, D.V.M.
Diplomate American College of Veterinary
  Internal Medicine
President
The Animal Emergency and Referral Center
Fort Pierce, Florida

William W. Muir III, D.V.M., Ph.D.
Diplomate American College of Veterinary
  Anesthesiology
Diplomate American College of Veterinary
  Emergency and Critical Care
Professor and Chairman
Department of Veterinary Clinical Sciences
College of Veterinary Medicine
The Ohio State University
The Ohio State University Veterinary Teaching
  Hospital
Columbus, Ohio

Keith W. Prasse, D.V.M., Ph.D.
Diplomate American College of Veterinary
  Pathology
Associate Dean
College of Veterinary Medicine
University of Georgia
Athens, Georgia

M. Judith Radin, D.V.M., Ph.D.
Diplomate American College of Veterinary
  Pathology
Assistant Professor
Department of Veterinary Pathobiology
College of Veterinary Medicine
The Ohio State University
Clinical Pathologist
The Ohio State University Veterinary Teaching
  Hospital
Columbus, Ohio

William A. Rogers, D.V.M., M.S.
Diplomate American College of Veterinary
  Internal Medicine
Veterinary Internal Medicine Consultation
  Clinic
Milford, Ohio

Robert G. Sherding, D.V.M.
Diplomate American College of Veterinary
  Internal Medicine
Professor and Head of Small Animal Medicine
Department of Veterinary Clinical Sciences
College of Veterinary Medicine
The Ohio State University
Columbus, Ohio

Justin H. Straus, D.V.M.
Diplomate American College of Veterinary
  Internal Medicine
Staff Internist
Oradell Animal Hospital
Oradell, New Jersey

Margaret S. Swartout, D.V.M.
Internal Medicine Specialty Practice
Knoxville, Tennessee

Patricia D. White, D.V.M., M.S.
Instructor
Department of Veterinary Clinical Sciences
College of Veterinary Medicine
The Ohio State University
Columbus, Ohio

Susan Winston, D.V.M.
Diplomate American College of Veterinary
  Ophthalmologists
Veterinary Ophthalmology Clinic
Norcross, Georgia

PREFACE

The strong positive response to the first edition of this book on the part of practicing veterinarians was both heartwarming and overwhelming. I had hoped to organize a book that would meet your needs and, in large part, you have assured me that my contributors and I were successful. You were also kind enough to offer me advice for improvements in the second edition. After much time and hard work on the part of the contributors and publisher, I am now happy to present this, the second edition of *Quick Reference to Veterinary Medicine*.

This edition, like the first, is designed primarily for veterinarians in practice. It has also turned out to be helpful for senior veterinary students entering the small animal clinics. The format is designed to guide you to a diagnosis, offer you help in choosing a mode of treatment, and provide you with guidelines for locating additional reference material. The book, as before, is in outline form, which means that the coverage of individual topics is not intended to be comprehensive. Instead, the outline promotes both ease and speed of use. The book can be approached either by using the table of contents to find an appropriate chapter and then skimming to the relevant section, or by consulting the index to quickly identify a specific page where information on a problem can be found.

As you will see, the book has some major additions, the two most important being a section on patients with polydipsia and polyuria, as well as a section on the interpretation of biochemical profiles. Polydipsia and polyuria remain among the most common complaints in small animal practice. In addition, they are complex problems to approach diagnostically. The addition of this chapter by Dr. Hansen offers a much needed guide to these patients. The other new chapter is Dr. Radin's discussion of the biochemical profile. Most veterinarians now routinely use biochemical profiles in patient evaluation. Among the most common questions asked on consultation calls is "I have this unexpected laboratory abnormality. What does it mean and where should I go from here?" I believe that this chapter will help you to answer those questions.

In addition to the new chapters, some of the material has been reorganized to make the book easier to use. I have also been lucky not only to keep many of the previous authors, but to add some new ones who have improved the overall quality of the book with their contributions. It has been a privilege to work with all of the contributors to this book. I believe they are not only good veterinarians, but are dedicated to advancing their profession.

As before, there is neither the time nor space to acknowledge all of the people who directly or indirectly contributed to this project. Certainly, Nancy Mullins and all of the people at J. B. Lippincott deserve both thanks for their help and credit for their support and patience. Thanks, too, to all of the veterinarians who took the time to provide encouragement and suggestions. The secretaries who helped prepare the manuscript, both here at OSU and elsewhere, deserve special thanks. I would also like to give credit to my parents, who continue to inspire me with their example. Finally, I would like to thank Terry, who provided support and encouragement, and was willing to give up the time from our life that was needed to complete this project.

I would hope that, as in the past, the veterinarians who use this book will offer suggestions for its improvement. This book is meant for you to use and to be of help to you. It can do that only if you continue to help in its maintenance.

William R. Fenner, D.V.M.

Contents

••

PART ONE

CLINICAL SIGNS AND CLIENT COMPLAINTS

CHAPTER ONE

Shock

William W. Muir III

....

Traditional approaches to the classification of shock either stress the importance of various etiologies, including hemorrhage, trauma, sepsis, allergies, and drug reactions, or emphasize the functional relationship between effective circulating volume, the heart, and peripheral vasculature. The latter rationalization ascribes shock to hypovolemia, cardiac failure, obstruction (high resistance) to blood flow, or distributive (low resistance) to blood flow. Although instructive, these attempts at categorization fall far short of providing the necessary knowledge required for a rational approach to therapy. Rather, an appropriate approach to shock emphasizes the temporal pathophysiologic processes responsible for the circulatory changes that may potentially lead to patient decompensation and death. This chapter defines shock and discusses (1) current thoughts regarding the pathophysiology of shock; (2) circulatory compensation and decompensation; (3) signs and symptoms; (4) the relevance of monitored physiological variables; and (5) the treatment of shock syndromes.

Definition of Shock

1. Shock is a maldistribution of blood flow resulting in inadequate delivery of oxygen and nutrients to tissues. Unevenly distributed microcirculatory blood flow causes ischemia, hypoxia, and acidosis, which disrupt cell function and eventually progress to cell death.

2. Common signs

A. Blood pressure is usually decreased, but can be increased or normal during shock.

B. Blood flow (cardiac output) is usually decreased, but can be increased or normal during shock.

C. Peripheral vascular resistance is usually increased, but can be decreased or normal during shock.

D. Heart rate is usually increased, but can be decreased or normal during shock.

Pathophysiology of Shock

When insulted by ischemia, hypoxia, or acidosis, a variety of host defense responses are initiated, including (but not limited to): (1) activation of the autonomic nervous system; (2) the release of various hormones; (3) activation of the immune system; (4) leukocytic release of microsomal enzymes, proteases, lipases, and oxygen free radicals; (5) activation of the arachidonic acid cascade; and (6) activation of the coagulation complement and kinin systems. The activation of these various processes is the basis for host defense mechanisms; although at times these processes may seem haphazard and diametrically opposed, they represent the body's attempt to protect cellular function and restore tissue perfusion. Extreme responses, however, may backfire, leading to "vicious cycles" and a further deterioration of cellular integrity. An overview of the processes that may occur with shock follows.

1. Increases in autonomic neural activity stimulate cardiac and respiratory centers, causing a variety of other effects.

    A. Increased heart rate

    B. Increased myocardial contractility

    C. Increased arteriolar vasoconstriction

    D. Increased alveolar ventilation

2. Neuroendocrine substances alter cardiovascular reactivity and metabolism.

    A. Catecholamines cause vasoconstriction, hyperglycemia, a reduction in the amount of insulin released, and elevated plasma concentrations of free fatty acids (FFA).

        1) False neurotransmitters (octopamine) are released which interfere with normal vasomotor control.

    B. Glucocorticoids elevate plasma glucose, and potentiate or antagonize vasoactive substances.

    C. Aldosterone enhances sodium and water reabsorption, as well as potassium excretion, and promotes vasoconstriction.

    D. The renin-angiotensin system increases the amount of epinephrine, glucocorticoid, and aldosterone released, enhances sympathetic nerve activity, and constricts blood vessels.

    E. Pancreatic hormones increase blood glucose and protein metabolism.

        1) Glucagon induces hyperglycemia.

        2) Insulin reduces plasma glucose and FFA concentrations.

        3) Insulin resistance and decreased metabolism occur during the late stages of shock attributable to any cause, and during endotoxic shock, resulting in elevated plasma concentrations of glucose and insulin.

    F. Antidiuretic hormone increases peripheral vascular resistance, decreases cardiac output, and causes the renal retention of body fluids.

    G. Adrenocorticotropic hormone increases glucocorticoid synthesis and release.

    H. Opioids (endorphins, enkephalins, and dynorphins) cause pain relief, vasodilation, and hypotension.

    I. Thyrotropin releasing hormone acts as a physiologic opiate and leukotriene antagonist and produces pressor effects.

3. The immune system is frequently activated but may be depressed during shock.

    A. Trauma, hemorrhage, and sepsis temporarily depress reticuloendothelial system phagocytic capacity.

    B. Decreases in plasma fibrinectin are associated with reduced phagocytic capacity and a predisposition to sepsis.

    C. The number of lymphocytes and lymphocytic responses decreases following trauma and sepsis.

    D. The number of antibody-forming cells in the peripheral blood decreases following trauma and sepsis.

    E. Complement activation, triggered by hemorrhage, trauma, and sepsis, has several effects.

        1) Release of peptides active in inflammation

        2) Facilitation of phagocytosis by opsonization

        3) Lysis of invading organisms

        4) Promotion of tissue damage by an attack on cell membranes

        5) Increase in capillary permeability

    F. Complement consumption

        1) Enhances the inflammatory process

        2) Promotes tissue damage

        3) Increases capillary permeability

4. Hypoxia, ischemia, and acidosis activate monocytes, macrophages, and leukocytes which, in turn, trigger a cascade of cellular reactant substances.

    A. Interleukin-1, a product of activated monocytes and macrophages, functions as a hormone-like messenger which

        1) Stimulates fever by initiating prostaglandin synthesis

        2) Stimulates the activation and release of neutrophils

        3) Initiates proteolysis in skeletal muscles

        4) Stimulates insulin and glucagon production

        5) Activates the immune system

    B. Activated leukocytes release lytic enzymes (proteases, lipases) and oxygen free radicals, resulting in

        1) Initiation of the complement cascade

2) Damage to cell membranes by lysosomal enzymes

3) The release of autocoids (histamine, bradykinin, and serotonin)

4) Localized vasoconstriction

5) Increased capillary membrane permeability

5. Arachidonic acid metabolism is activated, producing a number of biologically active cyclo-oxygenase and lipoxygenase products.

A. Prostacyclin relaxes vascular smooth muscle and inhibits platelet aggregation.

B. Thromboxane A_2 constricts vascular smooth muscle, releases lysosomes, and causes platelet and leukocyte activation and aggregation.

C. Leukotrienes, of which slow-reacting substance of anaphylaxis is a member, produce many detrimental effects.

1) Vasoconstriction

2) Bronchoconstriction

3) Increase capillary membrane

6. Cellular damage increases capillary membrane permeability, cardiac depressant, and vasoactive peptides that are responsible for activation of factor XII. Factor XII converts kallikreinogen to kallikrein, bradykinin, and other active peptides, resulting in vasodilation and increased capillary permeability.

A. Factor XII initiates the intrinsic system in the coagulation cascade.

1) Fibrin thrombi are formed, perpetuating hypoxia, acidosis, and tissue damage.

a) Fibrin split products are formed.

b) Thrombocytopenia develops.

c) Hemorrhage occurs.

Compensation and Decompensation

Most compensatory changes are initiated in order to sustain tissue oxygen supply and preserve cellular metabolism.

1. Hemorrhage decreases total blood volume, central blood volume, arterial pressure, cardiac output, and oxygen delivery.

A. Compensatory mechanisms include tachycardia, systemic and pulmonary vasoconstriction, and increased myocardial contractility.

B. Blood flow is preferentially redistributed to the heart, brain, and liver at the expense of the kidney, gut, and skin.

C. With decompensation, arterial pressure and cardiac output continue to decrease until death.

D. Prolonged intense vasoconstriction predisposes the patient to ischemia, hypoxia, and cellular acidosis.

2. Trauma (surgical stress) increases autonomic neural activity which, in turn, stimulates the cardiorespiratory centers.

A. Compensatory mechanisms include tachycardia, increased central blood volume and contractility, and decreased arterial pressure and peripheral vascular resistance.

B. If hypovolemia does not occur, cardiac output increases.

C. Respiratory alkalosis occurs secondary to increased ventilation.

D. The duration and magnitude of the traumatic event determine the onset of various decompensatory events.

1) Unresponsive tachycardia

2) Decreased arterial pressure (<60 mmHg)

3) Decreased cardiac output (<90 mL/kg/min)

4) Activation of neuroendocrine, immune complement, and arachidonic acid systems by cellular breakdown products and sepsis.

3. Cardiogenic shock decreases cardiac output, which activates various neuroendocrine and renal mechanisms designed to restore blood flow.

A. Compensatory mechanisms include tachycardia, vasoconstriction, and increased total and central blood volumes.

B. Peripheral vascular resistance increases.

C. Cardiac decompensation produced by progressive heart failure or an inability of the heart to keep pace with venous return results in tachycardia, arterial hypotension, elevated venous pressures, reduced cardiac output, pulmonary edema, and ascites.

4. Sepsis activates neuroendocrine, immune, arachidonic acid, and complement systems.

A. Compensatory responses include fever, chills, leukocytosis with or without hypotension, and tachycardia. Cardiac contractility and alveolar ventilation are increased.

B. Cardiac output is usually normal or increased, whereas systemic vascular resistance is decreased.

C. The hyperthermic response increases metabolic and circulatory demands.

D. Decompensation, which can take hours or minutes, is an extension of the above-mentioned hyperdynamic state. Progressive increases in tissue oxygen demand and maldistribution of blood flow eventually lead to ischemia, hypoxia, and acidosis.

E. Endotoxin damages endothelial cells and causes the release of vasoactive peptides, resulting in

    1) Activation of the complement cascade

    2) Activation of the coagulation system

    3) Activation of factor XII, producing bradykinin and the release of other autocoids

    4) Activation of the fibrinolytic system

        a) Formation of fibrin split products

        b) Consumption of coagulation factors

        c) Thrombocytopenia

5. Redistribution of body water from plasma, interstitial, and intracellular compartments occurs in response to hemorrhage, trauma, and depletional states.

A. Body fluid shifts following hemorrhage attempt to refill the plasma compartments and cause a delayed reduction in hemoglobin concentration.

B. Inappropriate fluid shifts following trauma, surgery, and depletional states lead to hypovolemia, excessive interstitial water, reduced intracellular water, and increased total body water.

    1) Peripheral edema may occur.

    2) Pulmonary complications are common.

Signs and Symptoms

The signs and symptoms of shock are indicative of exaggerated adrenergic responses, tissue ischemia, hypoxia, and acidosis, as well as the direct effects of circulating harmful and beneficial substances.

1. Acute hemorrhage causes marked activation of the autonomic nervous system; redistribution of blood to the heart, brain, and lung; and a shift of body fluids to the plasma volume.

    A. Depression, fainting

    B. Pale or white mucous membranes

    C. Decreased skin temperature

    D. Prolonged capillary refill time

    E. Tachycardia

    F. Oliguria

    G. Delayed reduction in hemoglobin

2. Severe physical or surgical injury increases autonomic neural activity, which stimulates central cardiac and respiratory centers and activates humoral mechanisms.

    A. History of trauma or surgery

    B. Physical evidence of injury (fractures, lacerations)

    C. Depression, collapse

    D. Signs of hemorrhage

    E. Tachypnea, respiratory distress

3. Heart failure gradually activates the autonomic nervous system, induces retention of electrolytes (Na^+, Cl^-) and water, and activates body neurohumoral mechanisms.

    A. Reduced exercise tolerance, depression or fainting

    B. Pale and cold mucous membranes

    C. Prolonged capillary refill time

    D. Tachycardia and arrhythmias

    E. Weak peripheral pulses

    F. Cardiac murmurs

    G. Oliguria

    H. Pulmonary edema and ascites

4. Localized or systemic infection, with or without bacteremia and endotoxemia, is associated with autonomic activation of the cardiorespiratory centers and the immune, coagulation, complement, and kinin systems, as well as the release of various hormones, prostaglandins, and vasoactive peptides.

A. Depression
B. Fever, chills
C. Warm skin and mucous membranes
D. Normal or red mucous membranes
E. Tachycardia
F. Weak pulses
G. Tachypnea
H. Oliguria
I. Leukocytosis or leukopenia
J. Thrombocytopenia

Monitoring

The purpose of monitoring is to provide vital information that is useful in evaluating patient trends, and to guide the course of therapy. A global approach to monitoring should be utilized, including a detailed medical history and meticulous physical examination supplemented by physiologic, laboratory, and radiographic information. Serial measurements are mandatory.

  1. Circulatory system monitoring should stress tissue perfusion, but must emphasize variables reflecting oxygen transport.
    A. Heart rate
    B. Heart and lung sounds
    C. Pulse pressure measurement
    D. Mucous membrane capillary refill time
    E. Mucous membrane color
    F. Temperature
    G. Packed cell volume and hemoglobin concentration
    H. Blood pressure measurement using
      1) Direct arterial or venous (central venous pressure [CVP]) catheters
      2) Indirect blood pressure cuffs or Doppler devices
    I. Electrocardiogram
    J. Blood gas and pH measurements
      1) Arterial blood gases are indicative of adequate oxygenation and ventilation.
      2) Venous blood gases and pH reflect tissue metabolic status and adequacy of blood flow (cardiac output).
  2. Respiratory system monitoring should evaluate alveolar ventilation and must stress arterial oxygenation.

    A. Mucous membrane color (cyanosis, ashen-grey color)
    B. Respiratory rate
    C. Thoracic radiographs
    D. Effort of breathing (dyspnea)
    E. Tidal volume
      1) Subjectively assessed by re-breathing from a bag (anesthetic machine)
      2) Ventilometer
    F. Blood gases and pH
      1) Arterial blood gases are used to assess oxygenation (Po_2) and ventilation (Pco_2).
  3. Extracellular fluid volume should be assessed continuously to ensure adequate tissue perfusion and to prevent overhydration.
    A. Skin turgor
    B. Mucous membrane color and capillary refill time
    C. Urinary output
    D. Urine sodium concentration
    E. Urine and plasma osmolality
    F. Responses of CVP to a fluid challenge
      1) Sudden increases in CVP (>5 mmHg) with small fluid infusions are indicative of too rapid an infusion rate, overtransfusion, or poor cardiac function.
  4. Laboratory evaluation may provide insights regarding tissue damage, infection, and prognosis.
    A. Hemogram (hematocrit, total protein, platelets)
    B. White cell counts
    C. Electrolytes (Na^+, K^+, Cl^-, Ca^{2+}) and anion gap
    D. Blood urea nitrogen and creatinine to evaluate renal function
    E. Tests of visceral organ damage
      1) Alanine transaminase (ALT) and alkaline phosphatase (ALP) measurements to test for liver damage
      2) Aspartate transaminase and lactic dehydrogenase measurements to test for general tissue damage
      3) Lipase or amylase measurements to test for pancreatic damage
    F. Lactate
      1) Excellent indicator of the severity of tissue acidosis and prognosis (normal value <15 mmol/L)

G. Blood gases and pH (see 2F)
H. Coagulation screening tests
   1) Clotting time
   2) Fibrin split products

Treatment

In general, the initial treatment for shock should be titrated, and should be aimed at correcting hypovolemia secondary to fluid losses or hemorrhage, restoring cardiac function secondary to heart failure, and correcting hypoxemia secondary to airway obstruction or ventilatory failure. Once life-threatening conditions are controlled, the therapeutic goal should then be to improve tissue metabolism by augmenting the compensatory mecha-

nisms that maintain perfusion and oxygen delivery and by eliminating infection. A five-step approach, based on the following order of priorities, should be instituted: (1) ventilation; (2) infusion of blood or fluids; (3) maintenance of cardiac function; (4) drug therapy to restore, maintain, and protect cellular function; and (5) surgical intervention, if necessary (Table 1-1) (see Chapter 9 for a discussion of cardiopulmonary resuscitation).

1. Fluid (crystalloid, colloid, blood) replacement and volume loading are guided initially by measurement of arterial pressures, CVP, heart rate, Hct, and total protein, and subsequently by urine volume and cardiac output.

   A. Balanced (physiologic) electrolyte, sodium-containing, crystalloid replacement

Table 1-1. **Drugs used for the treatment of shock***

Generic Name	Trade Name	Dosage and Route of Administration	Effect
Hypertonic saline (7.5%)	—	4 mL/kg	Cardiovascular support
Sodium bicarbonate	Sodium bicarbonate	.5 mEq/kg IV	Alkalinizing solution
Dextran	Gentra 70 Lomodex 70	10–20 mL/kg/d IV	Decreased platelet aggregation; blood volume expansion
Crystalloid	Lactated Ringer's Acetate Ringer's	20–40 mg/kg IV	Volume replacement
Dexamethasone	Decadron phosphate Dexamethasone sodium phosphate	3–6 mg/kg IV	Membrane stabilization Inhibited release of shock factors
Methyl prednisolone sodium succinate	Solu-Delta-Cortef	15–30 mg/kg IV	Membrane stabilization Inhibited release of shock factors
Lidocaine HCl	Xylocaine HCl	2–4 mg/kg IV (dogs) .5–1 mg/kg IV (cats) 50 μg/kg/min IV	Antiarrhythmic
Procainamide	Pronestyl	5–10 mg/kg IV 50 μg/kg IV	Antiarrhythmic
Nitroprusside	Nipride	.5–1 μg/kg/min IV	Vasodilation
Dopamine Dobutamine	Intropin Dobutrex	5 μg/kg/min IV (to effect)	Inotropes and blood pressure support
Phenylephrine	Neo-Synephrine	.01–.1 mg/kg IV (to effect)	Vasoconstriction
Gentamycin	Gentocin	3 mg/kg IM q6h	Antibiotic
Ampicillin	Omnipen	12–15 mg/kg IV or IM q6h	Antibiotic

* See text for discussion and additional modes of therapy.

solutions (acetate or lactated Ringer's) are used for replacement therapy.

1) Total dose may vary from 20 to 90 mL/kg in the dog and cat.

2) Severe hemorrhage requires rapid volume loading (40 to 90 mL/kg of a crystalloid).

3) The rate or volume of the fluid administered should be limited if CVP exceeds 10 cm H_2O.

4) Mean arterial blood pressure should be maintained at levels exceeding 80 mmHg. Systolic blood pressure should exceed 100 mmHg.

5) Administration of whole blood is indicated when the hemoglobin falls below 7 g/dL or when the Hct falls below 20%.

6) Colloid-containing solutions (Dextran 70) are indicated when total plasma proteins fall below 3.5 g/dL.

a) Dextran 70 is preferred.

b) Hemorrhagic diathesis, hypervolemia, and pulmonary edema are caused by rapid or overadministration of fluids.

7) Known quantities of blood loss are replaced 1:1 with blood or colloids, and 1:3 with crystalloid.

a) Base replacement (HCO_3^-) is indicated if stored blood is used (0.5 mEq/kg).

8) Fluids must be administered cautiously and monitored judiciously in patients demonstrating

a) Cardiac failure

b) Pulmonary disease

c) Gradual increases in CVP (>10 cm H_2O)

d) Renal failure

e) Sepsis

f) Postoperative and post-traumatic effects

B. Hypertonic sodium-containing solutions (7.5%, 2400 mosm/L) and hypertonic saline (7.5%) mixed with colloidal solutions (6% Dextran 70) are excellent for restoring volume and normal hemodynamics.

1) The basic pattern of cardiovascular response includes restoration of mean arterial blood pressure, cardiac output, acid-base equilibrium, and plasma volume expansion.

2) The dose of either solution is 4 mL/kg in the dog and cat.

2. Respiratory care consists of establishing a patent airway, suctioning the endotracheal tube, turning the patient from side to side, administering chest physical therapy, and avoiding fluid overload.

A. Low arterial Po_2 values (<60 mmHg) require elevation of the inspired oxygen concentration to 35% to 40%.

3. Metabolic acidosis is a frequent complication of shock and should be assumed to be present during or following periods of poor perfusion, hypoxia, or both.

A. Sodium bicarbonate is the best source for base replacement therapy.

B. Base replacement should be guided by measurement of venous blood gases and pH levels.

C. The dose of sodium bicarbonate is calculated by the following formula:

$$\begin{aligned}\text{Sodium bicarbonate needed (mEq)}\\= \text{Base deficit (mEq/L)}\\\times 0.3 \times \text{body weight (kg)}\end{aligned}$$

D. Base replacement should not exceed 1.0 mEq/kg/h when plasma pH values are unavailable.

4. Corticosteroids, although controversial, may be useful when used in pharmacologic doses early in septic and traumatic shock. They may not be beneficial in hemorrhagic shock, and may be harmful in cardiogenic shock.

A. Glucocorticosteroids stabilize lysosomal membranes; inhibit prostanoid production by inhibiting phospholipase A_2, thereby limiting activation of the arachidonic cascade; inhibit platelet aggregation; improve oxygen transport in peripheral tissues; and lower pulmonary vascular resistance.

B. When used early in septic shock, glucocorticosteroids, in combination with antibiotics, maximize survival.

C. Dosages of 30 mg/kg of methylprednisolone sodium succinate or 3 to 6 mg/kg of dexamethasone sodium phosphate must be administered for therapy to be effective.

5. Inotropic drugs, such as dopamine hydrochloride and dobutamine hydrochloride, are useful in patients with cardiac failure or reduced ventricular performance, and lidocaine or procainamide hydrochloride are useful in the treatment of ventricular arrhythmias.

A. Dopamine or dobutamine can be used to increase cardiac contractility and cardiac output at dosages of 3 to 5 μg/kg/min.

    1) Excessive dosages cause tachycardia and cardiac arrhythmias.

    2) Hypothermia and acidosis limit the response to catecholamine therapy.

B. Lidocaine and procainamide are usually effective for the acute therapy of ventricular arrhythmias (see Chapter 9 on cardiopulmonary resuscitation).

    1) Lidocaine: 2 to 4 mg/kg intravenously (IV) for dogs, and 0.5 to 1 mg/kg IV for cats, or at infusion rates of 30–60 μg/kg/min

    2) Procainamide: 5 to 10 mg/kg IV for both dogs and cats, administered at a rate of 50 μg/kg/min

6. Vasodilators and vasopressors are considered only after appropriate fluid therapy is administered, acid–base disorders are corrected, and inotropic drugs and other supportive measures have failed to restore circulatory homeostasis.

A. Decreased peripheral vascular resistance will decrease cardiac afterload and may increase cardiac output, tissue perfusion, and venous return.

B. Decreased cardiac afterload and preload may increase cardiac output and decrease pulmonary congestion.

    1) Nitroprusside, 0.5 to 1 μg/kg/min IV

C. Vasopressors are administered after careful patient evaluation and administration of adequate fluid therapy, and then only to maintain mean arterial blood pressure.

    1) Dopamine, > 5 μg/kg/min IV

    2) Phenylephrine hydrochloride, 0.01 to 0.1 mg/kg IV

7. Infection must be treated with appropriate antibiotics and surgical drainage, if required. Sepsis is a major complication following extensive trauma or surgery.

A. Markedly improved survival occurs with administration of glucocorticoid-antibiotic therapy.

B. Therapy should be guided by the results of culture and sensitivity testing.

C. Broad-spectrum antibiotics are preferred.

    1) Gentamicin, 3 mg/kg intramuscularly (IM) q6h

    2) Ampicillin, 12 to 15 mg/kg IV or IM q6h

    3) Alternatively, both of these drugs may be administered concomitantly.

8. Either oral or parenteral nutritional support is required because of the increased metabolic rates in post-traumatic and septic patients.

A. Hypertonic glucose (25%), together with amino acid solution (5.5%), supplies adequate calories and can be administered slowly through a central venous catheter.

    1) The caloric requirement for dogs is 150 kcal/kg/d.

    2) Metabolizable amino acid (TravaSol), 6 g, mixed with 150 kcal of energy (42 g of dextrose)

    3) For short-term (<24 hours) therapy, 1.0 g/kg/h of glucose is adequate.

B. Insulin (.1 to .3 U/g glucose) should be added to prevent hyperglycemia.

9. New therapeutic approaches that counter the progression to irreversible shock are continually being developed. Many produce transient beneficial hemodynamic and blood chemical effects. A decrease in mortality has not been demonstrated consistently.

A. Naloxone hydrochloride inhibits the hypotensive effects of endogenous opioids that are thought to be important in septic shock.

    1) Naloxone, .5 to 1 mg/kg IV

B. Antiprostaglandins may inhibit thromboxane production and improve survival.

    1) Flunixin meglumine, .1 to .3 mg/kg IV

C. Glucagon may restore smooth muscle reactivity to neurotransmitters and catecholamines in patients with septic and cardiogenic shock.

    1) Glucagon, .1 mg/kg IV

Suggested Readings

Muir WW, Bonagura J: Cardiovascular emergencies. In Sherding RG (ed): Medical Emergencies, pp. 37–94. New York, Churchill Livingstone, 1985.

Muir WW, DiBartola SP: Fluid therapy. In: Kirk RW (ed): Current Veterinary Therapy, VIII, pp. 28–40. Philadelphia, WB Saunders, 1983.

CHAPTER TWO

Lymphadenopathy

Alan S. Hammer and C. Guillermo Couto

Because of the dynamic nature of the reticuloendothelial and immunologic systems in animals, the lymph node is a constantly changing entity that responds to its antigenic environment. As such, lymphadenopathy may be the only sign of disease in a patient, and can be associated with a number of diseases ranging from infections to immune-mediated processes to neoplastic lesions. Lymphadenopathy can be a diagnostic aid in confirming and identifying a disease process or it can be a dilemma, depending on the method used to approach the patient. The importance of lymph nodes as antigen processors affords them a primary role in the immune system; indeed, they are one of the main sources of reticuloendothelial and immunologic cells for the body.

1. Lymph node anatomy, histology, and physiology

A. Histologic examination reveals that lymph nodes are composed of a capsule, subcapsular spaces, a cortical area, a paracortical area, and a medulla. Antigenic particles delivered to the node by afferent lymphatics are filtered through the subcapsular, trabecular, and medullary sinuses. In this way, the macrophages lining these sinuses can phagocytize the particles and present them to the lymphoid cells. Occasionally, if the particle burden is large, the macrophages may proliferate, forming clusters of so-called epithelioid cells that resemble undifferentiated metastatic carcinoma.

B. The cortex is composed principally of B lymphocytes arranged in lymphoid follicles. Primary follicles are those with small lymphocytes, whereas clusters of immature lymphocytes and macrophages are termed secondary follicles. The pale central areas of secondary follicles are referred to as germinal centers. The paracortical area is composed primarily of T cells. The medullary cords lie between the reticuloendothelial sinuses, and may be packed with plasma cells during an immune response. Lymph flows from the medulla to the hilar region, where the efferent lymphatics are located.

C. Filtration of lymph occurs as it percolates through the node. Retention of particulate materials on the surface of the macrophages allows for stimulation of antibody production through the interaction of these cells and the B and T lymphocytes. This reaction can be seen in the germinal centers of the secondary follicles and in the medullary area of the node. Lymphocyte trafficking involves mostly T cells and occurs through the postcapillary venules. It is this recirculating lymphocyte pool that accounts for the wide range of immunologic responses of the immune system.

D. The lymph nodes and the anatomic areas they drain in the dog and cat are listed in Table 2-1. The lymphatic pathways listed are among the most common, but structures certainly are not limited to drainage through just those pathways. The nodes most easily palpated in the normal dog and cat are the

Table 2-1. **Anatomical location of lymph nodes and drainage patterns**

Lymph Node	Structures Drained
Parotid	Eyelids and associated glands, external ear, parotid gland
Mandibular	All portions of the head not drained by parotid lymph node, including the oral cavity
Medial and lateral retropharyngeal	Parotid and mandibular lymph nodes, muscles of head and neck, paranasal sinuses, nasal cavity, hyoid apparatus, larynx, pharynx, oral cavity
Superficial cervical (prescapular)	Caudal portion of head, lateral surface of neck, thoracic limb
Deep cervical	Larynx, trachea, esophagus, thyroid
Axillary	Thoracic wall, thoracic limb, cranial end of mammary chain
Sternal	Diaphragm, mediastinum, pleura, thoracic wall, cranial end of mammary chain, pectoral muscles
Mediastinal	Sternal, tracheobronchial, and cervical lymph nodes; mediastinum; esophagus; heart; aorta; vertebrae
Tracheobronchial	Lungs, bronchi, esophagus, trachea, heart, mediastinum
Lumbar aortic	Lumbar vertebrae, adrenal glands, urogenital system
Medial iliac (sublumbar)	Pelvis, pelvic limb, urogenital system, caudal digestive tract, inguinal lymph nodes
Hypogastric	Thigh, pelvis, pelvic viscera, tail, lumbar region
Deep inguinal	Pelvic limb
Hepatic	Stomach, duodenum, pancreas, liver
Splenic	Esophagus, stomach, pancreas, spleen, liver, omentum, diaphragm
Cranial mesenteric	Jejunum, ileum, pancreas
Colic	Ileum, cecum, colon
Gastric	Esophagus, stomach, liver, diaphragm, peritoneum
Pancreaticoduodenal	Duodenum, pancreas, omentum
Popliteal	Pelvic limb
Femoral	Medial side of the pelvic limb
Superficial inguinal	Ventral abdominal wall, caudal mammary chain, prepuce, scrotum, pelvic limb

mandibular, prescapular, axillary, superficial inguinal, and popliteal nodes.

2. Definition of lymphadenopathy

   A. Lymphadenopathy is a change in the size or consistency of a lymph node. The area involved may be solitary, regional, or generalized. The pattern of distribution may be helpful in establishing the possible cause(s) of the lymphadenopathy.

   1) A soft consistency to the node usually indicates abscessation, necrosis, or hemorrhage.

2) Heat and pain may accompany acute inflammation or metastatic neoplasia.

3) A firmer-than-normal consistency is associated with hyperplasia and with infiltrative processes, such as leukemic or other neoplastic infiltrates.

3. Pathogenesis based on histologic and cytologic changes

A. Reactive lymphadenopathy, lymph node hyperplasia, and lymphadenitis

Lymph node enlargement occurs as a result of proliferation of normal cells or infiltration by normal or abnormal cells. Histologically and cytologically, the cell type involved can be useful in defining the type of lymph node pathology and response.

1) If normal lymphoreticular cells proliferate in a node, the term reactive lymphadenopathy is used. This reactive process occurs in response to infectious and immunologic stimuli, and is characterized by an increased number of large lymphocytes, lymphoblasts, plasma cells, and macrophages. This type of reaction can be seen following vaccinations, especially in younger animals.

2) A mild eosinophilic response may be seen in hyperplastic lymph nodes in response to skin diseases and pyoderma; increased numbers of mast cells may also be noticed.

3) If polymorphonuclear leukocytes or macrophages predominate in the lymph node infiltrate, then the term lymphadenitis is used. The lymphadenitis may be suppurative if neutrophils predominate, as in moist juvenile pyoderma (puppy strangles); granulomatous if macrophages are the predominant cell, as seen in fungal infections or diseases caused by the higher bacteria (e.g., Histoplasma, Mycobacterium); or pyogranulomatous if both neutrophils and macrophages are present, as is classically seen in feline infectious peritonitis and blastomycosis.

B. Neoplastic and non-neoplastic infiltrates

Infiltration by abnormal cells can cause lymphadenopathy. Neoplastic cells infiltrating lymph nodes fall into two categories: hemolymphatic and metastatic. Examples of the hemolymphatic neoplasms include lymphoma, acute lymphoblastic leukemia, chronic lymphocytic leukemia, myelocytic leukemia, and mast cell neoplasia. A metastatic infiltrate may be of any cell type (except for hemolymphatic cells), but typical examples include squamous cell carcinoma, mammary adenocarcinoma, oral melanoma, and various sarcomas. A form of non-neoplastic eosinophilic infiltrate occurs in the hypereosinophilic syndrome of cats.

Various causes of lymphadenopathy are listed in Table 2-2. Note that reactive lymphadenopathies and lymphadenitis are grouped together, and that neoplastic infiltrative disorders are listed as a separate category.

4. Evaluation of the patient with lymphadenopathy

In evaluating the patient with lymphadenopathy, it is important to carefully consider the history and physical examination, in addition to the laboratory and cytologic findings.

A. History

1) When evaluating the history, it is useful to keep in mind the animal's geographic location and the places it has visited. For example, Yersinia infections are endemic to the western United States, where they are manifested as sylvatic plague. Travel to the Pacific Northwest may expose the animal to salmon poisoning (*Neorickettsia helminthoeca*). Coccidioidomycosis is most common in the southwestern United States, whereas histoplasmosis and blastomycosis are endemic to the Mississippi and Ohio River Valleys. Certain areas of the southern subtropical United States have been associated with leishmaniasis.

2) Seasonal variations are also important to consider. For example, Rocky Mountain spotted fever occurs primarily in spring and summer.

3) Finally it is always important to question the owner about recent vaccinations and other associated signs, such as cough or diarrhea, which may aid in diagnosis.

B. Physical examination

On physical examination, the distribution pattern of the lymphadenopathy, the palpatory characteristics, and the presence of heat, pain, or fever are important features. The liver and spleen should also be evaluated for enlargement. Periodontal disease and gingivitis

Table 2-2. *Etiologies of lymphadenopathy*

1. Reactive lymphadenopathies, lymphadenitis, and non-neoplastic infiltrative diseases
  A. Infectious
    1) Bacterial
      Corynebacterium sp.
      Brucella canis
      Yersinia pseuodotuberculosis (subsp. *pestis*)
      Actinomyces
      Nocardia
      Mycobacteria
      Localized bacterial infection (periodontal disease, abscess, pyoderma)
      Streptococci (puppy and kitten strangles)
      Staphylococci
      Borrelia burgdorferi
    2) Mycotic
      Histoplasma capsulatum
      Blastomyces dermatitidis
      Coccidioides immitis
      Cryptococcus neoformans
      Sporothrix schenckii
      Candida
      Phaeohyphomyces
      Zygomyces
    3) Algal
      Prototheca
    4) Rickettsial
      Ehrlichia canis
      Neorickettsia helminthoeca
      Rickettsia rickettsii
    5) Parasitic
      Demodex canis
      Trypanosoma cruzi
      Babesia canis
      Leishmania donovani
      Hepatozoon canis
      Toxoplasma gondii
    6) Viral
      Infectious canine hepatitis
      Canine herpesvirus
      Canine viral enteritides
      Feline leukemia virus
      Feline infectious peritonitis
  B. Noninfectious
    1) Postvaccinal
    2) Immune-mediated
      Rheumatoid arthritis
      Polyarthritis (immune-mediated)
      Systemic lupus erythematosus
    3) Localized inflammation
    4) Mast cell infiltrate (non-neoplastic)
    5) Eosinophilic granuloma complex
    6) Hypereosinophilic syndrome
    7) Young animal
    8) Idiopathic
      a) Distinctive peripheral lymph node hyperplasia (secondary to retrovirus infection)
      b) Maine coon cat lymphadenopathy
      c) Plexiform vascularization of lymph nodes

(continued)

Table 2-2. (Continued)

2. Infiltrative lymphadenopathies
   A. Primary hematopoietic neoplasms
      1) Lymphosarcoma
      2) Malignant histiocytosis
      3) Leukemias
         a) Acute lymphoblastic
         b) Chronic lymphocytic
         c) Myelogenous
         d) Erythroleukemia
         e) Megakaryocytic
      4) Multiple myeloma
      5) Systemic mast cell disease
   B. Metastatic neoplasms
      1) Malignant melanoma
      2) Mammary adenocarcinoma
      3) Squamous cell carcinoma
      4) Perirectal adenocarcinoma
      5) Prostatic adenocarcinoma
      6) Primary lung carcinoma
      7) Fibrosarcoma
      8) Osteosarcoma
      9) Mast cell tumor
    10) Other

are important to note if submandibular lymphadenopathy is found. Common etiologies of so-called pseudolymphadenopathy include an excess of fat (most often in the popliteal and prescapular regions), mistaking the inguinal mammary gland for the superficial inguinal lymph node, and mistaking the salivary glands for lymph nodes. The areas draining a lymph node exhibiting solitary lymphadenopathy should be evaluated carefully for any signs of infection, inflammation, or neoplastic process.

   C. Hematologic findings

Hematologic changes in patients with lymphadenopathy can be very specific (e.g., in leukemias) or can be rather nonspecific.

   1) Anemia accompanying lymphadenopathy is commonly nonregenerative and may be attributable to chronic disease in inflammatory, infectious, or neoplastic disorders. Hemoparasitic lymphadenopathy is usually accompanied by regenerative anemia (except in chronic ehrlichiosis). The anemia may also be related to feline leukemia virus (FeLV), in which case an accompanying macrocytosis may be seen, associated with dyserythropoiesis. Finally, the anemia may be attributable to myelophthisis secondary to myeloproliferative diseases or neoplasia metastatic to the bone marrow.

   2) Thrombocytopenia may be seen in ehrlichiosis, Rocky Mountain spotted fever, FeLV infection, sepsis, leukemia, lymphoma, myeloma, and systemic lupus erythematosus.

   3) Leukocytosis is common in patients with lymphadenopathy and is usually an inflammatory neutrophilia with a left shift and monocytosis.

   4) In leukemic patients, circulating blasts may be seen.

   D. Biochemical findings

Biochemical findings of particular interest in patients with lymphadenopathy are hypercalcemia and hyperglobulinemia. Lymphoma and multiple myeloma are the diseases most commonly associated with hypercalcemia and generalized lymphadenopathy in dogs. However, blastomycosis and anal sac adenocarcinoma can also cause hypercalcemia and lymphadenopathy. If a monoclonal gammopathy is detected, in dogs, multiple myeloma, lymphoma, and ehrlichiosis should be suspected; in cats, monoclonal gammopathies occur in association with lymphoma and multiple myeloma. If a polyclonal gammopathy is found, mycotic infections, feline infectious peritonitis, lymphoma, and ehrlichiosis should be investigated as possible causes.

E. Radiographic findings

Radiographic evaluation of patients with lymphadenopathy may reveal sternal and hilar lymphadenopathy, mediastinal masses, hepatosplenomegaly, and iliac lymphadenopathy with ventral deviation of the colon. Further evaluation of the abdomen with ultrasonography may reveal hepatic or splenic changes, and mesenteric, iliac, or aortic lymphadenopathy.

F. Bone marrow findings

Bone marrow aspiration or core biopsies, or both, are indicated if hematologic abnormalities, such as cytopenias or circulating blasts, are present, or if a hematologic neoplasm is suspected. If no obvious cause of hypercalcemia can be found, a bone marrow aspirate may be helpful, as many dogs with lymphoma and hypercalcemia exhibit infiltration of the bone marrow with neoplastic cells.

G. Lymph node cytology

The procedure that is best able to provide significant diagnostic information in patients with lymphadenopathy is percutaneous lymph node aspiration. Using this technique, a diagnosis can be obtained in approximately 90% of the cases. When performing lymph node aspiration, the technique and choice of nodes are important.

1) Procedure for aspiration

The skin overlying peripheral lymph nodes is not usually clipped and scrubbed; however, aspiration of deeper nodes and body cavities does require surgical preparation. Large soft nodes often have necrotic or hemorrhagic centers; therefore, they should not be used for aspirates in a patient with generalized lymphadenopathy. The submandibular nodes usually have a component of reactive lymphadenopathy secondary to periodontal disease which may impair interpretation. A 12- or 20-cc syringe, a 25- or 22-gauge needle, coverslips, and stain are needed. The needle is inserted into the lymph node and 10 to 15 cc of negative pressure is applied two to three times. The needle is redirected several times to evaluate the node thoroughly.

All negative pressure must be released prior to withdrawing the needle or the cells will be aspirated from the hub of the needle into the barrel of the syringe and will be unretrievable for examination. The needle is then removed, the syringe filled with air, and the cells in the hub expelled onto coverslips for pull-smear preparation and staining.

2) Staining

Although there are innumerable staining procedures available, three techniques are commonly used. Wright's staining is probably the best; however, it requires good quality control and a fair amount of practice. There are several types of modified Wright's stain available as kits (Harleco's Diff Quik), and these yield more reproducible results and are easier to use. Lastly, new methylene blue, used as a wet mount on a dried smear, can be also utilized as a stain. It yields different qualitative results and complements the Wright's stain.

3) Cytologic findings

The normal lymph node is composed of 80% to 90% small lymphocytes with occasional macrophages, large lymphocytes, and plasma cells. In comparison, reactive lymph nodes have a higher number of large lymphocytes and immunoblasts, more plasma cells, occasional neutrophils, and mast cells. Lymphadenitis can be classified as suppurative if neutrophils predominate, granulomatous if macrophages are the dominant cell, and pyogranulomatous if there is a mixed population of macrophages and neutrophils. Cells that infiltrate lymph nodes include mast cells, eosinophils, and neoplastic cells, including carcinoma, sarcoma, and melanoma cells. Often, there is little or no lymphoid tissue seen if the tumor has replaced all of the lymph node. Lymphomas are characterized by a monomorphic population of immature lymphoid cells with a high nucleocytoplasmic ratio, multiple nucleoli, vacuolization, and a basophilic cytoplasm. Other myeloproliferative diseases involving the lymph node may resemble lymphomas, requiring further evaluation of peripheral blood and bone marrow to confirm a diagnosis.

H. Lymph node biopsy

    1) Indications

Biopsy samples of a lymph node are extremely helpful in cases in which fine needle aspirates prove to be nondiagnostic. A discussion of histopathology is beyond the purpose of this text, except to mention an example in which biopsy may be more useful than fine needle aspirate. Mast cells can be found occasionally in reactive lymph nodes, but one of the main differential diagnoses would also be regional mast cell tumor. If the lymph node is draining a mast cell tumor, the mast cells will appear in the sinuses and subcapsular spaces. If it is a reactive node, the mast cells will have a different distribution, with cells appearing throughout the node.

    2) Procedure

The biopsy procedure may be an excisional biopsy, a wedge biopsy, or a Tru-Cut biopsy. The advantages of an excisional biopsy are removal of malignant tissue in the case of a neoplasm and the availability of additional tissue to evaluate for architectural changes. The disadvantages are that it is an invasive procedure and involves the loss of one of the "immune barriers." Wedge biopsy, although similarly invasive, does leave some of the lymph node intact. The Tru-Cut biopsy is the least invasive of the three procedures, but is the most likely to miss a focal lesion or to yield insufficient tissue for adequate evaluation of the lymph node architecture.

  5. Selected causes of lymphadenopathy

The following sections briefly describe some of the most important and less common causes of lymphadenopathy. Table 2-3 classifies the various lymphadenopathies by region, cytologic grouping, and etiology.

    A. *Brucella canis* infections are classically associated with fetal resorption and abortion, vaginal discharge, testicular changes, and generalized lymphadenopathy. Discospondylitis can develop, and ocular signs, such as corneal edema and anterior uveitis, may be seen. Diagnosis is based on serologic findings or isolation of the organism.

    B. Juvenile pyoderma, or puppy strangles, can cause severe regional lymphadenitis with suppuration and painful nodes in the facial and cervical regions. A similar condition exists in cats and is caused by a Lancefield group G β hemolytic streptococci. Affected kittens have fever, diarrhea, and cervical lymphadenopathy, which later develops into abscesses.

    C. *Yersinia pseudotuberculosis* (subspecies *pestis*) is a zoonotic disease that is endemic to the southwestern United States rodent population and is manifested as sylvatic plague. In cats exposed to rodents with the disease, severe suppurative lymphadenopathy can occur, along with fever and lethargy. Usually the involved nodes are limited to one region. Diagnosis is based on culture results; patient isolation procedures should be instituted until culture results confirm or refute the tentative diagnosis.

    D. Actinomycosis is usually a localized pyogranulomatous infection of the tissues or body cavities. Effusion is common in the involved body cavities. So-called sulfur granules may be seen in the exudate. Osteomyelitis may be a presenting complaint. Regional lymphadenopathy may develop in the nodes draining the infected areas (e.g., in the sternal or tracheobronchial nodes of dogs with pyothorax).

    E. Nocardiosis may present as fistulous tracts, draining lymph nodes, osteomyelitis, or pyothorax. Multiple sites of infection are common. Again, the lymphadenopathy is confined to regional nodes draining the affected areas.

    F. Clinical signs of mycobacterial infections, including tuberculosis, are reflected by the organ system affected. Tuberculosis is most commonly associated with infected owners transmitting the organism to their pets. Bronchopneumonia, pulmonary nodule formation, and hilar lymphadenopathy are seen in affected dogs, and are associated with a nonproductive cough, fever, anorexia, and lethargy. Cats, which have a higher prevalence of intestinal involvement than do dogs, often exhibit diarrhea, vomiting, weight loss, and mesenteric lymphadenopathy. Various atypical mycobacterial infections of the skin and subcutaneous tissues have been reported in the dog and especially in the cat. Trans-

Table 2-3. **Patterns of lymphadenopathy by etiology**

	Regional	Thoracic	Abdominal	Generalized
Bacterial	Corynebacteria Yersinia Actinomyces Nocardia Mycobacteria Streptococci Staphylococci Borrelia	Actinomyces Nocardia Mycobacteria	Actinomyces Mycobacteria	Brucella Bacterial endocarditis Borrelia
Mycotic	Cryptococcus Sporothrix Zygomyces	Histoplasma Blastomyces Coccidioides	Histoplasma Coccidioides Zygomyces	Histoplasma Blastomyces Coccidioides Cryptococcus
Rickettsia				*Ehrlichia canis* *Rickettsia rickettsii* *Neorickettsia* *helminthoeca*
Parasitic	Demodex			Demodex Trypanosoma Leishmania

Viral		Feline infectious
		  peritonitis
		  (FIP)
			FIP	FIP
				Feline leukemia
				  virus (FeLV)

Noninfectious/
Non-neoplastic
	Localized
	  inflammation
				Vaccinations
				Arthritis
				  (rheumatoid,
				  polyarthritis)
				Systemic lupus
				  erythematosus
				Hypereosinophilic
				  syndrome
				Idiopathic

Neoplastic	Melanoma
	Mammary
	  carcinoma
	Squamous cell
	  carcinoma
	Fibrosarcoma
	Osteosarcoma
	Mast cell tumor
		Mammary
		  carcinoma
		Melanoma
		Lung carcinoma
		Fibrosarcoma
		Osteosarcoma
			Perirectal
			  carcinoma
			Prostatic
			  carcinoma
			Bladder carcinoma
			Intestinal
			  carcinoma
			Mast cell tumor
				Lymphoma
				Leukemias
				Malignant
				  histiocytosis

mission of the disease is thought to occur through soil-contaminated bites, punctures, and scratches.

G. *Blastomyces dermatitidis* is a dimorphic fungus that is disseminated primarily by environmental exposure. It usually affects the lungs, but generalized pyogranulomatous lymphadenitis, osteomyelitis, and skin lesions are also common. Anterior uveitis and chorioretinitis are also commonly seen.

H. *Histoplasma capsulatum* is another dimorphic fungus with specific geographic distribution. The pulmonary form is associated with parenchymal nodules and tracheobronchial lymphadenopathy. Often, the coughing and dyspnea accompanying this disease are secondary to the bronchial compression caused by the reactive hilar nodes. Disseminated histoplasmosis is associated with gastrointestinal (GI) or liver disease, or both. The diarrhea may be primarily large or small bowel in origin, or both. Mesenteric lymphadenopathy and splenomegaly are common. Other less common signs of histoplasmosis include peripheral lymphadenopathy, osteomyelitis, and central nervous system (CNS) and ocular involvement. In contrast to blastomycosis, in which the inflammation is pyogranulomatous, the changes associated with histoplasmosis are primarily granulomatous.

I. Cats with cryptococcosis usually present with upper respiratory signs, such as sneezing, nasal discharge, and chronic nasal masses. There may also be ocular, CNS, or skin involvement. Submandibular lymphadenopathy is common, and occasionally, peripheral lymphadenopathy may occur with widespread infection. In dogs, CNS and ocular signs are the most common presenting signs; mild peripheral lymphadenopathy may be present.

J. *Coccidioides immitis* is a soil organism restricted to the lower Sonoran life zone; it is transmitted mainly by inhalation of the arthrospores. Clinical signs of disseminated coccidioidomycosis are related to the pulmonary disease and may include fever, anorexia, and weight loss. Localized lymphadenopathy is common, but generalized lymphadenopathy occurs infrequently. Cardiac, CNS, and GI infection can also occur. Osteoproductive bone lesions involving primarily the appendicular skeleton may occur. The overlying skin may also be affected, which may help to differentiate this disease from primary bone neoplasms.

K. *Sporothrix schenckii* is a saprophytic soil organism that can be pathogenic when introduced via punctures and wounds. Cases in dogs and cats have involved primarily the skin, although occasional cases of systemic dissemination have been reported.

L. Zygomycoses, previously phycomycoses, are diseases caused by a variety of nonseptate fungal organisms that most often involve the GI tract. Vomiting or diarrhea may occur, and if oral or skin involvement is present, draining tracts with peripheral lymphadenopathy may be evident. Abdominal masses are palpable, and lesions may be detected by a barium GI series.

M. Prototheca is a rare algal organism causing disseminated disease in the dog and cat. Signs include bloody diarrhea, weight loss, blindness, and CNS lesions. Occasionally, cutaneous lesions have been reported.

N. Salmon poisoning is a disease caused by a rickettsial agent, *Neorickettsia helminthoeca*, carried by the trematode *Nanophyetus salmincola.* Three hosts are required in the trematode life cycle: snails, fish, and mammals or birds. Signs of infection become evident five to seven days after eating the fish and include fever, vomiting, diarrhea, and lymphadenopathy. A related disorder, Elokomin fluke fever, has similar clinical signs but is less severe.

O. *Ehrlichia canis* is a tick-borne rickettsial disease with an acute and a chronic phase. Clinically, the acute phase is transient and includes fever, oculonasal discharge, lymphadenopathy, and dyspnea. Thrombocytopenia may be present, and leukocytosis and monocytosis are characteristic. The chronic phase is characterized by a tendency to bleed secondary to thrombocytopenia; depression; weight loss; anemia or other cytopenias; and occasionally, CNS signs secondary to meningitis or hemorrhage. Polyclonal or monoclonal hyperglobulinemia is frequently present.

P. Rocky Mountain spotted fever is another tick-borne rickettsial disease with a seasonal pattern extending from April through September. Fever, anorexia, vomiting, diarrhea, lymphadenopathy, splenomegaly, oculonasal discharge, cough, and muscle or joint tenderness are often present. Petechial and ecchymotic hemorrhages may occur, and the bleeding diathesis may become clinically significant. Anterior uveitis and retinal hemorrhages are also features of this disease. Involvement of the cardiovascular, renal, or neurologic system is the most common cause of death.

Q. *Trypanosoma cruzi* is a hemoparasite transmitted by insect vectors of the Reduviidae family. Also known as Chagas' disease, the clinical signs include tachycardia, ascites, hepatomegaly, and occasionally, lymphadenopathy, diarrhea, and weight loss. Sudden death may also occur. This disease is primarily limited to the Gulf States and Central and South America.

R. Leishmaniasis is another flagellated arthropod-borne protozoan parasite. Dogs with visceral leishmaniasis typically have a history of living in an endemic area, such as near the Mediterranean. Weight loss, lymphadenopathy, and anemia may be evident. Cutaneous lesions commonly accompany this disease.

S. Dogs with demodicosis may have generalized lymphadenopathy due to the presence of deep pyoderma and parasite migration to the lymph nodes. The alopecia, scaling, and folliculitis along with finding the parasite on skin scrapings are diagnostic.

T. The immune-mediated arthritides may be associated with lymphadenopathy. These arthritides can be classified as either erosive or nonerosive. Rheumatoid arthritis is an erosive arthritis that affects primarily small breeds of dogs; the presence of rheumatoid factor in the serum is usually diagnostic. Nonerosive arthritides may be idiopathic, or may be associated with other diseases, such as various infectious diseases, systemic lupus erythematosus (SLE), or inflammatory bowel diseases. Patients with SLE may have renal, hematologic, dermatologic, articular, or neuromuscular abnormalities of immune pathogenesis. Various laboratory tests, such as the direct Coombs test, lupus erythematosus (LE) preparations, antinuclear antibody (ANA) tests, and immunofluorescent evaluation of biopsy material from affected sites, may be needed for diagnosis.

U. The eosinophilic granuloma complex affecting cats has three typical presentations. Eosinophilic ulcers (rodent ulcers) occur on the upper lip and nasal philtrum, eosinophilic plaques appear on the abdominal and flank regions, and linear granulomas occur on the posterior thigh and in the oral cavity.

V. There are reported cases of lymphadenopathy in cats, the pathogenesis and classification of which remain somewhat obscure.

1) The first series of cases involved a distinctive peripheral lymph node hyperplasia similar to that seen in cats with experimental FeLV infection. Most of the cats with clinical disease tested positive for the FeLV antigen. Other clinical signs included fever, lethargy, anorexia, and vomiting. A significant number of cats were anemic, and several were neutropenic.

2) Another series of cases involved young cats with marked generalized lymphadenopathy resembling lymphoma. Half of the cats in the series were Maine Coon cats, and all of the cats tested negative for FeLV antigen. Several histopathologic features of lymphoma were present, including loss of normal nodal architecture and a uniform population of cells in the paracortical areas. However, other features that were present were not compatible with malignant disease, including active germinal centers and a mixed population of cells in the sinuses. Except for the cat that was euthanized on presentation, the other cats had resolution of the lymphadenopathy and were alive 12 to 84 months after the diagnosis, indicating a disease entity distinct from lymphoma.

3) Lastly, plexiform vascularization of solitary cervical or inguinal nodes in cats has been described. Replacement of interfollicular pulp by a plexiform proliferation of small, capillary-sized vascular channels, as well as lymphoid atrophy, has been reported. The affected cats were asymptomatic at the time of presentation, and surgical removal of the affected nodes was followed by an uneventful recovery in most cats.

W. Of the neoplastic lymphadenopathies, the hematopoietic malignant processes are the most likely to cause generalized involvement. Lymphoma is the most common hemolymphatic neoplasm of the dog. In the multicentric form, there is a generalized lymphadenopathy, with nodes three to five times their normal size. Hepatosplenomegaly is a common occurrence, and anterior uveitis may be seen. The diagnosis can often be established on the basis of fine needle aspiration of affected nodes with typical cytologic findings. If there are hematologic changes, such as cytopenias or circulating blasts, other differential diagnoses, such as lymphoblastic leukemia or myelogenous leukemia, must be considered. Currently, treatment for multicentric lymphoma at this institution involves the use of cyclophosphamide, vincristine, cytosine arabinoside, and prednisone. Other forms of lymphoma include alimentary, mediastinal, ocular, CNS, cutaneous, and other extranodal forms.

X. Specific diagnosis of any of the leukemias listed in Table 2-2 requires bone marrow aspiration and, usually, special cytochemical stains. One form of leukemia worthy of note is chronic lymphocytic leukemia. In this disorder, mild peripheral lymphadenopathy is usually present, but fine needle aspirates are not diagnostic since they contain mostly well-differentiated lymphocytes. Diagnosis is based on the elevated numbers of circulating mature lymphocytes and the increased percentage of mature lymphocytes in the bone marrow. These dogs may do well for years with chemotherapy before succumbing to their disease. Occasionally, prolonged survivals are seen in untreated dogs.

Y. Multiple myeloma is a neoplasm of the plasma cells. It may be diagnosed by fulfillment of three of four criteria: monoclonal gammopathy, osteolytic bone lesions, increased numbers of plasma cells in bone marrow aspirates, and presence of Bence Jones proteinuria. Likewise, systemic mast cell disease is diagnosed by fulfillment of two of four criteria: presence of mast cells in liver or spleen, in lymph nodes, in bone marrow, and in peripheral blood or buffy coat smears. The majority of dogs with systemic mastocytosis have cutaneous involvement.

Z. One last hematopoietic neoplasm to consider in patients with lymphadenopathy and concomitant weight loss and anemia is malignant histiocytosis. Bone marrow aspiration supports the diagnosis when atypical, phagocytic histiocytes are noted. Spleen, liver, lungs, and lymph nodes are usually involved.

Suggested Readings

Greene CE: Clinical Microbiology and Infectious Diseases of the Dog and Cat. Philadelphia, WB Saunders Company, 1984

Lucke YM, Davies JD, Wood CM, et al.: Plexiform vascularization of lymph nodes: An unusual but distinctive lymphadenopathy in cats. J Comp Pathol 97: 109, 1987

Mooney SC, Patnaik AK, Hayes AA, et al.: Generalized lymphadenopathy resembling lymphoma in cats: Six cases (1972–1976). J Am Vet Med Assoc 190: 897, 1987

Moore FM, Emerson WE, Cotter SM, et al.: Distinctive peripheral lymph node hyperplasia of young cats. Vet Pathol 23: 386, 1986

Swindle MM, Narayan O, Luzarraga M, et al.: Pathogenesis of contagious streptococcal lymphadenitis in cats. J Am Vet Med Assoc 179: 1208, 1981

CHAPTER THREE

Fever of Unknown Origin

Kirk H. Haupt

A fever of unknown or undetermined origin (FUO) is a continuous, intermittent, or relapsing febrile disorder that remains undiagnosed following routine historical, physical, and laboratory evaluation. Fever is the primary finding in disorders of this kind. Other findings are usually nonspecific. The patient with an FUO typically has a chronic, occult disease process that is difficult to diagnose.

Basic Principles

Thermoregulation

1. Body temperature is controlled by a thermostatic mechanism (thermoregulatory center), located in the anterior hypothalamus, which under normal circumstances regulates the balance between heat gain and heat loss.
2. Changes in ambient and internal temperature are conveyed from peripheral and central thermoreceptors to the thermoregulatory center. In turn, the thermoregulatory center, as dictated by the thermostatic temperature setting or "set-point," initiates the appropriate physiologic responses to cause heat loss or heat gain.
    A. Heat loss is facilitated by cutaneous vasodilation, panting, sweating, a change of posture to increase body surface area (stretching out), and a cool environment. Cats spread saliva over their fur to facilitate heat dissipation.
    B. Heat gain results from heat production (through increased thyroxine and cate-

cholamine activity and shivering) and heat conservation (cutaneous vasoconstriction, piloerection, postural changes to decrease body surface area [e.g., curling up], and seeking a warm environment).

Fever Versus Hyperthermia

Hyperthermia is a general term for the nonspecific elevation of body temperature, whereas fever is a specific type of hyperthermia produced by the action of pyrogens.[14,18] It is important clinically to distinguish between true fever and other forms of hyperthermia, which will be termed nonpyrogenic hyperthermias in this chapter.

1. Fever
    A. True fever is caused by a variety of exogenous pyrogens, including infectious agents and their products, antigen/antibody complexes, antigens (via lymphokines from sensitized lymphocytes), and pharmacologic agents (Fig. 3-1).[7,8]
    B. Exogenous pyrogens do not produce fever directly; rather, they cause the release of endogenous pyrogen from phagocytic cells in the blood (neutrophils, eosinopils, and monocytes) and the tissues (Kupffer cells, alveolar macrophages, splenic sinusoidal cells, peritoneal lining cells, and other fixed macrophages).
    C. This endogenous pyrogen, a small protein, exerts a direct effect on the hypothalamus to reset the body thermostat to a higher set-point.

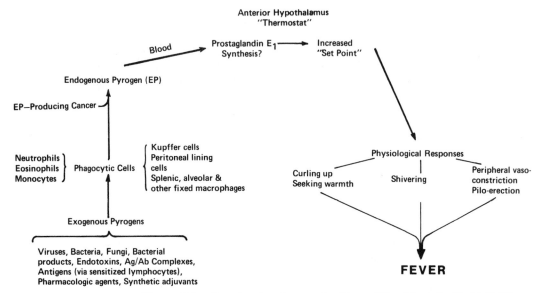

Figure 3-1. *Postulated pathogenesis of fever. (After Dinarello CA, Wolff SM: Pathogenesis of fever in man. N Engl J Med 298:607–612, 1978)*

D. By turning up the thermostat, physiologic responses for heat gain are activated to elevate the body temperature to correspond to the new hypothalamic setting (Figs. 3-1 and 3-2).

E. Endogenous pyrogen has been shown to induce the synthesis of prostaglandin E_1 (PGE_1), and it has been postulated that PGE_1 acts as a central mediator of fever. This is supported by the observation that salicylates

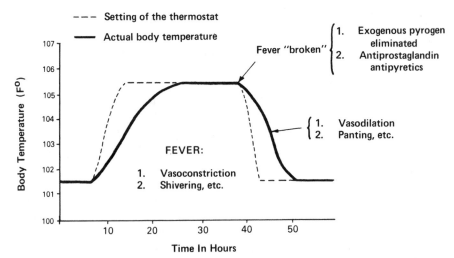

Figure 3-2. *The relationship of thermostat setting to body temperature in fever. (After Guyton CA: Body temperature, temperature regulation, and fever. In Guyton CA: Textbook of Medical Physiology, 4th ed. Philadelphia, WB Saunders, 1971)*

and similar antipyretics block prostaglandin synthesis, thereby lowering the thermostat set-point to reduce fever. Recent studies have downplayed the importance of PGE_2 as a central mediator of fever; this area is currently a subject of open investigation.[4]

F. Elimination of the exogenous pyrogen from the body, with subsequent reduced activity of endogenous pyrogen, causes the thermostat to be reset to a normal body temperature (Fig. 3-3). Physiologic mechanisms for heat loss are activated, allowing the body temperature to return to normal.

2. Nonpyrogenic hyperthermias

A. Nonpyrogenic hyperthermias may result from increased internal heat production (e.g., vigorous muscle contractions during exercise or convulsions) or from exposure to high ambient temperature (e.g., heat stroke). In these situations, the thermostat set-point is adjusted for a normal body temperature, but the physiologic responses to allow a corresponding heat loss are overwhelmed by the excess heat load (see Fig. 3-3). In some instances, the mechanisms for heat loss are depressed or functioning improperly. An example of the latter occurs when animals recovering from general anesthesia are placed on heating pads or in otherwise warm environments. General anesthesia depresses heat-loss mechanisms (particularly panting), predisposing the animal to nonpyrogenic hyperthermia.

B. Rarely, primary damage to the thermoregulatory center (e.g., tumors) will produce a severely impaired or nonfunctioning thermostat, incapable of responding to either hot or cold environments.[18] In these instances, nonpyrogenic hyperthermia may occur following exposure to hot environments.

C. Nonpyrogenic hyperthermias respond only to elimination of the cause, or to physical removal of the excess heat load by whole-body cooling.[17,18]

Etiology

The potential causes of FUO in small animals may be classified under the general headings of infections, immune-mediated disorders, neoplasms, miscellaneous conditions, and undiagnosed FUO.[9,11] (See Table 3-1.)

1. In accordance with the definition of FUO, febrile diseases in which the cause is readily

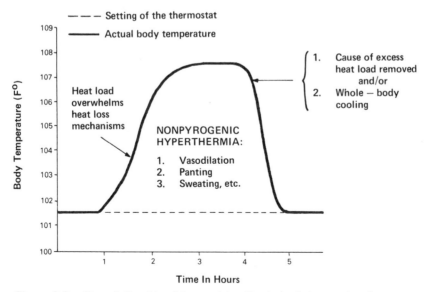

Figure 3-3. *The relationship of thermostat setting to body temperature in nonpyrogenic hyperthermia.*

Table 3-1. **Potential causes of fever of unknown origin (FUO) in small animals**

Infections

Systemic

Feline leukemia virus (FeLV)-related disease (viremia, cancer, secondary infection resulting from immunosuppression, immune complex disease)*

Feline immunodeficiency, virus (FIV)

Feline infectious peritonitis (FIP)*

Septicemia or bacterial endocarditis*

Mycosis (histoplasmosis, blastomycosis, cryptococcosis, coccidioidomycosis, nocardiosis, actinomycosis)*

Toxoplasmosis

Feline upper respiratory disease

Helminth migrations

Canine rickettsial diseases (ehrlichiosis [*Ehrlichia canis*], Rocky Mountain spotted fever [*Richettsia rickettsii*])

Canine hepatozoonosis

Canine Lyme disease (*Borrelia burgdorferi*)

Localized*

Subcutaneous or deep soft tissue abscess or cellulitis

Undetected foreign body at any site (plant awns, porcupine quills, needles, small sticks)

Urogenital tract infection (prostatitis or prostatic abscess, orchitis, pyelonephritis, perirenal abscess, endometritis or pyometra, emphysematous cystitis)

Abdominal infection (peritonitis, hepatic or pancreatic abscess, cholangiohepatitis, sublumbar abscess)

Thoracic infection (pulmonary or mediastinal abscess, pyothorax, pneumonia)

Bone infection (osteomyelitis, discospondylitis)

Central nervous system infection (meningitis, myelitis, encephalitis)

Phlebitis or thrombophlebitis (secondary to the use of intravenous [IV] catheters or caustic drugs)

Urinary catheter-induced infection (pyelonephritis, sepsis)

Postsurgical complication (falciform ligament infection; ovarian and uterine stump infections; postcastration rupture of prostatic abscess; pneumonia; osteomyelitis)

Immune-mediated Disorders

Systemic lupus erythematosus (SLE)

Rheumatoid arthritis (RA)

Idiopathic immune-mediated polyarthritis*

Idiopathic immune-mediated polymyositis*

Neoplasms

Primary fever (visceral lymphoma, leukemias)

Secondary causes

Infection (invasive alimentary and urogenital tract cancers, immunosuppression caused by cancer or cancer therapy)*

Tissue necrosis (hemangiosarcoma)

Functional neoplasms (thyroid tumors, pheochromocytoma)

(continued)

Table 3-1. (Continued)

Miscellaneous

Fictitious fever*

    Excitement or fear

    High ambient temperature or humidity, poor ventilation

    Exercise

    Exaggerated diurnal temperature variation

Drugs

    Tetracycline hydrochloride (in cats)*

    Dinitrophenol (DNP)

    Penicillin, streptomycin, sulfonamides, novobiocin, amphotericin B, quinidine, phenytoin, aspirin.[6,9]

Tissue necrosis or inflammation

    Pulmonary thromboembolism (dirofilariasis, hypoalbuminemia)*

    Torsions (spleen, testicle, uterus)

    Feline steatitis

    Nodular panniculitis

    Postsurgical inflammations (cystotomy urine leaks, falciform ligament necrosis, fractured femur repairs, reactions to catgut sutures)

Endocrine

    Hyperthyroidism (iatrogenic, thyroid tumors)

    Pheochromocytoma

Muscle tremors or tetany

    Hypocalcemia

    Intoxications

Pituitary-hypothalamic lesions (neoplasms, infarcts, trauma, inflammation, post-heat stroke)

Undiagnosed FUO

* Denotes the most common causes of FUO

---

determined by signs or laboratory findings are not considered in this discussion. For example, a bite-wound abscess often results in fever, but the diagnosis is apparent following a routine physical examination. FUO generally is the result of an occult disease.

2. Many cases of FUO are attributable to common diseases but are difficult to diagnose because they present atypically or have nonspecific signs.

3. In rare instances, the "fever" of unknown origin may not be true fever but, instead, a form of nonpyrogenic hyperthermia.

4. In human surveys, the etiologic distribution of FUO is as follows: 40% infections, 20% immune-mediated disorders, 20% neoplasms, 10% undiagnosed FUO.[9] A similar distribution might be expected in veterinary medicine.

Infections

1. Systemic and local infections constitute a large percentage of FUO cases.

2. Systemic infections, especially the FeLV, FIV and FIP viruses, are frequent causes of febrile, occult disease in cats.

3. Hidden, localized infections are a prominent consideration in dogs.

4. In some geographic areas (midwestern and southwestern United States), systemic mycotic infections are a significant cause of FUO.

5. Tick-borne rickettsial diseases that affect dogs have an increased prevalence in some geographic locations.

Immune-mediated Disorders

1. Fever often precedes the onset of other clinical signs in immune-mediated disorders.

2. SLE, RA, and idiopathic, immune-mediated polyarthritis and polymyositis are important considerations.

3. Immune-mediated fevers are recognized less frequently in cats than in dogs.

4. Immune complexes and antigens (via lymphokines from sensitized lymphocytes) act as exogenous pyrogens to cause immune-mediated fever.[2,8]

Neoplasms

1. Occult neoplasia is an important disease to rule out in cases of FUO, particularly in older patients.

2. Fever may occur as a primary response to cancer or as a secondary response to the complications of cancer.

3. Primary fever usually results from immune damage to neoplastic tissues. In some instances, cancer (e.g., lymphomas and renal cell carcinomas in humans) may produce pyrogenic agents with biologic properties similar to endogenous pyrogen (see Fig. 3-1).[7,10]

4. Secondary infection may be the most common cause of fever related to cancer. Infection is a potential complication of occult alimentary and urogenital tract cancers, secondary to destruction of serosal and epithelial barriers to bacterial invasion. Immunosuppression, caused both by malignant neoplasia (especially lymphoreticular and hematopoietic cancer) and by anticancer therapy, also predisposes an animal to infection.

5. Fever may also accompany spontaneous tissue necrosis of occult tumors.

6. Rarely, nonpyrogenic hyperthermia secondary to functional pheochromocytomas and thyroid tumors may present as an FUO (see section on Endocrinologic Hyperthermia in this chapter).

Fictitious Fever

1. Fictitious fever must be differentiated from true fever and other pathologic causes of hyperthermia. Fictitious fever is common in small animals owing to a number of factors that produce benign, nonpyrogenic hyperthermia.

2. Excitement- and fear-induced muscle tremors, cutaneous vasoconstriction, and piloerection cause heat gain, resulting in hyperthermia.

3. High ambient temperatures, increased humidity, and confinement within poorly ventilated enclosures (automobiles, cages) interfere with heat dissipation and produce an excess heat load which, when severe, can lead to heat stroke.

4. Exercise (increased muscle activity) often produces a heat load that exceeds the physiologic capacity to dissipate heat.

5. In normal animals, an exaggerated diurnal variation in body temperature may be confused with fever. Species most active during daylight have a peak temperature in the early afternoon and a low temperature early in the morning; in nocturnal animals, this rhythm may be reversed.[1] Dogs and cats have normal diurnal temperature variations of 37.9°C to 39.9°C (100.2°F to 102.8°F) and 38.1°C to 39.2°C (100.5°F to 102.5°F), respectively.

6. Consider or control for all of these factors when evaluating a patient's temperature critically. Generally, animals with fictitious fever have no other signs of systemic illness.

Drug-induced Hyperthermia

1. Drugs are an uncommon cause of FUO.

2. In cats, the exception is oral tetracycline hydrochloride, which occasionally causes true fever 24 to 48 hours after initial administration. As with most drug fevers, the probable mechanism is hypersensitivity.[2,11]

3. When an overdose of DNP is administered, rapidly fatal hyperthermia may occur as a result of an uncoupling of oxidative phosphorylation, resulting in the release of energy in the form of heat.[13] Because DNP toxicosis produces nonpyrogenic hyperthermia, severe elevations in body temperature will only respond to whole-body cooling. Paradoxically, toxic doses of aspirin can also uncouple oxidative phosphorylation and produce hyperthermia.

Tissue Necrosis and Inflammation

1. Tissue necrosis or inflammation in the absence of infection will occasionally cause FUO.
2. Examples in veterinary medicine include pulmonary thromboembolism, organ torsions, and steatitis in cats fed red tuna.
3. Tissue necrosis and inflammation cause true fever, but the source of the pyrogens is unknown.

Endocrinologic Hyperthermia

1. Hyperendocrinism resulting in nonpyrogenic hyperthermia is an uncommon cause of FUO.[16]
2. Hyperthyroidism associated with functional thyroid tumors and toxic administration of thyroid preparations may cause hyperthermia, presumably by accelerating the basal metabolic rate and increasing heat production.[16] Additional signs in cats with thyroid tumors include polydipsia, polyuria, polyphagia, voluminous stool, weight loss, and tachycardia.
3. Functional pheochromocytomas usually produce very nonspecific signs (weakness, panting, tachycardia, and occasionally, hyperthermia). The excess heat load results from a catacholamine-induced increase in metabolic thermogenesis and impaired heat dissipation secondary to cutaneous vasoconstriction.[16]

Muscle Tremors and Tetany

1. Vigorous muscle contractions produce nonpyrogenic hyperthermia.
2. Hypocalcemic dogs may present with hyperthermia; tetany is the presumed cause.[15]

Pituitary-hypothalamic Lesions

1. Lesions involving the thermoregulatory center in the anterior hypothalamus are rare.
2. Damage to the body's "thermostat" results in an inability to respond to hot or cold environments. Thus, nonpyrogenic hyperthermia or hypothermia may occur.

Diagnosis

1. Avoid launching into an extensive work-up of fever without first ruling out the most common, self-limiting viral and bacterial infections, or fictitious fever. Multiple temperature readings may be necessary to establish that hyperthermia is, in fact, a real finding.
2. FUO is potentially one of the most challenging diagnostic problems in veterinary medicine. The cardinal rule is to investigate every clue thoroughly, regardless of how subtle or insignificant it may seem.

History

1. Evaluate the history of the animal with the potential causes of FUO in mind. Valuable clues are sometimes seemingly minor historical points.
2. Consider the signalment—in particular, the age (occult neoplasia) and sex (genital-tract disease)—of the animal.
3. Ask appropriate questions to review each organ system; this may help to localize the disease process.
4. Specific questions should elicit the following historical information:
    A. History of previous wounds or injuries of infectious disease (predisposing the animal to local or systemic infections)
    B. Past and current geographic locations (systemic mycosis, dirofilariasis, rickettsial diseases)
    C. Exposure to other animals (communicable disease)
    D. Previous illnesses or death in the household (FeLV-related disease, FIP)
    E. Reproductive history (metritis)

F. Previous surgery (postsurgical, IV therapy, and urinary catheter complications; metastatic cancer)

G. Current drug therapy (drug fever)

H. Diet (steatitis)

5. The animal's response to a previous drug regimen may be useful information. For example, temporary or partial improvement while on antibiotics suggests a complicated bacterial infection.

Physical Examination

1. Repeated, thorough physical examinations often uncover previously overlooked or new abnormalities that develop as the disease progresses.

2. Careful inspection for the following physical findings may aid in the diagnosis:

A. Local areas of pain or swelling (especially muscle, joints, spine, kidneys, prostate, testicles, and abdomen)

B. Organomegaly (owing to neoplasia, mycotic disease, immune-mediated disorders, local bacterial infection)

C. Lymph node enlargement (local bacterial infection, metastatic neoplasia, mycotic disease, lymphosarcoma)

D. Previously undetected heart murmur (bacterial endocarditis)

E. Ocular manifestations of systemic disease (systemic mycosis, FeLV-related disease, FIP, canine distemper, toxoplasmosis, lymphosarcoma, metastatic neoplasia)

3. The magnitude of temperature elevation may be an important clue. In human medicine, true fevers rarely exceed 41.1°C (106°F);[3] in small animal medicine, this ceiling is probably around 41.6°C (107°F). Temperatures greater than 107°F are probably attributable to nonpyrogenic hyperthermia or fever with superimposed nonpyrogenic hyperthermia (such as occurs with convulsions). Fever curves are used to characterize febrile conditions as continuous, intermittent, remittent, or relapsing. They rarely correlate to a specific etiology, and are of little value in the diagnosis of FUO.[2]

Diagnostic Approach

1. The diagnostic approach for FUO varies according to the signalment, history, physical examination, and geographic area.

2. Table 3-2 summarizes the potentially useful procedures for diagnosing an FUO. "Starting Point in the FUO Work-up" lists those tests routinely performed in our hospital at the start of the work-up.

3. Serial hemograms are helpful in detecting the presence, severity, and progression of an inflammatory process in the body. True fevers, resulting from inflammation, are often accompanied by an immature neutrophilia. Mild to moderate nonregenerative anemias are frequently associated with chronic inflammatory disease and malignant disease. Rarely, a specific disease process may be detected (e.g., leukemia).

4. A complete biochemical profile may aid in localizing the disease process to an organ system.

5. Multiple urinalyses are useful in screening for urinary tract infections.

Table 3-2. **Diagnostic procedures for fever of unknown origin (FUO)**

Evaluation Techniques

Blood tests

    Serial hemograms

    FeLV (indirect fluorescent antibody) test

    Complete biochemical profile

    Serology—FeLV-ELISA, FIV, FIP, toxoplasmosis, histoplasmosis, blastomycosis, coccidioides, cryptococcosis, *Ehrlichia canis, Rickettsia rickettsii, Borrelia burgdorferi,* titers.

    Immune tests—lupus erythematosus (LE) cell preparation, antinuclear antibody (ANA) titer, Coombs' test, rheumatoid factor (RF)

    Serum protein electrophoresis

    Serum thyroxine (T_4) and triiodothyronine (T_3)

Urinalysis

Parasitology

    Fecal flotation and saline preparation

    Microfilaria tests

(continued)

Table 3-2. (Continued)

Cytology
    Lymph node aspirates
    Samples from arthrocentesis in multiple joints
    Bone marrow biopsy specimens
    Cerebrospinal fluid (CSF)
    Prostatic fluid or semen
    Body cavity specimens
    Masses
Culture and sensitivities
    Blood
    Bone marrow
    Urine
    Prostatic fluid or semen
    CSF
    Joints
    Areas of local involvement
Roentgenography
    Scout films of thorax and abdomen
    Contrast roentgenography
    Skeletal survey for osteolytic lesions
Miscellaneous
    Biopsy of masses, lymph node, muscle, joint
    Endoscopy, bronchoscopy, proctoscopy, laparoscopy
    Exploratory surgery—laparotomy, thoracotomy
Therapeutic trials
    Antibiotics
    Antiprostaglandin antipyretics
    Immunosuppression with corticosteroids, cytotoxic drugs

Starting Point in the FUO Work-up
General
    Hemogram
    Complete biochemical profile
    Urinalysis
    Scout films of thorax and abdomen
Canine
    Blood cultures
    Immune tests—LE cell preparation, ANA titer, Coombs' test, and RF
Feline
    FeLV (fluorescent antibody) test
    Serology—FeLV, FIV, FIP and toxoplasmosis titers

6. Scout roentgenograms of the thorax and abdomen are helpful in detecting localized disease in the body cavities or adjacent bony structures.

7. Serial aerobic and anaerobic blood cultures should be obtained in dogs to evaluate for possible bacterial endocarditis or sepsis. One author believes that the most rewarding results (i.e., positive cultures) are obtained by determining a temperature graph with rectal temperatures taken every two hours; the first blood cultures are collected when the temperature peaks or plateaus, and additional samples are harvested 30 minutes later.[9]

8. Dogs should undergo screening tests for immune-mediated disease (LE cell preparation, ANA titer, Coombs' test, and RF).

9. Test cats with FUO for FeLV, FIV, FIP, and toxoplasmosis.

10. Obtain culture and sensitivities for body fluids or tissues that are thought to be inflamed.

11. In some geographic areas, systemic mycotic and rickettsial serologic studies are useful.

12. Therapeutic trials should be administered with caution. "Shotgun" mixtures of antibiotics, steroids, and other drugs are contraindicated, as they are potentially harmful and only serve to confuse the clinical picture. Rather, broad-spectrum antibiotic therapy should be instituted initially because it is less risky, and because a bacterial etiology for FUO is common. Obtain bacterial culture samples before beginning a course of antibiotics. In selected cases, antiprostaglandin antipyretics may help to differentiate between true fever (in which case the temperature should decrease with treatment) and nonpyrogenic hyperthermic conditions (in which the temperature would remain unaffected). Immunosuppression (with corticosteroids and cytotoxic drugs) is reserved either for patients with confirmed immune-mediated disease or as a last resort following a concerted attempt at antibiotic therapy. Indiscriminate use of immunosuppression may produce catastrophic results in patients with occult infections.

Treatment

General Principles

1. The paramount goal in the management of any FUO disorder is to diagnose a treatable disease. Specific treatment of the underlying disease is the treatment of choice for hyperthermia.

2. Unfortunately, many animals with FUO have a poor or guarded prognosis upon diagnosis.

3. Treatment of the patient with undiagnosed FUO depends on the clinical circumstances. Immunosuppressive therapy should be reserved as a last resort. Multiple broad-spectrum or combination antibiotic regimens should be initiated in the event that the patient has an occult bacterial infection. Symptomatic antipyretic therapy may be necessary to reduce the fever to a tolerable level.

Symptomatic Reduction of Hyperthermia

1. Antipyretic therapy can be harmful to the patient with infectious disease. Hyperthermia may benefit the host by inhibiting viral replication, activating the host's defense mechanisms (particularly leukocyte function), and decreasing the availability and uptake of iron by microbes (iron is necessary for normal microbial growth and reproduction).[3] Hyperthermia, by causing the patient to feel ill, encourages inactivity and rest.

2. Conversely, hyperthermia contributes to anorexia, a critical factor in patients with prolonged illnesses. The energy required to "feed a fever" may be a considerable metabolic drain. Severe and prolonged hyperthermias (temperatures greater than 41.4°C) may result in brain damage or heat stroke.

3. The benefits and drawbacks of symptomatic treatment for hyperthermia should be weighed carefully. Body temperatures exceeding 41.1°C (106°F) are considered medical emergencies; aggressive attempts should be made to lower the temperature in such cases. However, the symptomatic treatment of less severe hyperthermias may eliminate a valuable clinical monitor. That is, by monitoring body temperatures that are unaffected by symptomatic treatment, the clinician may assess the severity and progression of the disease, as well as the response to specific therapy.

4. Modes of symptomatic treatment

A. A proper choice of treatment requires knowledge of the specific type of hyperthermia present—true fever or nonpyrogenic hyperthermia.[16,17,18,19] Although this information is frequently unavailable, most patients with FUO have true fevers.

B. The recommended treatment for true fever is antiprostaglandin antipyretics because of their ability to reset the hypothalamic thermostat set-point to a lower temperature and "break" the fever (see Fig. 3-2). Physical removal of heat from patients with true fever by means of whole-body cooling (i.e., ice water baths) is less effective and potentially harmful.[16,18] Physically removing heat from patients with active fevers causes an increased metabolic stress to produce heat, as the body strives to maintain the high temperature dictated by the thermostat set-point.

1) A list of antiprostaglandin antipyretics that are effective in the treatment of true fever in small animals follows. The salicylates (acetylsalicylic acid and sodium salicylate) are popular because they are reasonably safe and inexpensive. The toxic effects of salicylates include emesis, gastric ulceration, central nervous system (CNS) disturbances, and acid–base imbalances.[20,21] Toxicity is particularly a problem in cats. Because of their small size and slow hepatic clearance of salicylates, they are easily overdosed, even to the point of causing hyperthermia secondary to an uncoupling of oxidative phosphorylation.[22] The amount of aspirin administered to cats should never exceed the maximal recommended dose. Acetaminophen is well tolerated by dogs when administered in normal therapeutic doses, and has an antipyretic effect equivalent to that of aspirin.[5,6] However, hepatotoxicity occurs at high doses, and use of acetaminophen is contraindicated in patients with severe liver disease. Acetaminophen should never be administered to cats because of hematologic toxicity (methemoglobin formation). Dipyrone is a very effective antipyretic, but probably should be limited to short-term use because of the potential for leukopenia and agranulocytosis to develop. Other toxic effects associated with dipyrone include gastritis, increased tendency for bleeding, and serious hypothermia when administered with phenothiazines.[20] Flunixin meglumine is a potent antipyretic and analgesic that currently is not approved for use in small animals.

2) Phenothiazines are effective in treating true fever and are unique because they utilize both central and peripheral (vasodilatory) mechanisms to lower body temperature.[20]

Antiprostaglandin Antipyretic Dosages for the Cat and Dog

Acetylsalicylic acid (aspirin)
    Dog: 25–35 mg/kg PO q8h[21]
    Cat: 12.5–25 mg/kg PO q24h[22]
Sodium salicylate
    Dog: 10 mg/kg IV q8h
    Cat: 10 mg/kg IV q24h
Acetaminophen
    Dog: 10–15 mg/kg PO q8–24h[5]
    Cat: contraindicated
Dipyrone
    Dog and Cat: 25 mg/kg SQ, IM, IV, or PO q8h
Flunixin meglumine (Banamine®—Schering)*
    Dog: 0.5–1.0 mg/kg IM or IV, only once[12]
    Cat: not recommended

C. Whole-body cooling is the only effective method (aside from eliminating the cause) of reducing the body temperature of patients with nonpyrogenic hyperthermia, in whom an excess heat load exists with a normally set hypothalamic thermostat (see Fig. 3-3).[16,18]

1) Techniques include ice water baths and enemas, alcohol baths, and the use of fans.

2) To avoid hypothermia, discontinue these procedures when the temperature has been reduced to 39.4°C (103°F).

---

* Not approved for use in small animals

References

1. Andersson BE: Temperature regulation and environmental physiology. In Swenson MJ (ed): Dukes' Physiology of Domestic Animals, 8th ed, pp 1119–1134. Ithaca, Cornell University Press, 1970

2. Atkins E, Bodel P: Clinical fever: Its history, manifestations, and pathogenesis. Fed Proc 38:57–63, 1979

3. Bernheim HA, Block LH, Atkins E: Fever: Pathogenesis, pathophysiology, and purpose. Ann Intern Med 91:261–270, 1979

4. Cranston WI: Central mechanisms of fever. Fed Proc 38:49–51, 1979

5. Cullison RF: Acetaminophen toxicosis in small animals: Clinical signs, mode of action, and treatment. Compend Contin Educ Pract Vet 6:315–323, 1984

6. Davis LE: Fever. J Am Vet Med Assoc 175:1210–1211, 1979

7. Dinarello CA: Production of endogenous pyrogen. Fed Proc 38:52–56, 1979

8. Dinarello CA: Wolff SM: Pathogenesis of fever in man. N Engl J Med 298:607–612, 1978

9. Drazner FH: Diagnostic approach to patients with prolonged febrile illness. Compend Contin Educ Pract Vet 1:753–756, 1979

10. Freidman HH: Fever of Unknown Origin in Problem-Oriented Medical Diagnosis. Boston, Little, Brown & Co., 1975

11. Jacoby GS, Swartz MN: Fever of unknown origin. N Engl J Med 289:1407–1410, 1973

12. Jenkins WL, Stephens K: Some recent advances in pharmacotherapeutics. Proceedings, Amer An Hosp Assoc pp 557–563. Annual Meeting, Orlando, March 23–29, 1985

13. Legendre AM: Disophenol toxicosis in a dog. J Am Vet Med Assoc 163:149–150, 1973

14. Musacchia XJ: Fever and hyperthermia. Fed Proc 38:27–29, 1979

15. Sherding RG, et al: Primary hypoparathyroidism in the dog. J Am Vet Med Assoc 176:439–444, 1980

16. Simon HB: Daniels GH: Hormonal hyperthermia. Am J Med 66:257–263, 1979

17. Stern RC: Pathophysiologic basis for symptomatic treatment of fever. Pediatrics 59:92–98, 1977

18. Stitt JT: Fever vs. hyperthermia. Fed Proc 38:39–43, 1979

19. Wolff SM, Fauci AS, Dale DC: Unusual etiologies of fever and their evaluation. Annu Rev Med 26:277–281, 1975

20. Woodbury DM, Fingl E: Analgesics, anti-pyretics, anti-inflammatory agents, and drugs employed in the therapy of gout. In Goodman LS, Gilman A (eds): The Pharmacologic Basis of Therapeutics, 5th ed, pp 325–358. New York, Macmillan, 1975

21. Yeary RA, Brant RJ: Aspirin dosages for the dog. J Am Vet Med Assoc 167:63–64, 1975

22. Yeary RA, Swanson W: Aspirin dosages for the cat. J Am Vet Med Assoc 163:1177–1178, 1973

CHAPTER FOUR

Bleeding Disorders and Epistaxis

Justin H. Straus

Bleeding Disorders

1. Bleeding may be attributable either to a local lesion in an animal with normal hemostasis or to a defect in the hemostatic mechanism.

2. A careful history, physical examination, and use of laboratory information enable the clinician to make a diagnosis and develop an appropriate therapeutic plan.

3. The clotting mechanism is the result of three interdependent functions: vascular function, platelet function, and coagulation.

A. Vascular function—Blood vessel injury leads to local reflex vasoconstriction, decreased blood flow, and reduced escape of blood.

B. Platelet function—Blood vessel injury exposes collagen, elastin, and basement membrane. Platelets adhere to blood vessel walls and release their contents, bringing about platelet aggregation and platelet plug formation.

C. Coagulation (Fig. 4-1)

1) Blood vessel injury exposes collagen or other abnormal surfaces, leading to activation of factor XII and the intrinsic clotting system.

2) Tissue injury causes release of tissue thromboplastin (factor III) and activation of the extrinsic clotting system.

3) Both the intrinsic and extrinsic systems react with factors X and V in the presence of calcium and platelet factor three (PF_3) to convert prothrombin to thrombin.

4) Thrombin then converts fibrinogen to soluble fibrin monomer, which forms insoluble fibrin polymer (clot) in the presence of calcium, factor XIII, and thrombin.

4. Fibrinolysis begins after clot formation.

A. Plasminogen is converted to plasmin by activators found in blood vessel walls, body fluids, and most tissues.

B. Plasmin, a proteolytic enzyme, digests and dissolves the fibrin clot.

C. Fibrin and fibrinogen degradation products (fibrin and fibrinogen split products [FSPs] or fibrinolytic split products) are the end products of fibrin digestion. These products have anticoagulation properties.

Etiology

Thrombocytopenia

1. Decreased platelet production

A. Aplasia or hypoplasia of the bone marrow

1) Ionizing radiation

2) Chemical toxicity

3) Estrogen toxicity

4) Idiopathic disease

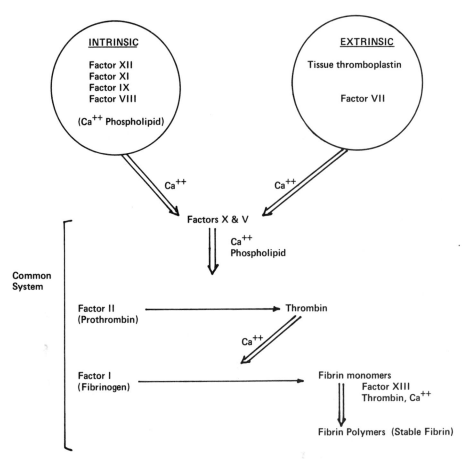

Figure 4-1. *Flow chart for clotting cascade*

B. Bone marrow infiltration or neoplastic proliferation
  1) Lymphosarcoma (LSA)
  2) Lymphocytic leukemia
  3) Myelogenous leukemia
C. Myelosuppressive drugs, such as cyclophosphamide
D. *Ehrlichia canis, E. platys, E. equi* infection
E. Ineffective platelet production
2. Increased platelet destruction by the reticuloendothelial (RE) system
A. Immune-mediated thrombocytopenia
  1) True autoimmune thrombocytopenia
  2) In conjunction with immune-mediated hemolytic anemia (IHA) or systemic lupus erythematosus (SLE)
  3) Secondary to antibody production against bacteria or viruses adsorbed to platelets
  4) Secondary to antibody production against drugs adsorbed to platelets (promazines, sulfonamides, aspirin, phenylbutazone, methimazole, propylthiouracil)
  5) Secondary to immune complexes adsorbed to platelets
B. Direct damage to platelets by bacterial exotoxins or endotoxins
3. Disorders of distribution
A. Splenic torsion
B. Hypersplenism (not yet described in dogs)
4. Increased platelet consumption
  A. Severe vasculitis
    1) Feline infectious peritonitis (FIP)

2) Endotoxemia

3) Some immune-mediated disorders

4) *Rickettsia rickettsii* infection

B. Disseminated intravascular coagulation (DIC)

C. Hypersplenism (not yet described in dogs)

Platelet Function Defects

1. Acquired

  A. Renal disease

  B. Cirrhosis

  C. Various malignant diseases

  D. Dysproteinemias (multiple myeloma)

  E. Drug-induced defect (aspirin, phenylbutazone, promazine-type tranquilizers, sulfonamides, nitrofurans, local anesthetics)

  F. Live-virus vaccine administration

2. Inherited

  A. Canine thrombocytopathy (basset hounds, foxhounds, Scottish terriers)

  B. Canine thrombocytopathy plus thrombasthenia (otter hounds)

Acquired Coagulation Disorders

1. Toxins (warfarin, diphacenone)

2. Severe liver disease

3. Vitamin K deficiency

4. DIC

Inherited Coagulation Disorders

1. Factor VIII deficiency (hemophilia A)

2. Factor IX deficiency (hemophilia B)

3. Factor VII deficiency

4. Factor X deficiency

5. Factor XI deficiency

6. Factor XII deficiency

7. Fibrinogen deficiency

8. Prothrombin complex deficiency

9. von Willebrand's disease (VWD)

History

1. Obtain precise information concerning the present and past bleeding episodes.

2. Ascertain whether the amount of bleeding is proportionate to the injury.

3. Question the owner about the type of bleeding (profuse or seeping), the source of hemorrhage, and its inception (spontaneous or initiated by minor trauma, severe trauma, or surgery).

4. With spontaneous hemorrhage, include specific questions about changes in urine or fecal color, episodes of weakness, unexplained lameness, or skin and mucous membrane hemorrhages.

5. Explore the possibility of pre-existing disease, such as neoplasia or renal or liver disease.

6. Characterize previous bleeding episodes according to age at onset, frequency, severity, and predisposing factors. Bleeding problems beginning at 6 months of age or younger often indicate a hereditary defect.

7. Investigate bleeding secondary to previous elective surgical procedures. Some animals with hereditary defects have survived these procedures without abnormalities detected by the owner or veterinarian.

8. Obtain a family history, if known, as it may be helpful.

9. Recall that spontaneous bleeding in two or more unrelated animals in the same house or neighborhood is highly suggestive of toxin or drug ingestion.

10. Investigate environmental factors, especially whether the animal is confined or allowed to roam, and the possibility of exposure to warfarin, aspirin, or other drugs and chemicals.

11. Obtain current use and history of drug administration. Estrogen injections may lead to a thrombocytopenia, and aspirin ingestion may result in a thrombopathia.

12. Obtain information about previous treatment of the bleeding disorder. This is essential because the failure of a proper therapeutic trial may eliminate certain etiologies. Previous blood transfusions necessitate the use of type A negative blood (DEA 1.1 and DEA 1.2 [dog erythroycte antigen]) or crossmatching.

13. Obtain a vaccination history as modified live-virus vaccines can cause a transient thrombocytopenia or platelet function defect.

Physical Examination

1. The clinical signs and severity of bleeding are often an indication of the location of the problem in the hemostatic mechanism.

2. Petechial hemorrhages usually indicate defects involving either platelets or blood vessels. Examine oral, penile, and vulvar mucous membranes, as well as the skin.

3. Large, deep hemorrhages into body cavities, muscles, or subcutaneous tissues usually indicate a defect in the intrinsic or extrinsic systems.

4. Epistaxis or melena is most likely caused by a platelet abnormality, although either may be seen with coagulation defects.

5. Joint pain from hemarthrosis usually indicates a clotting defect.

6. Ecchymoses and bruises of the skin are found with many hemostatic defects.

7. The animal should be thoroughly examined for evidence of trauma.

8. Icterus may be seen with hemolysis, primary liver disease, or bile duct obstruction. Thrombocytopenia along with immune-mediated hemolytic anemia, decreased production of clotting factors secondary to liver disease, and a reduction in the vitamin-K–dependent factors secondary to obstructive biliary disease may cause bleeding disorders and be associated with icterus.

9. Hematuria is often seen with thrombocytopenia.

10. If only one site of hemorrhage is present, a primary disorder of the involved system is likely.

11. Splenomegaly may be present if an immune-mediated disorder, hypersplenism, or splenic torsion is the cause.

Diagnostic Approach

1. Bleeding disorders often necessitate extensive laboratory tests and other ancillary services.

2. A thorough history and physical examination assist the clinician in choosing the appropriate tests for each patient.

3. A complete blood count (CBC) is essential for every animal with a bleeding disorder.

A. The packed cell volume (PCV) aids in determining the extent of the bleeding.

B. An increase in the total protein may be seen with dysproteinemias; a reduction in total protein is compatible with blood loss or possibly severe liver disease.

C. An elevated white blood cell (WBC) count may be associated with infection or inflammation. A decreased WBC count is often seen in endotoxemia secondary to sepsis.

D. If significant bleeding has occurred within the previous 72 hours, there is evidence of a regenerative anemia (polychromasia, anisocytosis) in most bleeding disorders.

E. Lack of signs of regeneration at this time suggests a primary problem that also causes a nonregenerative anemia (see etiology of nonregenerative anemias in Chapter 19).

F. Nonregenerative anemia, leukopenia, and thrombocytopenia may be seen in cases of aplastic anemia and bone marrow failure.

G. Increased numbers of nucleated red blood cells (RBCs) may be observed during regenerative anemias, but in the absence of reticulocytosis, they often indicate splenic dysfunction (such as hemangiosarcoma), bone marrow disease, or chronic hypoxia.

H. The peripheral blood smear may be used to make a rough estimate of the platelet count.

1) Fewer than 5 to 8 platelets per oil immersion field suggests thrombocytopenia.

2) Check for platelet clumping at the feathered edge.

3) Macroplatelets (large platelets) will be observed where there is an increased platelet turnover rate and rapid production (i.e., increased destruction).

4) Spherocytes and thrombocytopenia suggest IHA and immune-mediated thrombocytopenia.

5) Schistocytes and helmet cells, along with thrombocytopenia, suggest the presence of DIC.

Table 4-1. **Changes in tests evaluating hemostasis in specific coagulation disorders***

	Intrinsic System Activated Partial Thromboplastin Time (APTT)	Extrinsic System One-Stage Prothrombin Time (OSPT)	Fibrin Split Products (FSP)	Platelet Count	Bleeding Time
Factor VIII deficiency	↑	N	N	N	N
Factor IX deficiency	↑	N	N	N	N
Factor X deficiency	↑	↑	N	N	N
Factor VII deficiency	N	↑	N	N	N
Factor XI deficiency	↑	N	N	N	N
Factor XII deficiency	↑	N	N	N	N
von Willebrand's disease	↑ to N	N	N	N	↑
Warfarin poisoning and vitamin K deficiency	↑	↑	N	N	N
Disseminated intravascular coagulation (DIC)	↑ to N	↑ to N	↑	↓ to N	↑
Thrombocytopenia	N to Sl ↑	N	N	↓	↑
Platelet function defect	N	N	N	N to ↑	↑

* N = normal; ↑ = increased; ↓ = decreased; Sl ↑ = slightly increased. Normal FSP < 1 : 5.

Specific Tests to Evaluate Hemostatic Defects

1. Ideally, all three functions of the clotting mechanism should be evaluated. However, tests for platelet function and vascular defects are not routinely performed (Table 4-1).

2. For all bleeding disorders, the extrinsic and intrinsic systems and platelet numbers should be evaluated.

A. Intrinsic system—partial thromboplastin time (PTT), activated partial thromboplastin time (APTT), activated coagulation time (ACT), Lee White clotting time

1) Activated coagulation time is an easy in-house test to perform.

a) Materials—ACT tubes BD #6522, 37°C incubator, stopwatch

b) Blood is drawn from the jugular vein free of any tissue juices.

c) Then, 2 cc of blood is placed in the tube and the stopwatch is started. The tube is inverted five times and is then placed in the incubator.

d) After 60 seconds, the tube is checked every 15 seconds for evidence of a clot.

e) Normal canine: <120 sec

f) Normal feline: <90 sec

g) Controls should be performed periodically in every hospital to establish normal values.

B. Extrinsic system—one-stage prothrombin time (OSPT)

C. Platelet numbers—estimation from peripheral blood smear: quantification using a hemocytometer

1) Normal values are 150,000 to 400,000/mm³.

2) A value of less than 100,000/mm³ is usually clinically significant.

3) Spontaneous bleeding is not usually seen until the platelet count falls below 50,000/mm³, although this is extremely variable.

3. Tests evaluating the clotting cascade usually are normal or only slightly prolonged in cases of thrombocytopenia, unless the reduced platelet number is attributable to DIC.

4. Platelet function and numbers can be evaluated using the cuticle or the buccal mucosa bleeding time. The bleeding from severing of a toe nail through the cuticle under light anesthesia or from a controlled laceration of the buccal mucosa should cease in less than five minutes. The bleeding area should *not* be blotted.

5. A latex agglutination test is available to evaluate levels of FSPs.*

    A. An increase in FSPs indicates increased fibrinolysis.

    B. Increased FSPs may be associated with DIC or primary fibrinolysis.

6. Fibrinogen levels are sometimes decreased in DIC and primary hypofibrinogenemia.

7. The collection and preparation of blood samples are extremely important.

    A. Whenever possible, obtain samples before beginning treatment.

    B. During collection, take care to avoid introducing tissue juices that may lead to platelet clumping and false coagulation results.

    C. Collect samples from a large vein with a plastic syringe.

    D. Collect blood for platelet evaluation in ethylenediaminetetraacetate (EDTA) and perform tests within two hours of collection.

    E. For coagulation tests, mix nine volumes of blood with one volume of 3.8% (0.13 mol) sodium citrate in a plastic or siliconized tube. Use high-speed centrifugation (3000 rpm for 15 min) immediately after sample collection to separate the plasma. Then test or freeze it at −20°C. Submit blood samples from at least one normal patient at the same time because of variation in test values from different laboratories and periodically from the same laboratory.

8. Bone marrow biopsy is important in evaluating thrombocytopenia.

    A. Megakaryocyte number and morphology often distinguish between decreased production and the other causes of thrombocytopenia.

    B. A bone marrow biopsy is indicated in the diagnosis of thrombocytopenia when clotting tests are normal (eliminating DIC as the cause), unless macroplatelets are noted or an immune-mediated cause is suspected based on immunologic tests or previous response to therapy.

    C. Abnormal bleeding from the biopsy site is usually not a significant problem even in severe thrombocytopenias.

Other Laboratory Tests

1. Urinalysis (UA)

    A. Evaluates renal function

    B. Evaluates urinary tract as source of blood loss

2. Fecal analysis

    A. Evaluates gastrointestinal (GI) tract as source of blood loss

    B. Acholic feces are seen in cases of bile duct obstruction.

3. Blood chemistry profile

    A. Evaluates renal function

    B. May disclose evidence of liver disease

4. Chest and abdominal roentgenograms

    A. Blood loss into body cavities

    B. Roentgenographic evidence of neoplasia

    C. Possible splenic enlargement with immune-mediated disorders

5. PF$_3$ release test

    A. Detects the presence of antiplatelet antibody

    B. Is specific for immune-mediated thrombocytopenia

6. Coombs' test, antinuclear antibody (ANA) titer, lupus erythematosis preparation (LE prep) (used to evaluate the presence of immune-mediated disease)

7. Blood cultures, fungal titers, Ehrlichia titer, protein electrophoresis, and immunoelectrophoresis are indicated in specific diseases.

* Thrombo-Wellcotest, Burroughs Wellcome Company, Wellcome Research Division, Research Triangle Park, North Carolina

Treatment

1. For severe bleeding episodes from any cause, administer fresh-frozen homologous plasma, 6 to 10 mL/kg of body weight at a rate of 4 to 6 mL/min.

2. Give whole-blood transfusions, but make sure they are as fresh as possible; clotting factor activity diminishes rapidly after collection (10 to 20 mL/kg of body weight). One unit of fresh blood increases the level of platelets above the critical level of 20,000 in a medium-sized dog.

3. Administer RBCs or whole blood when the PCV falls below 20%.

4. Crossmatching for both dogs and cats is highly recommended. Because many dogs with bleeding disorders need multiple transfusions throughout their lifetimes, transfusion incompatibilities can be reduced by using DEA 1.1, DEA 1.2 negative blood.

5. Blood collected into plastic bags containing either citrate-phosphate-dextrose or acid-citrate-dextrose is preferred. These bags prevent the activation of platelets and factor XII: they also prevent the damage to platelets that occurs when nonsiliconized glass bottles are used.

6. Platelet-rich plasma (PRP) is prepared by either slow centrifugation (800 rpm for 5 to 10 min) or rapid spinning (1500 rpm for 2 to 3 min). Since platelets deteriorate rapidly, administer PRP within two hours after preparation.

7. Prepare plasma to be saved for transfusions of clotting factors by centrifugation of whole blood at 2500 to 3500 rpm for 15 minutes. The plasma is frozen at $-20°C$ in plastic containers. Store the remaining RBCs for 4 to 6 weeks at 4°C.

8. Cryoprecipitates of fresh-frozen plasma are very rich in factors I (fibrinogen) and VIII (5 to 15 times greater concentration). They are prepared by thawing frozen homologous plasma slowly at 4°C, and centrifuging the precipitate at 4°C. The precipitate is collected and refrozen at $-20°C$. The supernatant is also collected and saved for treatment of factor II, VII, IX, and X deficiencies. When using cryoprecipitates, thaw and dissolve them in 5% dextrose.

9. Avoid parenteral injections when possible. Intravenous and subcutaneous routes with small-gauge needles are preferred because large hematomas may develop after intramuscular injections.

10. Bleeding may be very difficult to control after placing jugular indwelling catheters. Recommend placement in the cephalic or saphenous veins.

11. Avoid or use cautiously any drugs that are known to interfere with hemostasis (e.g., aspirin, live-virus vaccines).

12. Feed the patient a soft diet to decrease injury to gums.

13. Eliminate all external and internal parasites.

14. Provide individual housing to minimize trauma.

15. Do not drain hematomas. In the case of rupture, pack them with antibiotic ointments and topical thrombin if available and apply pressure bandages. Observe the patient carefully for bandage discomfort. Close the wounds surgically.

Specific Platelet Disorders

Decreased Platelet Production

1. Because most causes of decreased platelet production also affect the myeloid and erythroid precursors, a peripheral blood smear discloses a simultaneous nonregenerative anemia and leukopenia.

2. Bone marrow biopsy reveals a reduction of megakaryocytes and erythroid and myeloid precursors.

3. In the cases of bone marrow infiltration or neoplastic myeloproliferation, abnormal cells are found.

4. Eliminate the underlying cause and provide supportive care.

    A. Discontinue all drugs unless the thrombocytopenia is known not to be drug-related or unless the drug is essential for the patient.

    B. You may need to administer whole blood or PRP.

    C. Please refer to treatment of aplastic anemia for recommendations concerning corticosteroids and immunosuppressive drugs (see Chapter 15).

D. Treatment for estrogen toxicity and *E. canis* infections is discussed under nonregenerative anemias.

E. Immune-mediated destruction directed at the platelet *and* megakaryocyte has been described in humans, and may present as decreased platelet production.

F. A rare disorder is ineffective platelet production, in which increased numbers of megakaryocytes are found in the bone marrow, and there is a marked decrease in peripheral platelet numbers.

Increased Platelet Destruction

1. Immune-mediated thrombocytopenia (IMT) results either when antibody is directed against the platelet membrane itself (true autoimmune type), or against viruses, drugs, or bacteria adhering to the platelet membrane, or when antigen-antibody complexes adhere to platelets.

2. These events result in accelerated removal of platelets by the reticuloendothelial macrophage system (RES), primarily the spleen. This is a likely occurrence because the spleen is both the major site of antiplatelet antibody production and a major phagocytic organ. Palpable splenomegaly may be detected, but it is not common.

3. Acute IMT is usually seen in younger animals, and is often preceded by a viral infection or vaccination by 1 to 2 months.

4. Diagnosis of true autoimmune idiopathic thrombocytopenia purpura, also referred to as ITP, is confirmed by a positive PF_3 test or by demonstrating autoantibody on megakaryocytes by direct immunofluorescent techniques. The specificity and sensitivity of the latter technique is unknown; the sensitivity of the PF_3 test has recently been questioned.

5. Careful consideration should be given to possible concurrent disease or drug administration in order to disclose the underlying etiology.

6. Therapeutic objectives are to control bleeding, treat underlying disease when present, increase platelet numbers (preferably

without transfusions), and administer supportive care.

7. All drugs should be discontinued unless it is certain that a drug-induced thrombocytopenia is not present, or unless the drug is essential for the well-being of the animal.

A. In most cases of drug-induced thrombocytopenia, recovery occurs two weeks after the drug is withdrawn. This disease entity can be very hard to differentiate from true autoimmune thrombocytopenia.

B. Bacterial infections should be treated with appropriate antibiotics.

C. Cats being treated for hyperthyroidism with methimazole or propylthiouracil should have their platelet counts monitored frequently.

8. Platelet numbers may be increased by use of corticosteroids, immunosuppressive drugs, or splenectomy.

A. Corticosteroids

1) This group of drugs initially suppresses phagocytic activity by the RES. It decreases platelet destruction, improves vascular integrity, and appears to stimulate platelet production or release from the bone marrow. Decreased antibody production does occur, but this is not significant until seven to fourteen days later.

2) Prednisone, 2.2 mg/kg, administered in divided doses b.i.d. for 7 to 10 days, is the initial drug of choice in IMT. Larger dosages may be needed in some cases.

3) After the platelet count has returned to normal, the drug is tapered slowly over a period of 8 to 12 weeks.

4) An increase in platelet numbers may not be seen until five to seven days after initiating corticosteroid administration.

5) Low-dose, alternate-day therapy may be needed in some cases.

B. Immunosuppressive drugs

1) These drugs are indicated when corticosteroids have proved to be ineffective; some clinicians believe they should be used immediately in severe cases, in conjunction with corticosteroids.

2) Vincristine has proved to be effective in cases of IMT that are refractory to corticosteroids.

a) Vincristine increases platelet production, so corticosteroid administration should be continued to decrease destruction.

b) There is some question as to whether these new platelets function 100% normally.

c) Dose: 0.5 mg/m^2 IV once weekly

3) Cyclophosphamide (50 mg/m^2 for 4 days of the week) or azathioprine (2.0 mg/kg daily) may also be effective.

4) Corticosteroids should be administered in conjunction with these drugs, but at reduced dosages to minimize side effects. The agents listed above must sometimes be administered on a long-term basis. The lowest possible dose of all drugs should be used.

5) CBCs on a periodic basis should be performed because of the myelosuppressive capabilities of these drugs.

C. Splenectomy

1) This procedure is indicated when:

a) Medical therapy fails to evoke a response.

b) Medical therapy results in undesirable side effects.

c) Recurrent episodes of thrombocytopenia occur.

d) Acute cases fail to respond to transfusions.

2) This procedure is highly effective in humans, but results have been variable in the dog.

3) Recently, splenectomy has been advocated by some clinicians relatively early in the treatment of IMT.

9. PRP or fresh blood transfusions may be needed in severe cases.

10. Platelet counts should be monitored closely until a normal value is attained; then, periodic evaluations will suffice.

11. Owners should be warned that exacerbations may follow remissions at any time, and are commonly more severe than the initial episode.

12. Estrus and pregnancy exacerbate platelet destruction, so ovariohysterectomy should be performed when platelet numbers have normalized.

Disorders of Distribution

1. Normally, one third of the circulating blood platelets are moving in and out of the spleen, so any cause of splenomegaly can decrease platelet numbers (i.e., LSA, hemangiosarcoma, mastocytosis).

2. A huge vascular tumor anywhere in the body may sequester platelets.

3. Splenic torsion

A. Animals with splenic torsion may present with depression, anemia, hemoglobinuria, splenodynia (painful spleen), and splenomegaly.

B. Thrombocytopenia is not a consistent finding. It may be attributable to sequestration in the spleen, or may be the result of vascular alterations secondary to localized DIC.

C. Treatment consists of correction of the splenic torsion.

D. The animal will have a guarded prognosis because death following surgery is not uncommon.

4. Hypersplenism is a recognized cause of thrombocytopenia in humans, but this syndrome has not yet been recognized in dogs. It is not truly a disorder of distribution because increased platelet consumption contributes to the thrombocytopenia.

Increased Platelet Consumption

1. In disorders in which a severe vasculitis is present, platelets adhere to damaged endothelium throughout the body and are consumed.

A. Vasculitis is a prominent feature of endotoxemia, FIP, Rocky Mountain spotted fever, and many immune-mediated disorders.

B. Treatment is directed at the primary disease process.

2. Platelets are consumed during the hypercoagulative state in DIC and as a result of vascular alterations (see pp. 46 and 47).

3. In cases of metastatic hemangiosarcoma, platelets are consumed when small hemorrhages occur secondary to DIC and while traversing through abnormal vascular spaces.

4. In all of these cases, the underlying disease process should be treated and supportive care provided.

Platelet Function Defects

1. Platelet function defects should be considered in animals with petechiae or persistent bleeding with normal or increased platelet numbers.

2. Congenital defects

A. Canine thrombocytopathy has been found in basset hounds, foxhounds, and Scottish terriers.

1) An autosomal dominant mode of inheritance results in homozygotes having a moderately severe bleeding tendency, and heterozygotes having only mild problems.

2) Decreased platelet aggregation and retention are found in association with normal clot retraction and prolonged bleeding time. Clotting parameters and the platelet count are normal.

3) Do not perform surgical procedures on these animals unless PRP or whole blood is administered before the procedure.

4) Transfusions to control spontaneous bleeding usually are not needed.

B. In otter hounds, a mixed defect similar to thrombocytopathy plus thrombasthenia (Glanzmann's disease) exists. Laboratory findings are similar to those in canine thrombocytopathy, except poor clot retraction is also found.

C. In VWD, a defect in platelet adhesion and aggregation in some cases is seen in association with a clotting factor abnormality. (See section on VWD later in this chapter).

3. Acquired defects

A. Guanidinosuccinic acid and other compounds that accumulate in the blood during the uremic state are believed to cause a platelet dysfunction that can be reversed by dialysis. Another contributing factor may be increased prostacyclin production by vascular endothelium in uremia, resulting in decreased platelet aggregation.

B. Dysproteinemias result in platelet dysfunctions by coating the platelet surface and preventing platelets from adhering normally.

C. Drug-induced platelet function defects have been known to be associated with the administration of aspirin, phenylbutazone, vincristine, promazine-type tranquilizers, sulfonamides, nitrofurans, and local anesthetics. Following a single dose of aspirin, platelet dysfunction may be present for seven to ten days, the life span of the platelet.

D. A defect in platelet function may persist for seven to ten days after injection of live-virus vaccines. A mild thrombocytopenia during the viremic phase may occur. Viral infections may cause similar changes.

E. Treatment for acquired platelet dysfunction consists of drug removal in the case of drug-induced defects and treatment of the underlying disease process when this is the cause.

Acquired Coagulation Disorders

Toxin Ingestion (Warfarin, Diphacinone, Pindone)

1. Warfarin and related compounds antagonize vitamin K action in the liver, resulting in the production of nonfunctional vitamin-K–dependent factors (II, VII, IX, X).

A. Vitamin K is converted to vitamin K epoxide when it catalyzes the carboxylation of the clotting factors II, VII, IX, and X, making them functional.

B. The enzyme Vit-K epoxide reductase catalyzes the reaction back to vitamin K.

C. Vitamin K antagonists block the action of Vit-K epoxide reductase.

D. Acarboxylated clotting factors poorly bind to calcium and phospholipids.

E. These acarboxylated clotting factors accumulate in the liver and enter the systemic circulation. Here, they are referred to as PIVKA (proteins induced by vitamin K absence or antagonists). The Thrombotest* assays PIVKA and, in Europe, has been found to be very sensitive to vitamin K absence or antagonism.

---

* Accurate Chemical & Scientific Corp. Westbury, NY

2. Clinical signs are extremely variable. Affected animals may exhibit acute collapse, dyspnea, joint pain, subcutaneous swellings, hematochezia, hematuria, oral and nasal bleeding, or severe bruising.

3. Results of tests assessing both the intrinsic and extrinsic clotting systems will be prolonged, and because factor VII has the shortest half-life of the vitamin-K–dependent factors, extrinsic system abnormalities may be noted first.

4. Bleeding may occur with a single massive exposure or multiple small-dose exposures.

5. Treatment involves administering vitamin K_1, providing supportive care, and inducing vomiting if the patient is seen soon after ingesting the toxin.

6. Vitamin K_1 (phytonadione—Aqua-MEPHYTON, Veta K_1®) is both the most potent and most rapidly acting form of vitamin K.

7. Diphacinones and the newer anticoagulants are more potent than Warfarin.

    A. If they are consumed or if the type of toxin ingested is unknown, then administer vitamin K_1, 5 mg/kg, SQ.

    B. In 6 to 12 hours, begin vitamin K, 2.5 mg/kg, administered in divided doses b.i.d. or t.i.d. for 14 to 28 days (see Chapter 28).

    C. If bleeding is initially severe, subcutaneous administration should be continued for 24 to 48 hours.

    D. If Warfarin is consumed, administer vitamin K_1 in an initial loading dose of 5 mg/kg SQ. Then begin a regimen of 2.5 mg/kg PO daily for seven days (see Chapter 28).

8. In severe bleeding episodes, vitamin K_1 may be given intravenously. Add 15 to 75 mg of vitamin K_1 to 5% dextrose to make a 5% suspension and administer over a six to eight hour period.

9. Subcutaneous injection with a small-gauge needle is recommended. Anaphylactic reactions have occurred in humans and dogs after IV administration.

10. Vitamin K_1 begins to reverse the low prothrombin level in 30 minutes. Six hours after administration, bleeding usually stops.

11. The half-life of Warfarin is 14.5 hours, resulting in a clinical effect lasting seven days. Administer oral vitamin K_1 (Mephyton tablets) 2.5 mg/kg for seven days.

12. Because the half-life of diphacenone is 4 to 5 days, its clinical effect can last for 30 days. Administer oral vitamin K_1, 2.5 mg/kg, for 14 days. Recheck the PT two to three days after the medication has been discontinued. If it is elevated, then continue the medication another two weeks.

13. Always check the OSPT two to three days after oral vitamin K_1 administration has been discontinued.

14. Supportive therapy in the form of whole-blood transfusions may be needed in severe cases of bleeding.

15. Warfarin poisoning should be considered in every small animal with a bleeding disorder; highly effective therapy is available.

16. If an animal is seen eating the toxic material, induce vomiting, administer a cathartic, and medicate with oral vitamin K_1, 1 mg/kg for seven days.

Severe Liver Disease

1. Clotting factors I, II, V, VII, IX, X, and XI are synthesized by the liver.

2. Hepatic tissue is very important in clearing the blood of FSPs that have anticoagulant properties.

3. A deficiency in clotting factors and the increased levels of FSPs result in the bleeding disorder. This may be complicated by DIC and a platelet function defect that is sometimes seen with severe liver disease.

4. In experimental studies, 80% of the hepatic tissue must be nonfunctional before bleeding will occur.

5. Bleeding tendencies may be seen in cases of severe jaundice in which either primary liver disease or biliary obstruction is the underlying problem.

    A. Bile salts are needed for the absorption of vitamin K, which is essential for the production of factors II, VII, IX, and X in the liver.

    B. In severe primary hepatic disease, the administration of vitamin K does not improve clotting times.

C. In the case of decreased vitamin K absorption secondary to obstructive biliary disease, vitamin K administration returns clotting times to normal within 48 hours.

D. OSPT is the test of choice.

6. In cases of hepatic failure, direct treatment of the underlying cause is indicated. In general, bleeding in these cases responds poorly to treatment unless there is an improvement in liver cell function.

Vitamin K Deficiency

1. A deficiency in vitamin K may result from obstructive biliary disease, malabsorptive states, and long-term intestinal antibiotic administration with reduced bacterial synthesis.

2. Treat by correcting the underlying problem and administering vitamin K_1 (see section on warfarin poisoning earlier in this chapter).

Disseminated Intravascular Coagulation (DIC)

1. DIC is an intermediary mechanism secondary to a wide variety of disorders. A new term to describe this state is intravascular coagulation and fibrinolysis syndrome (ICF).

A. Excessive activation of the clotting mechanism results in fibrin clot formation throughout the microcirculation.

B. This leads to depletion of clotting factors, platelets, and fibrinogen; activation of the fibrinolytic system; and increased levels of FSPs, the combination of which leads to a bleeding diathesis.

C. Widespread organ dysfunction results from obstruction of the microcirculation.

2. DIC may be acute or chronic, localized or generalized. It is always secondary to an underlying disease process.

3. Any disease process that results in endotoxin release, vasculitis, stasis of blood flow, hypotension, exposure of blood to abnormal surfaces, or release of tissue thromboplastin has the capability of initiating DIC.

A. The magnitude, duration, and extent of the insult determines whether DIC develops and whether the acute fulminating form with

a short course, a subacute form, or a chronic form develops.

B. Diseases associated with secondary DIC include:

    1) Septicemia

    2) Endotoxemia

    3) Malignant diseases (disseminated hemangiosarcoma; malignant lesions involving the thyroid gland, mammary gland, or nasal epithelium)

    4) Liver disease

    5) Amyloidosis

    6) Viruses (infectious canine hepatitis, FIP, herpesvirus)

    7) Severe infections

    8) Gastric dilatation, volvulus syndrome

    9) Shock from any cause

    10) Hemorrhagic gastroenteritis

    11) Obstetrical problems

    12) Heat stroke

    13) Heartworms (caval syndrome)

4. History

A. In chronic DIC, recurrent minor episodes of bleeding are noted. The animal may have a history of nonspecific weight loss and lethargy.

B. Acute DIC is accompanied by a sudden onset of bleeding. Signs may be related to organ dysfunction from microcirculation obstruction.

C. In both forms, the history also reflects the primary disease process.

5. Physical examination

A. The chronic form of the disease may only disclose evidence of mild bleeding.

B. In acute DIC, almost any abnormality may be found, depending on the extent of the impaired microcirculation. The animal may be presented before the bleeding diathesis develops.

C. Findings also reflect the underlying disease process.

D. Oozing and hematoma formation at venipuncture sites are seen in both acute and chronic DIC.

6. Laboratory examination may reveal any of the following:

A. A peripheral blood smear may reveal microangiopathic hemolysis (i.e., schistocytes, helmet cells); signs of a regenerative anemia; thrombocytopenia; or macroplatelets. However, RBC fragmentation may also occur in Heinz-body anemias, iron deficiency anemias, and structural defects of the heart and large blood vessels.

B. A platelet count may reveal thrombocytopenia of varying degrees in almost all cases.

C. Clotting test results may be prolonged, normal, or even shortened.

1) Overproduction of clotting factors may occur to compensate for continuous consumption of factors.

2) Factors V and VIII are usually decreased in DIC, which may result in more severe prolongation of tests that evaluate the intrinsic system.

D. Fibrinogen levels may be decreased (acute DIC), or normal to increased (chronic DIC).

E. In tests of fibrin or fibrinogen degradation products, concentrations less than 1 to 5 are normal for the dog. However, negative test results do not rule out DIC.

F. Low antithrombin III levels are found in 85% of DIC cases. Assays are not yet available for use in veterinary practice.

G. Blood chemistry profile changes reflect damage to specific organ systems.

H. There is no single test that is pathognomonic for DIC.

7. Treatment

A. Initial treatment should be directed at the underlying factors and the primary disease process.

1) Improve organ perfusion with vigorous fluid therapy to eliminate and prevent capillary stasis.

2) Correct metabolic acidosis, hypoxia and dehydration (if present).

3) Treat infection with broad-spectrum antibiotics.

4) Use surgery, radiation therapy, or chemotherapy to treat malignant diseases.

5) Corticosteroids may be contraindicated in animals with DIC, except in endotoxic shock for which they have been shown to be beneficial. These drugs decrease RES function; in DIC, they may decrease the clearance of FSPs.

6) Consider using mannitol or diuretics to prevent renal shutdown after volume expansion has been accomplished.

B. Only use heparin before treating the underlying disease process when bleeding is life-threatening.

1) Heparin therapy itself may be life-threatening in the face of poor clotting ability or if a high risk for bleeding exists, as with surgery. If no definitive primary disease is identified, heparin therapy is the treatment of choice.

2) Antithrombin III (AT III) is a naturally occurring anticoagulant made by the liver. It binds with activated forms of factors II, IX, X, XI, and XII.

3) In the presence of heparin, the rate of neutralization of these factors is increased, especially activated factors II and X. Since AT III is consumed during DIC, transfusions are almost always indicated, together with heparin therapy, in order to increase the levels of AT III.

4) The dosage in the dog is 150 to 250 U/kg SQ t.i.d.; in the cat, the dosage is 50 to 100 U/kg SQ. Therapeutic levels are thought to be attained when the PTT is 1.5 times the pretreatment level. Other clinicians advocate a dosage of 75 U/kg SQ t.i.d.

5) Protamine sulfate combines with heparin and neutralizes it. The dosage is 1 mg of protamine sulfate per 100 U of heparin, administered IV over a period of 10 minutes. If one hour has passed since the heparin administration, then the dose is reduced by 50%.

6) Continue heparin therapy as long as it is useful in preventing bleeding. Platelet numbers increase slowly over a few days, whereas fibrinogen increases more rapidly. After heparin is discontinued, monitor these parameters frequently to determine whether excessive coagulation is again occurring.

C. RBC, clotting factor, and platelet replacement

1) Clotting factor and platelet replacement prior to anticoagulation therapy with heparin may accelerate the coagulopathy.

2) Use whole-blood transfusions with caution if heparinization has not approached completion.

D. Miscellaneous treatment regimens

1) Platelet function inhibitors, such as aspirin, may be useful in chronic DIC. If administered along with anticoagulants, a synergistic effect occurs, and the dose of anticoagulant must be decreased.

2) Inhibitors of fibrinolysis, such as epsilon aminocaproic acid, are contraindicated in DIC.

Inherited Bleeding Disorders

Factor VIII Deficiency

1. Factor VIII deficiency (hemophilia A, classic hemophilia) is the most common inherited defect in dogs, but is rarely seen in cats.

2. It is X-chromosome–linked, so affected animals are usually males; heterozygote females are asymptomatic carriers.

3. Bleeding may be severe, moderate, or mild, depending on the degree of factor VIII deficiency.

4. Bleeding problems usually occur near weaning age.

5. Laboratory findings

  A. Decreased factor VIII activity (<20%)

  B. Normal or increased concentrations of factor-VIII–related antigen

  C. Test results of intrinsic clotting system are abnormal

  D. Test results of extrinsic clotting system are normal.

  E. Platelet numbers and bleeding times are normal.

  F. Heterozygote females have 40% to 60% factor VIII activity.

6. The plasma defect is not corrected by transfusion with normal serum.

7. Treatment—Administration of fresh-frozen plasma at a rate of 6 to 10 mL/kg t.i.d. for three to five days, or until the bleeding stops

Factor IX Deficiency

1. Factor IX deficiency (hemophilia B, Christmas disease) is X-chromosome–linked, but much more rare than hemophilia A.

2. It has been diagnosed in a family of British short-haired cats and cairn terriers, black and tan coonhounds, St. Bernards, French bulldogs, Alaskan malamutes, cocker spaniels, and an old English sheepdog.

3. It is clinically similar to factor VIII deficiency.

4. Laboratory findings

  A. Decreased factor IX activity

  B. Heterozygote females have 40% to 60% of factor IX activity.

  C. Test results of intrinsic clotting system are abnormal.

  D. Test results of extrinsic clotting system are normal.

  E. Platelet numbers and bleeding times are normal.

5. Transfusion with normal serum corrects the defect.

6. Treatment—Administration of fresh-frozen plasma at a rate of 6 to 10 mL/kg b.i.d. for three to five days, or until the bleeding stops

Factor VII Deficiency

1. Documented in beagles and a malamute

2. Autosomal dominant mode of inheritance

3. Bleeding tendency is minor; increased bruising is evident.

4. Laboratory findings

  A. Decreased factor VII activity (1% to 4% in homozygotes; 50% in heterozygotes)

  B. Test results of intrinsic clotting system are normal.

  C. Test results of extrinsic clotting system are abnormal.

  D. Platelet numbers and bleeding times are normal.

5. Associated with this defect is an increased susceptibility to generalized demodicosis.

6. Transfusion therapy is usually not required.

Factor X Deficiency

1. Documented in cocker spaniels

2. Autosomal incompletely dominant mode of inheritance

3. Bleeding tendency is usually severe in young dogs and mild in adult dogs.

4. The trait appears to be lethal in the homozygous state.

5. Homozygotes may be stillborn or may die early in life from intrathoracic, intra-abdominal, or umbilical bleeding.

6. Heterozygotes have minor problems that are exacerbated by surgery.

7. Laboratory findings

  A. Decreased factor X activity (18% to 65% in heterozygotes)

  B. Test results for both intrinsic and extrinsic clotting systems are markedly prolonged in the homozygous state, and mildly prolonged in heterozygotes.

  C. Platelet numbers and bleeding times are normal.

8. No response is seen with vitamin K therapy.

9. Treatment—Administration of fresh-frozen plasma at a rate of 6 to 10 mL/kg daily for three to five days, or until the bleeding stops

Factor XI Deficiency

1. Diagnosed in springer spaniels and Great Pyrenees

2. Autosomal incompletely dominant mode of inheritance; heterozygotes are asymptomatic.

3. Bleeding tendency may be minor or severe.

4. Hemorrhage within 24 hours of surgery is the hallmark of the disease.

5. Laboratory findings

  A. Decreased factor XI activity (1% to 10% in homozygotes; 25% to 60% in heterozygotes)

  B. Test results of intrinsic clotting system are abnormal.

  C. Test results of extrinsic clotting system are normal.

  D. Platelet numbers and bleeding times are normal.

6. Treatment—Administration of fresh-frozen plasma at a rate of 6 to 10 mL/kg daily for three to five days.

Von Willebrand's Disease (VWD)

1. VWD is an inherited disease characterized by diminished factor VIII activity, a platelet function defect, and decreased production of von Willebrand's factor (vWf).

2. Inheritance is autosomal and incompletely dominant. The disease has been observed in many breeds of dogs.

3. vWf is synthesized by vascular endothelium and megakaryocytes. Its functions are:

  A. To bind factor VIII in a complex, and act as a carrier for this factor in plasma in order to stabilize it.

  B. To mediate platelet adhesion to the subendothelium of the injured blood vessels.

4. vWf is found in plasma of hemophiliac patients. Transfusion with this plasma results in an increase in factor VIII activity.

5. A decrease in factor VIII (VIII:C) activity is measurable, along with a decrease in factor VIII antigen (VIII:Ag).

  A. Routine clotting tests evaluating the intrinsic pathway are usually not diagnostic.

  B. Specialized assays are available to measure factor (VIII:C), factor (VIII:Ag), and the vWf antigen (vWf:Ag).*

6. The prolonged bleeding time is attributable to the platelet function defect, and can be measured using the cuticle bleeding and buccal mucosal bleeding times. Clot retraction and platelet aggregation are usually normal. However, defective platelet aggregation may be seen in response to the administration of ristocetin.

7. Morbidity is high and mortality is low, with the bleeding diathesis varying from mild to moderate. Bleeding is exacerbated by surgery and trauma. Hematochezia, melena, hematuria, or subcutaneous hematomas may be seen. Prolonged estrual bleeding is common. The clinical severity of VWD decreases in severity with each pregnancy in females, and with age in both sexes.

8. Diagnosis is based on measurement of factor VIII coagulant activity.

  A. Factor VIII coagulant activity: normal—60% to 72%

* Jean Dodds, New York State Department of Health, Albany, NY

B. The severity of the clinical signs depends on the percentage of coagulant activity.

1) <10%—severe signs
2) 10% to 20%—moderate signs
3) 20% to 25%—mild signs
4) 50% to 60%—normal

9. Treatment—Whole-blood transfusions are effective.

A. Dogs with VWD can synthesize their own factor VIII for 24 hours after a transfusion. Fresh-frozen plasma will correct the factor VIII abnormality.

B. The platelet function defect is corrected, but only transiently, after fresh whole-blood transfusion.

C. Hypothyroidism may exacerbate the bleeding tendencies of dogs with VWD, and should be investigated as a possible contributing factor. Dr. Jean Dodds believes that every animal with VWD should be treated with thyroid replacement therapy.

D. The vasopressin analogue desmopressin (DDAVP) has been found to increase the release of VWF from endothelial stores in normal dogs.

1) Studies are underway to evaluate its effects in dogs with VWD.

2) Administration of DDAVP, 1 μg/kg SQ, to donor dogs 30 minutes before phlebotomy has significantly increased vWf:Ag concentrations.

Other Deficiencies

1. Factor XII deficiency has been found in a clinically normal cat and in a miniature poodle. Test results of the intrinsic clotting mechanism were prolonged. This defect is normal in some lower mammalian and nonmammalian species. No treatment is required.

2. Fibrinogen deficiency has been diagnosed in a collie and in St. Bernards. It is inherited as an autosomal incompletely dominant trait. Test results of both the intrinsic and extrinsic clotting systems are markedly prolonged. Whole-plasma, equivalent to 6 to 10 mL/lb of body weight, is administered once a day for three to five days, or until the bleeding stops.

3. A prothrombin complex deficiency has been found in boxers.

4. Dysfibrinogenemia has been documented in a collie and a boxer.

·················
Epistaxis

Epistaxis may result from a primary nasal problem, or it may be secondary to a bleeding disorder.

Etiology

1. Trauma
2. Foreign bodies (e.g., grass awns, wood splinters)
3. Infection
  A. Bacterial
  B. Mycotic
4. Benign polyps
5. Malignant neoplasia
  A. Adenocarcinoma
  B. Squamous cell carcinoma
  C. Fibrosarcoma
  D. Osteosarcoma
  E. Chondrosarcoma
6. Allergy
7. Bleeding disorders
  A. Multiple myeloma
  B. Other (see preceding section of Bleeding Disorders in this chapter)

History

Historical and physical examination findings pointing to nasal hemorrhage suggest only that the problem is within the nasal cavity. A history of melena, hematuria, or subcutaneous hemorrhage suggests a primary bleeding disorder.

1. Question the extent and duration of bleeding to help quantify the blood loss.
2. A chronic mucopurulent nasal discharge followed by one episode of epistaxis points to a primary abnormality of the nasal cavity.
3. Attempt to rule out trauma as a cause.

4. Question the owner about the dog's environment, as running through tall grass increases the likelihood that a foreign body is present.

5. Investigate historical evidence of concurrent disease, as epistaxis may just be a manifestation of another problem resulting in presentation of the patient to the veterinarian.

6. It is not uncommon for epistaxis to be the presenting complaint in cases of multiple myeloma, with or without the hyperviscosity syndrome.

7. Bilateral epistaxis increases the likelihood that a bleeding disorder is present.

Physical Examination

1. Perform a thorough physical examination to rule out the possibility that a primary disease process is causing a secondary epistaxis.

2. Search carefully for signs of bleeding tendencies.

3. An elevated body temperature may be indicative of an infectious process.

4. Evidence of trauma may be found.

5. Examine the nose and mouth very carefully for masses, discharges, and erosions and fluctuations in the palate.

6. Perform a fundic examination; look for evidence of bleeding or hyperviscosity (engorged blood vessels).

Initial Laboratory Examination

1. The CBC may reveal a leukocytosis and significant left shift, indicative of inflammatory disease.

2. The presence of a regenerative anemia, together with only one acute episode of epistaxis, suggests previous blood loss; this must be investigated.

3. Thrombocytopenia may be evident on examination of the peripheral smear.

4. An elevation of the plasma protein is suggestive of multiple myeloma.

5. Melena should be able to be detected one to two days after an episode of epistaxis because blood is inevitably swallowed by the patient.

6. A blood chemistry profile and UA are usually unremarkable unless a concurrent disease process is present.

7. History, physical examination findings, and the initial laboratory evaluation enable the clinician to determine whether the problem is primarily in the nasal cavity or is secondary to another disorder. If a secondary disease process (e.g., a bleeding disorder) is suspected, specific laboratory tests should be performed to investigate the numerous possibilities.

Examination Under Anesthesia

1. Anesthesia is required for further evaluation of a primary nasal problem.

2. Prior to administering an anesthetic, obtain chest roentgenograms and look for metastases or evidence on an infectious pulmonary disease process.

3. Examine the oral and nasal cavities carefully and take skull roentgenograms.

4. Perform a nasal flush, culture the material obtained for bacteria and fungi, and stain for microscopic examination. Often, specimens large enough for histopathologic exam are obtained.

Treatment

1. Acute epistaxis often subsides with cage rest.

2. Cold packs may be placed over the animal's nose.

3. Tranquilization, especially the phenothiazine tranquilizers with their alpha-blocking effect to lower blood pressure, is very useful. However, tranquilizers are contraindicated in cases of severe bleeding in which hypovolemia is possible, and in debilitated animals.

4. Diluted epinephrine (1 : 50,000) instilled into the nares is sometimes useful when only capillary bleeding is present. It has a short duration of action.

5. To prevent aspiration, place the heads of unconscious animals below chest level.

6. You may have to pack the nares and caudal nasal cavities in cases of severe bleeding. Monitor recovery from anesthesia very carefully.

7. Treatment of the underlying disease process is essential.

    A. Use appropriate antibacterial and antifungal drugs to treat infectious processes.

    B. Surgery, chemotherapy, or radiotherapy may be useful for specific neoplasms.

    C. Specific chemotherapy is available for the treatment of multiple myeloma.

    D. Foreign body removal or fracture repair may be necessary.

    E. In cases of severe or persistent bleeding, monitor the PCV and total protein; a blood transfusion may become necessary.

Suggested Readings

Badylak SF, Dodds WJ, Van Fleet JF: Plasma coagulation factor abnormalities in dogs with naturally occurring hepatic disease. Am J Vet Res 44: 2336–2340, 1986

Breitschwerdt EB: Infectious thrombocytopenia in dogs. Compend Contin Educ Pract Vet 10: 1177–1190, 1988

Campbell KL, George JW, Greene CE: Application of the enzyme-linked immunosorbent assay for the detection of platelet antibodies in dogs. J Am Vet Med Assoc 88: 68–71, 1985

Couto CG: Hematologic abnormalities in small animal cancer patients. Part I. Red blood cell abnormalities. Compend Contin Educ Pract Vet 6: 1059–1065, 1984

Davenport DJ, Breitschwerdt EB, Carakostas MC: Platelet disorders in the dog and cat. Part I. Physiology and pathogenesis. Compend Contin Educ Pract Vet 4: 762–772, 1982

Davenport DJ, Breitschwerdt EB, Carakostas MC: Platelet disorders in the dog and cat. Part II. Diagnosis and management. Compend Contin Educ Pract Vet 4: 788–796, 1982

Dodds WJ: von Willebrand's disease in dogs. Mod Vet Pract 65: 681–686, 1984

Feldman BF, Handagama P, Lubberink AAME: Splenectomy as adjunctive therapy for immune-mediated thrombocytopenia and hemolytic anemia. J Am Vet Med Assoc 187: 617–619, 1985

Feldman BF, Maderwell BR, O'Neill S: Disseminated intravascular coagulation: Antithrombin, plasminogen, and coagulation abnormalities in 41 dogs. Am J Vet Med Assoc 179: 151, 1981

Greene CE: Disseminated intravascular coagulation in a dog; A review. J Am Anim Hosp Assoc 11: 674–687, Sept/Oct 1975

Greene CE, Harvey JW: Canine ehrlichiosis. In Greene CE (ed): Clinical Microbiology and Infectious Diseases of the Dog and Cat. Philadelphia, WB Saunders, 1984, 545

Green RA: Activated coagulation times in monitoring heparinized dogs. J Am Vet Res 41: 1793–1797, Nov 1980

Green RA: Hemostasis and disorders of coagulation. Vet Clin North Am [Small Anim Pract] 11: 289–317, 1981

Green RA: Hemostatic disorders. In Ettinger SJ (ed): Veterinary Internal Medicine. 3rd ed, Vol 2: 2246–2264. Philadelphia, WB Saunders, 1989.

Harvey JW, Simpson CF, Gaskin JM: Cyclic thrombocytopenia induced by a rickettsia-like agent in dogs. J Infect Dis 137: 182–188, Feb 1978

Jain NC, Finkl JG (eds): Clinical hematology. Vet Clin North Am 11: 2, 1981

Jain NC, Switzer JW: Autoimmune thrombocytopenia in dogs and cats. Vet Clin North Am 2: 421–434, 1981

Johnson GS, Schlink GT, Fallon RK, et al: Hemorrhage from the cosmetic autoplasty of Doberman pinschers with von Wildebrand's disease. Am J Vet Res 46: 1335–1340, 1985

Johnstone IB: Inherited defects of hemostasis. Compend Contin Educ Pract Vet 4: 483–488, 1982

Joshi BC, Raplee RG, Powell AL, Hancock F: Autoimmune thrombocytopenia in a cat. J Am Anim Hosp Assoc 15: 585–588, Sept/Oct 1979

Kirk RW (ed): Current Veterinary Therapy VII. Philadelphia, WB Saunders, 1980

Kirk RW (ed): Current Veterinary Therapy VIII. Philadelphia, WB Saunders, 1983

Kirk RW (ed): Current Veterinary Therapy IX. Philadelphia, WB Saunders, 1986

Kociba GJ: The diagnosis of hemostatic disorders. Vet Clin North Am 6: 609–623, 1976

Kotter CA: Immune thrombocytopenia purpura. Med Clin North Am 64: 761, 1980

MacEwen EG, Withrow SJ, Patnaik AK: Nasal tumors in the dog. Retrospective evaluation of diagnosis, prognosis, and treatment. J Am Vet Med Assoc 170: 45–48, Jan 1, 1977

McDougal BJ: Allergic rhinitis—A cause of recurrent epistaxis. J Am Vet Med Assoc 172: 545–546, Sept 15, 1977

McMillan R: Chronic idiopathic thrombocytopenia purpura. N Engl J Med 304: 1135, 1981

Mount MC, Feldman BF, Buffington T: Vitamin K and its therapeutic importance. J Am Vet Med Assoc 180: 1354–1356, 1982

Norris AM: Intranasal neoplasms in the dog. J Am Anim Hosp Assoc 15: 231–236, Mar/Apr 1979

Peterson ME, Dodds J: Factor IX deficiency in an Alaskan malamute. J Am Vet Med Assoc 174: 1326–1327, June 15, 1979

Schalm OW, Jain NC, Carroll EJ: Veterinary Hematology, 3rd ed. Philadelphia, Lea & Febiger, 1975

Sherding RG, Dibartola SP: Hemophilia B (factor IX deficiency) in an old English sheepdog. J Am Vet Med Assoc 176: 141–142, Jan 15, 1980

Thomason KJ, Feldman BF: Immune-mediated thrombocytopenia: Diagnosis and treatment. Compend Contin Educ Pract Vet 7: 569–576, 1985

Thorn GW, Adams RD, Braunwald E, Isselbacher KJ, Petersdorf RG: Harrison's Principles of Internal Medicine, 8th ed. New York, McGraw-Hill, 1977

Weiss RC, Dodds WJ, Scott FW: Disseminated intravascular coagulation in experimentally induced feline infectious peritonitis. Am J Vet Res 41: 663, 1980

Wilkins RJ, Hurwitz AI, Dodds WJ: Immunologically mediated thrombocytopenia in the dog. J Am Vet Med Assoc 163: 277–282, Aug 1, 1973

Williams DA, Maggio-Price L: Canine idiopathic thrombocytopenia: Clinical observations and long-term follow-up. J Am Vet Med Assoc 185: 660–663, 1984

Withrow SJ: Diagnostic and therapeutic nasal flush in small animals. J Am Anim Hosp Assoc 13: 704–707, Nov/Dec 1977

CHAPTER FIVE

Obesity and Cachexia

Margaret S. Swartout

Obesity

Obesity may be defined as an increase in body weight to a level above that which is normal for an animal's size and body type.

Incidence

1. It has been estimated that 24% to 44% of pet dogs are obese.

A. The highest incidence of obesity is seen in Labradors, cairn terriers, cocker spaniels, dachshunds, Shetland sheepdogs, and collies.

B. Obesity is more likely to occur in dogs owned by obese owners than in those owned by nonobese owners; it is also more prevalent in dogs owned by middle-aged or elderly clients than in those owned by younger owners.

1) Decreased exercise opportunities are provided by the owner.

2) Increased food intake occurs as a result of the animal's boredom.

C. Obesity is more likely to occur in older dogs than in younger ones owing to the former's decreased metabolic rate, lean body mass, and physical activity level, all of which contribute to a reduction of 20% in caloric need (as compared to that of younger dogs).

D. Gender and reproductive status

1) Female dogs are more likely to be obese than male dogs.

2) Neutered dogs are more likely to be obese than intact dogs.

a) Neutering decreases roaming behavior and energy expenditure.

b) The habits of dog and owner dictate that the same diet is likely to continue after neutering, resulting in an energy surplus and weight gain.

E. The owner's feeding practices may contribute to obesity, as with the provision of table scraps, treats, and ad libitum feeding; the interpretation of hunger as a sign of good health; and the provision of food as an expression of caring.

2. It has been estimated that 6% to 12% of pet cats are obese.

A. The incidence of obesity in cats is lower than in dogs because cats are better able to control their energy balance on ad libitum feeding regimens. In those cats that control their energy balance poorly, ad libitum feeding practices may contribute to obesity.

B. The feeding of a very palatable canned gourmet cat food often contributes to obesity in cats.

C. Obesity is generally seen in older adult cats who are less active, and in neutered cats.

Effects of Obesity

When an animal's body weight is 15% or more above normal, it is predisposed to many medical problems.

1. Orthopedic disease

  A. Animals that are overweight are more prone to joint injury and secondary degenerative joint disease.

2. Cardiopulmonary problems

  A. Compression of the chest wall and trachea by fatty tissue can contribute to hypoventilation, collapsing trachea, increased incidence of tracheobronchial disease, and cor pulmonale.

  B. Excess body tissue results in additional demands for oxygen and increased cardiac work load.

  C. Compromise of the cardiopulmonary system may result in exercise intolerance.

3. Obese animals are more prone to heat intolerance owing to insulation with subcutaneous fat.

4. Obese animals have an increased incidence of dystocia.

5. Surgical difficulty and anesthetic risk are both increased in the obese animal.

6. Obesity followed by prolonged anorexia (as a result of some stressful event or illness) may lead to idiopathic hepatic lipidosis in cats, resulting in the death of most of the animals so affected.

7. Obesity may increase an animal's chance of developing diabetes mellitus.

8. Obesity can decrease the response to infectious disease in dogs.

9. Obesity may increase the incidence of pyodermas.

10. Obese dogs may be predisposed to pancreatitis.

11. A higher incidence of feline urologic syndrome is found in obese cats.

12. Obese animals have an unappealing appearance and may be lethargic. These factors may be of great importance to the owner and should not be underestimated as a motivation for pursuing a weight loss program.

Etiologic Considerations

1. Causes of pathologic obesity to be ruled out include:

  A. Hypothalamic or pituitary lesion or dysfunction

  B. Endocrine imbalances

  1) Hyperadrenocorticism
  2) Hypothyroidism
  3) Insulinoma

  C. These causes are responsible for a small number of cases of obesity.

  D. Pseudo-obesity secondary to edema, peritoneal effusion, or gross hepatomegaly/splenomegaly can often be misinterpreted as obesity.

2. Physiologic obesity is attributable to energy intake in excess of that utilized in an otherwise healthy animal.

  A. Inadequate exercise

  B. Excess caloric intake

Diagnostic Approach

History

1. A pet's obesity is usually not recognized by the owner. The veterinarian generally notes the condition when the pet is presented for routine immunizations or for problems secondary to the obese condition.

2. Determine the type, amount, and frequency of exercise.

3. Determine the type, quantity, schedule, and caloric value of the diet fed.

  A. Foods of high palatability, efficient utilization, and high caloric density are most likely to contribute to obesity.

  B. Ad libitum feeding increases the incidence of obesity.

4. Water consumption

  A. Increased water consumption may be seen with hyperadrenocorticism, but is observed uncommonly with hypothyroidism.

  B. Central nervous system (CNS) disturbances that cause obesity may cause increased water intake.

5. Reproductive history

  A. A history of anestrus, irregular heat cycles, or infertility may be associated with endocrine disturbances.

  B. Obese animals may have experienced dystocia.

6. Behavioral history

  A. Animals that are heat seekers may be hypothyroid.

B. Animals with insulinomas often exhibit episodic seizures and weakness.

C. CNS lesions contributing to obesity can also result in behavioral changes.

Physical and Neurologic Examination

1. Recognition of obesity
   A. Gross obesity is obvious.
   B. Objective evaluations
   1) Weight charts for breeds are available, but the best guideline is the animal's nonobese weight ascertained from previous medical records.
   2) The amount of tissue overlying the rib cage can be a useful parameter:
      a) Too thin—ribs easily seen
      b) Normal—ribs barely seen and easily felt
      c) Too fat—ribs cannot be seen, and a distinct layer of fat can be palpated
   3) An obese animal can have a pendulous abdomen, areas of fatty deposition (pads) over the tailhead and hips, and a waddling walk. A normal dog should have an indentation behind the rib cage with light fleshiness over the hips when viewed from above, and a trim, firm stomach.

2. Evaluation of hair coat and skin
   A. A bilaterally symmetrical alopecia in the absence of inflammation or pruritus is suggestive of endocrine disease.
   B. Skin fold pyodermas may be associated with physiologic obesity.
   C. Skin infections can be seen with hyperadrenocorticism and hypothyroidism.
   D. Calcinosis cutis is sometimes noted with hyperadrenocorticism.
   E. Hyperpigmentation can be seen with both hyperadrenocorticism and hypothyroidism.

3. Neurologic abnormalities
   A. Pituitary or hypothalamic disorders may cause obesity, the signs of which may include:
      1) Visual deficits with or without normal pupillary light reflexes
      2) Seizures, circling
      3) Personality changes

B. Peripheral nerve and muscle abnormalities have been associated with endocrine disease.
   1) Peripheral neuropathy has been noted in animals with hyperadrenocorticism, hypothyroidism, and insulinoma.
   2) Dogs with hyperadrenocorticism and hypothyroidism may demonstrate polymyopathy and may exhibit a slow, stilted gait.

Diagnostic Aids

1. Hematology
   A. Animals with hyperadrenocorticism may demonstrate mature neutrophilia, eosinopenia, lymphopenia, and sometimes, high red blood cell (RBC) parameters.
   B. Hypothyroid animals may have a normocytic, normochromic anemia.

2. Serum biochemical studies
   A. Hyperadrenocorticism results in moderate to severe increases in serum alkaline phosphatase levels, along with mild to moderate elevations in alanine aminotransferase, cholesterol, and occasionally, glucose levels.
   B. Animals with hypothyroidism may demonstrate increased serum cholesterol levels.
   C. Fasting hypoglycemia may be noted in patients with insulinoma.

3. Urinalysis
   A. There may be a mild to marked decrease in urine specific gravity in animals with hyperadrenocorticism.
   B. Glycosuria may occasionally, and ketonuria may rarely be demonstrated in animals with hyperadrenocorticism.
   C. Animals with hyperadrenocorticism have a high incidence of urinary tract infections (UTIs), although examination of the urine sediment may not reveal inflammatory changes.

4. Endocrinologic testing
   A. Serum triiodothyronine and thyroxine (T_3–T_4) analysis should be performed, and a thyroid-stimulating hormone test should be considered in order to rule out hypothyroidism.
   B. A low-/high-dose dexamethasone suppression test should be performed to

evaluate the animal for the presence and type of hyperadrenocorticism.

Treatment

1. Rule out and treat causes of pathologic obesity. A weight reduction program should be instituted for physiologic obesity. Secondary disease prevention and the anticipated improvement in appearance as a result of weight loss should be emphasized to the owner.

2. General approaches to weight reduction

   A. Increased exercise

   B. Decreased caloric intake

      1) Caloric restriction at home

      2) Starvation under veterinary supervision

   C. Pharmacologic intervention

3. Specific weight reduction regimens

   A. Increased exercise

      1) Two 10- to 15-minute brisk walks per day are recommended for dogs if constraints upon exercise are not advisable (e.g., owing to severe cardiopulmonary disease, locomotion problems, or gross obesity).

      2) Cats can also be taken for supervised walks, and the whole family can become involved in providing increased opportunities for play.

      3) The exercise program should be maintained once the optimal weight has been attained.

   B. Caloric restriction program for dogs

      1) Obtain complete client cooperation and commitment.

      2) Give the client explicit explanations and written instructions.

      3) Weigh the dog and set a weight loss goal, estimating the time required to reach that goal. With a recommended decrease in caloric intake to 60% to 65% of the maintenance requirement (Table 5-1), body weight should decrease 3% per week for the first six weeks, then 2% per week after eight weeks.

      4) The daily ration should be divided into three to six feedings per day.

      5) Instruct the owner to keep the dog out of the rooms where food is prepared or eaten by the family.

      6) Diet specifics

         a) Dogs will not lose weight if the diet contains scraps, snacks, or sweets. Asking the owner to record everything (including amounts) that the dog eats may preclude cheating.

         b) As a general rule, the tactics employed in selecting a diet include:

            i. The dog should take in a reduced amount of energy and maintain an adequate intake of protein, while increasing satiety.

            ii. The diet should be 35% to 45% lower in caloric density than the dog's previous dietary intake.

            iii. Fat should be restricted to less than 10% dry matter.

            iv. Protein should be supplied at a minimum of 4.0 g/kg of body weight per day.

            v. Replace digestible carbohydrate with indigestible fiber, such as cellulose flour or vegetables, so that fiber is more than 15% dry matter.

         c) Specially formulated reducing diets, such as Prescription Diet r/d®* or Special Diet O®†, or a homemade reducing diet can be used. Reduced-calorie weight-maintenance foods, such as Fit-N-Trim®‡, Cycle-3®§, and w/d®* can also be used in the correct caloric proportions. Special diets may be easier for some owners and pets to accept, as the amount of food in the bowl may change very little, if at all. However, special diets may connote a "quick fix" to some owners, rather than a commitment to a long-term solution.

---

* Hill's Pet Products, Inc., Topeka, KS 66601

† Cadillac Pet Foods, Inc., Pennsauken, NJ 08110

‡ Ralston Purina Co., St. Louis, MO 63188

§ Gaines Professional Services, P.O. Box 9001, Chicago, IL 60604

Table 5-1. **Energy requirements of dogs***

Body Weight		Estimated kcal/kg/d Body Weight		Estimated kcal/lb/d Body Weight	
(kg)	**(lb)**	**Adult Maintenance**	**Growing Puppies**	**Adult Maintenance**	**Growing Puppies**
0.5	1.1	136	272	62	124
1.0	2.2	134	268	61	122
1.5	3.3	122	244	55	110
2.0	4.4	111	222	50	100
2.5	5.5	105	210	48	96
3.0	6.6	100	200	45	90
3.5	7.7	96	192	44	88
4.0	8.8	93	186	42	84
4.5	9.9	91	182	41	82
5	11.0	88	176	40	80
6	13.2	84	168	38	76
7	15.4	81	162	37	74
8	17.6	78	156	35	70
9	19.8	76	152	34	68
10	22.0	74	148	34	68
15	33.1	67	134	30	60
20	44.1	62	124	28	56
25	55.1	59	118	27	55
30	66.1	56	112	25	50
35	77.2	54	108	25	50
40	88.2	53	106	24	48
45	99.2	51	102	23	46
50	110.2	50	100	23	46

* Adapted from data compiled by the National Academy of Sciences, National Research Council (From The Basic Guide to Canine Nutrition, 4th ed, 1977, reprinted by permission of Gaines Professional Services)

d) Smaller amounts of good-quality commercial or balanced homemade diets may be used instead.

e) Canned green beans, canned carrots, or boiled yellow winter squash without salt or butter can be used as a physical filler with any of the diets to increase satiety.

f) Vitamin and mineral supplementation is recommended if the ration does not afford an adequate supply.

g) The dog should be weighed weekly by the clinician. If the dog does not lose weight, decrease the amount fed by 20%.

h) A graph of the dog's body weight should be kept, with daily entries being made by the owner. If the owner is unable to weigh the dog, a daily record of the girth measurement at the level of the xiphoid should be kept; alternatively, the owner may be invited to bring the dog in to the veterinary hospital to be weighed as often as is necessary.

i) Once a satisfactory weight has been reached, the dog should be placed on a regulation maintenance, low-calorie maintenance, or reducing diet at caloric levels that prevent weight fluctuation. Ask the owner to weigh the dog weekly. If the body weight begins to increase, decrease the amount fed by 10% to 20%.

   j) Perform a follow-up examination one month and three months later.

   k) Caloric reduction in a hospital setting may convince an owner who is having difficulty withholding treats that weight loss is possible for the dog.

   C. Caloric restriction program for cats

   1) Weigh the cat and establish an optimal body weight (Table 5-2), communicating this information to the owner. As a rule of thumb, a healthy, nonobese cat should weigh 3.5 to 4.5 kg (8 to 10 lb). Cats of common domestic breeds that weigh more than 5.5 kg (12 lb) are usually overweight.

   2) Estimate the time required to reach the optimal weight; this usually takes about 12 weeks. At a 30% to 40% rate of caloric restriction, the expected weight loss is $\frac{1}{2}$ pound after one week, one pound after four weeks, and more than three pounds by 12 weeks.

   3) Obtain an accurate history of the cat's eating and environmental patterns, including diet, amount and type of snacks, and whether the cat is left outdoors unsupervised.

Discourage snacks and the attainment of food outside the house. Attempt to maintain the existing feeding schedule.

   4) Diet specifics

   a) Caloric intake should be 65% to 70% of the maintenance requirement for optimal body weight (see Table 5-2).

   b) A reduction in the amount of maintenance food fed can be attempted, but this may be difficult to maintain, as hungry cats tend to annoy their owners. A reducing diet that physically fills the cat but is restricted in calories (by replacing fat and digestible carbohydrates with undigestible fiber) is helpful. Palatability is retained if dietary protein levels are maintained.

   i. Feline r/d®* is generally required in amounts of $\frac{1}{4}$ to $\frac{1}{2}$ can per cat per day.
   ii. A homemade feline reducing diet can be used.
   iii. A vitamin and mineral supplement may be used if the diet does not contain adequate supplies.

   5) Total veterinarian–client cooperation, explicit instructions, and weekly hospital

* Hill's Pet Products, Inc., Topeka, KS 66601

Table 5-2. **Daily food requirements of cats according to age***

Age or Condition	Expected Weight		Daily Calories Body Weight		Daily Ration	
	kg	lb	kcal/kg	kcal/lb	g	oz
Newborn	0.12	0.26	380	172	30	1.1
5 weeks	0.5	1.1	250	113	83	2.9
10 weeks	1	2.2	200	91	133	4.7
20 weeks	2	4.4	130	59	173	6.1
30 weeks	3	6.6	100	45	200	7.1
Adult	4.5	9.9	80	36	240	8.5
Adult (pregnant)	3.5	7.7	100	45	233	8.2
Adult (lactating)	2.5	5.5	250	113	416	14.7
Neuter Male	4	8.8	80	36	213	7.5
Neuter Female	2.5	5.5	80	36	133	4.7

* From The Basic Guide to Canine Nutrition, 4th ed, 1977, reprinted by permission of Gaines Professional Services

weight determinations are necessary. Have the owner keep a graph of the cat's weight.

6) Once the optimal weight has been reached, prescribe a good-quality maintenance or weight loss ration at a level that just maintains the cat's optimal weight. Recheck the cat's weight one and three months later, and at six-month intervals thereafter. The owner should continue to weigh the cat weekly and record the weight. If it increases by more than 10% over the optimal weight, reinstitute the weight reduction diet and program.

D. Starvation program for dogs

1) In a few instances in which an owner cannot maintain a caloric reduction program because of the difficulty and frustration associated with the program, starvation conducted within the veterinary hospital may be proposed as an alternative. Ketosis and metabolic acidosis are less severe in the dog than in humans.

2) The disadvantages of a starvation program include some tissue damage, vitamin and mineral deficiencies, mild initial diarrhea with loss of sodium and water, perceived inhumane treatment, and the possibility that the dog may not start eating again after optimal weight has been achieved.

3) Procedure for weight loss via starvation

a) Hospitalization

b) Complete physical examination and testing to rule out endocrine and metabolic disorders

c) Complete withdrawal of all food

d) Vitamin and mineral supplements, with water given ad libitum

e) When the desired weight is reached, the dog is gradually (over a period of two to three days) introduced to a good commercial dog food in an amount needed for maintenance, and is then sent home.

f) The animal is seen and weighed weekly for several weeks, and the amount fed is adjusted accordingly.

4) The results may be successful and gratifying for the client, avoiding the frustrating and possibly unsuccessful experience with home weight-reduction programs. How-

ever, the weight loss may also be temporary because the owner has not participated in the program, and may gradually revert to old feeding habits.

E. Starvation programs are contraindicated in cats owing to the increased risk of hepatic lipidosis in once-obese cats that do not eat for prolonged periods of time.

F. Pharmacologic control of hunger or weight loss is of no benefit in animals, and is associated with many side effects. Therefore, such an approach is not recommended.

G. Prevention of obesity

1) It is most important to prevent obesity during growth. Ad libitum feeding is discouraged.

2) Discourage snacks, table-feeding, and human food.

3) Encourage regular exercise.

4) A lifetime adjustment in feeding habits is needed.

··················
Cachexia

Cachexia may be defined as a profound decrease in body weight to a level less than what is normal for an animal's size and body type.

Etiologic Considerations

1. Inadequate nutrition

A. Starvation

1) Inadequate caloric or nutritional intake

2) Inappropriate diet

B. Gastrointestinal (GI) parasitism

C. Inability to digest and absorb nutrients

1) Maldigestion

2) Malabsorption

D. Loss of calories

1) Protein-losing nephropathy

2) GI abnormalities

2. Neoplasia

3. Metabolic disorders

A. Heart failure
B. Chronic renal disease
C. Chronic liver disease
D. Endocrine diseases
    1) Diabetes mellitus
    2) Hyperadrenocorticism
    3) Hypoadrenocorticism
    4) Hyperthyroidism
  4. Chronic infectious disease
    A. Systemic fungal diseases
    B. Feline infectious peritonitis (FIP)
    C. Diseases associated with feline leukemia virus (FeLV)
    D. Rickettsial diseases (ehrlichiosis and Lyme disease)

Effects of Cachexia

1. Protein-calorie malnutrition with resulting GI digestive and absorptive abnormalities
2. Hypoalbuminemia, decreased plasma protein, and altered plasma protein binding of drugs
3. Decreased hemoglobin production and anemia
4. Decreased resistance to bacterial infection
5. Poor wound healing with increased incidence of decubital ulcers
6. Growth retardation

Diagnostic Approach

History

In general, animals with cachexia have chronic abnormalities. The related problems are often subtle, and may have been present for so long that the owner may consider them to be normal for that animal. Specific historical information may help the examiner to concentrate on investigation of a specific body system.

  1. Nutritional history
    A. Decreased food intake and weight loss
      1) Inadequate caloric or nutritional intake
      2) Environmental disturbance(s) causing anorexia, especially in cats
      3) Neurologic disorder
      4) Illness or treatment results in cases of malaise, anorexia, or nausea
    B. Increased appetite and weight loss
      1) Hyperthyroidism
      2) Hyperadrenocorticism
      3) Diabetes mellitus
      4) Maldigestion
  2. Gastrointestinal history
    A. Unusual nature of stools
      1) Voluminous, soft, odoriferous stools
        a) Maldigestion
        b) Hyperthyroidism
      2) Intermittently watery to firm stools, or constant diarrhea
        a) Malabsorption
        b) GI parasitism
        c) Metabolic disorders (e.g., renal or liver diseases; hypoadrenocorticism)
      3) Melena
        a) GI parasitism
        b) GI neoplasia
        c) GI diseases resulting in malabsorption
        d) Metabolic disorders (renal or liver diseases; hypoadrenocorticism)
    B. Vomiting
      1) GI inflammatory diseases, and gastric or high intestinal neoplasia
      2) Metabolic diseases (renal or liver diseases, diabetic ketoacidosis, and hypoadrenocorticism)
  3. Respiratory history
    A. Dyspnea
      1) Pleural effusion
        a) FIP
        b) Lymphosarcoma
        c) Hypoalbuminemia
        d) Heart failure
        e) Pulmonary infections
        f) Chylothorax
        g) Pyothorax
        h) Diaphragmatic hernia
      2) Intrathoracic masses
        a) Lymphosarcoma
        b) Thymoma
        c) Heart base tumor
      3) Pulmonary edema

    a) Heart failure
    b) Uremia
    c) Hypoalbuminemia
    d) Infections
  B. Cough
    1) Heart failure, especially in dogs
    2) Heartworm disease
    3) Heart base tumor
    4) Hilar lymphadenopathy
    5) Pulmonary infections
4. History of limping
  A. Mycotic osteomyelitis
  B. Neoplastic bone lesions
  C. Septic or immune-complex arthritis
5. History of blindness or other ocular disorders
  A. Diabetic cataracts
  B. Intraocular, CNS, or generalized neoplasia
  C. Some infectious diseases (systemic mycoses, FIP, ehrlichiosis)
  D. Hypertension associated with renal disease
  E. Hepatic encephalopathy
  F. CNS disorder
6. History of polyuria and concomitant polydipsia
  A. Hyperthyroidism
  B. Hypoadrenocorticism
  C. Hyperadrenocorticism
  D. Diabetes mellitus
  E. Chronic renal and liver disease
  F. Rarely, heart failure
7. History of pseudo-obesity
  A. Peritoneal effusion
    1) Hypoproteinemia
    2) Portal hypertension
      a) Right heart failure
      b) Liver disease
    3) Abdominal neoplasia
  B. Extreme hepatomegaly/splenomegaly
  C. Subcutaneous edema
    1) Liver disease with decreased production of albumin
    2) Protein-losing nephropathy and hypoalbuminemia
    3) Protein-losing enteropathy and hypoproteinemia
    4) Right heart failure

Physical Examination

A complete physical examination is essential in evaluating animals with cachexia. Significant findings may include the following:

  1. Mass lesions may be noted with neoplasia, adenomatous thyroid hyperplasia, and osteomyelitis.
  2. Peritoneal effusion may be secondary to hypoproteinemia, portal hypertension, abdominal neoplasia, or FIP.
  3. Dyspnea and cough may be attributable to pleural effusion, pulmonary edema, heart failure, pneumonia, or neoplasia (pulmonary and intrathoracic).
  4. Limb masses may be the result of neoplasia or infection involving the bony skeleton. Joint swelling can be associated with septic or immune-complex arthritis.
  5. Neurologic abnormalities may be associated with neoplasia, mycotic diseases, FIP, and ehrlichiosis involving the CNS.
  6. In some cases, no abnormalities are seen.

Diagnostic Aids

  1. Obtain baseline laboratory data.
    A. Complete blood count (CBC), including white blood cell (WBC) differential cell count
    B. Serum biochemistry profile
      1) Total protein
      2) Renal function tests
      3) Liver-associated enzymes
      4) Electrolytes
    C. Urinalysis
      1) Specific gravity determination
      2) Screening for protein, glucose, and ketones
      3) Sediment examination
  2. Perform thoracic and abdominal radiography to identify:
    A. Masses and other evidence of neoplasia
    B. Organomegaly
    C. Effusions
    D. Lytic and/or proliferative bone lesions

Specific Disorders

Inadequate Nutrition

Starvation

1. Lack of adequate food and calories
  A. Starvation from neglect
  B. Inability to take in food as a result of other animals' aggression (need to feed separately)
  C. Physical infirmity preventing:
    1) Ambulation to food
    2) Prehension, mastication, or swallowing of food
  D. Inadequate nutrition during periods of stress (e.g., during pregnancy, or when exposed to extreme or prolonged cold)
2. Lack of proper and appropriate food
  A. Owner's harmful feeding practices may result in undernutrition or malnutrition.
    1) Human food offered in a poorly balanced dietary regimen
    2) Feeding of fad diets
  B. Inappropriate long-term use of restricted-nutrient diets
3. Mobilization of body fat and muscle protein depletion, with utilization to meet energy requirements
4. Starvation can be diagnosed on the basis of the history.
5. Laboratory findings include decreased serum albumin concentrations, increased serum alkaline phosphatase activity, and decreased hematocrit values.
6. Treatment consists of feeding adequate amounts of a well-balanced diet and, initially, provision of a vitamin and mineral supplement.

Significant GI Parasitism

1. Common among young animals
2. Can cause problems in animals of all ages
3. Common clinical signs
  A. Diarrhea
  B. Vomiting
  C. Unthriftiness

4. Cachexia may be attributable to parasitic nutrient and blood consumption.
5. Treatment consists of appropriate administration of anthelmintics.

Maldigestion and Malabsorption

1. Maldigestion may result from an inability to digest dietary nutrients. Exocrine pancreatic insufficiency (EPI), which occurs infrequently in cats, may be attributable to:
  A. Pancreatic acinar atrophy
  B. Chronic relapsing and acute pancreatitis
  C. Functional EPI secondary to starvation or malabsorption, resulting in protein-calorie malnutrition
2. Malabsorption may result from chronic small intestinal disease and mucosal abnormalities, resulting in an inability to absorb dietary nutrients.
  A. Diffuse chronic inflammatory bowel disease
  B. Lymphangiectasia
  C. Lymphosarcoma
  D. Histoplasmosis and other mycotic intestinal diseases
  E. Villous atrophy (e.g., gluten enteropathy, other causes)
  F. Lactase and mucosal biochemical defects
  G. Chronic giardiasis and other parasitic diseases
  H. Small intestinal anaerobic bacterial overgrowth
3. Anorexia may also produce cachexia through maldigestion and malabsorption.
  A. Malaise and nausea
  B. Vitamin and electrolyte abnormalities secondary to diarrhea, malabsorption, and vomiting
    1) Fat-soluble vitamins, folic acid, vitamin B_{12}, and calcium are the most important deficiencies.
    2) Hypokalemia can contribute to inappetence.
  C. Impaired assimilation of nutrients owing to maldigestion or malabsorption

Clinical Signs

1. Maldigestion

    A. Voluminous and greasy stools

    B. Voracious appetite, pica, coprophagia

    C. Occasional flatulence

2. Malabsorption

    A. Fluid to semisolid episodic or constant diarrhea

    B. Vomiting

    C. Inappetence

    D. Abdominal discomfort

    E. Borborygmus and flatulence

    F. Hypoproteinemia (pitting edema, ascites, or hydrothorax, generally seen when serum albumin is $\leq$1.5 g/dL)

Diagnostic Aids

1. Obtain baseline laboratory data, including:

    A. Results of fecal flotations for parasitic ova

    B. Saline smears with fresh feces to test for protozoal parasites

2. Other tests that are useful in defining type, area of involvement, and etiology of GI disease include:

    A. Fecal fat examination

    B. Serum trypsin-like immunoreactivity

    C. N-benzoyl-L-tyrosyl-para-aminobenzoic acid test

    D. D-xylose absorption test

    E. Plasma turbidity test

    F. Serum B_{12} and folate determinations

    G. Bacteriologic culture of intestinal aspirates

    H. Nitrosonaphthol test

3. Survey radiographs and contrast studies are helpful in the detection of mass lesions, obstructions, and other GI abnormalities.

4. Endoscopic or surgical biopsy with histologic examination may be needed to establish a diagnosis.

Treatment

1. Pharmacologic intervention

    A. Pancreatic enzyme replacement therapy should be instituted in animals with EPI.

    B. Although there is no indication for the routine use of antibiotics in animals with diarrhea, tetracycline, tylosin, or chloramphenicol are indicated for treatment of bacterial overgrowth.

    C. Metronidazole may be used to treat giardiasis.

    D. Immunosuppressive drugs can be useful in treating some inflammatory bowel disorders and lymphangiectasia.

    E. Gastrointestinal lymphosarcoma should be treated with chemotherapy.

2. Dietary intervention

    A. Small, frequent meals (three to four per day) should be provided for animals with maldigestion or malabsorption disorders.

    B. A diet low in fat, such as i/d®* or r/d®*, should be fed to animals with maldigestion disorders.

    C. For malabsorption, a highly digestible diet that is low in fat and lactose, and that contains high-quality protein, is advised. R/d®*, i/d®* or d/d®* may be used. Alternatively, a homemade diet, formulated with a 4 : 1 ratio of carbohydrate to protein and using rice or potatoes as a carbohydrate source, and low-fat cottage cheese, yoghurt, eggs, or lean broiled chicken or lamb as a protein source, may be used.

    D. For gluten enteropathy, a trial of d/d®*, i/d®*, or Eukanuba®‡ is appropriate.

    E. Eukanuba®†, Science Diet®*, or Advanced Nutrition Formula (ANF)‡ can be helpful in immunoproliferative enteropathy affecting basenjis.

    F. Food hypersensitivity or eosinophilic gastroenteritis may be treated with a trial of d/d®*, rice, and chicken or lamb.

    G. If malabsorption is severe, elemental diets, such as Vivonex®§ or Portagen®‖, may be needed.

    H. Medium-chain triglycerides (MCT oil®‖) may be added to the diet of animals with lymphangiectasia, anaerobic bacterial overgrowth, or other malabsorption disorders as a source of fat calories that are absorbed directly into the portal system.

    I. Cats with intestinal problems fare best

---

* Hill's Pet Products, Inc., Topeka, KS 66601

† The Iams Co., Dayton, OH 45414

‡ Ross-Wells Division of Beatrice Foods Co., Mequon, WI 53092

§ Norwich Eaton Pharmaceuticals, Inc., Norwich, NY 13815

‖ Mead Johnson & Co., Evansville, IN 47721

on high-fat diets, such as c/d®*. Alternative diets to try include lamb, chicken, Iams®†, Science®*, and Tender Vittles®¶. As cats have a low tolerance for starch, it should be restricted in the diet.

J. A vitamin and mineral supplement should be provided.

1) Injectable fat-soluble vitamins, and oral water-soluble vitamins and vitamin K should be used.

2) Empiric doses of vitamin B_{12} (500 μg/mo parenterally) and folate (5 mg PO/d) have been given to dogs with chronic GI disease with some success.

Prognosis

1. The prognosis for animals with EPI secondary to acinar atrophy and pancreatitis is good with proper diagnosis and treatment.

2. The prognosis for animals with maldigestion can be good to poor, depending on the etiology. Proper diagnosis and treatment can significantly prolong good quality of life for many affected animals.

Neoplasia

Clinical Approach

1. Any animal in whom there is weight loss of unexplained origin warrants a complete examination of all body systems for evidence of a neoplastic process.

2. Identify the type of neoplasia.

A. Cytologic examination of fine needle aspiration specimen

B. Histologic examination of surgical or endoscopic biopsy material

3. Thoroughly evaluate the patient.

A. Perform complete hematologic and biochemical examinations. Associated abnormalities that may cause clinical signs and may be life-threatening include:

1) Cytopenias

2) Gammopathies

3) Hypercalcemia

4) Hypoglycemia

5) Disseminated intravascular coagulation

6) Other paraneoplastic disorders

¶ Cadillac Pet Foods, Inc., Pennsauken, NJ 08110

B. Search for evidence of metastasis by physical examination and with thoracic and abdominal radiographs.

1) Aspiration or biopsy of lymph nodes, bone marrow, and other organs may aid in the detection of metastasis.

2) This information will also facilitate the staging of the neoplasia. Staging of the tumor generally correlates with prognosis, except in hematopoietic tumors.

Treatment

Therapeutic recommendations can be made based on the type of malignant lesion, the presence or absence of metastasis, staging of the neoplasm, associated abnormalities, and the patient's physical status.

1. Surgery is one of the primary treatments for tumors.

A. Optimally, it is used to excise a primary tumor and adjacent healthy tissue margins without causing irreparable injury to the patient.

B. Noncurative reduction of large tumor masses may result in clinical improvement, and may augment the effectiveness of adjuvant therapeutic regimens.

2. Chemotherapy involves the use of antineoplastic agents to destroy tumor tissue.

A. It is used for widely disseminated or metastatic disease, as well as for other tumors that are not surgically excisable, and for those that prove to be refractory to irradiation and other therapeutic regimens.

B. Tumor cells are more sensitive to the drugs used than are normal cells.

C. Maximal efficacy and minimal side effects are attained by the use of a combination of chemotherapeutic drugs, as each drug has its own peculiar differences in mechanisms of action and limitations of tolerance.

3. Radiation therapy

A. This type of therapy involves the use of ionizing radiation to damage or kill malignant cells.

B. It can be administered by an external beam or from a source placed on or within the patient.

4. Immunotherapy attempts to stimulate the body's defense system to kill tumor cells.

5. Hyperthermia

A. Therapeutically induced local or whole-body hyperpyrexia (40° to 43°C) results in cellular damage or death of tumor.

B. Immunogenicity of some tumor cells may be augmented, increasing the patient's immune response against the cancer.

6. Miscellaneous

A. Antiplatelet therapy may help control metastasis.

B. Monoclonal antibodies may aid cancer therapy by selective delivery of therapeutic agents to tumor cells, induction of passive immunotherapy, and neutralization of the hormones responsible for paraneoplastic syndromes.

Cachexia Secondary to Cancer

1. Inadequate food intake

A. Result of cancer-associated malaise, nausea, and anorexia.

B. The side effects of the anticancer therapy itself (pain from surgery, stomatitis from radiation therapy, and so on) may decrease food intake.

2. Abnormal metabolism of the patient with cancer

A. Abnormal absorption, utilization, and metabolism of nutrients.

B. Tumors may increase the metabolic rate of the patient.

3. Treatment

A. Cure or control of the underlying malignant disease, if possible.

B. Feeding a variety of foods in several small, frequent meals may help to increase caloric intake.

C. For animals requiring parenteral hyperalimentation, low-carbohydrate and high-protein solutions are recommended because of the changes in energy metabolism and nitrogen balance that are thought to occur in affected animals.

Prognosis

Although the prognosis for the cure of many types of malignant neoplasia is poor, proper therapy can significantly prolong a pet's good quality of life. Multimodality approaches, using appropriate combinations of treatment methods, can achieve high remission rates with some tumor types.

Metabolic Disorders

Cardiac Cachexia

Etiologic Considerations

1. Heart disease, a common condition in domestic dogs and cats, may be caused by a variety of disorders.

A. Acquired diseases of the myocardium and the atrioventricular valves

B. Heartworm disease

C. Congenital anomalies

D. Pericardial disease

E. Neoplasia

2. Heart failure may result when heart or pericardial disease results in a diminution of cardiac performance to a degree that compensation can no longer occur.

3. Subsequent activation of the renin-angiotensin system and release of antidiuretic hormone results in:

A. The retention of sodium and water

B. Excess intravascular fluid volume, which increases cardiac work load and congestion

4. Cardiac cachexia has been attributed to several different entities.

A. Anorexia secondary to:

1) Malaise

2) Acute change of diet, or poor palatability of food

3) Loss of potassium and B vitamins

4) Nausea and vomiting consequent to digitalis overdose

B. Malabsorption of nutrients may occur secondary to pooling and stasis of visceral blood, with possible development of a protein-losing enteropathy.

C. A catabolic state develops secondary to protein and energy deficits.

D. Poor perfusion results in peripheral tissue hypoxia and weakness.

Clinical Signs

1. Cough, especially in dogs

2. Dyspnea

3. Restlessness, especially when recumbent

4. Episodes of syncope

5. Cyanosis

6. Polyuria and polydypsia

7. Pseudo-obesity secondary to ascites or subcutaneous edema

Diagnostic Aids

Characterization of heart and associated problems should be attempted utilizing routine radiography, hematologic studies, electrocardiography, echocardiography, and angiography, when indicated.

Treatment

1. Pharmacologic intervention

   A. Digitalis glycosides

      1) To improve myocardial contractility

      2) These drugs may cause the side effects of vomiting and diarrhea, which may, in turn, result in fluid and electrolyte abnormalities.

   B. Diuretics

      1) To increase renal excretion of sodium and water

      2) Long-term administration of diuretics has been associated with increased excretion of potassium, magnesium, zinc, iron, and water-soluble vitamins.

   C. Vasodilators reduce cardiac afterload or preload.

   D. Antiarrhythmic drugs promote more normal cardiac pump function.

2. Dietary intervention

   A. The goals of dietary management of cardiac patients include:

      1) Decreased cardiac work load

      2) Maintenance of lean body weight so that cachexia or obesity do not occur

      3) Provision of adequate calories, protein, vitamins, and minerals

      4) Maximization of the palatability of the diet

   B. Sodium restriction

      1) A sodium intake of 30 mg/kg/d is recommended in patients with mild heart disease and early congestive states (210 mg/100 gr dry food matter).

      2) For animals diagnosed as having moderate heart failure, 13 mg/kg/d may be administered (100 mg/100 gr dry food matter).

      3) More stringent sodium restriction may be needed in cases of severe heart failure.

      4) Some water softeners add sodium to the drinking water.

   C. Adequate amounts of protein

      1) Dogs need 14% to 18% protein in diet dry matter.

      2) Cats should receive a relatively greater proportion of protein (25% to 45% in diet dry matter).

      3) Protein sources (eggs, chicken, or pork) provide high-quality and easily digestible protein.

   D. Adequate energy must be provided to prevent muscle catabolism. After protein needs are met, carbohydrates and fats should be added to meet caloric demand (see Tables 5-1 and 5-2).

   E. B vitamin requirements are greater in affected animals than in healthy animals. Brewer's yeast (1 g/kg) or a B-complex vitamin preparation may be provided if the diet is not supplemented.

   F. Calcium, potassium, and magnesium are important in heart muscle function.

      1) Supplementation of potassium with dietary sources (e.g., bananas, molasses) is considered the safest method.

      2) Mineral supplementation may be provided if not supplied adequately in the diet.

   G. Taurine deficiency has been associated with dilated cardiomyopathy in cats. Oral taurine supplementation (500 mg PO b.i.d.) has been suggested for affected cats with low serum taurine concentrations.

   H. Specific diets

      1) Prescription Diets (canine and feline) h/d* and Special Diet (canine) H®† provide the sodium restriction necessary for moderate to severe heart failure, as well as vitamin and mineral supplementation. Taurine has been added to feline h/d®*.

      2) Animals with mild heart failure may be fed the prescription diets described above, along with commercial dog food

---

* Hill's Pet Products, Inc., Topeka, KS 66601

† Cadillac Pet Foods, Inc., Pennsauken, NJ 08110

(those with a moderate sodium content—350 to 400 mg/100 mg dry weight) to increase palatability. Prescription Diet k/d* provides the salt restriction necessary for mild heart disease, and may be tried by itself.

    3) Homemade diets may be substituted.

    I. Fostering acceptance of dietary changes by pet.

    1) Warm foods to volatilize odors.

    2) Switch diet slowly, over the course of four to five days.

    3) Feed small amounts frequently.

    4) Add flavor enhancers in small amounts.

    a) Garlic powder

    b) Salt substitutes containing potassium chloride

    c) Honey and molasses

    d) Low-sodium butter, which is especially enjoyed by cats

    e) Low-sodium cottage cheese, especially for cats

    f) Boiled lean meat

    5) Drugs to increase the appetite may be tried.

    a) Diazepam, 0.1 to 0.5 mg IV for anorectic cats, which can be followed by an oral dose of 1 to 2 mg/cat to maintain appetite stimulation.

    b) B vitamins

Prognosis

The prognosis for heart disease, heart failure, and the control of cardiac cachexia may be good to poor, depending on the etiology and on the owner's compliance with medication and dietary regimens. Existence of concurrent renal or hepatic disease, or both, will affect the prognosis.

Renal Failure Cachexia

Etiologic Considerations

1. Renal disease results in renal failure (RF) when there is a loss of >75% of nephron function as a result of:

    A. Interstitial disease

    B. Glomerular disease

    C. Tubular disease

    D. Vascular abnormalities

    E. Congenital anomalies

    F. Neoplasia

2. The remaining nephrons must handle the excretion or retention of water and solutes, which was previously handled by all of the renal mass.

    A. Each nephron undergoes an increase in glomerular filtration rate (GFR), despite a decrease in total kidney GFR. A high protein intake contributes to glomerular hyperfiltration.

    B. The result is glomerulosclerosis, eventual nephron loss, and deterioration of renal function.

    C. Solute retention occurs (e.g., increased blood urea nitrogen [BUN]), with retained protein catabolites contributing significantly to the production of clinical signs of RF.

    D. There is concomitant loss of fluids and solutes (e.g., polyuria).

3. Parathyroid hormone (PTH)

    A. Increased serum concentrations promote bone demineralization.

    B. Increased levels of PTH may contribute to the clinical signs of uremia.

4. An inability to excrete gastrin results in increased gastric acid production, gastroenteritis, GI ulceration, and vomiting.

5. Anemia may be the result of:

    A. Decreased renal erythropoietin production

    B. Shortened life span of red blood cells

    C. GI blood loss

6. Hypertension is common in dogs (and also occurs in cats) with RF and glomerular disease secondary to:

    A. Inadequate sodium homeostasis

    B. Other hormonal and neurological phenomena

7. Polyuria and anorexia may result in hypokalemia.

8. Water-soluble vitamin deficiencies may occur secondary to polyuria.

9. Cachexia in association with RF may be attributable to several factors:

    A. Anorexia secondary to:

    1) Malaise

    2) Nausea, gastritis, and vomiting

    3) Oral ulceration and discomfort

4) Impaired taste acuity

5) Loss of B vitamins and potassium

B. Impaired intestinal digestion and absorption of proteins and carbohydrates

C. Impaired tubular reabsorption of amino acids

D. Loss of protein via GI hemorrhage or proteinuria in glomerular disease

E. Peripheral insulin resistance, which may contribute to increased energy demands

F. Soft tissue catabolism as a result of inadequate energy intake and protein loss

Clinical Signs

The clinical signs of RF may be nonspecific, vague, and insidious.

1. Polyuria and polydypsia

2. Unthrifty appearance

3. Halitosis, stomatitis, and oral ulcers

4. Vomiting and diarrhea

5. Dehydration

6. Neurologic disturbances

7. Blindness

8. Pathologic fractures

9. Edema and ascites

10. Coagulopathies

11. Dyspnea and coughing

Diagnostic Aids

Diagnosis of RF is facilitated by urine biochemical studies, survey and contrast radiography, ultrasonography, and renal biopsy with histopathologic examination.

Treatment

1. Rectify the underlying cause.

2. Pharmacologic intervention

A. Cimetidine

1) Decreases gastric acid production

2) Reduces circulating PTH and phosphorus concentrations

B. Antiemetics to decrease vomiting

C. Phosphorus restriction to slow the progression of RF

1) Aluminum hydroxide phosphorus binders, when given with meals, decrease intestinal phosphorus absorption.

2) Dietary phosphorus restriction must be instituted concomitantly.

D. Administration of antihypertensives and gradual sodium restriction (to 0.2% to 0.3% in dietary dry matter) are instituted if hypertension or the nephrotic syndrome is diagnosed.

E. Anabolic steroids promote erythropoiesis.

3. Dietary intervention

A. Goals of dietary management in RF

1) Meet all of the animal's nutritional needs so that cachexia is minimized.

2) Control dietary input so that intake does not exceed the animal's ability to utilize or excrete it.

B. A copious supply of fresh water should always be available.

C. Adequate energy supplies must be provided. Caloric requirements in animals with RF may be greater than in normal animals.

1) Dogs with RF require 70 to 100 kcal/kg/d. The recommended caloric intake for cats with RF is 70 to 80 kcal/kg/d.

2) An insufficient caloric intake will result in the catabolism of body soft tissue and will worsen azotemia.

D. Control of dietary protein is important.

1) Decreased protein intake may slow the progression of renal damage.

2) Decreased protein intake will decrease the circulating end-products of protein metabolism that cause azotemia.

3) Insufficient provision of essential amino acids will result in body protein catabolism.

4) Restricted amounts of protein that is of high biological quality and is easily digestible, such as egg and milk proteins, are recommended.

a) Dogs should be provided with 2.0 to 2.2 g/kg of protein per day.

b) The requirement for cats may be higher; a value of 3.3 to 3.8 g/kg daily has been suggested.

c) Animals with severe RF may require more stringent protein restriction.

5) If an animal has glomerular disease with proteinuria, additional amounts of high-quality protein may be required to replace the protein that has been lost.

a) The amount of extra protein needed can be determined by performing a 24-hour urine albumin analysis; alternatively, it may be estimated from a urine spot sample protein/creatinine ratio.

b) The extra protein provided should be of high biological quality, such as that derived from eggs (2 g protein/egg).

6) Generally, diets containing restricted quantities of high-quality protein will also be low in phosphorus.

E. Fats (especially in cats) and carbohydrates (which dogs like) may be used to provide the bulk of calories.

F. Vitamin D and calcium are not routinely supplemented owing to the risk of soft tissue mineralization.

G. A B vitamin supplement (not protein-containing brewer's yeast) and 50 to 100 mg of vitamin C daily may be beneficial.

H. Specific diets

1) Canine and feline Prescription Diet k/d®*, and Special Diet N®† provide protein, phosphorus, and sodium restriction, as well as vitamin supplementation. Prescription Diet u/d®* may be used in cases of severe RF.

2) Homemade diets with appropriate vitamin supplementation can also be used successfully.

I. Alleviate anorexia and improve palatability.

1) Feed multiple, frequent meals.

2) Warm food to volatilize odors.

3) Flavor food with chicken fat or broth.

4) Fry food in unsalted butter (especially for cats).

5) Carbohydrates will enhance the flavor of canine diets.

6) Provide potassium-rich foods and B vitamins, if needed.

Prognosis

Although RF is often inexorably progressive, proper dietary and medical regimens can slow deterioration and perceptibly improve the animal's quality of life.

---

* Hill's Pet Products, Inc., Topeka, KS 66601
† Cadillac Pet Foods, Inc., Pennsauken, NJ 08110

Hepatic Cachexia

Etiologic Considerations

1. The liver is responsible for the metabolism and utilization of nutrients from the GI tract, and for detoxifying drugs and toxins. Compromise of these functions can be caused by a number of disorders.

A. Hepatocellular disease

B. Biliary disease

C. Portosystemic vascular anomalies

D. Neoplasia

2. Hepatic encephalopathy may be caused by cerebral effects secondary to toxins and false neurotransmitters.

A. Toxins, such as ammonia, mercaptans, short-chain fatty acids, indole, skatol, biogenic amines, and gamma-aminobutyric acid, are absorbed from the GI tract.

B. Alterations in body amino acid metabolism result in increased levels of circulating aromatic amino acids and decreased branched-chain amino acids.

3. Ascites and subcutaneous edema may form as a result of increased portal hypertension, hypoalbuminemia, and salt and water retention.

4. Coagulopathies, secondary to decreased hepatic synthesis of coagulation factors and antithrombin III, may be evident.

5. GI hemorrhage, secondary to increased bile-acid–stimulated gastrin secretion and GI ulceration, may result in anemia.

6. Polyuria with concomitant polydipsia is attributable to decreased medullary hypertonicity, changes in intrarenal hemodynamics, and increased sensitivity of portal vein osmoreceptors.

7. Cachexia-producing factors

A. Anorexia

1) Secondary to toxins in the CNS

2) Secondary to nausea, gastroenteritis, and vomiting

3) Hypokalemia owing to anorexia, polyuria, use of diuretics, and vomiting

4) Vitamin deficiencies secondary to anorexia, and decreased hepatic conversion and storage

B. Decreased hepatic synthesis of albumin is accompanied by blood protein loss via bleeding.

C. Malabsorption of fat and fat-soluble vitamins may occur as a result of insufficient hepatic bile salts or bile duct obstruction.
D. Abnormal carbohydrate and fat metabolism
E. Catabolism of soft tissue to meet body demands

Clinical Signs

Many clinical signs associated with hepatic failure may be episodic and exacerbated by a high-protein meal. Hypersalivation is commonly seen in cats.

Diagnostic Aids

1. Specialized tests of hepatic function, such as the ammonia tolerance test, preprandial and postprandial serum bile acids, plasma amino acids, and sulfobromophthalein or indocyanine green dye excretion tests, are indicated.
2. A liver biopsy, determination of hepatic copper content, radiographic contrast study of portal venous and liver blood flow, or measurements of portal venous pressure may render a definitive diagnosis and suggest the proper mode of therapy.

Treatment

1. Treatment of the underlying cause
2. Surgical ligation of congenital portosystemic shunts
3. Medical treatment for hepatic failure
    A. Lactulose and neomycin may be used to decrease the bacterial production of ammonia and other toxins in the intestine.
    B. Bleeding should be controlled by the elimination of GI parasites and cimetidine; vitamin K_1 may be needed in cases of biliary obstruction.
    C. For ascites or edema, the use of furosemide or spironolactone diuretics is recommended, along with low-sodium diet.
4. Dietary intervention
    A. Goals
        1) Reduce the clinical signs associated with hepatic encephalopathy.
        2) Reduce the role of liver function in:
            a) Gluconeogenesis
            b) Amino acid deamination

            c) Lipid metabolism
        3) Provide conditions for optimal hepatic regeneration, if that is possible.
    B. Provide adequate calories (see Tables 5-1 and 5-2).
    C. Protein
        1) Reasons for changing quantity and type
            a) Reduce blood ammonia and other encephalopathic toxins which are by-products of protein degradation.
            b) Provide a more normal balance of plasma amino acids.
            c) Provide adequate protein necessary for hepatic regeneration, albumin production, and prevention of body catabolism.
        2) Specific recommendations
            a) Provide 1.4 to 2.2 g/kg/d of protein for dogs.
            b) Supply food in several divided amounts during the day.
            c) Cottage cheese is a good source of protein that is high in biologic value.
                i. It provides the correct ratio of branched-chain to aromatic amino acids.
                ii. High digestibility provides less substrate for ammonia production by intestinal bacteria.
    D. Fats
        1) Small amounts of fat (4% to 6% dry weight for dogs) are essential, and will provide essential fatty acids and fat-soluble vitamins.
        2) Palatability and caloric content of food are increased with the addition of fats.
        3) Excessive amounts may aggravate encephalopathy by adding short-chain fatty acids.
        4) The use of MCT oil is contraindicated.
    E. Carbohydrates provide the bulk of the calories.
        1) Should be easily digestible
        2) Boiled macaroni or white rice are recommended.
    F. Potassium supplementation for hypokalemia should be in the form of foods, if possible.

G. Sodium intake should be restricted if edema or body cavity effusions are noted.

H. Fat-soluble and B-complex vitamins, as well as minerals, should be supplemented.

I. Lipotrophic agents containing methionine are contraindicated in hepatic insufficiency, as they may precipitate or worsen hepatic encephalopathy.

J. Arginine insufficiency has been suggested as one of the possible causes of idiopathic hepatic lipidosis in cats. Although arginine is available in eggs, these must be fed with caution as they contain methionine and may worsen hepatic encephalopathy.

K. Bedlington terriers and other dogs affected with excessive hepatic copper must be fed a low-copper diet. Organ meats, shellfish, nuts, and chocolate should be avoided. Owners are advised to feed lean beaf, cottage cheese, and vitamin-mineral supplements without copper.

L. Specific diets

1) Prescription Diets (canine and feline) k/d®* and u/d®* and Special Diet N®† provide restricted amounts of protein of high biologic value, as well as vitamin supplementation.

2) Homemade diets are often fed successfully, as well.

3) Vitamin and mineral supplements should be provided.

4) Palatability of the food may be increased by:

a) Warming the food

b) Providing multiple small meals

c) Using carbohydrates as flavor enhancers for dogs

Hyperthyroidism

1. Hyperthyroidism is a disorder affecting mature cats that is caused by an excess of circulating T_4 and T_3, usually as a result of adenomatous hyperplasia involving either both lobes or a single thyroid lobe.

2. Thyroid hormones exert stimulatory actions, resulting in increased energy metabolism. Excessive circulating thyroid hormones may affect many organs and drive the sympathetic nervous system.

3. Cachexia

A. Excessive levels of circulating thyroid hormones produce a catabolic state.

B. Cats often exhibit voracious appetite, but are unable to utilize calories sufficiently to prevent body wasting.

1) Patients may vomit (after eating very quickly), and have diarrhea (possibly as a result of increased intestinal motility), so that what is eaten is not utilized properly.

2) Malabsorption and excessive fecal fat may occur.

Clinical Signs

1. Polyphagia

2. Hyperactivity

3. Tachycardia and arrhythmias

4. Polyuria and polydipsia

5. Diarrhea and voluminous frequent stools

6. Panting

7. Fever

8. Occasional anorexia

Diagnostic Aids

1. Serum T_3 and T_4 analysis should be performed.

2. Electrocardiograms and echocardiograms are performed to determine the presence of associated cardiac abnormalities.

3. Thyroid scanning with pertechnetate ($^{99m}TcO_4$) is performed to examine functioning thyroid tissue.

Treatment

1. Surgical thyroidectomy or radioactive iodine (I^{131}) treatments are curative.

2. The antithyroid drugs methimazole and propylthiouracil are used for stabilization prior to definitive therapy; alternatively, they may be used for long-term noncurative control of hyperthyroidism.

3. Associated myocardial abnormalities or arrhythmias should be treated appropriately.

4. Good quality food of high caloric value should be provided frequently.

* Hill's Pet Products, Inc., Topeka, KS 66601
† Cadillac Pet Foods, Inc., Pennsauken, NJ 08110

Hypoadrenocorticism

1. Hypoadrenocorticism causes illness and cachexia uncommonly in dogs and rarely in cats. It may be caused by:
    A. Primary adrenocortical insufficiency
    B. Decreased pituitary adrenocortico-tropic hormone (ACTH) production
2. The related physiologic abnormalities are attributable to inadequate secretion of mineralocorticoids and glucocorticoids.
3. Mineralocorticoid deficiency causes:
    A. Hypotension secondary to impairment of sodium conservation
    B. Arrhythmias owing to the inability to excrete potassium
4. Glucocorticoid deficiency causes:
    A. Anorexia and vomiting
    B. Lethargy
    C. Metabolic changes
    D. An inability to respond appropriately to stress
5. Cachexia is attributable to:
    A. Anorexia and vomiting
    B. Metabolic changes secondary to glucocorticoid deficiency
        1) Impaired gluconeogenesis
        2) Impaired fat metabolism and utilization
        3) Liver glycogen depletion

Clinical Signs

1. Depression
2. Weakness
3. Vomiting and diarrhea
4. Shaking
5. Polyuria and polydipsia

Diagnostic Aids

Diagnosis is facilitated by an ACTH stimulation test assessing serum cortisol concentrations.

Treatment

1. Mineralocorticoids and glucocorticoids
2. Dietary intervention
    A. Sodium chloride (NaCl) must be provided at a dose of 0.5 to 5 g/d (1 tablespoon of table salt = 3.5 g of NaCl).
    B. Good quality food should be provided.

Diabetes Mellitus

Diabetes mellitus (DM) is a disease of absolute or relative insulin deficiency that is seen more commonly in dogs (females > males) than in cats (males > females).

Etiologic Considerations

1. Common causes
    A. Chronic relapsing pancreatitis resulting in fibrosis and loss of the beta cells in islets of Langerhans
    B. Canine juvenile DM results from atrophy of islet cells.
    C. Feline DM is usually associated with islet amyloid deposition.
2. Non–insulin-dependent DM is rare in animals.
3. Insulin deficiency, aggravated by glucagon excess, results in:
    A. Impaired movement of glucose into many tissues, as well as glycogenolysis, resulting in fasting hyperglycemia
    B. Release of free fatty acids from peripheral tissues
    C. Release of gluconeogenic amino acids from the muscles
4. Polyuria with associated polydipsia is attributable to osmotic diuresis.
5. Ketoacidosis
    A. Increased levels of serum and urine ketones occur as a result of fatty acid breakdown.
    B. As ketones accumulate, metabolic acidosis develops.
    C. Vomiting, diarrhea, and sodium wasting result in dehydration.
6. Total body potassium deficits
    A. Osmotic diuresis
    B. Vomiting
    C. Anorexia
    D. Loss of muscle mass
7. Cachexia associated with DM
    A. Anorexia secondary to:
        1) Malaise
        2) Nausea and vomiting
        3) Hypokalemia
    B. Patients are unable to use carbohydrate sources.
    C. Lack of insulin results in catabolism of soft tissues to meet energy demands.

1) Mobilization of triglycerides for energy needs

2) Breakdown of body proteins for gluconeogenesis

Clinical Signs

1. Polyuria and polydipsia
2. Polyphagia
3. Vomiting and diarrhea
4. Hepatomegaly
5. Cataracts in dogs
6. Icterus (more prevalent in cats than in dogs)
7. Obesity or cachexia
8. Polyneuropathy (cats may have plantigrade stance)
9. Ulcerative dermatosis

Diagnostic Aids

1. A serum amylase/lipase analysis and abdominal radiography should be performed if pancreatitis is suspected.
2. Glucose tolerance testing can aid in the diagnosis of atypical DM.
3. Glycosylated hemoglobin, serum hormone, and immunoreactive insulin determinations may aid in the assessment of the hard-to-control diabetic patient.

Treatment

1. Pharmacologic intervention
  A. Injectable insulin
  B. Concurrent pancreatitis and EPI must be managed, if present.
    1) Pancreatitis is managed with fluid therapy and food restriction
    2) EPI is managed as described earlier in this chapter under maldigestion
2. Dietary intervention
  A. Consistency in diet timing, quantity, and quality is important.
    1) One-quarter to one-half the daily ration is provided in the morning after the insulin injection.
    2) The remainder of the food is fed in the afternoon or evening when the previously injected insulin is judged to be at its peak serum concentration.
  B. No snacks are permitted.
  C. Specific diets

    1) A good quality commercial food can be used. A high-protein, low-carbohydrate, and low-fat diet is ideal.
    2) A history of pancreatitis or EPI may dictate the use of a low-fat diet.
  D. Potassium replacement via food sources is optimal. In a critical care situation, it may be included (as KCl or K_3PO_4) with the intravenous fluids.
  E. Vitamin and mineral supplementation may be beneficial.
  F. Hypoglycemic insulin reactions can be treated with corn syrup or honey (4 tablespoons/10 kg body weight). If the animal cannot swallow, these substances can be rubbed on the patient's gums during transport to the veterinarian.
3. Exercise should be of the same type, duration, and timing each day.

Prognosis

An uncomplicated case of diabetes will generally respond well to diligent owner care. The prognosis for complicated DM is dependent on the animal's coexisting problems.

Infectious Diseases

Cachexia Associated with Chronic Illnesses

1. Anorexia
  A. Chronic malaise
  B. Vitamin, mineral, and electrolyte deficiencies secondary to anorexia and organ system involvement
  C. Nausea and vomiting with gastrointestinal involvement
  D. CNS involvement
2. Fever increases metabolic rate and catabolism.
3. Other pathophysiologic abnormalities associated with organ dysfunction (e.g., gastrointestinal malabsorption, protein-losing nephropathy, and the like).
4. Treatment
  A. Rectify the underlying problem.
  B. Provide supportive care.
5. The diet provided should be of good quality, with vitamin and mineral supplementation when appropriate.

Systemic Mycoses

The systemic mycoses are fungi that infect animal species causing generalized, often nondescript, clinical illness. These agents include *Histoplasma capsulatum*, *Blastomyces dermatiditis*, *Cryptococcus neoformans*, *Coccidioides immitis*, and *Aspergillus*. Dogs are more frequently affected than cats by most mycoses, but cats have a higher incidence of cryptococcosis. Disseminated aspergillosis is rare, and generally occurs as an opportunistic infection in immunosuppressed pets.

Clinical Presentation

1. Coughing and dyspnea
   A. Pneumonia
   B. Pleural effusion
2. Coccidioidomycosis may result in heart failure.
3. Chronic sinusitis and rhinitis can occur in blastomycosis, aspergillosis, and cryptococcosis.
4. Organomegaly
5. Chronic diarrhea, malabsorption, and protein-losing enteropathy may be seen with histoplasmosis, coccidioidomycosis, and aspergillosis.
6. Liver involvement (histoplasmosis, coccidioidomycosis) may be evidenced by icterus or hypoalbuminemia.
7. Genitourinary tract involvement can result in orchitis, prostatitis (blastomycosis, coccidioidomycosis), and renal disease (cryptococcosis, coccidioidomycosis).
8. Lameness, joint swelling, and pathologic fractures are presenting features of mycotic osteomyelitis.
9. Draining skin lesions are evident in some affected animals.
10. Ocular disease may be seen.
11. Neurologic signs may be seen in any of these diseases, but are reported most frequently in cases of cryptococcosis.

Diagnostic Aids

1. CBC
   A. Mild nonregenerative anemias (of chronic disease)
   B. Leukocytosis with a left shift
   C. Monocytosis
2. Serum biochemical studies
   A. Total serum protein values may be low, normal, or increased.
   B. Hypercalcemia is a rare manifestation of blastomycosis.
   C. Increased liver enzymes or bilirubinemia may be noted if the liver is affected.
   D. Azotemia may be noted in animals with renal involvement or dehydration, or both.
3. Urinalysis
   A. Inflammatory changes and proteinuria may be noted when the prostate or kidneys, or both, are affected.
   B. Proteinuria may also be attributable to immune-complex glomerulonephritis.
   C. Organisms can be identified in urine sediment.
4. Radiologic examination
   A. Thoracic radiographs demonstrate pulmonary, pleural, cardiac, and pericardial abnormalities.
   B. Abdominal radiographs demonstrate organomegaly, and a GI barium series may suggest wall thickening or mucosal irregularities.
   C. Bony lesions may be lytic or prolific.
5. Cytology
   A. Most rapid and least costly method of diagnosis
   B. Samples should be obtained from:
      1) Nasal, cutaneous, and draining lymph node exudates
      2) Impression smears of biopsies and rectal scrapings
      3) Aspirates of lymph nodes, subcutaneous nodules, bone lesions, affected organs, bone marrow, tracheal wash, and ocular aqueous or vitreous material
      4) Cerebrospinal fluid (CSF)
6. Biopsy
   A. Surgical, endoscopic, or laparoscopic
   B. In animals without any obvious organ involvement but with suspected systemic mycoses, biopsy of a lymph node may provide a diagnosis.
7. Cultures
   A. Utilize material obtained for cytologic and biopsy studies

B. Use a commercial microbiologic laboratory only.

8. Serology

A. Agar gel immunodiffusion

B. Complement fixation

C. Latex agglutination

Treatment

1. Amphotericin B

A. Fungicidal and fungistatic polyene antibiotic with immunoadjuvant effects.

B. Dose: 0.1 to 1.0 mg/kg/d IV infusion in 5% dextrose given three times a week to a total dose of 4 to 25 mg/kg, depending on the organism and the patient's status.

C. Side effects

1) Nephrotoxicity

a) Determine pretreatment BUN values.

b) Prior to each treatment, repeat BUN. If BUN >50 to 60 mg/dL, discontinue treatment until it is <40 mg/dL.

c) Methods advocated to decrease nephrotoxicity:

    i. Infuse mannitol at 1 g/kg IV along with administration of the amphotericin B.

    ii. Place the animal on a slow IV drip of 0.9% saline prior to initiation of drug therapy.

2) Hypokalemia may occasionally warrant potassium supplementation.

2. Ketoconazole

A. Ketoconazole is a primarily fungistatic imidazole antibiotic, with some immunomodulant activities.

B. Administer the drug orally (with food), 10 to 30 mg/kg in divided doses t.i.d.

C. Mild side effects

1) Anorexia

2) Vomiting

3) Increased liver enzyme values

4) Reversible

D. More powerful imidazole antibiotics, such as itraconazole, may be available soon.

3. Flucytosine

A. Fluorinated pyrimidine which may be fungicidal or fungistatic

B. Dosage: 100 to 150 mg/kg/d PO in doses divided q.i.d. (a lower dose range is recommended for cats)

C. Low toxicity

D. Used in conjunction with another drug to prevent the emergence of resistant fungal strains

4. Specific treatment regimens

A. Avoid steroids.

B. Ketoconazole is used whenever possible, as it has relatively low toxicity and it is easy to administer.

1) For coccidioidomycosis:

a) Administer ketoconazole for 6 to 12 months.

b) A few animals require medication indefinitely.

2) For histoplasmosis and blastomycosis:

a) Continue treatment with ketoconazole for a minimum of three months, and 30 days beyond resolution of clinical signs.

b) If the disease is fulminant, a combination drug regimen of ketoconazole and amphotericin B should be initiated.

    i. Begin amphotericin B and ketoconazole together.

    ii. Administer amphotericin B at the dose indicated earlier until a cumulative dose of 4 to 8 mg/kg is reached.

    iii. Ketoconazole therapy should be continued after discontinuation of amphotericin B therapy.

3) For cryptococcosis:

a) A combination of amphotericin B and flucytosine has been found to have a synergistic effect.

    i. Administer flucytosine for one to four months, or until there are no clinical signs of disease.

    ii. Administer amphotericin B until a cumulative dose of 10 mg/kg has been reached.

    iii. Adjust the flucytosine dosage by dividing the daily dose by the increased serum creatinine value if azotemia occurs.

b) Ketoconazole has been shown to be effective in the treatment of feline cryptococcosis.

4) For aspergillosis:

    a) Ketoconazole, amphotericin B, or flucytosine therapy can be tried.

    b) A regimen of debridement of nasal lesions and flushing with povidone-iodine solution, along with administration of thiabendazole, has been recommended by some.

Prognosis

The prognosis is poor without treatment. The prognosis is guarded to good if treatment is instituted, depending on the disease and organ system involvement. Relapses may occur.

Feline Infectious Peritonitis

FIP is caused by a coronavirus infection that causes variable clinical disease. Animals that develop clinical FIP generally have a progressively debilitating, and usually fatal, disease.

Clinical Presentation

1. FIP has been noted to occur most commonly in cats between six months and five years of age.

2. Fever, depression, anorexia, and weight loss are consistent features.

3. Other clinical signs vary with the type of disease manifestation.

    A. The effusive form is expressed as polyserositis with peritoneal effusion and abdominal distention, or pleural effusion and dyspnea.

    B. The noneffusive form consists of an insidious pyogranulomatous infection and inflammation localized to one or more organ systems, with various manifestations.

    1) When the kidney is affected, renomegaly and signs of RF result.

    2) Involvement of the liver is manifested by icterus and hepatic encephalopathy.

    3) Pancreatitis may occur, with vomiting, diarrhea, and possible DM.

    4) Enlargement of the spleen and mesenteric lymph node has been reported as well.

    5) Granulomatous pneumonia

    6) Involvement of the heart or pericardium results in heart failure.

    7) Ocular abnormalities

    8) CNS disease with ensuing behavioral changes and seizures

4. The associated "Kitten Mortality Complex" consists of reproductive failure and kitten mortalities.

Diagnostic Aids

1. CBC

    A. Nonregenerative anemia

    B. An absolute neutrophilia is common

    C. Leukopenia, lymphopenia, and eosinopenia sometimes occur.

    D. Disseminated intravascular coagulopathy

2. Serum biochemical studies

    A. Often reveal an increased plasma protein (>7.8 g/dL), with serum fibrinogen levels >400 mg/dL

    B. Other abnormalities are related to the organ system affected.

3. Cytologic examination often reveals characteristic proteinaceous, pyogranulomatous exudate.

    A. Abdominal or pleural fluid

    B. CSF

    C. Aqueous humor

4. Serology

    A. Indirect fluorescent antibody (IFA) most commonly used.

    B. Titers are difficult to interpret.

    1) A positive coronavirus titer can result from exposure to the FIP virus in the recent or far past.

    2) A positive titer can also result from infection with feline enteric coronavirus.

Treatment

The majority of cats clinically affected with FIP die. Palliative therapy is aimed at decreasing the harmful response of the cat's immune system.

1. Immunosuppressive drugs (e.g., prednisone, melphalan)

2. Abdominal or pleural effusions may have to be drained.

Diseases Related to Feline Leukemia Virus

FeLV is a retrovirus associated with a number of clinical syndromes, including lymphosarcoma, nonregenerative anemias, myeloproliferative diseases, and immune-mediated disorders.

Clinical Presentation

1. Young kittens are more susceptible than are adult cats. Latent infections may be reactivated at a later time.
2. Clinical signs vary with the type of organ system involvement.
    A. Lymphosarcoma
        1) Organomegaly
        2) Lymphadenopathy
        3) RF
        4) GI abnormalities
        5) Ocular abnormalities
        6) CNS signs
        7) Dyspnea with thymic lymphosarcoma
    B. Hematopoietic abnormalities
    C. Ulcerative mucocutaneous disorders
    D. Immune-mediated polyarthritis
    E. Immune-mediated glomerulonephritis
    F. Fever of unknown origin
    G. Chronic infections
    H. "Fading kitten syndrome" (thymic atrophy)
    I. Fetal resorption, abortion, infertility

Diagnostic Aids

1. CBC
    A. Nonregenerative anemia
    B. Atypical leukopenia
    C. Pancytopenia
    D. Leukemias
    E. Hemolytic anemia
    F. Cyclic hematopoiesis
    G. Opportunistic hemobartonellosis
2. Biochemical changes relate to organ system defects.
3. Other tests to assess organ system abnormalities may be employed (e.g., urinalysis, radiographic and ultrasonographic procedures).
4. Cytology can quickly provide a diagnosis.
    A. Aspirates of bone marrow, lymph nodes, affected organs, and pleural fluid
    B. Impression smears of biopsies of affected tissues
5. Tests to detect FeLV group specific antigens:
    A. IFA ("Hardy test")
    B. Enzyme-linked immunosorbent assay (ELISA)
6. Feline oncornavirus-associated cell membrane antigen (FOCMA) test detects antibodies directed against tumor surface antigens.

Treatment

1. Controversial
2. Chemotherapy
3. Transfusions
4. Antibiotics for infections
5. Anabolic steroids

Prevention

1. Cats with positive results on FeLV testing should be isolated from other cats.
2. Cats that test negative for the FeLV should be vaccinated.

Prognosis

The prognosis for healthy FeLV-positive cats is fair to guarded. For FeLV-positive sick cats, the prognosis is poor.

Canine Ehrlichiosis

Etiologic Considerations

The causative agent of canine ehrlichiosis is the rickettsia *Ehrlichia canis*, which is transmitted by the brown dog tick, *Rhipicephalus sanguineus*.

Pathophysiology

1. Three disease phases
    A. In the acute phase, organisms enter the mononuclear leukocytes and the lymphoreticular tissue, producing vasculitis.
    B. The subclinical phase is associated with elimination of the organism in immunocompetent dogs.
    C. The chronic phase affects those animals in which there rickettsial elimination has been ineffective.
2. German shepherd dogs are at increased risk for the disease.

Clinical Signs

1. Fever
2. Oculonasal discharge
3. Anorexia

4. Dyspnea
5. Lymphadenopathy
6. Splenomegaly
7. Neurologic signs
8. Cyanosis
9. Depression
10. Pale or congested mucous membranes
11. Abdominal tenderness
12. Bleeding tendencies
13. Ocular inflammation and blindness
14. Subcutaneous edema

Diagnostic Aids

1. Hematology
   A. Thrombocytopenia
   B. Variable RBC and WBC numbers
2. Serum biochemical studies
   A. Increased alanine transferase (ALT) and serum alkaline phosphatase (SAP)
   B. Mild icterus
   C. Increased serum globulins
   D. Possible hypoalbuminemia
3. Coagulation studies
   A. Prolonged bleeding time
   B. Poor clot retraction time
4. Urinalysis
   A. Proteinuria may exist with immune-complex glomerulonephritis.
5. Cytology
   A. A CSF tap may be performed if there are neurologic signs of disease.
     1) Mild increase in CSF proteins
     2) Mononuclear pleocytosis
   B. Identification of intracytoplasmic organism inclusions in tissue or bone marrow aspirates
6. The IFA test is highly sensitive and specific for *E. canis*.

Treatment

1. Treat animals with suspected disease that have positive antibody titers.
2. Administer oxytetracycline or tetracycline HCl, 22 mg/kg PO t.i.d. for 21 days.
3. Doxycycline, 5 to 10 mg/kg PO s.i.d. for a period of seven to ten days may be more efficacious.

Prevention

1. Control tick populations by spraying kennels and dipping dogs every one to two weeks.
2. Long-term tetracycline administration (6.6 mg/kg PO s.i.d.) for nine months is advised in epizootic areas so that ticks will pass through a generation cycle, thereby eliminating the infection.

Prognosis

The prognosis is good to poor, depending on the stage of the illness and the severity of clinical signs.

Suggested Readings

Barlough JE, Stoddart CA: Feline infectious peritonitis. Cornell Feline Health Center Info Bull 6: 1–6, 1984

Basic Guide to Canine Nutrition. Chicago, Gaines Pet Foods Corporation, 1977.

Bauer JE: Nutrition and liver function: Nutrient metabolism in health and disease. Compend Contin Educ Pract Vet 8(12): 923–931, 1986

Breitschwerdt EB, Waltman C, Hagstad HV, et al: Clinical and epidemiologic characterization of a diarrheal syndrome in Basenji dogs. Am Vet Med Assoc 180(8): 914–920, 1982

Chiapella AM: Treatment of intestinal disease. Vet Clin North Am 13(3): 567–584, 1983

Cotter SJ: Feline viral neoplasia. In Greene CE (ed): Clinical Microbiology and Infectious Diseases of the Dog and Cat, pp 490–513. Philadelphia, WB Saunders, 1984

Crow SE, Oliver J: Cancer cachexia. Compend Contin Educ Pract Vet 3(8): 681–686, 1981

DeBruijne JJ, Lubberink AMME: Obesity. In Kirk RW (ed): Current Veterinary Therapy VI, pp 1068–1070. Philadelphia, WB Saunders, 1977

Ettinger SJ: Body weight. In Ettinger SJ (ed): Textbook of Veterinary Internal Medicine, 2nd ed, pp 100–102. Philadelphia, WB Saunders, 1983

Feldman EC, Peterson ME: Hypoadrenocorticism. Vet Clin North Am 14(4): 751–766, 1984

Greene CE, Harvey JW: Canine ehrlichiosis. In

Greene CE (ed): Clinical Microbiology and Infectious Diseases of the Dog and Cat, pp 545–561. Philadelphia, WB Saunders, 1984

Jacob AI, Canterbury JM, Gavellas G, Lambert PW: Reversal of secondary hyperparathyroidism by cimetidine in chronically uremic dogs. J Clin Invest 67: 1753–1759, 1981

Lewis LD: Obesity in the dog. J Am Anim Hosp Assoc 14: 402–409, 1978

Lewis LD, Morris ML, Hand MS: Small Animal Clinical Nutrition III. Topeka, Kansas, Mark Morris Associates, 1987

Macy DW: Systemic mycoses. In Morgan RV (ed): Handbook of Small Animal Practice, pp 963–973. New York, Churchill Livingstone, 1988

Newberne PM: Overnutrition on resistance of dogs to distemper virus. Fed Proc 25: 1701–1710, 1966

Osborne CA, Polzin DJ: Conservative medical management of feline chronic polyuric renal failure. In Kirk RW (ed): Current Veterinary Therapy VIII, pp 1008–1019. Philadelphia, WB Saunders, 1983

Peterson ME: Feline hyperthyroidism. Vet Clin North Am 14(4): 809–826, 1984

Peterson ME: Hyperadrenocorticism. Vet Clin North Am 14(4): 731–749, 1984

Pion PD, Kittleson MD, Rogers QR, Morris JG: Myocardial failure in cats associated with low plasma taurine: A reversible cardiomyopathy. Science 237: 764–768, 1987.

Polzin DJ, Osborne CA: Conservative medical management of canine chronic polyuric renal failure. In Kirk RW (ed): Current Veterinary Therapy VIII, pp 997–1007. Philadelphia, WB Saunders, 1983.

Ralston SL: Dietary management of chronic cardiac disease. Proceedings, Ninth Annual Kal-Kan Symposium, October, 1985, pp 63–67

Strombeck DR, Schaeffer MC, Rogers QR: Dietary therapy for dogs with chronic hepatic insufficiency. In Kirk RW (ed): Current Veterinary Therapy VIII, pp 817–821. Philadelphia, WB Saunders, 1983

Tams TR: Canine protein-losing gastroenteropathy syndrome. Compend Contin Educ Pract Vet 3(2): 105–118, 1981

CHAPTER SIX

Lameness

James M. Fingeroth

Definitions

Lameness is the clinical sign associated with perceived pain from an extremity in animals. Lameness is also induced when there is structural/functional impairment of an extremity. Lameness may be further characterized as either weight-bearing or non–weight-bearing.

1. Non–weight-bearing lameness
   A. Limb bone fractures are the most common cause of this type of lameness.
   B. The affected limb is usually carried with the joints in flexion as the animal moves.
2. Weight-bearing lameness
   A. Synonymous with a limp
   B. The animal will use the limb to a variable degree (ranging from merely touching the toes to the ground to very subtle dysfunctions) during locomotion.

Orthopedic Examination

1. Although the veterinarian and the owner alike are generally drawn toward the most obvious problem, it is important for clinicians to discipline themselves to perform a complete orthopedic examination, including all portions of the musculoskeletal system. This will help the veterinarian avoid missing other related or unrelated abnormalities.
2. The orthopedic examination should be performed systematically. No part of a limb should be "skipped," as even minor injuries, such as incomplete fractures in a phalanx, can induce a significant degree of lameness.
3. Visual examination and direct palpation may reveal soft tissue or joint swelling which may help to localize the source of lameness.

Procedure

General Observation

1. If the animal is ambulatory, the first part of the examination should be to observe the patient walking slowly, then briskly, then trotting. This is especially important when the complaint involves a subtle, weight-bearing lameness.
2. Certain gait abnormalities are characteristic, if not pathognomonic, for certain diseases, and the astute clinician, familiar with these patterns of lameness, can frequently diagnose the problem as the animal is initially led into the examining room.

Manual Examination

1. With the animal standing, the limbs are first palpated and assessed for certain factors, such as muscle mass, asymmetry, and swelling.
2. Clinicians should work slowly and calmly, attempting to soothe the patient as they proceed with their examination. The

more relaxed the patient, the more information the orthopedist can obtain during the examination.

3. The animal is then placed in lateral recumbency.

Forelimb

1. Manus

A. The manus should be squeezed firmly and the patient observed for a pain response or crepitus. Normally, animals do not object to such manipulation unless there is an injury or disease present.

B. If a pain response is observed, the pads, nails, and digits should be checked carefully and individually, including a range of motion test for each digit.

1) Suspected phalangeal or metacarpal fractures can be confirmed radiographically.

2) Foreign bodies may be extremely difficult to identify unless a draining tract is present or the material is radiolucent.

3) Tumors may occur in the digits (e.g., squamous cell carcinoma), producing lysis, proliferation, or both in the affected bones.

2. Carpus

A. The carpus should be tested for:

1) Range of motion in the dorsal/palmar plane

2) Response to direct palpation

3) Crepitus

4) Medial/lateral stability in full extension

B. Normally, the carpus can be flexed nearly 180 degrees without restriction or pain. There is normally some amount of varus (medial) and valgus (lateral) bending present, as well as some cranial/caudal translation. When a carpal problem is thought to be the source of lameness, these normal degrees of motion should be kept in mind.

3. Antebrachium

A. The radius and ulna should be palpated and stress should be applied to evaluate the animal for axial instability or crepitus.

B. The elbow should be put through a complete range of motion.

1) Extension and flexion should be done with some force to elicit any pain response or crepitus that was not observed during casual flexion/extension.

2) Reaction to pronation and supination should also be assessed.

3) Medial/lateral stability with the elbow fully extended should be checked.

4) Squeezing the medial and lateral epicondyles may elicit a pain response if elbow pathology is present.

C. The brachium is examined by direct palpation. By squeezing directly on the humeral diaphysis (rather than on the overlying muscles), a pain response may be elicited in the presence of humeral disease (such as panosteitis).

Shoulder

1. Full extension, flexion, abduction, adduction, and rotation should be tested for a pain response, crepitus, or instability.

2. An important caveat is to remember that the elbow should be held in as neutral a position as possible when examining the shoulder. For example, maximum flexion or extension of the shoulder is often performed by grasping the antebrachium as a lever. This places the elbow in a corresponding position of flexion or extension, and if elbow pathology is present, a painful elbow may be misdiagnosed as a shoulder lameness.

3. The scapula is palpated to assess the animal for supraspinatus or infraspinatus atrophy, fractures, or evidence of serratus ventralis injury.

4. Finally, the axilla should be palpated for the presence of masses or pain. Tumors, such as neurofibrosarcomas and lipomas, frequently occur in this region and may induce lameness because of pain or mechanical interference with limb function.

Hindlimb

1. The examination of the hindlimb is performed similarly to that of the forelimb.

2. The pes is examined in the same fashion as the manus.

3. The tarsus should be stressed to test the integrity of the collateral ligaments, calcanean tendon, and plantar ligament.

4. The crus is palpated for deformity, instability, or crepitus in the tibia or fibula.

5. The calcanean tendon and gastrocnemius muscle bellies are examined for integrity.

Stifle

1. Examination of the stifle should commence with palpation to assess this area for any evidence of joint effusion.

2. With the limb in extension, the patella should be grasped and stressed medially and laterally in order to determine whether there is a tendency to luxate.

3. While in extension, the medial and lateral collateral ligaments should be tested.

4. An attempt to produce a cranial drawer sign should be performed with the limb in several positions between full extension and full flexion.

    A. The presence of this sign, except in very young patients with immature ligaments, is pathognomonic for rupture of the cranial cruciate ligament.

    B. Excessive internal rotation is also found in most dogs with stifles deficient in cranial cruciate integrity.

    C. If a drawer sign is found, critically assess whether it involves the cranial or caudal drawer sign, or both. Caudal drawer motion is indicative of injury to the caudal cruciate ligament, and although most often this occurs in conjunction with a cranial ligament tear, it has also been reported as an isolated injury.

    D. Dogs that are well-muscled (especially in the hamstrings), very tense, or that have sustained only partial tears of the cranial cruciate ligament may have little or no drawer sign found during the orthopedic examination. In the case of the latter, such drawer as is present is often found only with the stifle in flexion.

    E. If a cruciate ligament injury is suspected but not confirmed during routine examination, sedation or general anesthesia may be required to complete the analysis.

5. Medial meniscal injury frequently accompanies complete tears of the cranial cruciate ligament, and is thought to be the major source of pain in those animals so affected. Occasionally, a "click" is heard or palpated as the stifle is put through a range of motion. Although suggestive of a meniscal tear, this sign is neither 100% sensitive nor specific; in other words, some dogs without clicks will have a meniscal injury, whereas others with an audible click will be found not to have any meniscal injury at arthroscopy or surgery. The cause of a click in these latter cases is unknown.

6. Animals with stifle pain often walk with a non–weight-bearing lameness of the affected limb. Characteristically, these patients will carry the limb in a very flexed position, with no attempt to touch the toes to the ground. Subtle injuries, however, such as partial tears of the cranial cruciate ligament or injuries to the long digital extensor tendon, may result in only an intermittent weight-bearing lameness, and are somewhat difficult to diagnose.

Femur, Thigh, and Hip

1. The femur and surrounding thigh muscles should be palpated similarly to the other long bones.

2. Examination of the hip is initially performed indirectly by observation of the gait, assessment of relative thigh muscle mass, and questioning of the owner with respect to how the animal sits, lies, rises, walks, and runs. Direct examination of the hip begins with putting the joint through a range of motion. By grasping the stifle, the hip can be flexed, extended, abducted, adducted, and rotated internally and externally. Pain, crepitus, or instability should be recorded.

3. When coxofemoral luxation is suspected, several clues may be derived from palpation or observation before radiographs are ordered.

    A. First, observe the animal's gait. Animals with craniodorsal luxations will typically walk with a non–weight-bearing lameness, with the toes just barely off the ground. The limb will be externally rotated, causing the toes to deviate laterally. Dogs with ventral luxations will often touch the toes to the ground, but will bear only minimal weight. These animals will hold the limb internally rotated, with the toes deviated medially.

    B. With the femur held approximately perpendicular to the pelvis, a depression can be palpated with the thumb between the greater trochanter and the ischiatic tuberosity.

The hip is then externally rotated, causing the trochanter to rotate caudally. In a reduced hip, this caudal movement of the trochanter will displace the examiner's thumb from the depression (the so-called *thumb test*). In the presence of a craniodorsal luxation, the trochanter does not enter this depression, and in some cases, the thumb will be perceived to sink more deeply as the gluteal muscles and external rotators are twisted medially toward the pelvis. With a ventral luxation, the trochanter is usually depressed and difficult to palpate at all until the hip is reduced.

C. Another way of examining a patient for the presence of a hip luxation is to place the animal in dorsal recumbency, holding the femurs side by side, perpendicular to the table surface. By observing the height of the stifles above the table surface, any discrepancy between the two sides will be readily apparent. A relatively lower stifle indicates dorsal displacement of the femoral head out of the acetabulum. It is not necessary to grasp the limbs and extend them to gain this information. Extension of a dislocated hip induces pain, and often the animal will struggle when this is attempted. The method advocated here is usually well-tolerated by the patient and yields exactly the same insight.

4. Instability of the hip, often indicative of dysplasia, is evaluated by performance of the *Ortolani test.*

A. With the animal in lateral recumbency and the femur held perpendicular to the pelvis by grasping the stifle, the femur is gently pushed in a dorsal direction. The opposite hand rests on the pelvis to prevent the patient from sliding, and the thumb of this hand rests on the greater trochanter. If instability is not obvious, the femur can be adducted slightly to exacerbate any tendency for the femoral head to subluxate laterally. If the femoral head is felt (via the thumb on the trochanter) to lift out of the acetabulum, this is termed *Barlow's sign.* This sign is frequently not observed in dysplastic dogs, as they are already subluxated when the Ortolani test is initiated. However, a relaxation of the dorsal pressure, accompanied by pressure on the trochanter or abduction of the femur, will often allow the maximally subluxated femoral

head to drop back down to a variable degree into the acetabulum. This is usually felt, often heard, and is sometimes visible from a substantial distance away. This is termed a positive *Ortolani sign* (note the distinction between Ortolani's test and Ortolani's sign), and can be graded for severity. Dysplastic hips may not exhibit a positive Ortolani sign, and this may be because the acetabulum is too shallow or the round ligament too redundant to allow any reduction of the subluxation.

B. Another test for hip instability is to attempt to lift the femoral head straight laterally out of the acetabulum by using the femoral shaft as a handle. This movement can again be palpated by placement of the thumb on the greater trochanter. A positive test is called a *Barden's sign,* and should be recorded in millimeters of movement.

Pelvis

1. The lateral aspect of the pelvis is difficult to assess unless there is an obvious deformity or mass. The groin area should be palpated for masses.

2. The medial aspect of the pelvis can be examined by digital rectal palpation. The entire inner wall and floor of the pelvis should be swept with a gloved finger, looking for masses, crepitus, or displaced bone fragments. During the course of the rectal examination, the lumbosacral junction and sciatic nerves may also be checked. Spondylosis may be palpated, and a pain response to direct pressure may be elicited.

3. Tumors, such as neurofibrosarcomas, can invade the sciatic nerves as they course medially along the pelvic wall towards the ischiatic notch, causing tremendous pain and lameness.

The orthopedic examination is completed by repeating the extremity evaluation on the contralateral forelimb and hindlimb.

Inconclusive Findings

Failure to identify a musculoskeletal abnormality as the source of lameness in a patient suggests two major possibilities: (1) a musculoskeletal problem is present, but was missed during the examination; or (2) the problem is not an orthopedic one per se.

1. The former may occur when a very subtle lesion exists. The best insurance against missing such a lesion is to perform an orthopedic examination systematically, as described.

2. The most common nonorthopedic cause of lameness is referred pain to an extremity, called a *root signature.* An infiltrative or compressive mass affecting the proximal portion of a peripheral nerve or the nerve roots supplying that nerve may be perceived consciously as discomfort emanating from the distal receptor region of the nerve. Hence, a compressed nerve root in the spine may be felt as a pain or dysesthesia in a digit, causing the patient to limp or hold the limb elevated off the ground. This is commonly observed in dogs with lateral or ventrolateral extrusions of cervical intervertebral disks from C3–4 to T1–2. Similar signs can be seen in a hindlimb if nerve roots supplying the cauda equina or lumbosacral plexus are affected. A careful neurologic and spinal examination should be performed in an attempt to confirm the presence of a root signature.

Quick Reference for Common Causes of Lameness

Although the spectrum of diseases that can produce lameness is unlimited, some entities are very common and show up regularly in veterinary practices. The following is offered as a quick guide to some of the key differential diagnoses to be considered when lameness is localized to a particular part of an extremity.

Fracture

1. Most fractures are caused by trauma, and are accompanied by swelling and instability.
2. Traumatic fractures in skeletally immature animals frequently involve growth plates. Injuries to or in the vicinity of growth plates, or subsequent rigid fixation, may lead to

premature closure of the growth plate. If the patient still has significant growth potential, this could ultimately result in limb deformity. Early correction of any recognized deformity is essential.

3. Even with closed fractures, there is often substantial soft tissue injury around the bone. Because the blood supply to the bone is dependent on these soft tissues, it is imperative to include soft tissue injury management in the overall treatment plans. In young animals, femoral fractures in particular may be accompanied by tremendous shredding, hemorrhage, and swelling of the overlying quadriceps femoris muscle group. Resultant compartment syndrome can lead to degeneration of the muscles and replacement by nonfunctional scar tissue (contracture), leading to a nonfunctional limb.

4. Be very wary of animals that are presented for evaluation of a fracture without a sufficient history of trauma. Animals with normal bone do not usually sustain major fractures going down stairs or running in the yard. In such cases, suspect the possibility of a *pathologic* fracture, one in which the injured bone was preweakened. Major causes for pathologic fracture include metabolic bone disease (e.g., renal disease, starvation) and neoplasia. Treatment must be directed toward the underlying process, as well as the fractured bone itself.

5. When obtaining radiographs of limbs with fractured bones, be sure to include the joint above and joint below. Obtain two views perpendicular to each other.

6. Assess both the patient and the radiographs for evidence of an open (compound) fracture. Open fractures represent orthopedic emergencies.

Joint Diseases

Arthritis

Arthritis is usually classified as inflammatory or noninflammatory. Inflammatory arthritides include septic arthritis and immune-mediated arthritis. Noninflammatory arthritis includes primary and secondary degenerative joint disease.

Inflammatory

1. Septic arthritis

A. Septic arthritis can occur as a result of direct penetrance by microorganisms into the joint from the outside, or hematogenous seeding of the synovium.

B. Affected joints are usually swollen, warm, and painful. Lameness may be weight-bearing or non–weight-bearing.

C. Radiographic evidence of subchondral bone erosion may be seen in severe or sub-acute to chronic cases.

D. Cytologic, physiochemical, and micro-biologic analyses of synovial fluid should be performed.

E. Treatment is based on debridement, drainage, lavage, and systemic use of appropriate antimicrobial drugs.

2. Immune-mediated arthropathy

A. Immune-mediated arthropathies often represent local manifestations of a systemic disease. Patients may exhibit generalized malaise, anorexia, fever, or leukocytosis. These latter clinical signs may occur concomitantly with lameness or may precede any lameness by days, weeks, or months.

B. These diseases may produce an erosive or nonerosive arthritis, as visualized by radiography.

1) *Erosive arthritis* is usually attributable to rheumatoid disease.

2) *Nonerosive arthritis* may be the result of systemic lupus erythematosis (SLE), but in veterinary medicine is usually idiopathic.

C. Definitive diagnosis of immune-mediated joint disease is based on synovial biopsy. Histologic and immunochemical analysis of biopsy samples should yield conclusive data, including such findings as immunoglobulin deposition on basement membranes, presence of lupus erythematosus (LE) cells in the biopsy sample, and characteristic inflammatory responses.

D. Positive rheumatoid factor (RF), or the finding of LE cells in peripheral blood, is a suggestive finding, but false-positive results are possible.

E. Treatment is based on appropriate immunosuppression, using corticosteroids, cytotoxic chemotherapeutic drugs, and gold salts. Symptomatic relief is sometimes achieved with nonsteroidal anti-inflammatory drugs (NSAIDs), such as aspirin, but with much less reliability than in people. End-stage arthritis is treated by arthrodesis, excision arthroplasty, or joint replacement.

Noninflammatory

1. Degenerative joint disease (DJD; osteoarthritis) is usually secondary to abnormal joint biomechanics.

2. Primary DJD (in which no antecedent cause is identified) is an uncommon cause of clinical disability in veterinary patients. Any cause of joint surface incongruity (previous fracture, dysplasia, infection, etc.) can lead to wear and tear on cartilage surfaces.

3. Because Mother Nature abhors unstable joints, the body strives to restore closefitting surfaces. This is accomplished through fibrosis and osteophytosis. As articular cartilage is worn and eroded, the subchondral bone bears an increasing load, leading to sclerosis and collapse of the joint space. Each of these features are typical hallmarks of DJD.

4. Although radiographic evidence of DJD is common in many joints, not all degenerate joints are associated with clinical lameness. Therefore, other causes of lameness should be ruled out, and a specific pain response to manipulation of the affected joint should be elicited before implicating DJD as the cause of clinical disability in a patient.

5. Treatment is based on rest, regular and moderate exercise, and analgesics. Osteoarthritis that is unresponsive to conservative treatment may be managed surgically by excision arthroplasty, arthrodesis, or joint replacement.

Osteochondrosis

1. Osteochondrosis is a syndrome characterized by abnormal (usually delayed) endochondral ossification. The disease can affect articular (epiphyseal) or metaphyseal growth plates, and can occur in any part of the body. Various species are affected, and different species and breed patterns are recognized.

2. Because cartilage is devoid of an independent blood supply, it is dependent on diffusion of nutrients and waste products from and to the synovial fluid, or from nearby metaphyseal or epiphyseal vessels. If endochondral ossification is delayed or arrested, the cartilage model becomes too thick, resulting in necrosis of central portions. The affected portion of the cartilage loses its normal mechanical integrity and becomes vulnerable to collapse or cracking with normal stresses. The result may be failure of the affected part to unite properly with the metaphysis (e.g., ununited anconeal process), or easy separation of the unaffected part from the main part of the bone (e.g., fragmented coronoid process). When the epiphyseal growth plate is affected, the result is collapse and fissuring of the overlying articular cartilage.

3. Fissuring may produce a loose flap of cartilage overlying the bed of necrotic tissue more deeply, a process termed *osteochondritis dissicans (OCD)*. Inflammation in OCD is attributable to leakage of breakdown products and enzymes from the necrotic cartilage into the synovial fluid.

4. The cause of osteochondrosis is not known, but is probably multifactorial. Genetics, nutrition, and activity seem to play major roles. Relative overnutrition of calories, protein, or certain minerals, such as calcium, is probably a more common cause than is undernutrition. Large, rapidly growing animals are usually much more affected than small animals.

5. Treatment depends on the location and severity of the osteochondrosis lesion.

Metabolic Bone Diseases

Hypertrophic Osteodystrophy

1. Hypertrophic osteodystrophy (HOD) is a disease affecting skeletally immature, usually large breed dogs. The lesion occurs in the growth plates of long bones, typically the radius. The exact pathogenesis is unknown, but genetics and nutrition appear to be important factors.

2. Affected dogs present with lameness and metaphyseal swelling, and are often systemically ill (fever, inappetance, lethargy). The illness in some dogs is especially severe and can be fatal. The disease is usually bilateral.

3. The radiographic hallmark is the presence of a transverse radiolucent line parallel and proximal to the physis.

4. The clinical course may be cyclical.

5. Treatment is aimed at analgesia and control of fever. Some veterinarians advocate treatment with ascorbic acid (vitamin C) based on apparent clinical response. There are no accepted studies that lend credence to this theory, although it is possible that there are two forms of HOD, one of which is ascorbate-responsive. Rest and nonsupplemented balanced nutrition are probably the major means of limiting the disease and preventing acute recurrence.

Panosteitis

1. Panosteitis is most commonly seen in German shepherds, but can affect other breeds. Most patients are affected between the ages of 6 and 18 months, but occasionally, older dogs with no previous history of panosteitis will develop the disease. The disease is usually self-limiting and cyclical in nature.

2. Although "shifting leg lameness" is typically described in animals with this disease, it is not uncommon for only a single extremity to be clinically affected in a cyclical fashion. Affected dogs usually present with a weight-bearing lameness that is exacerbated by heavy exercise. Clinical diagnosis is based on signalment, history, and a finding of excruciating pain on palpation of the diaphyses of affected bones.

3. It may take as long as three to four weeks for typical radiographic changes (increased mottled density of the medullary canal, starting in the region of the nutrient foramen; periosteal new bone) to become apparent.

4. Treatment is limited to rest, analgesics, and proper diet. Some dogs do not improve with analgesic therapy. Most dogs recover fully from the disease by the time they are one to two years of age.

Osteopenia/Osteoporosis/Osteomalacia

1. *Osteopenia* is the radiographic impression of relatively decreased bone density, regardless of cause.

A. Generalized osteopenia requires a 50% reduction of bone density before it can be so appreciated with routine roentgenograms.

2. By contrast, *osteoporosis* is a histologic finding of decreased bone tissue. Because bone is a dynamic tissue that is continuously being formed and resorbed, a relative outstripping of new bone production by resorption will result in osteoporosis. Unlike human females, dogs do not usually develop osteoporosis with age. Disuse, stress, protection, and hyperparathyroidism are the most common causes of osteoporosis in animals.

3. Failure of bone matrix (osteoid) mineralization is termed *osteomalacia.* In immature animals with vitamin D deficiency, the condition is called rickets. Renal disease is probably the most common cause of osteomalacia in adults. General starvation is occasionally seen in young puppies fed extremely poor diets.

4. Osteopenia (whether attributable to osteoporosis or osteomalacia) itself is usually not a painful condition, although patients with hyperparathyroidism may have clinical signs of generalized discomfort. Osteopenia can predispose the patient to pathologic fractures, and may make application of internal fixation devices difficult. Treatment for osteopenia depends on the underlying cause.

Hypertrophic Osteopathy

1. Hypertrophic osteopathy (HO) used to be called hypertrophic pulmonary osteoarthropathy (HPOA), then hypertrophic osteoarthropathy. The current nomenclature recognizes that lesions other than pulmonary or even thoracic masses can be associated with the syndrome, and that the disease affects the bones but not the joints.

2. Affected patients present with nonedematous, painful, firm swellings of the limbs. Frequently, all extremities are affected. Usually, the distal limbs (manus, pes) are affected, but in severe cases, the lesions can extend to include the scapulae or pelvis. Patients are often febrile.

3. On radiographic examination, the disease is characterized by the presence of diffuse, radiating, periosteal new bone formation along the shafts of the affected bones.

4. A search should be made for a mass lesion elsewhere that may be triggering a neurohumeral reaction. HO has been seen in dogs with neoplastic and non-neoplastic thoracic lesions. It has also been reported in dogs with abdominal tumors, particularly masses involving a portion of the urinary conduit. The exact pathogenesis is unknown.

5. Treatment is directed at the underlying primary (mass) lesion. HO may regress after removal of the inciting cause, but not all animals exhibit radiographic improvement.

Infection (Osteomyelitis)

Osteomyelitis, like septic arthritis, can occur as a result of direct penetration of bone by microorganisms, or by hematogenous seeding. The presence of avascular soft tissues or bone, and dead space (as can occur after open reduction of fractures) increases the risk that contaminating microorganisms will be able to colonize and infect the area.

1. Types

A. Acute osteomyelitis causes non–weight-bearing lameness, pain, warm swelling, and systemic signs of illness (fever, leukocytosis, inappetence). Mycotic infections of bone may be accompanied by other clinical signs of systemic mycosis. Early, vigorous antimicrobial therapy may be successful in treating acute osteomyelitis.

B. Chronic osteomyelitis implies that colonization by microorganisms has been achieved, and has outstripped the host's defense mechanisms.

2. Signs of infection

A. Affected animals may be presented for a variety of clinical signs, the most common being an intermittent weight-bearing lameness. Other signs, such as draining sinuses, leukocytosis, fever, or general illness are less common, and their absence does not rule out the diagnosis of chronic osteomyelitis.

B. Any organism can cause osteomyelitis, but the most common in dogs are *Staphylococcus, Streptococcus,* and *Escherichia coli.*

C. The radiographic appearance is variable. If a sequestrum is present, it will appear as a dense bone fragment with absent periosteal or endosteal reaction.

3. Treatment. Chronic osteomyelitis represents the equivalent of an abscess in the bone. Treatment, therefore, is similar to treatment for any abscess, including debridement, drainage, and second intention healing.

4. Culture. Cultures should be obtained from the depths of the wound or from obviously necrotic or infected tissues. Draining tracts should not be cultured at the site of the cutaneous sinus or cloaca since erroneous results are likely.

5. Fractures. If a metal implant is in place for fracture fixation, it should not be removed until the fracture is healed or the implant is no longer serving a useful mechanical role. Fractures can heal in the face of infection as long as stability and blood supply are maintained. After fracture healing, the implants should be removed to prevent them from acting as safe harbors for resistant microorganisms.

Neoplasia

Bone tumors may be primary or secondary, malignant or benign. Animals with bone tumors usually present with lameness that is initially weight-bearing, but may become non–weight-bearing. Clinical signs are often progressive, and the course of disease (especially with primary malignant bone tumors) is frequently rapid (days to weeks). Some animals with bone tumors are presented because of an acute onset of pain and non–weight-bearing lameness. Often, these patients have suffered a pathologic fracture in the region of the tumor.

Osteosarcoma

1. Osteosarcoma (OSA), also known as osteogenic sarcoma, is the most common bone tumor occurring in dogs. It most often affects middle-aged to older giant breed dogs. It usually arises in the metaphyseal zones of long bones; the most common sites of occur-

rence are the distal radius, distal femur, proximal humerus, and distal tibia. However, it can arise anywhere, including the flat bones of the appendicular skeleton (scapula; pelvis), mandible, calvarium, and spine.

2. The radiographic appearance and biological aggressivity are extremely variable, and depend in part on the site of origin. Generally, long bone osteosarcoma is a highly malignant, rapidly destructive, early metastasizing disease. Although only about 10% of dogs with OSA will have radiographic evidence of pulmonary metastasis at the time of initial diagnosis, about 90% will be dead at the end of one year of follow-up, usually because of metastatic pulmonary disease. Osteosarcoma of the flat bones and skull may be less biologically aggressive.

3. Treatment is aimed at both local and systemic control.

A. Local control seeks to eradicate the primary tumor. This is usually achieved through amputation. Local control can also be achieved in some cases by tumor sterilization using regional chemotherapy and irradiation, followed by en bloc resection of the affected bone and replacement with an allograft (limb salvage techniques).

B. Systemic control is based on chemotherapy. New protocols, using such drugs as cis-platin®, have shown considerable promise for improvement of long-term survival statistics compared to local control alone or older chemotherapy regimens.

4. Many owners are disinclined toward amputation because of anticipated problems in ambulation or behavior. It should be stressed to such owners that:

A. Dogs frequently have already learned to walk on three limbs, and that the affected limb represents only a heavy, painful, and useless appendage.

B. Dogs are usually not adversely affected psychologically by amputation and, in fact, may be in better spirits once the source of pain and disability is removed.

Fracture-associated Sarcoma

1. Fracture-associated sarcoma (FAS) is thought to be a variant of osteosarcoma that is seen in previously fractured limbs. Usually, there is a history of some form of internal fixation device being used, but not always. The incidence of this disease is quite low, but may be increasing as more dogs undergo open reduction and internal fixation of fractures.

2. The exact etiology is unknown, but is likely to involve chronic stimulation of osteoblasts. Chronic low-grade infection, corroded metal, and other factors are implicated in causing a long-term stimulus to bone turnover, which may ultimately lead to neoplastic transformation.

3. FAS differs from typical OSA in that it often arises in the diaphyseal region of a long bone, rather than the metaphysis. Because it is an uncommon disease, the biologic nature of the tumor is unknown, although it may be as aggressive (in terms of local destruction or metastasis) as classic OSA.

Chondrosarcoma

1. Chondrosarcoma (CSA) is more common in the axial skeleton (maxilla; nasal cavity) than in the appendicular skeleton.

2. Like OSA, chondrosarcomas of the limbs tend to arise in the metaphyseal regions.

3. Chondrosarcomas frequently mineralize, but their matrix is devoid of osteoblasts or osteoid.

4. CSA appears to be less systemically aggressive than OSA, and early amputation may lead to fairly prolonged survival.

Fibrosarcoma

1. Fibrosarcoma (FSA) is a tumor that usually arises in the soft tissues and secondarily invades the bone.

2. The extent of soft tissue swelling is frequently greater than that which occurs with either OSA or CSA.

3. Although OSA and CSA typically demonstrate both proliferative and lytic changes on radiographs, FSA is almost always purely lytic in its appearance.

4. Wide excision (e.g., proximal amputation) is indicated to decrease the risk of local recurrence.

Synovial Cell Sarcoma

1. Synovial cell sarcoma (SCS) is a malignant neoplasm that arises in periarticular soft tissues, or in similar tissues in bursae and tendon sheaths.

2. As the tumor enlarges, it secondarily invades the adjacent structures (bones and joints). Of all the previously mentioned tumors, only SCS is frequently observed to involve structures on both sides of a joint, with destruction of bone on either side.

3. Any joint can be affected, but the stifles and elbows have had the highest reported prevalence.

4. Because the tumor is relatively uncommon, its propensity for distant metastasis is not well documented in animals.

Squamous Cell Carcinoma

1. Squamous cell carcinoma (SCC) is probably the most common tumor that involves the phalanges and metacarpals (metatarsals). Dogs with digital SCC are often presented for what initially seems to be paronychia, but which fails to respond to the usual modes of therapy.

2. Treatment is digital amputation or irradiation, or both.

Multiple Myeloma (Plasmacytoma)

1. Multiple myeloma (plasmacytoma) is a form of lymphoma in which a clone of immunoglobulin-producing B lymphocytes (plasma cells) undergoes malignant transformation.

2. Clusters of tumor cells may reside in the bone marrow, producing multifocal "punched out" lesions on radiographs of affected bones.

3. Lesions can occur anywhere and may involve multiple sites in the body. Sites of active marrow activity in adults (spine, flat bones, metaphyses) are the most common locations for myeloma bone lesions. Affected animals may be presented for pathologic fractures.

4. Because the disease is systemic, local treatment (e.g., amputation) is contraindicated. Appropriate systemic chemotherapy (prednisone, melphalen, etc.) often causes remission of the disease and, in some cases, regression of bone lesions has been documented.

Metastatic Tumors of Bone

1. Metastatic tumors of bone can occur with a wide variety of epithelial and mesothelial primary malignant lesions. In general, bony metastasis is far less commonly seen in animals than in humans.

2. The most common metastatic bone tumors reported are mammary and prostatic carcinomas. The latter may invade bone by distant hematogenous seeding, or by direct extension via lymphatics and venules. The lumbar spine, pelvis, and proximal femurs are predilected sites for spread of prostatic carcinoma.

3. Treatment consists of appropriate systemic chemotherapy, and is often short-lived in efficacy or unrewarding.

Bone Cysts

1. Bone cysts are sometimes diagnosed radiographically when a relatively uniform expansile lytic area is found. True bone cysts, which are benign, are usually diagnosed in young dogs and are fluid-filled.

2. Biopsy is essential to rule out malignant disease that has the radiographic characteristics of a cyst.

3. Treatment includes curettage, drainage, and some form of limb support as the lesion heals.

Cancellous grafting does not appear to enhance the healing rate of treated bone cysts.

Osteocartilagenous Exostoses

1. Osteocartilagenous exostoses may be single or multiple. They occur in skeletally immature animals and cease growth with closure of other growth plates in the body. They represent ectopic centers of endochondral ossification.

2. Continued growth of an exostosis after an animal matures is cause for concern (indicating possible malignant transformation).

3. The pathologic effects of exostoses are almost always attributable to mechanical interference with a joint or in the spine because of nerve root or spinal cord compression.

4. Treatment involves resection of the mass.

Neuromuscular Diseases

A wide variety of peripheral nerve, muscle, or neuromuscular junction lesions can cause lameness in animals. These are discussed in Chapter 17.

Regional Lameness

The following is presented to offer the clinician a list of common differential diagnoses for lameness localized to a specific region. The list is not comprehensive, and its use depends on the performance of an accurate orthopedic examination to identify the source of pain or disability.

Digits—nail avulsion, fracture, foreign body, pyoderma, tumor
Manus/Pes—fracture, foreign body, tumor, hypertrophic osteopathy
Carpus—fracture, luxation, hyperextension, immune-mediated arthritis

Note: Young dogs (especially of large breeds) are occasionally presented because of profound laxity in the carpal or tarsal joints, or both. The laxity may be so severe that the puppy walks on the distal antebrachium or distal crus in a completely palmargrade or plantargrade stance. Usually, there is no pain or radiographic abnormality found in affected joints. The cause is probably related to nutrition, and may represent asynchronous maturation of bones and ligamentous structures. Although it is tempting to treat these animals by placing the affected limb in a supportive splint or cast, this usually fails to resolve the problem and may, in fact, delay recovery. The strengthening of ligaments and tendons, much like bones, depends on reorientation of collagen along lines of stress. Affected dogs should, therefore, be allowed to bear weight as normally as possible, unless secondary injuries are occurring. The animal's diet should be investigated carefully; if found to be too rich in protein, calories, vitamins, or minerals, it should be changed to a well-balanced, unsupplemented adult dog food. The laxities usually improve spontaneously with this treatment in four to eight weeks.

Antebrachium—fracture, tumor (distal radius, OSA), bite wounds, growth deformity

Elbow—ununited anconeal process, fragmented coronoid process, OCD, fractures, luxation, synovial cell sarcoma

Brachium—fracture, panosteitis, tumor (proximal humerus, OSA)

Shoulder—fracture, luxation, OCD, tumor, bicipital bursitis

Axilla—lipoma, neurofibrosarcoma, brachial plexus avulsion

Scapula—fracture, serratus ventralis avulsion, rib injury, tumor

Tarsus—as for carpus; severe shear wounds/open fractures, OCD, calcanean tendon laxity or calcaneal fracture

Crus—fracture, tumor, tibial tuberosity avulsion

Stifle—ruptured cranial cruciate ligament, meniscal tear, avulsed popliteal tendon, avulsed or displaced long digital extensor tendon, collateral ligament injury, patellar luxation, OCD, immune-mediated arthritis, synovial cell sarcoma

Thigh—fracture, tumor (proximal and distal femur, OSA), quadriceps contracture, panosteitis

Hip—dysplasia, Legg-Calvé-Perthes disease (avascular necrosis), fracture, tumor, infection, luxation

Pelvis—fracture, tumor, metastasis

Suggested Readings

Arnoczky SP (ed): Muculoskeletal system. In Slatter DH (ed): Textbook of Small Animal Surgery. Philadelphia, WB Saunders, 1985

Brinker WO, Piermattei DL, Flo, GL: Handbook of Small Animal Orthopedics and Fracture Treatment. Philadelphia, WB Saunders, 1983

deLahunta A, Habel RE (eds): Applied Veterinary Anatomy. Philadelphia, WB Saunders, 1986

CHAPTER SEVEN

Intermittent Weakness

Ronald Lyman

General Principles

1. A primary complaint of intermittent weakness can arise from a pathologic process in one of several body systems.

2. It is desirable, but often not possible, to attempt diagnosis during a "symptomatic" period.

3. In general, the clinician should consider metabolic, cardiopulmonary, neurologic (affecting the central nervous system [CNS]), generalized motor unit disorders, orthopedic, and articular causes of this problem.

4. In some cases, combinations of causes contribute to the signs (e.g., polyneuropathy and polymyopathy in toxoplasmosis).

5. The clinician must be alert to the tendency for clients to rationalize signs as relating to the normal aging process, or some antecedent trauma. Owners often complain that their pet has a "problem with its hips."

6. The reader is referred to other chapters for additional information on many specific causes discussed in this chapter.

Etiology

Metabolic Causes

1. Hypoglycemia (see Chapter 25)
2. Hypokalemia (see Chapter 24)
3. Hyperkalemia (see Chapter 24)
4. Hypothyroidism (myxedema) (see Chapter 15)
5. Hyponatremia (see Chapter 24)
6. Hypernatremia (see Chapter 24)
7. Hypercalcemia (see Chapter 24)
8. Hypocalcemia (see Chapter 24)
9. Hyperosmolality (see Chapter 24)
10. Anemia of nonhemorrhagic origin (see Chapter 17)
11. Glucocorticoid-deficient hypoadrenocorticism (see Chapter 14)
12. Hyperviscosity syndrome (see Chapter 24)
13. Hypophosphatemia (see Chapter 24)
14. Hypomagnesemia (see Chapter 24)

Cardiopulmonary Problems

1. Cardiac arrythmias (see Chapter 9)
  A. Sinus arrest ("sick sinus syndrome")
  B. Second- or third-degree heart block
  C. Ventricular tachycardias
  D. Atrial fibrillation or flutter
2. Congenital heart disease (see Chapter 9)
  A. Patent ductus arteriosus (PDA)
  B. Pulmonic stenosis (PS)
  C. Aortic stenosis (AS)
  D. Tetralogy of Fallot
  E. Atrial septal defect (ASD)
  F. Ventricular septal defect (VSD)
3. Cardiomyopathy (see Chapter 9)
4. Acquired valvular disease (see Chapter 9)
  A. Mitral insufficiency
  B. Tricuspid insufficiency
  C. Vegetative endocarditis
5. Pericardial effusions (see Chapter 9)
6. Dirofilariasis (see Chapter 9)
7. Congenital pulmonary disease
  A. Hypoplastic trachea

B. Upper airway stenosis (nares, larynx, soft palate)

8. Acquired pulmonary/pleural disease (see Chapter 9)
   A. Pulmonary alveolar infiltrates
   B. Pulmonary interstitial infiltrates
   C. Pleural effusions
   D. Tracheal collapse
   E. Upper airway obstruction (e.g., laryngeal paresis)

9. Anemia secondary to hemorrhage or blood loss (see Chapter 4)
   A. Coagulopathies
   B. Hemorrhage from gastrointestinal (GI) ulcerations
   C. Hemorrhage from neoplasms

10. Thromboembolism
   A. Cardiomyopathy
   B. Dirofilariasis
   C. Neoplasia
   D. Nephrotic syndrome
   E. Bacterial endocarditis

Orthopedic Causes

1. Diseases of large breed, growing canines
   A. Panosteitis
   B. Hypertrophic osteodystrophy (HOD)
   C. Osteochondritis dessicans (OCD)
2. Osseous neoplasia (primary or metastatic)
3. Osteomyelitis
4. Fractures (pathologic)
5. Ligamentous or soft tissue injury (e.g., ruptured anterior cruciate ligaments)

Articular Causes

1. Nonerosive idiopathic polyarthritis
2. Nonerosive polyarthritis associated with drug use
3. Polyarthritis associated with systemic lupus erythematosus (SLE)
4. Polyarthritis associated with chronic infectious disease (e.g., ehrlichiosis)
5. Polyarthritis associated with bacterial endocarditis
6. Rheumatoid arthritis (RA)
7. Degenerative osteoarthritis

Neurologic Causes Involving the CNS

1. Cerebrum (see Chapter 17)
   A. Epilepsy
   B. Neoplasia
   C. Inflammatory disease
   D. Narcolepsy
   E. Myxedema associated with hypothyroidism
2. Spinal cord
   A. Congenital spinal cord lesions
      1) Atlanto-occipital subluxation
      2) Hemivertebrae
      3) Spina bifida
      4) Leukosdystrophy of young rottweilers
      5) Myelopathy of young Afghans
      6) Spinal muscular atrophy of Brittany spaniels
   B. Other spinal cord lesions
      1) Degenerative myelopathy of German shepherds (geriatric)
      2) Caudal cervical vertebral instability/malformation (Dobermans, Great Danes)
      3) Lumbosacral instability
      4) Intervertebral disk extrusions
      5) Neoplasia of the spinal cord or canal
      6) Discospondylitis
      7) Meningitis/myelopathy of infectious etiology
         a) Canine distemper
         b) Ehrlichiosis
         c) Lyme's disease
         d) Rocky Mountain spotted fever
         e) Cryptococcosis
         f) Coccidiodomycosis
         g) Blastomycosis
         h) Candidiasis
         i) Histoplasmosis
         j) Phaeohyphomycosis
         k) Toxoplasmosis
         l) Feline infectious peritonitis (FIP)
         m) Feline leukemia virus (FeLV)
         n) Feline immunosuppressive virus-related disease (FIV)
      8) Meningitis of unknown etiology
         a) Reticulosis

b) Granulomatous meningo-encephalitis

c) Eosinophilic meningo-encephalitis

Generalized Motor Unit Disorders

1. Peripheral neuropathies
  A. Idiopathic polyradiculoneuritis (coonhound paralysis)
  B. Distal polyneuropathy of Doberman Pinschers
  C. Progressive axonopathy of boxers
  D. Giant axonal neuropathy of German shepherds
  E. Brachial plexus neuropathy
  F. Cauda equina compression
  G. Toxoplasma polymyositis/polyneuropathy
  H. Diabetic polyneuropathy
  I. Polyneuropathy associated with hypothyroidism
  J. Toxic neuropathy
    1) Lead
    2) Vincristine
    3) Organophosphates
    4) Hexacarbons (paint solvents)
  K. Ischemic neuropathy
    1) Vasculitis
    2) Thromboembolism associated with feline cardiomyopathy
  L. Paraneoplastic neuropathy
  M. Neuropathy associated with chronic infection (e.g. ehrlichiosis)
  N. Traumatic neuropathies
    1) Traction of the cauda equina associated with tail-pulling in cats
    2) Brachial plexus avulsion
2. Diseases of the neuromuscular junction
  A. Tick paralysis
  B. Myasthenia gravis
  C. Botulism
  D. Coral snake venom
3. Myopathies (see Chapter 17)
  A. Congenital
    1) Dermatomyositis of collies
    2) Myopathy of Labrador retrievers
    3) Myopathy of Irish terriers/golden retrievers
    4) Myotonia in chow chows

    5) Canine x-linked muscular dystrophy (golden retrievers)
  B. Acquired
    1) Myopathy associated with hyperadrenocorticism
    2) Toxoplasma polymyositis
    3) Idiopathic polymyositis
    4) Eosinophilic polymyositis
    5) Nutritional myopathy
4. Unclassified
  A. Episodic weakness of young Burmese cats

Clinical Approach

1. The signalment may suggest appropriate differential diagnoses.
  A. Congenital lesions in the young
    1) Hypoplastic trachea—chow chows
    2) Hemivertebrae—English bulldogs
    3) Atlantoaxial subluxation—Yorkshire terriers/small breeds
    4) Panosteitis—large breeds
    5) PDA—German shepherds
    6) AS—boxers
    7) PS—German shepherds
    8) Tetralogy of Fallot—keeshonds
    9) Dermatomyositis—collies
  B. Other lesions
    1) Sick sinus syndrome—miniature schnauzers
    2) Intervertebral disk extrusion—dachshunds
    3) Degenerative myelopathy—geriatric German shepherds
    4) Caudal cervical vertebral malformation/instability—Doberman Pinschers, Great Danes
    5) Distal polyneuropathy—Doberman Pinschers
    6) Diabetic polyneuropathy—felines
    7) Idiopathic polyradiculoneuritis—shepherd types
    8) Hemangiosarcoma—German shepherd
    9) Myxedema—Doberman Pinscher
    10) Cardiomyopathy—Doberman Pinschers, Persian cats

History

1. The following information should be obtained:

A. Client's description of the "episodes"

1) Episodes lasting seconds support a diagnosis of cardiopulmonary disease.

2) Episodes lasting one to five minutes are indicative of a seizure disorder.

3) Episodes associated with excitement or feeding suggest a diagnosis of narcolepsy.

B. Vaccinations

C. Dietary habits/frequency of feeding

D. Exposure to toxins (lead, organophosphates, rat poisons, ethylene glycol)

E. Current drug therapy (trimethoprim/sulfa combinations, insulin, aminoglycosides)

F. Trauma

G. Knowledge of littermates/line

H. Heartworm prevention

I. Travel history

J. Description of stools

K. Previous fever

L. GI signs

M. Respiratory signs

N. Lameness

O. Urinary signs

Physical Examination

1. A complete physical examination is essential in diagnosing the underlying disorder.

A. Auscultation with concurrent pulse determination

1) Pulse deficits with a rapid heart rate suggest arrhythmia.

2) Absence of femoral pulses indicates possible thromboembolism.

3) A slow heart rate suggests hypoadrenocorticism or cardiac arrhythmia.

B. Determination of mucous membrane color/presence of petechiae

C. Fundic examination

1) Chorioretinitis (FeLV, FIP, canine distemper, toxoplasmosis, fungal disease)

2) Retinal hemorrhage (coagulopathy, ehrlichiosis)

D. Deep palpation of the long bones

1) Pain may be indicative of panosteitis, HOD, or fractures.

E. Joint manipulation/palpation

1) Pain or swelling suggests articular causes.

F. Deep muscle palpation

1) Pain may indicate myopathy of neuropathy.

G. Spinal palpation

1) Pain indicates possible spinal cord disease.

H. Abdominal palpation

1) For detection of mass effects, peritoneal effusions

I. Jugular pulses suggest right-sided heart failure associated with dirofilariasis.

J. Neurologic examination

1) Generalized depression of the reflexes may indicate generalized motor unit disease related to a metabolic disorder.

2) A finding of dysfunction of asymmetrical cranial nerves V sensory and/or VII motor suggests a cerebral lesion.

3) Ataxia or conscious proprioceptive deficits indicate a possible neurologic lesion.

4) Abnormal spinal reflexes suggest a neurologic lesion.

5) General weakening with exercise supports a diagnosis of myasthenia gravis, hypoglycemia, or an electrolyte disorder.

Ancillary Diagnostic Tests

1. Routine baseline data include the following:

A. Complete blood count (CBC)

B. Biochemical profile with a valid fasting glucose determination

C. Electrolytes (serum)

D. Urinalysis

E. Heartworm (HW) test (consider occult HW antigen test)

F. Fecal flotation/occult blood tests

G. Routine, single electrocardiogram (ECG)

H. Thoracic roentgenograms

2. If metabolic causes are suspected, consider performing the following tests:

A. Triiodothyronine (T_3), thyroxine (T_4), thyroid-stimulating hormone (TSH) stimulation, thyroid releasing hormone (TRH) stimulation

B. Adrenocorticotropic hormone (ACTH) stimulation

C. Serum osmolality determination

D. Insulin/glucose ratio determination

E. Serum protein electrophoresis

3. If cardiovascular causes are suspected, the following tests may be helpful:

A. Repeated ECGs or Holter monitoring (continuous ECG)

B. Thoracic ultrasonography

C. Angiograms

D. Serial blood cultures (if bacterial endocarditis is suspected)

1) Obtain culture samples during fevers, if possible.

4. If neurologic causes are suspected, the following tests should be considered:

A. Electroencephalogram (EEG), cerebrospinal fluid (CSF) evaluation, skull radiographs for cerebral lesions

B. Magnetic resonance imaging (MRI) or computed tomography (CT) scanning for cerebral or spinal cord lesions

C. Plain spinal radiographs, CSF evaluation, electromyography (EMG), and myelogram for spinal lesions

D. Cultures, serologic studies, and titers performed on serum and/or CSF for infectious causes of neurologic disease if the EEG or CSF examination indicates inflammation

5. If generalized motor unit disease is suspected, consider performing the following tests:

A. Serum creatinine phosphokinase (CPK) determination

B. Clinical Tensilon test

C. EMG with electrodiagnostic edrophonium chloride test

D. Muscle and/or nerve biopsy

E. Measurement of serum acetylcholine receptor antibody levels.

6. If orthopedic disease is suspected, consider obtaining radiographs of the involved bones.

7. If articular disease is suspected, the following studies may be helpful:

A. Radiographs of the involved joints

B. Palpation of joints (with animal anesthetized)

C. Joint taps, cultures, cytologic studies

D. Serologic studies for diseases associated with articular signs (antinuclear antibody [ANA], lupuserythematosus [LE] prep, ehrlichiosis, Lyme's disease, rheumatoid factor)

8. If peritoneal effusion, pleural effusion, pericardial effusion, or abdominal masses are suspected, ultrasonography is indicated, and cytologic study with culture of the fluid is appropriate.

Clinical Signs, Treatment, and Prognosis in Animals with Intermittent Weakness

1. The reader is referred to the appropriate chapters for a discussion of cardiovascular (Chapter 9), neurologic (Chapter 17), orthopedic (Chapter 6), glucose (Chapter 22), electrolyte (Chapter 25), and pulmonary disorders (Chapter 9).

2. A discussion of articular causes of intermittent weakness, including degenerative osteoarthritis and rheumatoid arthritis, is found in Chapter 6. In this chapter, nonerosive polyarthritis is discussed, as are generalized motor unit diseases (myopathies are presented in Chapter 17).

Nonerosive Polyarthritis

This cause of intermittent weakness, which is primarily recognized in dogs has several probable etiologies.

Clinical Signs

1. The patient usually has intermittent fever concurrently with intermittent weakness.

2. Multiple sites of joint pain are noted, especially upon flexion and extension of the carpus or tarsus.

3. Visible or palpable joint swelling may be present, but is often not recognizable.

4. Roentgenograms will not show bony proliferation or lytic lesions, but may demonstrate joint effusion.

5. The diagnosis rests on evidence of inflammation upon cytologic study of more than one joint aspirate.

6. Cells may be primarily neutrophilic, or mixed with mononuclear cells.

7. If culture results are positive for bacteria or mycoplasma, or if organisms are positively identified on cytological examination, septic polyarthritis is diagnosed. (Most cases are found not to be septic.)

8. Positive blood culture results and/or vegetations on cardiac valves detected by ultrasonographic imaging support a diagnosis of polyarthritis associated with bacterial endocarditis.

9. The results of serologic examination for Lyme disease, Rocky Mountain spotted fever, or ehrlichiosis may be positive, supporting these diagnoses.

10. A chronic infection (e.g., pyometra) may accompany polyarthritis.

11. Doberman Pinschers are particularly susceptible to nonerosive polyarthritis secondary to sulfa/trimethoprim combination drug use.

12. Positive results from ANA serologic tests, LE prep, or other evidence of multiple-system, immune-mediated disease support a diagnosis of polyarthritis associated with SLE.

13. Most cases are found to be idiopathic.

Treatment

1. If a positive culture, vegetative cardiac valve, or infectious cause is demonstrated, long-term use of appropriate antibiotics is the treatment of choice.

2. If a site of chronic infection has been identified, resolution of the infection should be attempted (e.g., in pyometra).

3. If drug use is a suspected etiology, discontinue the drug(s) in question. Improvement should be noted within a few days.

4. Idiopathic nonerosive polyarthritis, or those cases associated with SLE, should be treated with immunosuppressive dosages of prednisone, the dosage of which can be tapered over a period of months if a good result is obtained.

5. Other immunosuppressives (e.g., azathioprine/cyclophosphamide) may be necessary.

6. Hemapheresis may result in improvement in refractory cases (when available).

Prognosis

1. The prognosis is good in most idiopathic or drug-induced cases.

2. There is a fair to poor prognosis in cases associated with SLE. Immunosuppressive therapy may be tapered in these cases, but it is not advisable to discontinue therapy altogether.

3. Prognosis is variable in cases associated with infectious agents.

Generalized Motor Unit Disorders

Idiopathic Polyradiculoneuritis ("Coonhound Paralysis")

Clinical Signs

1. Any signalment is possible, but adult shepherd mixes are most commonly seen in this author's practice.

2. Weakness is gradually progressive over a period of 2 to 14 days, and usually proceeds in a caudal to cranial fashion in the body.

3. Spinal reflexes become depressed. Cranial nerves may become involved, but the disease usually spares segments above the cervical region.

4. Deep pain sensation remains intact. Most patients do not appear to be in pain, but some exhibit spinal pain on palpation.

5. There may be a history of recent (<2 weeks) exposure to a racoon bite, or antecedent illness, injury, surgery, or vaccination.

6. A spinal tap may reveal increased amounts of protein, but normal numbers of cells (albuminocytologic dissociation).

7. An EMG (at least five to seven days after onset) typically reveals abnormal insertional activity (positive waves and/or fibrillations). Polyphasic M-waves may be seen. Evoked potential amplitude and motor nerve conduction velocities may or may not be decreased. Repetitive stimulation is normal.

Treatment

1. These cases usually gradually resolve with appropriate nursing care and treatment of complicating factors (e.g., pneumonia, urinary tract infection, decubiti).

A. Frequent turning

B. Physical therapy

C. Soft, clean bedding

2. Corticosteroids, immunosuppressives, and hemapheresis have been suggested, but have not been definitively shown to alter the clinical course of the disease.

3. If raccoon exposure was possible, the client must be warned that future exposures will likely result in longer episodes and more serious (or even fatal) weakness.

4. The clinician must be alert to the possibility of rabies in these cases, and should have the brain of the animal examined in the case of a fatality.

Prognosis

1. Prognosis is fair to good in most cases, although occasionally, a fatality will occur.

2. At the time the weakness reaches a plateau, then begins to improve, a good prognosis can be given.

Miscellaneous Peripheral Neuropathies

Other causes of peripheral neuropathies are listed in this chapter on page 95.

Clinical Signs

1. Peripheral neuropathies may be recognized by intermittent weakness and individual associated signs. Neurologic examination usually reveals depressed spinal reflexes.

2. EMG examination often reveals abnormal insertional activity in multiple motor units, with polyphasic M-waves, slow motor unit conduction velocities, and normal repetitive stimulation.

3. Nerve biopsy may reveal nerve fiber degeneration and depletion, paranodal or segmental demyelination, short intercalated internodes, and myelin ovoids and balls (e.g., in toxoplasma polymyositis/polyneuropathy).

4. Muscle biopsy in animals with pure polyneuropathy reveals typical neurogenic diffuse fiber atrophy.

5. Specific causes often have hallmark features.

A. Feline diabetic neuropathy affects geriatric cats with concurrent diabetes mellitus detected on ancillary diagnostic testing. These cats most often improve neurologically as their diabetes is controlled, and often revert to a diabetic remission.

B. Toxic neuropathies are heralded by a history of exposure to the offending agent (e.g., vincristine, organophosphates).

C. The initial signs of progressive axonopathy affecting boxers begin at one to two months of age.

D. An animal found to have metastatic neoplasia during the routine diagnostic workup of intermittent weakness may have paraneoplastic polyneuropathy if EMG examination indicates a neuropathy.

E. Peripheral neuropathy may be a concurrent problem in hypoglycemia associated with an insulin-secreting neoplasia.

F. The suggested readings and Chapter 16 provide additional information on other causes of peripheral neuropathy.

G. The prognosis of animals with peripheral neuropathy varies, and is dependent on the prognosis for treatment of the specific cause of the disorder.

Diseases of the Neuromuscular Junction

Tick Paralysis

Clinical Signs

1. Tick paralysis is the most frequent and easily diagnosed disease affecting the neuromuscular junction. It is most common in dogs, but rare in cats.

2. It is caused by the neurotoxin of the saliva in engorged female ticks, which are usually present around the head and neck of the host animal, and usually of the species *Dermacentor variabilis.*

3. Weakness proceeds in a caudal to cranial fashion, with spinal reflexes becoming depressed. The clinical course is one to four days in duration.

4. If the tick is particularly close to a cranial nerve, that nerve may be noticeably weaker.

5. Death (secondary to respiratory paralysis)

may occur if the tick is not removed or does not fall off the host.

6. Insertional activity on EMG is normal. A decreased amplitude or lack of conduction (no M-waves) may occur. No decremental response can be seen.

7. No improvement would be expected on a clinical Tensilon test.

Treatment

1. The offending tick(s) must be physically removed. Check inside the ear canals, between the toes, and everywhere else.

2. Judicial use of insecticide shampoo or dip should be considered.

Prognosis

1. If the diagnosis is correct, improvement within 24 hours and rapid recovery should occur.

Myasthenia Gravis

Clinical Recognition

1. Myasthenia gravis classically presents as weakness following exercise in young adult canines. The disease is rare in cats.

2. A congenital variant exists as an inherited disease reported in Jack Russell terriers.

3. The adult disease is caused by immune-mediated destruction of acetylcholine receptors, and is often self-limiting.

4. It sometimes is accompanied by megaesophagus and regurgitation, which is life-threatening.

5. Dogs with myasthenia gravis rarely have thymomas.

6. A clinical edrophonium chloride test (1 to 10 mg intravenously [IV]) should produce dramatic, temporary improvement in strength.

7. An EMG will reveal normal insertional activity and nerve conduction velocity, but a decremental response on repetitive stimulation.

8. This decremental response is temporarily reversed after IV administration of edrophonium chloride.

9. Serum acetylcholine receptor antibody levels can be assayed. (They are increased in

adult-onset myasthenia gravis.) These levels should be reviewed periodically.

Treatment

1. Pyridostigmine bromide, a long-acting cholinesterase inhibitor (Mestinon), is the drug of choice. Dosage is empirical.

2. If weakness persists or recurs, the dosage may be increased, then decreased from the baseline level (overdose or underdose will result in weakness).

3. Alternatively, IV edrophonium chloride, administered in conjunction with the baseline dosage of Mestinon, would help to determine whether more or less drug should be given orally.

    A. If the patient weakens or does not strengthen after IV administration of edrophonium chloride, decrease the oral dosage.

4. Beware of the possibility of pneumonia in patients with myasthenia gravis and megaesophagus, and treat accordingly.

5. Follow these patients with serial thoracic radiographs to screen for a slow growing thymoma. Resect the thymoma if found.

6. Immunosuppressive drugs may be beneficial in poorly responsive cases without pneumonia from megaesophagus.

Prognosis

1. Most dogs with adult-onset myasthenia gravis achieve a spontaneous remission if megaesophagus is not a life-threatening problem.

2. Dogs with congenital myasthenia gravis do not currently respond well to treatment.

Botulism Toxicity

Clinical Signs

1. Botulism toxicity, which is a rare disease in canines, is caused by the toxin of *Clostridium botulinum.*

2. It typically progresses rapidly to generalized lower motor neuron tetraparesis, with cranial nerve involvement and paralysis of respiratory muscles.

3. An EMG may reveal failure to conduct evoked potentials. Insertional activity is usually normal.

Treatment

1. Supportive care and time
2. Antitoxin is available, but may not be beneficial.

Prognosis

1. Poor

Coral Snake Venom Toxicity

Clinical Signs

1. Coral snake venom blocks conduction across the neuromuscular junction.
2. A visual sighting of the snake is necessary to establish the diagnosis in this rapidly progressive lower motor neuron tetraparesis.
3. The snake must actually cause an abrasion by "chewing" on the victim in order for inoculation of the venom to take place.

Treatment

1. Antivenom is available and effective if administered soon after the snake bite occurs.
2. Supportive care of a tetraparetic patient is necessary.

Prognosis

1. The prognosis guarded to poor.
2. Recovery of normal strength is possible if the patient survives.

Myopathies

A listing of myopathies is included in this chapter on page 95. Additional information is available in Chapter 16.

Unclassified Causes of Intermittent Weakness

A family of Burmese cats in Australia with intermittent weakness and neck ventroflexion has been described. The cause, clinical course, and treatment are as yet unclear. However, owing to the clinical similarities to thiamine deficiency and partial response in some of the cats to supplementation, the author has suggested chronic thiamine supplementation for such patients.

Suggested Readings

Armstrong PJ: Problem: Hypoglycemia. American College of Veterinary Internal Medicine Forum Proceedings, pp 2-103 to 2-109, Washington, DC, 1986

Averill DR: Degenerative myelopathy in the aging German shepherd dog: Clinical and pathologic findings. J Am Vet Med Assoc 162: 1045–1051, 1973

Barsanti JA, Walser M, Hatheway CL, et al: Type C botulism in American foxhounds. J Am Vet Med Assoc 172: 809–913, 1978

Blauch BS, Cash WC: A brief review of narcolepsy with presentation of two cases in dogs. J Am Anim Hosp Assoc 11: 467–472, 1975

Braund KG, Blagburn BL, Toivio–Kinnucan M, et al: Toxoplasma polymyositis/polyneuropathy. A new clinical variant in two mature dogs. J Am Anim Hosp Assoc 24: 93–97, 1988

Bryette DS, Feldman EC: Primary hypoparathyroidism in the dog. J Vet Intern Med 2(1): 7–14, 1988

Chrisman CL: Differentiation of tick paralysis and acute idiopathic polyradiculoneuritis in the dog using electromyography. J Am Anim Hosp Assoc 11: 455–458, 1975

Chrisman CL: Diseases of peripheral nerves and muscles. In Ettinger SJ (ed): Textbook of Veterinary Internal Medicine: Diseases of the Dog and Cat, pp 459–494. Philadelphia, WB Saunders, 1975

Cockrell BY, Herigstad RR, Flo GL, et al: Myelomalacia in Afghan hounds. J Am Vet Med Assoc 162: 362–365, 1973

Cork LC, Griffin JW, Munnell JF, et al: Hereditary canine spinal muscular atrophy. J Neuropathol Exp Neurol 37: 209–221, 1979

Cowell RL, Tyler RD, Clinkenbeard KD, et al: Ehrlichiosis and polyarthritis in three dogs. J Am Vet Med Assoc 192(8): 1093–1095, 1988

Cummings JF, Lorenz MD, deLahunta A, et al: Canine brachial plexus neuritis: A syndrome resembling serum neuritis in man. Cornell Vet 63: 589–617, 1973

Duncan ID: Etiology and classification of peripheral neuropathies. American College of Veterinary Internal Medicine Forum Proceedings, pp 325–329, San Diego, 1987

Fenner WR (ed): Quick Reference to Veterinary Medicine, pp 223–233. Philadelphia, JB Lippincott, 1982

Greene CE, Lorenz MD, Munnell JF, et al: Myopathy associated with hyperadrenocorticism in the dog. J Am Vet Med Assoc 174: 1310–1315, 1979

Griffiths IR, Duncan ID: Myotonia in the dog: A report of four cases. Vet Rec 93: 184–188, 1978

Hayes MA, Creighton SR, Boysen BG, et al: Acute necrotizing myelopathy from nucleus pulposus embolism in dogs with intervertebral disk degeneration. J Am Vet Med Assoc 173: 289–295, 1978

Jones BR, Anderson LJ, Barnes GRC, et al: Myotonia in related chow chow dogs. N Zealand Vet J 25: 217–220, 1977

Kelly MJ: Myasthenia gravis. Calif Vet 33: 25–26, 1979

Kelly MJ: Problems, diagnosis: Periodic weakness—Metabolic etiologies. American College of Veterinary Internal Medicine Forum Proceedings, pp 81–82, San Diego, 1985

Kelly MJ, Hill JR: Canine myxedema stupor and coma. Compend Contin Educ Pract Vet 6(12): 1049–1055, 1984

Knecht CD, Oliver JE, Redding RG, et al: Narcolepsy in a dog and a cat. J Am Vet Med Assoc 162: 1052–1053, 1973

Kornegay JN: Canine muscle disease. American College of Veterinary Internal Medicine Forum Proceedings, pp 5-33 to 5-40, Washington, DC, 1986

Kramer JW, Hegreberg GA, Bryan GM, et al: A muscle disorder of Labrador retrievers characterized by deficiency of type II muscle fibers. J Am Vet Med Assoc 169: 817–820, 1976

Krum SH, Cardinet GH, Anderson BC, et al: Polymyositis and polyarthritis associated with systemic lupus erythematosus in a dog. J Am Vet Med Assoc 170: 61–64, 1977

Lorenz MD, Cork LC, Griffin JW, et al: Hereditary spinal muscular atrophy in Brittany spaniels: Clinical manifestations. J Am Vet Med Assoc 175: 833–839, 1979

Mason K: A hereditary disease in Burmese cats manifested as an episodic weakness with head nodding and neck ventroflexion. J Am Anim Hosp Assoc 24: 147–151, 1987

Miller MM, Soave O, Dement WC: Narcolepsy in seven dogs. J Am Vet Med Assoc 168: 1036–1038, 1976

Oliver JE, Selcer RR, Simpson S: Cauda equina compression from lumbosacral malarticulation and malformation in the dog. J Am Vet Med Assoc 173: 207–214, 1978

Pedersen NC, Pool RC, Castles JJ, et al: Noninfectious canine arthritis: Rheumatoid arthritis. J Am Vet Med Assoc 169: 295–303, 1976

Pedersen NC, Weisner K, Castles JJ, et al: Noninfectious canine arthritis: The inflammatory nonerosive arthritides. J Am Vet Med Assoc 169: 304–310, 1976

Ribas JL, Braund KG: Fungal infections of the CNS in dogs and cats. American College of Veterinary Medicine Forum Proceedings, pp 5-19 to 5-25, Washington, DC, 1986

Ross LA: Disorders of sodium metabolism. American College of Veterinary Medicine Forum Proceedings, pp 2-111 to 2-117, Washington, DC, 1986

Scott DW, deLahunta A: Eosinophilic polymyositis in a dog. Cornell Vet 64: 47–56, 1974

Strombeck DR, Krum S, Meyer D, et al: Hypoglycemia and hypoinsulinemia associated with hepatoma in a dog. J Am Vet Med Assoc 169: 811–812, 1976

Tarvin G, Prata RG: Lumbosacral stenosis in dogs. J Am Vet Med Assoc 177: 154–159, 1980

Weller RE: Cancer-associated hypoglycemia in companion animals. Compend Contin Educ Pract Vet 7(5): 437–443, 1985

Zaki FA, Prata RG, Kay WJ: Necrotizing myelopathy in five Great Danes. J Am Vet Med Assoc 165: 1080–1084: 1974

Zaki FA, Prata RG: Necrotizing myelopathy secondary to embolization of herniated intervertebral disk material in the dog. J Am Vet Med Assoc 169: 222–228, 1976

CHAPTER EIGHT

Polyuria and Polydipsia

Bernard Hansen

••

Polyuria and polydipsia are common client complaints in small animal practice. Because a wide variety of disorders involving many different organ systems may result in these findings, a consistent and systematic approach is desirable when attempting diagnosis.

Definitions

1. Measures of concentration

   A. *Osmolality* refers to the number of particles of solute per kilogram of solvent. Thus, 1 mol of a nondissociable substance dissolved in 1 kg of water has an osmolality of 1.0 (1000 mosm).

   B. *Osmolarity* refers to the number of particles of solute per liter of solution.

   C. Because physiologic solutions are rather dilute, the two measures are almost identical. In clinical terms, however, osmolality is used more often.

   D. Osmolality is measured by measuring changes in the freezing point or vapor pressure of a solution. Plasma osmolality may be estimated by measuring the major osmoles in plasma:

$$P_{osm} = 1.86(Na + K) + BUN/2.8$$
$$+ \text{Glucose}/18 + 9$$

where 1.86 accounts for the anions associated with sodium and potassium, blood urea nitrogen (BUN) and glucose are measured in mg/dL, and a factor of 9 is added to account for miscellaneous minor osmoles present in plasma. Normal serum osmolality in the dog is 280 to 307 mosm/kg.

   E. *Effective osmolality*, or *tonicity*, refers to solutes that do not cross cell membranes. Urea is not an effective osmole because it readily enters cells, whereas sodium chloride (NaCl) or glucose are effective osmoles as they do not. Thus, a solution of urea that is isosmotic with plasma is the physiologic equivalent of distilled water, and is very hypotonic with respect to cells. An intravenous infusion would rapidly cause hemolysis.

2. *Specific gravity* is the ratio of the weight of a given volume of a solution to that of an equal volume of distilled water. The value depends upon the number, size, and weight of particles in the solution, and is estimated clinically with a refractometer. For solutions with particles of low molecular weight and size (e.g., normal urine), the specific gravity tends to vary linearly with osmolality.

3. *Diuresis* or *polyuria* refers to urine flow that is increased above the normal range of 24 to 41 mL/kg/d (dogs) or 22 to 30 mL/kg/d (cats).

4. *Solute diuresis* is an increase in urine flow that is caused by excessive excretion of a solute not reabsorbed within the renal tubules. Examples include mannitol, radiographic dyes, and glucose. Urine osmolality is equal to or higher than that of plasma.

5. *Water diuresis* refers to an increase in urine flow that is secondary to decreased reabsorption of water in the collecting tubules. Urine osmolality is hyposmotic to plasma.

6. *Polydipsia* refers to a prolonged state of excessive thirst. The normal water maintenance needs of dogs and cats are approximately 45 to 80 mL/kg of body weight/day. Because water requirements are proportional to body surface area, as opposed to body weight, larger dogs require less water per kilogram of body weight than do small dogs and cats. Consumption of more than 100 mL/kg of body weight/day under moderate environmental conditions is considered abnormal.

Normal Regulation of Water Balance

1. Thirst

A. Regulation of thirst is achieved via a complex system of receptors that includes circumventricular organs near the third ventricle of the brain which mediate osmolar stimuli. Hypovolemia and hypotension also stimulate thirst, as does dryness of the oropharyngeal mucous membranes. In normal humans, oropharyngeal dryness and cultural and social determinants of drinking behavior are probably the most important determinants of daily water intake. Water balance and free water excretion under euvolemic conditions are maintained primarily by the antidiuretic hormone–renal axis. Thirst becomes important as a control of water balance only when maximal renal water conservation is inadequate to maintain plasma osmolality and circulating blood volume within normal limits. The role of thirst in water balance in other species is poorly understood, but may be similar to that in humans.

2. Antidiuretic hormone (ADH) (vasopressin)

A. Antidiuretic hormone is a nine-aminoacid peptide that is synthesized by neurons in the supraoptic and paraventricular nuclei of the hypothalamus. The axons of these cells terminate in the posterior lobe of the pituitary (neurohypophysis), where ADH is stored and later released in response to appropriate stimuli. Additionally, some axons deliver ADH to the cerebrospinal fluid (CSF) or portal capillaries of the median eminence at the third ventricle. This characteristic accounts for preservation of osmoregulation in the presence of destructive lesions of the pituitary gland.

B. The major physiologic stimuli for ADH release are an increase in plasma osmolality and a decrease in the effective arterial blood volume (an unmeasurable entity describing effective tissue perfusion). Increases in plasma osmolality of as little as 1% to 2% above 280 mosm/kg stimulate ADH release, whereas similar reductions in osmolality cause low or undetectable concentrations. Pressure-sensitive receptors, primarily those of the carotid sinus and left atrium, are also important regulators of ADH release. Animals with reduced effective arterial blood volume (secondary to shock, congestive heart failure, etc.) secrete ADH even in the presence of normal or low plasma osmolality.

C. Minor stimuli for ADH release include pain, anxiety, hyperthermia, nausea, hypoglycemia, hypoxemia, and certain drugs.

3. Mechanism of urine concentration
Two important conditions must be met for formation of concentrated urine:

A. A hypertonic renal medullary interstitium must exist. Steps A through F in Figure 8-1 illustrate the sequence of events in renal reabsorption of solute and water.

1) The primary event in the generation of medullary hypertonicity is the active transport of NaCl out of the lumen of the thick portion of the ascending limb of the loop of Henle. This section of the tubule is relatively impermeable to water; hence, the tubular fluid is dilute as it enters the cortical portion of the ascending limb and the connecting segment.

2) Under the influence of ADH, the cortical connecting segment and cortical portion of the collecting duct are permeable to water, allowing it to be reabsorbed down its concentration gradient. Because cortical blood flow is high, the reabsorbed water is removed rapidly and does not appreciably dilute the tonicity of the cortical interstitium. Urea remains behind in the tubule and is further concentrated.

3) As tubular fluid moves down the collecting duct into the medullary intersti-

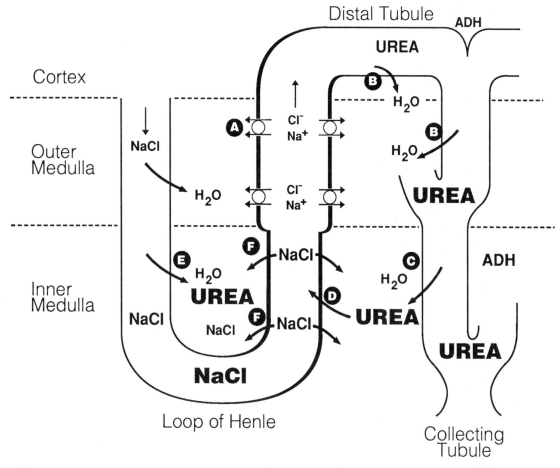

Figure 8-1. *The countercurrent hypothesis identifies the roles of sodium chloride and urea transport in the generation of concentrated urine. See text for details. (Adapted from Jamison RL, Maffly RH: The urinary concentration mechanism. N Engl J Med 295: 1059–1067, 1976. Reprinted with permission from The New England Journal of Medicine.)*

tium, it encounters a progressively greater osmotic gradient across the duct wall. Under the influence of ADH, the duct is permeable to both water and urea, and both are reabsorbed into the medullary interstitium. In the absence of ADH, the connecting segment and the collecting duct are relatively impermeable to water and urea, and the final osmolality of the urine is somewhat low. In dogs, the final urine osmolality may be as low as 50 mosm/kg.

4) Some of the reabsorbed urea reenters the loop of Henle, primarily in the thin ascending limb. This recycling of urea allows for maintenance of the high medullary concentrations of urea that contribute greatly to the generation of the medullary concentration gradient. The blood supply to the renal medulla (the vasa recta) is similarly arranged in a "hairpin" configuration; this allows for removal of reabsorbed water from the medullary interstitium with minimal removal of interstitial solute. In the absence of ADH, urea is lost in the urine and medullary tonicity is considerably reduced.

5) The hypertonic medullary interstitium induces water reabsorption from the thin descending loop of Henle. This segment is relatively impermeable to NaCl and urea. By the time filtrate reaches the deep hairpin turn, the concentration of NaCl is very high, and filtrate osmolality is similar to that of the medullary interstitium.

6) The thin ascending limb is relatively impermeable to water, very permeable to NaCl, and moderately permeable to urea. As fluid enters this segment, NaCl diffuses passively out of the lumen down its concentration gradient, and some urea enters the lumen down its concentration gradient. As a result, the tubular fluid is more dilute than that in the interstitium when it enters the thick portion of the ascending limb.

7) Approximately 70% of the filtrate leaving the glomerulus is reabsorbed isosmotically in the cortical proximal tubule. An additional 5% to 10% of th filtered water is reabsorbed in the thin descending portion of the loop of Henle. Hence, only about 20% of the filtered water enters the ascending limb of the loop of Henle, and it is reabsorption of this relatively small fraction of filtrate that is controlled by ADH.

8) The corticomedullary osmotic gradient may be lost under several conditions, including:

a) Loss of more than two-thirds of the functional nephrons

b) Prolonged diuresis of any etiology resulting in removal of medullary urea and sodium. (See section on medullary solute washout, page 109.)

B. ADH must be produced normally, and a functional collecting tubule response to ADH must exist.

Etiology

Conditions Resulting in Polyuria Secondary to Solute Diuresis

1. Glucosuria

A. Hyperglycemia in excess of the maximal renal glucose reabsorptive capacity

Table 8-1. *Causes of polyuria and polydipsia*

Solute diuresis
    Diabetes mellitus
    Renal tubular glucosuria
    Primary renal insufficiency or failure
    Postobstructive diuresis
Water diuresis
    Central diabetes insipidus
    Nephrogenic diabetes insipidus (congenital)
    Apparent psychogenic polydipsia
    Pyometra
    Hypoadrenocorticism
    Hyperadrenocorticism
    Hepatic failure
    Polycythemia
    Hypercalcemia
    Potassium depletion nephropathy
    Renal medullary solute washout
Iatrogenic causes
    Intravenous fluid therapy
    Excessive salt supplementation
    Drugs

(about 180 mg/dL) results in glucosuria. Tubular fluid glucose is an effective osmole and counters water reabsorption in the nephron distal to the proximal tubule, resulting in solute diuresis.

B. Primary renal glucosuria occurs secondary to a defect in proximal tubular reabsorption of glucose. This may be accompanied by defective reabsorption of phosphorus, amino acids, and electrolytes, as in the Fanconi-like syndrome described in basenji dogs.

2. Renal insufficiency

A. Renal insufficiency is associated with the loss of more than two-thirds of the functional nephrons, and is characterized by polyuria and secondary polydipsia. Primary renal failure occurs when more than 75% of nephron function is lost; it is further characterized by azotemia. The polyuria probably results from several factors:

1) Disruption of medullary architecture and loss of nephrons results in a failure to maintain a normal medullary concentration gradient. Because the animal must excrete the same daily solute load as a normal animal, the surviving nephron population is subjected to a solute (osmotic) diuresis.

2) Other factors include increased medullary blood flow and relative unresponsiveness of the collecting tubules to ADH. Cats with reduced nephron mass appear to retain greater concentrating ability than do dogs, even after the development of azotemia, and are often not polyuric until severe loss of function has occurred.

3. Postobstructive diuresis

A. A diuresis of several days' duration is often seen following relief of prolonged urethral obstruction. This syndrome is usually self-limiting, and is seen most commonly in male cats. Relief of the obstruction allows for renal excretion of accumulated metabolic wastes. Of these, urea is the most important osmotically, and excretion of large quantities of this compound results in an osmotic diuresis that lasts as long as significant plasma concentrations are present. Additionally, there may be transient tubular defects that impair the reabsorption of water and possibly, sodium, thus creating both water and osmotic diuresis.

Conditions Resulting in Polyuria Secondary to Water Diuresis

1. Central diabetes insipidus (CDI)

A. CDI is a rare disease characterized by a failure of the hypothalamus-neurohypophysis to secrete ADH in sufficient amounts to allow renal conservation of water. The inability to secrete ADH results in the production of large volumes of urine—up to 10 times the normal amount. There is no defect in the animal's thirst mechanism, and compensatory polydipsia occurs. The kidneys are functionally and anatomically normal, although the prolonged polyuria may result in loss of medullary solute. There appears to be no sex or familial predisposition. Affected dogs are generally middle-aged, although diabetes insipidus has been reported in dogs younger than 1 year of age. Causes in the dog include:

1) Hypothalamic-pituitary neoplasia

2) Cranial trauma

3) Visceral larva migrans

4) Cerebral inflammatory disease

B. History

1) Voluminous polyuria and insatiable polydipsia are the primary clinical signs. Nocturia and pollakiuria with incontinence secondary to the massive urine volume are common. The owner may note that the urine is unusually clear.

2) Onset is usually abrupt.

3) Signs referable to central nervous system (CNS) involvement at other locations are sometimes noted, including seizures, disorientation, visual disturbances, and incoordination.

C. Physical findings

1) Often normal

2) Focal neurologic deficits (hypothalamic syndrome) may be present.

3) The urinary bladder may be very large.

4) Generally, affected dogs are not dehydrated unless they are denied access to water.

2. Nephrogenic diabetes insipidus (NDI)

A. This term has been ascribed by some to any disease process that interferes with the generation, maintenance, or utilization of the renal corticopapillary concentration gradient. However, this definition is all-inclusive of disorders of water balance except CDI. A more descriptive and restricted definition includes only those disorders that result in an inability of the collecting duct epithelium to respond to ADH with an appropriate increase in water permeability.

1) Congenital NDI

a) A rare disease characterized by an intrinsic collecting duct defect resulting in an inability to respond to ADH. The defect involves the generation of cyclic adenosine monophosphate (cAMP), an essential biochemical intermediate in the hydro-osmotic response to ADH.

b) History and physical examination findings are identical to those of CDI, with the exception that polyuria and polydipsia are present since birth.

2) Acquired NDI

a) This group of disorders has been described in humans and other species. The most common causes include potassium depletion, hypercalcemia, and drugs. Clinically significant polyuria may not be present.

b) Because the electrolyte disturbances result in other renal anatomic and functional lesions, they will be discussed separately.

c) The drugs associated with collecting duct hyporesponsiveness to ADH in a variety of species include:

    i. Lithium
    ii. Demeclocycline
    iii. Methoxyflurane
    iv. Amphotericin B
    v. Gentamicin
    vi. Cisplatin
    vii. Propoxyphene
    viii. Isophosphamide
    ix. Clonidine
    x. Guanabenz
    xi. Colchicine
    xii. Vinca alkaloids

3. Apparent psychogenic polydipsia

A. Psychogenic or compulsive polydipsia is a poorly described disorder of water balance that is probably much more common than either CDI or NDI.

B. The history and physical examination findings are often similar to those of diabetes insipidus. The polydipsia may begin after some unusual or stressful event in the dog's life, such as moving, being kenneled, or being otherwise confined.

C. The pathophysiology of the disorder is unknown; however, it is likely that, in many dogs, it results from voluntary initiation of polydipsia as a result of some stressor or boredom. Once polydipsia has resulted in prolonged polyuria, loss of renal medullary solute and impaired concentrating ability may serve to perpetuate the problem. It is quite possible that some of these dogs have, instead, acquired defects in their subconscious thirst regulation, as has been described in humans. The nature and incidence of primary thirst disorders associated with polydipsia in dogs are unknown.

4. Pyometra

A. Polyuria and polydipsia are seen in approximately one third of dogs with pyometra.

B. Initially, renal water conservation ability may be normal; however, as the disease progresses with development of bacterial infection, a marked impairment of concentrating ability develops and the urine specific gravity value is usually 1.003 to 1.007. Hence, the ability to dilute the urine remains intact.

C. Interference of collecting tubule response to ADH by *Escherichia coli* endotoxin is thought to be an important mechanism of the polyuria.

5. Adrenal cortex disorders

A. Hypoadrenocorticism is occasionally associated with polyuria and polydipsia. The chronic renal loss of sodium seen with this disorder may result in loss of the corticopapillary osmotic gradient, thus impairing urine concentrating ability.

B. Hyperadrenocorticism is commonly associated with polyuria and polydipsia. Cortisol augments the delivery of filtrate out of the proximal tubule and interferes with the action of ADH at the collecting tubule, resulting in a water diuresis and compensatory polydipsia.

6. Chronic liver disease

A. Many dogs with chronic liver disease develop polyuria and polydipsia. There are likely to be several reasons:

1) Reduced metabolic capacity of the diseased liver may result in elevated plasma concentrations of glucocorticoids and aldosterone. The increased aldosterone concentrations promote sodium retention and compensatory polydipsia.

2) Reduced conversion of ammonia to urea results in a smaller daily load of urea for excretion. As urea is important for renal medullary osmotic gradient formation, this impairs the ability to concentrate the urine. Hyperammonemic encephalopathy may cause compulsive polydipsia in some dogs.

3) Hypokalemia frequently accompanies severe liver disease in dogs and impairs renal water conservation.

7. Primary polycythemia

A. Polydipsia and polyuria have been seen in approximately half of the dogs with primary polycythemia.

B. The mechanism is unknown; however, suppression of ADH release has been demonstrated in humans. Hypothalamic hypoxia secondary to hyperviscosity and reduced blood flow may play a role.

8. Hypercalcemia

A. Polyuria and polydipsia are often the first clinical signs noted in dogs with hypercalcemia.

B. Often, polyuria is present before any demonstrable reduction in glomerular filtration rate (GFR) is present. Possible mechanisms include impaired NaCl transport in the loop of Henle, increased medullary blood flow with loss of medullary solute, and impaired action of ADH at the collecting tubule.

C. Chronic calcium nephropathy is characterized histologically by calcium deposition and interstitial inflammation. With time, irreversible structural damage becomes widespread enough to result in renal failure and solute diuresis.

9. Potassium depletion nephropathy

A. Hypokalemia may develop as a result of prolonged gastrointestinal losses, anorexia, chronic liver disease, or potassium-losing renal disease.

B. Hypokalemia may result in renal dysfunction characterized by reduced GFR, impaired urine concentrating ability, impaired acid–base regulation, and derangements in the renal handling of sodium.

C. The magnitude of the concentration defect is dependent upon the severity and duration of potassium loss.

D. Impaired concentrating ability is associated with loss of medullary interstitial solute, impaired release of ADH, and impaired tubular response to ADH.

10. Medullary solute washout

A. Loss of medullary solute (sodium, chloride, and urea) results from prolonged water or osmotic diuresis, or from impaired tubular handling of sodium. Diuresis increases tubular flow rate and decreases the amount of sodium and urea that can be reabsorbed. Additionally, medullary blood flow is increased, which tends to remove medullary solute.

B. Once the corticopapillary osmotic gradient is lost, the ability to concentrate urine is severely impaired. Loss of medullary tonicity causes a reduced urine concentration, even in the presence of excessive ADH.

Iatrogenic Causes of Polyuria and Polydipsia

1. Intravenous fluid therapy
2. Dietary salt supplementation
3. Drug therapy
  A. Diuretics
  B. Glucocorticoids
  C. Drugs causing acquired NDI

Clinical Evaluation

1. Most dogs and cats with polyuria and polydipsia are diagnosed based on history, physical examination, and routine laboratory testing (Fig. 8-2). For many of these disorders, polyuria/polydipsia is only one of several coexisting abnormalities in the patient and may be relegated to minor importance.

2. Many owners misinterpret increased frequency of urination (pollakiuria) as increased urine output. Careful questioning is essential, and measurement of actual urine output may be helpful in differentiating between these conditions.

3. Before assuming that an animal is indeed polyuric or polydipsic, the animal's daily consumption of water or urine output should be measured and analyzed. In otherwise apparently healthy animals, this should be done by the owner at home. The home may be the ideal location, as this assesses the animal's consumption or output in a familiar environment and measurements are not affected by the stresses of hospitalization.

Laboratory Tests to Evaluate Urinary Concentrating Ability

1. Endogenous creatinine clearance test

A. This test is to determine renal GFR, as well as quantitative estimations of solute or protein excretion. The test is indicated in the evaluation of polydipsia and polyuria in order to diagnose renal insufficiency in polyuric, nonazotemic dogs. Cats appear to retain significant urine concentrating ability until there

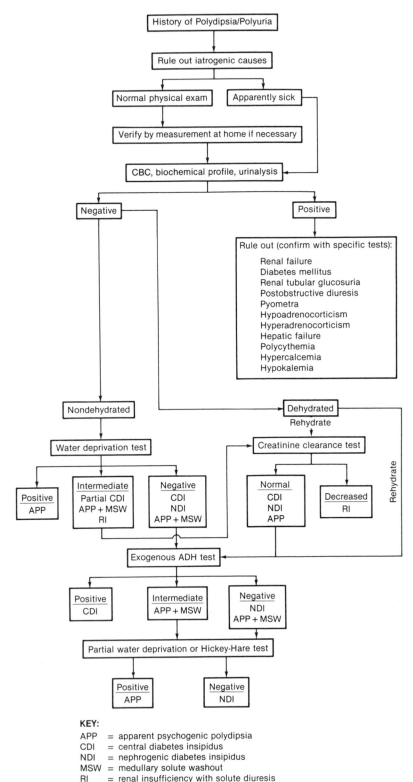

Figure 8-2. *Approach to the polyuric patient. (*APP, *apparent psychogenic polydipsia;* CDI, *central diabetes insipidus;* NDI, *nephrogenic diabetes insipidus;* MSW, *medullary solute washout;* RI, *renal insufficiency with solute diuresis)*

is severe loss of renal function. Hence, there may be a poor correlation between GFR and the presence or absence of an obligatory solute diuresis. In dogs, it may be best to perform this test prior to water deprivation testing in order to avoid the risk of dehydration and renal ischemic injury that could occur in these animals.

    B. Technique

        1) Empty the urinary bladder and discard the urine. Catheterize the bladder, if necessary, to empty it.

        2) Record the time the bladder is emptied.

        3) Carefully weigh (kg) the patient.

        4) Collect *all* urine voided during the test. Ideally, the test should last for 24 hours to maximize accuracy; however, it may be completed within as short a period as six hours if careful urine collection is performed. Allow the animal free access to water, but do not offer food during the collection period. If a metabolic cage is used, ensure that water is not spilled onto the cage floor.

        5) Obtain a serum sample at the midpoint of the collection period. Alternatively, a sample may be taken at the beginning and end of the collection period, in which case equal aliquots of serum are mixed together and assayed. Assay the serum to determine creatinine and osmolality values. If desired, assays for sodium, potassium, chloride, phosphate, urea, albumin, and globulin levels may be performed to assess renal fractional excretion of these substances.

        6) Empty the bladder at the end of the study and add this urine to the previously collected urine. Catheterization is necessary in males, whereas many female dogs will empty their bladders well voluntarily.

        7) Record the time the urine is collected.

        8) Weigh (kg) the animal again.

        9) Mix all urine well, and carefully measure the total volume. Submit an aliquot of urine to the laboratory for creatinine and osmolality determinations. If desired, assay additionally for sodium, potassium, chloride, phosphate, urea, albumin, and globulin levels.

    C. Interpretation

        1) The endogenous creatinine clearance is calculated by the following formula:

$$C_{cr} = \frac{urine_{cr} \times V}{serum_{cr} \times BW}$$

where V equals urine flow rate in mL/min and BW equals average body weight in kg.

        2) Published normal values for dogs have included 2.98 +/− 0.96 mL/min/kg, 3.7 +/− 0.77 mL/min/kg, and 2.53 +/− 0.95 mL/min/kg.

        3) In dogs, there is a consistent tendency for solute diuresis once renal function has declined by two thirds. Thus, creatinine clearance values of less than 1 to 1.5 mL/min/kg might reliably be expected to be associated with polyuria.

        4) Calculation of the clearance of free water provides further information for differentiating between solute and water diuresis. Clearance of free water may be calculated from the following formula:

$$C_{H_2O} = V - C_{osm}$$

where V equals urine flow rate in mL/min, C_{osm} equals osmolar clearance, and C_{H_2O} equals free water clearance.

The value for V is obtained as a direct measure, and C_{osm} is calculated by this formula:

$$C_{osm} = \frac{urine_{osm} \times V}{serum_{osm}}$$

The urine excreted during the collection period may be viewed as consisting of two components: urine required to excreted solutes isosmotic to plasma, and the excess of solute-free water. If the urine is isosmotic with plasma, C_{osm} equals V and C_{H_2O} equals zero. If the urine is hyperosmotic with respect to plasma, V is less than C_{osm} and C_{H_2O} is a negative value representing the amount of solute-free water that has been reabsorbed by the kidneys. If the urine is hyposmotic to plasma, V is greater than C_{osm} and C_{H_2O} is a positive value describing the amount of free water that has been excreted by the kidneys.

  2. Water deprivation testing

    A. The primary indication is evaluation of renal water conservation ability in animals that have had systemic diseases ruled out by history, physical examination, and routine serum and urine testing.

B. Hydration status must be monitored very carefully during the test period. Contraindications for testing include those animals with:

1) Azotemia

2) Dehydration

3) Extreme polyuria (a relative contraindication)

C. Technique

1) Allow the animal to urinate and obtain an accurate body weight (kg).

2) Withhold water but allow free access to dry food. Feeding provides a source of urea, which is needed for maximal renal concentrating ability.

3) Empty the bladder 6 to 12 hours after starting the test to rid the bladder of residual urine produced prior to the onset of the test.

4) Monitor patient hydration and urine concentration by measuring as many of the following parameters as possible:

a) Urine specific gravity

b) Urine osmolality

c) Serum osmolality

d) Urine/serum osmolality (U_{osm}/P_{osm}) ratio

e) Total plasma protein

f) Creatinine and BUN

g) Body weight (kg)

h) Skin pliability

5) Discontinue testing at the first sign of adequate urine concentrating ability or dehydration.

6) The indicators of adequate urine concentrating ability in normal dogs at the time they approach 5% dehydration, as determined by body weight loss, are:

a) Urine specific gravity exceeding 1.025. Most (95%) normal dogs (with no prior polyuria) increase their urine specific gravity to a value exceeding 1.048. Dogs with preexisting polyuria may have variable degrees of medullary solute loss that prevents maximal concentration; however, many of these dogs will still be able to achieve a urine specific gravity of 1.025.

b) The range of urine osmolality in normal dogs is 1768 to 2739 mosm/kg.

c) The U_{osm}/P_{osm} ratio in normal dogs ranges from 5.7 to 8.5.

7) Dogs with some impairment of renal concentrating ability may not be able to concentrate their urine above a specific gravity of 1.025. Values above 1.025 suggest that the hypophyseal–renal axis is capable of responding to a degree that would limit polyuria. Dogs with psychogenic polydipsia should be able to raise their urine specific gravity above this value unless they have coexisting disease or loss of medullary solute.

8) Indicators of dehydration

a) Acute weight loss is the "gold standard" indicator of dehydration. If the animal loses ≥5% of its body weight, the test should be discontinued.

b) An increase in plasma total solids above the baseline is suggestive of dehydration.

c) Changes in packed cell volume (PCV) are unreliable.

d) Skin pliability changes are very subjective and unreliable. Interpretation is influenced by experience, the examiner's knowledge of the animal's skin pliability before the test started, the amount of subcutaneous fat present, and the location on the body where pliability is assessed.

e) Creatinine and BUN values are rarely elevated during the course of properly executed water deprivation testing.

f) Extreme dehydration secondary to pure water loss may cause signs of hyperosmolarity (lethargy progressing to coma, trembling, salivation, and seizures). Severe loss of both sodium and water may cause signs of hypovolemia (tachycardia, weak pulse, cool extremities, weakness, depression).

3. Repositol ADH response test

A. Indicated to differentiate CDI from NDI and other disorders following negative water deprivation test results

B. Technique

1) Administer 5 U of vasopressin tannate oil suspension (Pitressin Tannate* in oil, Parke-Davis) intramuscularly (IM).

---

* Pitressin Tannate may be unavailable at this time.

2) A decrease of urine volume and thirst should be seen within two to four hours.

3) Empty the dog's bladder seven to eight hours after administration to remove any residual urine present in the bladder at the onset of the test period.

4) Collect urine samples (by catheter, if necessary) 9 and 12 hours after administration.

C. Interpretation

1) Normal dogs will show a peak response to reposital ADH at 9 to 12 hours, and will increase their urine specific gravity to a value of 1.028 to 1.057.

2) Dogs with hyposthenuria (urine specific gravity of 1.001 to 1.007) whose urine specific gravity increases to more than 1.012 following ADH injection have a significant response, suggesting either partial or complete CDI.

3) In dogs with long-standing polyuria and loss of renal medullary solute, the response to one injection may not be diagnostic. In these dogs, repeated injections at 24- to 48-hour intervals for several days may result in a progressive rise in urine specific gravity. During this period, the dog should be provided with high-protein food with adequate sodium to provide solute for the medullary interstitium.

4. Aqueous ADH response test

A. Like the reposital ADH test, this test is indicated to differentiate CDI from NDI and other disorders. However, it can be completed in less time than the reposital ADH test.

B. Technique

1) Empty the urinary bladder by indwelling catheterization.

2) Administer 10 mU of aqueous ADH/kg of body weight intravenously (IV) over a period of 60 minutes. Five units of fresh aqueous ADH is added to 1 liter of dextrose 5% in water and is administered at a rate of 2 mL/kg over a period of 60 minutes.

3) Collect urine samples 30, 60, and 90 minutes following initiation of the IV infusion. Empty the bladder completely at each collection.

C. Interpretation

1) Normal dogs that are water-loaded

at the onset of the infusion achieve a urine specific gravity of 1.012 to 1.033.

2) Dogs with hyposthenuria (urine specific gravity of 1.001 to 1.007) whose urine specific gravity increases to more than 1.012 following ADH infusion have a significant response, suggesting either partial or complete CDI.

3) Dogs with medullary solute loss may have an intermediate response, as with the reposital ADH test.

5. Partial water deprivation test

A. The partial water deprivation test is indicated to help differentiate those dogs with diabetes insipidus from those with medullary solute washout secondary to other diseases.

B. Technique

1) The dog's unrestricted 24-hour water intake should be measured by the owner at home and averaged over several days.

2) Once the daily water intake is known, the owner should be instructed to reduce the amount available to the dog to a quantity that is 5% to 10% less than the average daily consumption for three to five days. The dog's normal diet should be continued. The amount of daily water supplied to the dog should never be less than 45 cc/kg/d (the minimum daily maintenance requirement of normal dogs). Water should be set out in several portions over the day to prevent the dog from consuming the day's supply too rapidly, thereby leaving it with none for a portion of the day.

3) Each morning, the owner should weigh the dog carefully. In addition, the owner should be taught to recognize signs of dehydration and report them, along with any significant weight loss, to the clinician.

4) Gradual restriction of water intake, coupled with provision of protein (for urea production) and salt in the diet, should allow reestablishment of a corticomedullary osmotic gradient over a period of several days. This process may be augmented in some dogs by the administration of reposital ADH every 24 to 48 hours. These dogs must be carefully evaluated for signs of both water deprivation and water toxicity.

6. Hickey-Hare test

A. The Hickey-Hare test has been

adapted from human medicine for use in dogs as an alternative to water deprivation testing. It is indicated for the differentiation of polydipsic disorders with renal medullary solute washout from diabetes insipidus after negative results have been obtained from exogenous ADH testing. It is based on the principle that the IV administration of hypertonic saline solution should induce hypothalamic ADH release in response to the increase in plasma osmolality, resulting in reduced urine flow.

    B. Technique

      1) Water loading is accomplished by administering 20 mL/kg of tepid water via a stomach tube.

      2) Place an indwelling urinary catheter, empty the bladder, and measure urine flow (mL/min).

      3) Administer a 2.5% NaCl solution IV at the rate of 0.25 mL/kg/min for 45 minutes.

      4) Record the urine volume every 15 minutes during, and for 45 minutes after, completion of the infusion.

      5) Serum osmolality should be measured at the beginning and end of the infusion.

    C. Interpretation

      1) The normal response is a decrease in the rate of urine production throughout the test. In pituitary or diabetes insipidus or NDI, there should be either no change or an actual increase in urine flow. In other disorders complicated by medullary washout, the administration of NaCl should help to reestablish the corticomedullary osmotic gradient and allow for reduction of urine flow, as well as an increase in urine osmolality.

      2) Serum osmolality should rise by the end of the infusion to document that there was an effective stimulus for endogenous ADH release.

      3) Hypertonic saline infusions may be contraindicated in animals with cardiopulmonary disorders. Animals that are incapable of decreasing their urine output may develop significant hypernatremia (hyperosmolality) with signs that include lethargy progressing to coma, trembling, salivation, and seizures. Treatment includes administration of a loop diuretic and IV 5% dextrose in water.

Suggested Readings

Breitschwerdt EB: Clinical abnormalities of urine concentration and dilution. Compend Contin Educ Pract Vet 3(5): 414–422, 1981

Grauer GF: The differential diagnosis of polyuric-polydipsic diseases. Compend Contin Educ Pract Vet 3(12): 1079–1085, 1981

Hardy RM: Disorders of water metabolism. Vet Clin North Am 12(3): 353–373, 1982

Hardy RM, Osborne CA: Water deprivation and vasopressin concentration tests in the differentiation of polyuric syndromes. In Kirk RW (ed): Current Veterinary Therapy VII. Philadelphia, WB Saunders, 1980

PART TWO

SYSTEMS DISTURBANCES

CHAPTER NINE

Cardiovascular and Pulmonary Disorders

John D. Bonagura and Larry Berkwitt

•••

Certain problems are associated with cardio-vascular or pulmonary disease, including historical, physical, and laboratory abnormalities.[10,40,41,95] Examples of the presenting history of affected animals include chronic sneezing, coughing, and syncope. Heart murmurs, pulmonary crackles, and tachypnea are typical examples of physical problems. Laboratory or roentgenologic disorders, such as hypoxemia and increased pulmonary densities, are also attributable to disease of the heart or lung. In many instances, signs of cardiovascular and pulmonary disease are so similar that an etiologic diagnosis can be obtained only after completing a thorough clinical work-up. The purpose of this chapter is to offer the practicing veterinarian a framework for determining the cause of problems related to cardiovascular or pulmonary dysfunction. For clarity of discussion, we have divided these disorders arbitrarily into historical, physical, and laboratory or roentgenologic problems.

Treatment of these problems is based on identification of the underlying etiology. Our point of emphasis in this chapter is establishment of a correct diagnosis. Principles of treatment are described; however, the reader is urged to consult other sources for more detailed descriptions of therapy. To this end, most of the references concern therapeutic approaches to specific cardiovascular or pulmonary disorders. We have included a table of drug dosages as a general guideline (see Table 9.1). In all cases, the clinician should consult the manufacturer's pharmaceutical information and other pertinent published data before administering any drug.

Historical Problems

Sneezing, Nasal Discharge, and Epistaxis

Definitions and Causes

1. Sneezing, nasal discharge, and epistaxis are signs of disease located within the nasal cavity and paranasal tissues.[10,26,40,101] These problems may be associated with concurrent lower respiratory tract disease or be a symptom of coagulopathies or another systemic disease.

2. Sneezing is a reflex act initiated by irritation of the cilia within the nasal cavity. It is frequently accompanied by a nasal discharge. Acute paroxysmal sneezing is often attributable to infection, intranasal foreign material, allergy, hemorrhage, or injury. Chronic sneezing can be caused by immotile cilia syndrome and cleft palate in neonates, swallowing disorders, previous trauma, foreign bodies, allergic rhinitis, infectious disease, tooth root abscess, osteomyelitis, parasites,

(text continues)

117

Table 9-1. **Approximate doses of drugs commonly used to treat cardiopulmonary disorders**

Antiarrhythmic drugs

Propranolol	0.04–0.06 mg/kg (IV)
	Cat: 2.5–5 mg q8h (orally)
	Dog: 2–1 mg/kg q8h
Lidocaine	Dog: 2–8 mg/kg (IV) over a 10 minute period
	Dog: 25–75 (occasionally up to 100) μg/kg/min at constant rate of intravenous infusion
	Cat: 0.25–0.75 mg/kg (IV) over a 3–5 minute period
Procainamide	Dog: 2 mg/kg (IV) up to a maximum total dose of 20 mg/kg over a 30 minute period
	Dog: 8–20 mg/kg (IM, orally) every 6–8 hours
	Cat: 3–8 mg/kg (IM, orally) every 6–8 hours
Quinidine sulfate or gluconate	Dog: 6–16 mg/kg q8h to q6h (IM, orally)
Tocainide	Dog: 10–20 mg/kg
Phenytoin	Dog: 50–100 mg (IV)
	Dog: 8–15 mg/kg q8h (orally)
Digitalis	See below
Diltiazem	Dog: 0.5–1.3 mg/kg (orally) q8h
	Cat: 0.5–2 mg/kg (orally) q8h
Verapamil	Dog, cat: 0.05 mg/kg, every 10–30 minutes to a maximum cumulative dose of 0.15 mg/kg (IV)
Rapid oral digitalization	Dog: 0.02–0.06 mg/kg divided q12h for one day
Rapid IV digitalization	0.01–0.02 mg/kg; administer $\frac{1}{2}$ of calculated dose IV; wait 30–60 min and administer $\frac{1}{4}$ of dose; wait 30–60 min and administer remaining dose, if necessary
Digitoxin (dog)	
Oral maintenance	0.04–0.1 mg/kg divided q12h to q8h
Rapid IV digitalization	0.01–0.03 mg/kg; administer as per digoxin
Furosemide (Lasix) q6–8 h	2–4 mg/kg (IV, IM, SQ, orally); repeat q12h or q8h if needed
Hydrochlorothiazide	2–4 mg/kg (orally), once or twice daily
Chlorothiazide	20–40 mg/kg

Drugs used to treat heart failure and pulmonary edema

Oxygen therapy	40%–60% (avoid 60% for 24 hours)
Morphine sulfate	Dog: 0.1–0.25 mg/kg (IV, IM, SQ)
Acepromazine	Cat: 0.1–0.5 mg/kg (SQ)
Aminophylline	6–10 mg/kg (IV<SQ, orally) q8h
Digitalis glycosides	
Digoxin loading dose	Dog: 0.0055–0.011 mg/kg (IV) q1h to effect to a maximum total dose of 0.02 mg/kg (with ECG monitoring) (IV only). Begin oral therapy 12h later; oral method–twice the maintenance dose for 24–48 hours (see below)

(continued)

Table 9-1. *(Continued)*

Digoxin maintenance dose	Dog: 0.0055–0.011 mg/kg q12h; or 0.22 mg/mater sq body surface area q12h Cat: Elixer (0.05 mg per ml) 0.0035–0.0055 mg/kg once or twice daily; Tablet (0.125 mg) ¼ tablet once or twice daily
Digitoxin	Dog: 0.02–0.03 mg/kg q8h
Furosemide	Dog: 2–6 mg/kg; repeated q8–12h as needed (IV, IM, SQ, orally) Cat: 1–4 mg/kg; repeated q12h as needed (IV, IM, SQ, orally)
Spironolactone	2–6 mg/kg daily
Triamterene	2–4 mg/kg daily
Dobutamine (Dobutrex)	Dog: 2.5–20 μg/kg/min, constant rate IV infusion Cat: 2.5–10 μg/kg/min, constant rate IV infusion
Dopamine (Intropin)	2–10 μg/kg/min
Nitroglycerine ointment (2%)	⅛–1 inch cutaneously, q8–12h
Sodium nitroprusside (Nipride)	5–20 μg/kg/min at a constant rate of infusion
Hydralazine (Apresoline)	1–3 mg/kg q12h, orally (initial dose 0.5 mg/kg and titrate)
Prazosin (Minipress)	0.5–2 mg/kg q12h to q8h
Captopril (Capoten)	1–2 mg q12h to q8h
Amrinone (Inocor)	Dog: 1–3 mg/kg, IV followed by 30–100 μg/kg/min infusion

Drugs used in pulmonary medicine

Bronchodilators	
Aminophylline	See above
Quibron (theophylline plus guaifenesin)	Dose for theophylline: 6–10 mg/kg q8h to q6h
Terbutaline	1.25–5 mg q12h to q8h
Cough suppressants	
Dextromethorphan (Parlam)	2mg/kg q8h to q6h
Dihydrocodeinone (Hycodan)	Dog: 1.25–10 mg q12h to q8h
Dihydrohydroxycodeinone (Percodan)	Dog: 1.25–10 mg q12h to q8h
Codeine	Dog and cat: 1–2 mg/kg q12h to q8h
Butorphanol	

Drugs used for cardiopulmonary arrest

Sodium bicarbonate	0.5–1 mg/kg (IV)
Epinephrine HCl (Adrenaline)	Intracardiac 6–20 μg/kg, IV 0.05–0.2 mg/kg
Dopamine HCl (Intropin)	2–10 μg/kg/min(IV)
Metaraminol	1–5 mg/kg (IV)
Atropine sulfate	0.02–0.04 mg/kg
Crystalloid fluids	20–40 ml/kg
Doxapram HCl (Dopram)	1–4 mg/kg(IV)
Mannitol (20%)	1–2 g/kg(IV)
Antiarrhythmic drugs	See above

Key: *IV*, intravenously; *IM*, intramuscularly; *SQ*, subcutaneously; *IC*, intracardiac polyps, tumors of the paranasal passages, polycythemia, or paraneoplastic syndromes. Acute diseases may lead to secondary chronic nasal disease. This occurs in some cats with viral (Herpes-induced) upper respiratory disease, particularly if they are immunosuppressed by feline leukemia virus (FeLV), T-lymphotrophic virus (FIV), or feline infectious peritonitis (FIP) virus. Cryptococcosis is a serious cause of chronic nasal disease in the cat. Although cryptococcosis does occur in the dog, nasal aspergillosis and Penicillium species are more important causes of chronic nasal disease in this species. Other causes of chronic sinusitis in the dog include lymphoplasmacytic infiltration[21] and infection with rhinosporidium[2,34] and capillaria.[37] Anatomical malformation with inadequate sinus or choanal drainage, as well as nasopharyngeal polyps,[40] have been recognized in cats as causes of sneezing, nasal discharge, or stertorous breathing.

3. Nasal discharges are characterized by type, duration, and symmetry (unilateral or bilateral).

A. Discharges can be characterized as serous, mucopurulent, serosanguineous, or hemorrhagic (epistaxis). Serous discharges are caused by foreign material, allergic disease, or viral infections. Mucopurulent and serosanguineous discharges generally indicate a subacute or chronic process caused by foreign bodies, infectious diseases, or neoplasia. Lower respiratory tract infection can cause bilateral mucopurulent nasal discharges, or may lead to secondary sinusitis. Epistaxis is associated with trauma, infection, neoplasia, hypertension, or coagulopathies. Patients with thrombocytopenia, platelet function disorders, polycythemia, or dysproteinemias often present with epistaxis. Violent sneezing from intranasal foreign material may also lead to epistaxis of short duration with minimal reduction in the packed cell volume (PCV). Conversely, coagulopathies can evoke prolonged bleeding with development of moderate to severe anemia.

B. Nasal discharges can be unilateral or bilateral. Unilateral discharges are caused by lesions involving one side of the nasal septum; the etiology of these may include foreign bodies, early infection, or neoplasia. Bilateral discharges come either from the lower respiratory tract, as with pneumonia, or from diffuse nasal and sinus disease. Causes of bilateral discharge include coagulopathies, chronic bacterial or fungal infections, osteomyelitis, and neoplasia.

C. In clinical practice, the duration and character of the nasal discharge often dictate whether symptomatic treatment or a detailed medical work-up will be undertaken. Obvious causes of acute nasal discharge and sneezing, such as trauma, inhalation of foreign particulate matter, and feline or canine upper respiratory infections, are usually treated symptomatically. Chronic discharges should alert the clinician to the probability of polyps, neoplasia, fungal infection, a foreign body, periodontal abscess, osteomyelitis, or chronic sinus infection, allergy, or immunosuppression. These patients should undergo a thorough medical evaluation.

Clinical Diagnostic Approach

1. The physical examination reveals important clues to the cause of nasal cavity disease. Animals with nasal discharges usually sneeze, gag, and retch, and may cough as a result of postnasal drip. Descending lobar pneumonia may develop. Conjunctivitis and epiphora are common and may be unilateral, involving the affected side. Cats with chronic Herpes infection can have ocular involvement such as corneal ulceration, conjunctivitis, and chemosis. Additional signs of etiological importance include fever, contagion, lymphadenopathy, swelling or deviation of the skull, enlargement of the tonsils, sanguineous nasal discharge, and systemic signs of disease. In particular, neurologic signs suggest the possibility of extension of nasal sinus disease through the cribriform plate into the brain. In many cases, physical abnormalities dictate a thorough medical work-up. Conversely, with classical, acute signs of allergy or of upper respiratory viral infection, symptomatic treatment is recommended as a prudent course.[40,77]

2. Hematologic evaluation

A. The results of a complete blood count

(CBC) may be abnormal, but are usually non-specific. Polycythemia vera can lead to sneezing or epistaxis because of alterations of the microcirculation, including capillary engorgement and altered platelet function. Anemia may be present in chronic systemic disease and may accompany epistaxis. Leukocytosis suggests stress or inflammation, which can be secondary to trauma, infection, or neoplasia.

B. Elevation of the serum protein in nondehydrated patients, particularly the globulin fraction, is compatible with inflammatory disease. A monoclonal gammopathy secondary to myeloma or lymphoreticular disease may lead to platelet function abnormalities and subsequent epistaxis. Polyclonal (or monoclonal) gammopathy can be found in animals with chronic Ehrlichia infection or with heartworms; with the latter, pulmonary thrombosis may cause transient hemoptysis and epistaxis.

C. A bleeding profile, platelet count, and platelet function studies are indicated for the evaluation of epistaxis. Thrombocytopenia should be followed up with serologic studies for Ehrlichia, Rocky Mountain spotted fever, disseminated intravascular coagulation, and immune disease.

D. Other hematologic tests, such as immunodiffusion titers for cryptococcosis, aspergillosis or penicillium, elisa testing for FeLV/FIV and biochemical profiles to screen for systemic disease, may be indicated.

3. Radiographic studies—Roentgenograms of the skull, taken with the animal anesthetized, are always indicated in chronic nasal disease.[40] Ventrodorsal, open-mouth, lateral, and frontal sinus views are required for a thorough evaluation. Prominent abnormalities include increased fluid density, asymmetry, swelling or mass lesions, loss of turbinate structure, and bone destruction.

A. Increased fluid density is compatible with infection, hemorrhage, foreign bodies, polyps, or neoplasia (particularly when densities are localized to the caudal nasal cavity).

B. Loss of turbinate detail, swelling, and bone destruction are suggestive of neoplasia, although chronic inflammation can also cause these signs.

C. The teeth roots should be evaluated carefully for abscessation.

D. Bone lysis is an indication for nasal endoscopy with biopsy or surgical exploration of the nasal cavity and sinuses.

4. Nasal cavity examination, nasal flush cytology, culture and sensitivity of the nasal discharges, and biopsy are generally accomplished after skull roentgenography to prevent artifacts in the x-ray films.

A. An otoscope speculum and light source or an arthroscope are used to examine the rostral nasal cavities because occasionally, a foreign body or fungal growth may be found this way. A dental mirror or, in larger dogs, a retroflexed fiberoptic endoscope, is used to evaluate the caudal nasal passages for mass lesions, foreign bodies, or choanal obstruction.

B. A cotton swab or flushing of the nasal passages may be used to obtain samples for cytology and culture.[40,63,101] Consider using small biopsy forceps to obtain mucosal tissue samples, or use a trephine to enter the nasal cavity or sinus to obtain biopsy material. The collection of these samples is guided by radiography.[13]

C. The nasal discharge is cultured for both bacteria and fungi, and is stained with India ink to screen for *Cryptococcus neoformans*. Vigorous flushing with sterile saline may temporarily improve a chronic nasal condition by opening the airway and removing exudate.

D. Probe the periodontal space for an oronasal fistula in dogs with dental disease (particularly the canine teeth).

5. Fine-needle aspiration cytology of enlarged regional lymph nodes can be revealing.

6. Some cases of chronic nasal discharge cannot be diagnosed or treated without surgical exploration of the nasal cavities. During surgery, samples are taken for culture and histopathologic examination. At times, nasal aspergillosis can be diagnosed only by the detection of invading hyphae in tissue sections. Tumors, including polyps, carcinomas, fibrosarcomas, and osteosarcomas, are diagnosed by biospy. Polyps may be removed by this technique. If neoplasia is not suspected, the infected mucosa can be surgically removed, drainage established, or drainage tubes placed for further therapy.

Treatment

1. The management of acute nasal passage disease is directed toward the primary etiology and symptomatic therapy.[1,13,21,26,37,40,77,101]

2. Treatment of chronic fungal infections includes medical and surgical therapy. Various antifungal agents, including amphotericin B, thiabendazole, iodines, ketoconazole and other imidizoles, and flucytosine, have been used in the management of nasal aspergillosis or cryptococcosis.

3. Treatment of malignant nasal tumors can be discouraging, but various combinations of surgery, chemotherapy, and radiation therapy have been employed with radiation therapy often the most effective method.[1,26]

4. The treatment of chronic nasal disease can be successful only if a definitive diagnosis is established.

5. Surgery is successful for treating polyps and pharyngeal drainage problems in cats.

6. Antihistamines and prednisolone are used in the treatment of allergic rhinitis and lymphoplasmacytic rhinitis.

Cough

Definition

1. Coughing is a reflex act that can be initiated throughout the respiratory system, from the pharynx to the bronchioles.

2. Specific cough receptors are present in the pharynx, larynx, tracheobronchial tree, and small airways.

3. Coughing can also be initiated by abnormalities of the pleura, pericardium, or diaphragm; however, pleural effusions seldom cause coughing in the dog and cat.

4. The sites for reflex coughing are limited in number; however, the possible causes of the stimulation of the cough reflex are extensive. If possible, the list of diagnostic possibilities should be narrowed by determining the probable site of cough stimulation through the history and physical examination.

Then the diagnosis may be substantiated through appropriate ancillary tests. The following is a partial list of lesions that can lead to either coughing or respiratory distress (dyspnea) in animals.

Etiology of Cough or Respiratory Distress (Dyspnea)

Diseases of the Upper Airways[7,38,47,50,75,84,90,91,94]

Sinusitis with postnasal drainage
Pharyngeal inflammation
Upper airway obstruction
    Redundant soft palate (often associated with stenotic nares); nasopharyngeal polyps
    Laryngeal paralysis, collapse, or eversion of the sacules
    Tracheal collapse, obstruction (intraluminal, mural, or extraluminal compression), or rupture
Mediastinal mass with compression of the trachea
Esophageal diseases leading to aspiration of esophageal contents or dilatation of the esophagus with compression of the trachea
Hilar lymphadenopathy causing compression (tumor, fungal infection, granulomatous diseases)
Filaroides osleri infection
Tracheitis
Chondromatous hematoma of the trachea or bronchus
Left atrial enlargement leading to bronchial compression
Collapse of a major bronchus

Disease of the Lower Airways[3,6,8,17,23-25, 27,33,41,46,51,58,61,67-69,73,79,90,91,96,99]

Bronchial obstruction, irritation, or inflammation secondary to:
    Bronchitis of any cause (infectious, allergic, irritant)
    Lungworms (Filaroides species, Aleurostrongylus, Paragonimus, Capillaria)
    Allergic bronchial disease, including bronchial asthma
    Environmental irritants
    Bronchiectasis as a result of chronic bronchitis

Bronchial obstruction from:
  Collapse
  Compression (heart, tumor, lymph
    node)
  Congenital hypoplasia
  Foreign body
Pulmonary edema secondary to left heart
  failure or a noncardiogenic cause[46,96]
Dirofilariasis[24,25]
Infectious pneumonia, pulmonary abscess, or
  granuloma[90,91]
Immunologic disease of the lung (including
  "allergic" pneumonitis, pulmonary
  infiltrates of eosinophils)
Pulmonary neoplasm[5,8,26]
Pulmonary microlithiasis
Pulmonary hemorrhage
Aspiration pneumonia
Granulomatous lung diseases

Pleural Space Disease*[11]

Pleural effusion
Pneumothorax
Diaphragmatic hernia
Pleural fibrosis

Other Pulmonary Diseases or Contributing Lesions

Pulmonary vascular disease (emboli, DIC,
  heartworms)[24]
Pulmonary fibrosis from alveolitis, Cushing's
  disease, aging, or secondary to other
  pulmonary diseases[17,28,31]
Restrictive pulmonary diseases:[17,31]
  Pulmonary fibrosis
  Abnormal chest conformation
  Obesity
  Abdominal masses

Miscellaneous Causes of Hyperpnea or Respiratory Distress

Altered hemoglobin (anemia,
  methemoglobinemia)
Acidosis
Elevated body temperature (fever, heat stroke)
Neuromuscular weakness
Pain
Shock
Head trauma, central nervous system (CNS)
  disease

* A rare cause of cough

Hyperthyroidism
Cushing's disease[28]
Hypothyroidism (laryngeal paresis)[94]

Clinical Diagnostic Approach

1. In the differential diagnosis of cough, the following predispositions according to breed should be considered: toy breeds, tracheal collapse; small breeds, chronic bronchitis and chronic mitral valve disease; giant breeds, acquired cardiomyopathy; boxer dogs, heart base and pulmonary neoplasms, and cardiomyopathy; brachycephalic breeds, obstructive upper airway disease. Intact female dogs are predisposed to metastatic mammary carcinoma. Younger animals are more likely than older ones to be affected with pulmonary viral infection. Pleural effusion is common in cats. Obesity complicates or predisposes animals to respiratory diseases. When the patient has both cough and significant dyspnea, the initial diagnostic evaluation centers on the cause of respiratory distress (see below). The minimum data base for cough varies depending on the duration of coughing, the presence of systemic signs, and findings on physical examination. Obvious contagious diseases (like infectious tracheobronchitis) or mechanical problems (like tracheal collapse) seldom require major work-ups for accurate diagnosis. In other cases, a more extensive work-up is indicated, including thoracic roentgenograms, CBC, microfilaria examination, fecal flotation and sedimentation, culture and cytology of sputum, and serum chemistries.

2. Medical History

A. The animal's environment is important because some conditions, such as those associated with systemic mycoses, dirofilariasis, and foxtail awns, are endemic to geographic regions. In some areas, environmental pollutants may be important. Outside and working dogs may be exposed to mosquitoes, foreign bodies, and thoracic trauma.

B. Previous illness, therapy, or the animal's response to therapy may modify the diagnosis or treatment plan.

C. Exposure to other animals or disease vectors is an important consideration for infectious pulmonary disease. For instance, cats that hunt may acquire lungworms. Infectious tracheobronchitis is common in kenneled dogs.

D. The vaccination history and record of prophylaxis (e.g., heartworm preventative) should be obtained.

E. A complete description of the cough and associated breathing patterns should be noted.

1) Ascertain the onset and duration, progression, precipitating events, and type of cough; any associated nasal discharges or wheezing; the animal's ability to sleep at night; the effect of exercise and excitement; the relationship of the cough to eating, if any; and the character of any sputum.

2) Various etiologies may produce similar coughs. The cough associated with mechanical obstruction is often noted only with exercise or excitement. The animal is otherwise well and rests quietly, although obstructive noises or snoring may be heard. These are typical of soft-palate, laryngeal, or tracheal collapse or obstruction. The coughs are very loud (honking) and paroxysmal.

3) The cough associated with chronic bronchitis or pneumonia is also worsened by exercise or excitement, and may also be prominent in the morning when the animal attempts to expectorate accumulated mucus and exudate. Often, the pneumonic patient is febrile. Animals with bronchial collapse or compression, or with small airway disease, may also wheeze. The owner frequently will describe the cough as "dry," but notes that the animal retches and "tries to vomit" after a paroxysm of coughing. Because the animal swallows expectorated material, the character of the sputum may not be known. Dogs with aspiration pneumonia have a history of emesis or regurgitation, whereas in cats, a history of treatment with mineral oil may be elicited.

4) Coughs associated with other diseases of the pulmonary parenchyma (e.g., heartworm disease or tumor) frequently are dry and nonproductive. Exercise intolerance and weight loss may also be noted.

5) The cardiac cough is dry or moist, worsened by exercise, and associated with respiratory distress, nocturnal pacing, and orthopnea. It is often productive as edema accumulates, and may be associated with wheezing or "bubbling" noises.

6) Hemoptysis (coughing up of blood), which must be distinguished from hematemesis (inquire about abdominal press movements), is unusual in animals. Hemoptysis is usually associated with pulmonary embolus (heartworm), neoplasia, trauma, foreign body, granuloma, fulminant congestive heart failure, or coagulopathy, although there are other possible causes, such as infection.[6]

7) Coughing after eating or drinking may be caused by upper airway obstruction, laryngeal or pharyngeal paralysis; or esophageal disease with secondary aspiration.

F. If tachypnea or respiratory distress constitutes the principal complaint, the circumstances in which it occurs should be determined (e.g., after exercise, at all times, etc.). It should be noted that some dogs do not cough even under appropriate circumstances for a cough reflex (e.g., with aspiration pneumonia or early pulmonary edema). They may, however, demonstrate difficult breathing. Brachycephalic breed dogs have dyspnea as a result of their breeding.

G. The history should also elicit information about the general health of the animal because some causes of cough involve systemic disease and significant loss of body condition. Examples are systemic mycotic infections, heart disease, and pulmonary neoplasia.

3. A general physical examination is important because some causes of cough and dyspnea involve multisystemic disorders. The clinician should pay particular attention to the cardiopulmonary system, but should not ignore other systems.

A. Complete a careful cardiovascular examination. Listen for murmurs, gallops, and arrhythmias. Absence of auscultatory abnormalities in small breed dogs virtually rules out left-sided heart failure. In cats and in canine breeds prone to cardiomyopathy, murmurs may not be present, and apical gallop rhythms may be the only signal of heart failure.

B. Examine the mucous membranes, ocular fundus, lymph nodes, skin, mammary glands, abdomen, and esophagus (if palpable) because multisystemic or secondary pulmonary diseases are important considerations in chronic cough or dyspnea. Assess the swallowing and gag reflexes as dysphagia may lead to aspiration.

C. Examine the respiratory system with care.

1) Evaluation of the oral cavity, larynx, and upper tracheobronchial tree may require sedation or anesthesia, particularly if the clinician wishes to visualize the airways with an endoscope or bronchoscope.[7,65,94] Use light planes of anesthesia to evaluate the motor function of the larynx and pharynx. The arytenoids should move when stimulated manually.

2) Gain upper airway visualization, including the nares and pharynx, by direct visualization or endoscopy.

3) Palpate the trachea for deviation, masses, and collapse.

4) Evaluate the lower respiratory tract by means of the history, auscultation[10,17,60] and ancillary tests, such as thoracic roentgenography. Pulmonary crackles strongly suggest small airway diseases, such as bronchitis, pulmonary fibrosis, or pulmonary edema. Referred obstructive sounds often may be localized to specific areas in the upper respiratory tract.

5) Use percussion to detect the dull areas over pleural effusion, mass lesions, or atelectasis, and the hyperresonance of pneumothorax.

6) Observe ventilatory patterns.

a) Inspiratory dyspnea usually indicates upper airway obstruction, restrictive disease, lung fibrosis, or pleural effusion.

b) Expiratory dyspnea is common in lower airway disorders.

c) Both inspiratory and expiratory dyspnea are typical of heart failure (edema), masses or obstruction at the carina, and chronic bronchitis.

7) Inability to compress the feline cranial thorax or identification of Horner's syndrome in a dyspneic patient suggests a mediastinal mass.

4. Thoracic roentgenograms are essential in all cases of chronic cough.[5,12,41,62,88,89]

A. Evaluation of the cardiac silhouette, great vessels, pulmonary circulation, and veins is particularly important if heart failure, heartworm disease, or pulmonary embolism are suspected. Pulmonary edema and compression of the left mainstem bronchus by an enlarged left atrium are two common cardiac mechanisms for chronic cough (see section on cardiomegaly that follows). However, over-interpretation of cardiac changes frequently misleads the clinician to an erroneous diagnosis of heart failure. Most dogs with chronic respiratory disease have apparent moderate cardiomegaly on radiographic examination (cor pulmonale) but do *not* have heart failure.

B. Good quality dorsoventral and lateral roentgenograms are needed to evaluate the lungs, mediastinum, lymph nodes, and pleural space. If obstructive pulmonary signs are present, obtain both inspiratory and expiratory lateral films because intrathoracic collapse of the trachea and bronchi typically occurs during expiration, and inspiratory films are essential to study the lungs. Fluoroscopy may be needed to document dynamic airway collapse. Left and right lateral views may be needed to delineate some thoracic mass lesions.

C. If pleural effusion is detected in a coughing patient, suspect concomitant bronchopulmonary disease (see section on Pleural Effusion that follows).

D. Increased pulmonary densities are noted and defined by:

1) Intrapleural or intrapulmonary location

2) Distribution (e.g., cranioventral, multifocal, right lobar, perihilar, disseminated)

3) Pattern of density (i.e., alveolar, interstitial linear or nodular, peribronchial, or mixed)

4) Presence or absence of airway collapse or obstruction

5) Presence or absence of mediastinal widening or density changes (see section on increased pulmonary densities that follows)

6) Evidence for lymphadenopathy (e.g., fungal diseases, lymphoma, granulomatous disease)

5. CBC abnormalities may suggest infection, inflammation, or necrosis. Eosinophilia in the absence of intestinal or ectoparasitism suggests the possibility of heartworm disease, lungworms, allergic bronchitis, lymphoma, granulomatous disease, or pulmonary infiltrates with eosinophils ("allergic" pneumonitis).

6. Obtain a blood microfilaria test in areas where heartworm is endemic. Perform heartworm tests antigen (enzyme-linked immunosorbent assay [ELISA]) in patients suspected of having occult (microfilaria-negative heartworm disease.

7. Use direct fecal smears and special sedimentation methods, along with fecal flotation, to screen for lungworms, when appropriate.

8. Obtain serum chemistries to evaluate other body systems.

9. Based on analysis of the data base just outlined, determine a specific diagnosis or complete additional tests. Valuable ancillary studies are listed below.

A. Serum tests, including titers for aspergillosis, systemic fungi, FIP, and antinuclear antibody, are indicated in select cases. FeLV and FIV ELISA tests, lupus erythematosus (LE) cell preparation, and other immunologic studies may be useful.

B. If clinical signs and prior laboratory test results inadequately explain chronic cough or abnormal pulmonary densities, obtain a transtracheal aspiration sample.[30,32,41,52,53] This technique is imperative for the diagnosis of unexplained alveolar and bronchointerstitial disease, and for qualifying the causes of bronchitis and pneumonia. Culture and evaluate the aspirate for cytologic abnormalities. Typical patterns of inflammation include

1) Mucopurulent (typical of chronic bronchitis)

2) Suppurative (typical of bacterial bronchitis or bronchopneumonia)

3) "Allergic" (typical of allergic, parasitic, and some fungal and lymphoreticular pulmonary diseases)

4) Neoplastic (tumor cells obtained)

5) Mixture of inflammatory cells (e.g., allergic inflammation with secondary infection)

C. If pleural effusion is present, perform thoracentesis (see section on pleural effusion that follows).[11]

D. Fluoroscopy is useful in demonstrating dynamic collapse of a major airway when it cannot be shown by routine x-ray films.

E. Direct visualization of the upper airways, trachea, and bronchi is indicated when intraluminal masses, foreign body, *Filaroides oseri* nodules, or other causes of unexplained airway obstruction are suspected.[65] Rigid or fiberoptic endoscopes with suitable brushes and biopsy instruments are used. Bronchoalveolar lavage[17] using a wedged bronchoscope is performed to document alveolitis as a cause of pulmonary fibrosis. Differential cell counts of the aspirate can document alveolar disease.

F. Cytologic evaluation of conjunctival membranes (for distemper inclusions), skin ulcers (for systemic fungi), and enlarged lymph nodes (for infection or neoplasia) can be useful.

G. Cytologic examination of the lung by percutaneous needle aspiration or by lung biopsy via a minithoracotomy or bronchoscope is indicated in disseminated pulmonary disease (especially interstitial disorders) that is unexplained by previous noninvasive test results. Where appropriate, explore singular localized lung lesions surgically with the intent of removing and performing biopsy on the affected tissue.

H. Esophagoscopy is useful in diagnosing an esophagotracheal fistula.

I. An electrocardiogram (ECG) or echocardiogram[22,66,93] may suggest cor pulmonale or heart disease.

J. Perform other tests, including bronchography, pulmonary arteriography, radioisotope pulmonary scanning, and pulmonary function tests, only after consultation with appropriate specialists.

Treatment[4,17,23,24,33,38,39,46,47,49,54,58,67,69,72,73,76,78,90,91,94,96]

1. There are numerous potential causes of cough. It is necessary to identify a specific etiology to provide optimal therapy.

2. Treat acute coughs of infectious origin

with rest, inhalation of humidified air, antibiotics (in bacterial infections), and cough suppressants (in viral tracheobronchitis associated with nonproductive coughing). In bacterial bronchopneumonia, initiate specific antimicrobial therapy based on culture results.[51] Maintenance of hydration is essential, and administration of expectorants and bronchodilators may be useful in bronchitis and pneumonia. Culture cases of lingering acute tracheobronchitis by transtracheal aspiration and administer systemic doses of gentocin via a cold water nebulizer and face mask. This is particularly beneficial for *Bordetella bronchiseptica* infection.

3. Place obese patients with obstructive airway disorders on restricted calorie diets. Redundant soft palate can be resected and collapsing trachea can be treated surgically with a prosthesis.[38] Many cases of intrathoracic tracheal collapse have concomitant bronchitis, and the collapse responds partially to bronchodilators, prednisone, and cough suppressants.[17] Evaluate animals with chronic bronchitis by tracheal wash or bronchoscopy, and administer appropriate antibiotics, bronchodilators, and intermittent corticosteroids (if indicated by cytologic evaluation). Some patients benefit from expectorants and nebulization of humidified air. Minimizing environmental stresses, reducing exercise, and relieving exogenous cervical pressure (collars) facilitate successful medical therapy. Treat dogs with a compressed left mainstem bronchus for congestive heart failure, if it is present. The authors have used vasodilator and diuretic therapy in these patients to reduce mitral regurgitation and left atrial size, with associated diminution of the cough.

4. Treat other disorders based on elucidation of the primary cause.

Respiratory Distress

1. Respiratory distress, often called dyspnea or difficult breathing, can occur during inspiration or expiration. Dyspnea usually results from significant pulmonary or cardiovascular disease, and dictates a thorough yet gentle examination of the affected animal.

2. The causes of respiratory distress and/or tachypnea can be classified simply.

   A. Major airway obstruction or compression

   B. Small airway obstruction or narrowing

   C. Pulmonary edema or parenchymal disease

   D. Pleural space disease or intrapleural mass lesion

   E. Restrictive interstitial lung or thoracic disease

   F. Pulmonary vascular disease

   G. Miscellaneous causes of dyspnea or tachypnea (e.g., right-to-left cardiac shunt)

A more complete list of causes is provided in the previous section on cough.

Clinical Diagnostic Approach[7,10,11,47,54,60,62,65,67,72,88,94]

1. Animals with respiratory distress must be handled with care because struggling can result in respiratory arrest.

2. The initial clinical examination is outlined in Table 9-2. A systematic approach is mandatory to locate the anatomic source of difficult breathing so that effective treatment may be initiated. For example, obvious laryngeal stridor may indicate laryngeal paralysis that can be managed temporarily by tracheal intubation or tracheostomy. Similarly, the clinical identification of pleural effusion or pneumothorax indicates the need for thoracocentesis. Table 9-2 lists a scheme for ruling out the most common causes of dyspnea.

3. Frequently, patients must be stabilized before roentgenograms or other tests are performed. Initial management steps include[72]

   A. Thoracocentesis if pleural effusion or pneumothorax is suspected

   B. Sedation if restraint is difficult

   C. Oxygen and cage rest

   D. Reduction of stress and handling

   E. Tracheal intubation or tracheostomy[47] if life-threatening dyspnea is laryngeal or pharyngeal in origin

   F. Parenteral bronchodilators[76] (aminophylline) if bronchitis, asthma, tracheal collapse, or pulmonary edema is the tentative diagnosis

Table 9-2.   **Evaluation of the dyspneic patient**

Clinical Parameter	Comments
Patient medical history/ observation of patient	May give clue to etiology
Psychic component	Determine level of anxiety, ability to handle stress
Degree of dyspnea	Necessity for intermediate therapy, ability to obtain diagnostic information
Pattern of ventilation	Helps demonstrate origin of dyspnea
Chest excursion	Rule out rib fracture, flail chest, tension pneumothorax
Inspiratory dyspnea	Rule out effusion, pneumothorax, pulmonary edema, upper airway obstruction, lung fibrosis or interstitial infiltration
Expiratory dyspnea	Rule out lower airway diseases, pulmonary edema
Mucous membranes Cyanosis	Rule out airway obstruction, diffusion barrier (edema), ventilation/perfusion mismatch, shunt
Pallor	Rule out anemia, decreased cardiac output, shock
Brownish	Rule out methemoglobinemia
Physical examination	
Body temperature	Rule out infection, sepsis, heat stroke, ↑ work of breathing
Oral examination (sedation may be needed)	Rule out pharyngeal-laryngeal obstruction (dyspnea relieved by tracheal intubation)
Cardiac auscultation	Rule out murmurs, gallops, arrhythmias, muffled sounds (may be obscured by respiratory noises)
Pulmonary auscultation/percussion	Evaluate level of abnormality
Increased sounds (obstructive noises, crackles, and rhonchi)	Rule out obstruction of large airways, pulmonary infection, bronchitis, asthma, pulmonary edema, interstitial disease
Decreased sounds	Rule out pleural effusion, pneumothorax, mass lesions
Other findings	Rule out other signs of heart failure and other abnormalities that accompany disorders causing acute dyspnea
Thoracic roentgenograms	
Cardiac chambers and great vessels	Rule out heart disease (congenital and acquired)
Pulmonary vasculature and parenchyma	Rule out extracardiac signs of heart failure and other primary or secondary pulmonary disorders
Pleural space	Rule out pleural effusion, pneumothorax, diaphragmatic hernia

* From Bonagura JD: Pulmonary edema. In Kirk RW (ed): Current Veterinary Therapy III. Philadelphia, WB Saunders, 1980

G. Parenteral furosemide and venodilator therapy, if pulmonary edema is suspected[96]

H. Short-acting glucocorticoids (or epinephrine) if feline asthma is likely[66,69]

I. Corticosteroids if edematous soft palate is the cause of the dyspnea

4. Following initial patient stabilization, appropriate diagnostic tests are selected based on the patient's signalment, history, and physical examination. These tests are identical to those previously described in the section on cough.

5. Definitive therapy is always dependent on establishment of an anatomic and etiologic diagnosis.

Syncope

1. *Syncope* is a short period of unconsciousness related to disturbances in cerebral function.

2. Syncope usually results from diminished cerebral blood flow secondary to reduced cardiac output or a cerebrovascular accident (CVA).

3. Syncope also occurs secondary to disruptions in cerebral function caused by hypoglycemia or hypoxemia.

4. In veterinary medicine, syncope is often related to disorders of

A. Cardiovascular function

B. Pulmonary function or oxygen-carrying capacity (anemia)

C. Metabolism

5. Primary neurologic disorders, such as epilepsy, narcolepsy, or cataplexy, must be distinguished from true syncope (see Chapter 17).

Etiology

1. Cardiovascular causes of syncope are most important in veterinary medicine.

A. Cardiac rhythm disturbances (arrhythmias) can result in sudden reductions in cardiac output. Rhythm disturbances are classified as abnormalities of impulse formation or impulse conduction.

1) Abnormalities of impulse conduction include atrioventricular (AV) blocks and atrial standstill secondary to hyperkalemia or muscular disease. Second- and third-degree AV blocks cause ventricular bradycardia and Adams-Stokes syncope.

2) Abnormalities of impulse formation include sick sinus syndrome, sinoatrial arrest, and ectopia. Disorders of sinus impulse formation are most common in miniature schnauzers, dachshunds, cocker spaniels, and brachycephalic breed dogs. Supraventricular and ventricular tachyarrhythmias, such as paroxysmal atrial or ventricular tachycardia, occur secondary to many diseases and can lead to syncope. Persistent atrial standstill (silent atrial) is recognized in veterinary practice. Atrial fibrillation occasionally causes syncope. For specific electrocardiographic features of these disorders, see the section on cardiac arrhythmias that follows.

B. Organic heart disease causes syncope from decreased cardiac output, activation of vasodepressor reflexes, or hypoxemia secondary to cardiac shunt, pulmonary edema, or pleural effusion. Syncope may occur only after excitement, exercise, or violent coughing. Causes include

1) Congenital heart diseases, such as subvalvular aortic stenosis, pulmonary stenosis, and tetralogy of Fallot

2) Acquired heart diseases, such as heartworm disease, cardiomyopathy, pericardial effusion, and chronic valvular disease

3) Intra-atrial tumors that obstruct atrioventricular blood flow

C. Syncope associated with cerebrovascular disease is rare, although strokes have been known to occur with bleeding disorders, hyperproteinemia, hypertension, and severe atherosclerotic disease caused by hypothyroidism.

D. Acute hemorrhage results in hypotension and may lead to syncope.

E. Syncope associated with vasovagal or vasodepressor responses are poorly defined in animals, but may be associated with obstructive pulmonary disease (in brachycephalic breeds), abnormal baroreceptor function, or CNS lesions.

2. Pulmonary causes of syncope usually are related to obstructive disease or coughing. Obstructive disorders, including tracheal collapse and chronic bronchitis, lead to hypoxemia. Violent coughing can cause syncope, possibly from the untoward effects of high intrapleural pressure on venous return, cerebrospinal fluid (CSF) pressure, and arterial blood flow.

3. Other causes of syncope include anemia and metabolic disorders in which hypoglycemia develops. Recurrent hypoglycemia occurs in conjunction with inadequate nutrition (in working dogs), glycogen storage diseases (in puppies), liver disease and hepatic tumors, insulin overdose, and functional beta-cell tumors or B-cell hyperplasia of the pancreas. CNS hypoxia that is caused by pronounced anemia may lead to collapse or syncope.

4. Systemic disorders resulting in profound

weakness are sometimes confused with syncopal episodes. Hypoadrenocorticism, hypokalemia, bleeding abdominal hemangiosarcoma, neuromuscular diseases, and other systemic illnesses often cause hypotension and collapse, but are less likely to be associated with the loss of consciousness or the abruptness of the true syncopal attack.

5. Some drugs induce secondary orthostatic hypotension and may cause fainting. This should always be considered if the patient is receiving medication. Diuretics, alpha-adrenergic blockers (like promazine tranquilizers), and vasodilator drugs used in the management of heart failure are examples of potentially hypotensive agents.

Clinical Diagnostic Approach

1. The signalment and history are important. Certain breeds have genetic predispositions to particular cardiovascular or pulmonary diseases. For example, cardiac rhythm disturbances, like ventricular tachycardia, are common in boxer dog cardiomyopathy. Obstructive airway disease occurs frequently in brachycephalic breeds. Ascertain the circumstances associated with syncope (e.g., whether the episode is related to coughing or exertion). Obtain a medication history.

2. Seizure activity is usually ruled out by the history and neurologic work-up.

A. Syncope is distinguished from seizures, hepatic encephalopathy, and narcolepsy by obtaining a careful description of the event, completing a neurologic examination, and obtaining appropriate ancillary information (e.g., blood ammonia levels). Typical syncope is associated with vigorous activity, is short-lived (seconds), usually does not cause tonic–clonic convulsions or facial fits, and is not associated with an aura. Postictal behavior, which is typical of epilepsy, does not occur with syncope unless there is secondary ischemic injury to the CNS. It is common, however, to observe opisthotonos, crying, transient foreleg rigidity, and urination during a syncopal episode.

3. Particular attention should be directed to the physical examination. The clinician should search for objective signs of cardio-vascular disease, particularly murmurs, gallop rhythms, arrhythmias, and signs of congestive heart failure. Examine the respiratory system for obstruction, and the mucous membranes for cyanosis or pallor. Record the character and quality of the arterial pulse. Undertake a thorough neurologic examination to discern neurologic deficits. Rule out volume depletion leading to hypotension.

4. Obtain suitable laboratory and special studies, including:

A. An ECG—a 24-hour, tape-recorded ECG (Holter monitor)—may be required (see section on cardiac arrhythmias that follows).[93]

B. Thoracic roentgenogram or fluoroscopic study to evaluate pulmonary structure and dynamics

C. Echocardiogram to rule out cardiomyopathy, pericardial effusion, or cardiac tumor

D. Fasting blood glucose

E. PCV and total serum protein values

F. Other tests that may be necessary to diagnose or rule out etiologies described earlier include blood microfilaria examination, arterial blood gas tensions, blood ammonia, serum electrolytes, cholesterol, serum triiodothyronine (T_3) and thyroxine (T_4) determinations, spinal fluid analysis, and electroencephalogram.

Treatment

1. Specific and effective treatment is aimed at correction of the underlying etiology.

2. For cardiovascular syncope, antiarrhythmic drugs, a cardiac pacemaker, or agents useful in the management of heart failure may be indicated.[16,18,71,85–87,93,97] Readjust dosages of potentially hypotensive drugs. Manage hypotension or acute hemorrhage with intravenous infusions of balanced electrolyte solution or whole blood.

3. Treat syncope secondary to pulmonary disorders with airway maintenance; oxygen; bronchodilators, such as aminophylline or terbutaline hydrochloride; and mild sedation with diazepam, phenothiazine tranquilizers, or barbiturates. Cough suppressants (hydrocodone) may be needed for cough syncope. Specific medical or surgical therapy should be directed at the underlying etiology.

Miscellaneous Historical Disorders

Tiring, Exertional Weakness, and Fatigue

Tiring, exertional weakness, and fatigue are abnormalities common to cardiopulmonary disorders and abnormalities of other body systems. The cardiopulmonary/differential diagnosis of this problem is discussed elsewhere in this chapter.

Regurgitation

Regurgitation of solid food is a sign of esophageal disease, and is discussed in Chapter 10. Vascular ring anomalies are important considerations in the differential diagnosis of regurgitation in the young animal.

Hemoglobinuria

Pigment changes in the urine are covered in Chapter 23. Hemoglobinuria secondary to DIC and RBC trauma is a feature of the postcaval syndrome of canine heartworm disease.

Stunted Growth, Weight Loss, and Cachexia

Stunted growth, weight loss, and cachexia are nonspecific signs of disease that are frequently noted in animals with congenital heart disease, dirofilariasis, systemic mycosis, pulmonary neoplasia, and granulomatous diseases and chronic heart failure caused by valvular and myocardial disease.

Physical Problems

Abnormal Arterial Pulse

The normal femoral pulse occurs between the first and second heart sounds. It is quick to rise, decays gradually, and is easily palpated in most animals. It is caused by the pulse pressure and characteristics of blood flow in the cardiovascular system. Abnormalities of the arterial pulse include absent pulse, pulse deficit, irregular amplitude pulse, hypokinetic pulse, and hyperkinetic pulse (Fig. 9-1).

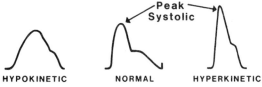

Figure 9-1. *Arterial pressure pulse waves. The configurations of typical arterial pulse waves are shown. Factors, such as stroke volume, rate of rise of arterial systolic pressure, pulse pressure, peak systolic arterial pressure, and aortic wall compliance, all influence the arterial pulse wave form. Other factors (such as heart rate, characteristics of the arterial system, state of hydration, and body configuration) also affect the subjective analysis of the arterial pressure pulse.*

Absent Pulses

1. Absent pulses typically indicate a terminal aortic thrombus associated with feline cardiomyopathy, a hypercoagulable state (e.g., renal amyloidosis with hypoproteinemia), or bacterial endocarditis. Arterial obstruction can be caused by a tumor, or rarely, by an intra-arterial foreign body (bullet), fungal, or tumor embolus.

2. Obesity may render the femoral pulses imperceptible in the cat.

3. The pulse is absent during *severe* hypotension or cardiac arrest.

Pulse Deficit and Irregular Amplitude Pulse

1. A pulse deficit is present when there are more first heart sounds than there are arterial pulses.

2. A pulse deficit usually indicates irregular ventricular filling and hypodynamic contractions caused by cardiac arrhythmia. Typical causes of pulse deficits are atrial fibrillation, premature beats, and ventricular tachycardia.

3. Irregular amplitude pulses occur when ventricular stroke volume changes on a beat-to-beat basis. This irregularity is usually associated with cardiac arrhythmias, although it can be present in normal animals with sinus arrhythmia and in animals with dyspnea and respiratory distress.

4. Variable intensity pulses are also described in pericardial disease (pulsus paradoxus) and ventricular failure or severe plasma volume depletion (pulsus alternans). Pulsus paradoxus refers to variations in pulse intensity related to phases of ventilation. Pulsus alternans is an alternating intensity pulse that occurs with severe heart failure, marked volume depletion, general anesthesia, or ventricular bigeminy.

5. Unexplained pulse deficits or irregularities should be documented and further characterized by an ECG.

Hypokinetic Arterial Pulse

1. A hypokinetic or weak arterial pulse is usually caused by a reduced stroke volume, with compensatory increases in peripheral resistance.

2. A hypokinetic arterial pulse is present in low-output heart failure from any cause (e.g., dilated cardiomyopathy).

3. Peripheral vasoconstriction secondary to hypovolemia and small stroke volume (e.g., in Addison's disease or shock) causes weak pulses.

4. The typical arterial pulse of aortic stenosis is weak and slow to rise (pulsus parvus et tardus).

5. Tachyarrhythmias (e.g., ventricular tachycardia) may cause weak pulses.

Hyperkinetic Arterial Pulse

1. The bounding or hyperkinetic arterial pulse occurs as a result of increases in stroke volume or cardiac output. Lowered peripheral resistance and shunts lead to high-output states (see Fig. 9-1). Abnormal pathways for blood flow permit rapid run-off of blood and lead to a wide pulse pressure and hyperkinetic pulse.

2. The bounding pulse is normal in some animals. Anxiety and sympathetic discharge predipose animals to this finding.

3. Abnormalities causing large left ventricular stroke volumes with opportunity for abnormal blood run-off include patent ductus arteriosus (PDA) and aortic insufficiency.

4. Bradycardia, an example being complete AV block, is associated with large stroke volumes, a long diastolic period for run-off, and a resultant bounding pulse.

5. Hyperkinetic pulses related to reduced peripheral resistance and high cardiac output are present in anemia, thyrotoxicosis, exercise, and fever.

6. Hypertension can be associated with hyperkinetic pulses, but this is quite variable.

Abnormal Venous Distention and Venous Pulse

Venous Distention

1. In the normal standing animal, jugular pulsations are frequently noted at the thoracic inlet. These right-sided dynamics are related sequentially to atrial filling and ventricular filling (atrial emptying). If the head is elevated, with the mandible held parallel to the floor, it is unusual to note jugular pulsations that extend more than one third of the distance up the neck. In the normal animal, the jugular vein does not remain distended.

2. Persistent distention of the jugular vein is related to abnormalities of the heart, pericardium, cranial mediastinum, or central circulatory blood volume.

3. Persistent distention of the jugular vein should be investigated by thoracic roentgenography and cardiac ultrasonography. Causes of elevated jugular venous pressure include right-sided heart failure, pericardial disease, a mediastinal mass that obstructs the cranial vena cava, and hypervolemia.

Abnormal Jugular Venous Pulse

1. The jugular pulse must be distinguished from transmission of the carotid pulse. If the pulse persists after light digital pressure is applied to the jugular vein at the thoracic inlet, the pulse origin is the carotid artery. The jugular pulse is occasionally prominent in normal puppies and in animals with anemia. Pathologic jugular pulsations caused by right heart failure may be accentuated by gentle abdominal compression (hepatojugular reflex).

2. Pathologic jugular pulses are related to

A. Resistance to right ventricular filling secondary to pulmonary stenosis, pulmonary hypertension, heartworm disease, cardiomyopathy, or chronic left heart failure. These are giant A waves.

B. Simultaneous contraction of the atria and ventricles (cannon A waves) caused by atrioventricular dissociation (AV block, ventricular tachycardia) or extrasystoles

C. Tricuspid insufficiency (giant C-V waves)

D. Elevated venous pressure with accentuation of normal venous pressure changes, which occurs in right ventricular failure, pericardial disease, and hypervolemia

Systemic Hypertension

1. Elevation of arterial blood pressure is being recognized with increasing frequency in small animal practice. Values exceeding 180 mmHg (systolic) and 100 mmHg (diastolic) are probably abnormal in the resting, non-tachycardiac pet. Since blood pressure is difficult to evaluate without direct-needle puncture of the femoral artery or the use of Doppler or oscillometric equipment, many cases of hypertension go undetected.

2. The most important cause of hypertension is chronic renal disease, which is covered in more depth in Chapter 12.

3. In addition to chronic glomerular and tubulointerstitial renal diseases, systemic hypertension is associated with Cushing's disease, hyperaldosteronism, pheochromcytoma, hyperthyroidism and administration of vasoconstricting drugs, such as those used for treatment of some forms of urinary incontinence.

4. Target organs of systemic hypertension include the kidneys (increased vascular injury), eyes (retinal detachments and hemorrhage), brain (vascular accident), and heart (left ventricular hypertrophy).

5. Management of systemic hypertension requires further definition in animals; however, a typical treatment regimen includes a sodium-restricted diet and administration of a diuretic (either furosemide or hydrochloro-

thiazide) and a vasodilator. Captopril or enalapril are most often used in cats, whereas prazosin has been most effective (in the authors' experience) in the dog. Other antihypertensive medications, including beta-blockers, labetalol, and hydralazine merit consideration in refractory cases.

Auscultable Cardiac Arrhythmia[16,18,35,85–87,93,97]

Normal Cardiac Rhythms

1. Normal cardiac rhythms in dogs and cats are sinus rhythm and sinus arrhythmia (irregular sinus rhythm). Normal heart rates vary widely according to age, breed, body weight, level of anxiety, endocrine status, and body temperature. Sinus rhythms usually result in a normal electrical activation sequence and produce related first and second heart sound. Sinus tachycardia is expected in neonates and cats, and may arise from excitement, exercise, fever, pain, hyperthyroidism, and anemia.

2. Sinus arrhythmia causes cyclic, recurrent changes in heart rate, intensity of heart sounds, and arterial pulse. It is normal in the dog, but is generally not auscultated in the normal cat.

3. The following auscultatory findings suggest a cardiac rhythm disturbance: premature sounds, absence of expected sounds, marked variation in sound intensity, splitting of heart sounds, and abnormal or variable heart rate.

Abnormal Cardiac Rhythms

1. Abnormal sinus rhythms are suggested by changes in the rate of the first and second heart sounds. Sinus bradycardia causes a slow, regular S_1-S_2 rhythm, whereas sinus tachycardia is characterized by a rapid, regular S_1-S_2 cadence. Sinus block and sinus arrest are characterized by pauses devoid of heart sounds. In classical sick sinus syndrome, periods of sinus bradycardia and sinus arrest may alternate with sinus or atrial tachycardia.

2. Premature beats are easily detected by

the presence of early first and soft second heart sounds. A pause generally follows the premature beat. It may be difficult to differentiate between premature atrial, junctional, and ventricular beats by auscultation, but premature ventricular beats cause splitting of the heart sounds owing to asynchronous ventricular activation.

3. Atrial fibrillation is characterized by a rapid, irregular heart rate with variable-intensity heart sounds and arterial pulse deficit. Often, the second sound is difficult to hear.

4. Paroxysmal supraventricular or ventricular tachycardia is characterized by a sudden burst of rapid heart rate that ends abruptly. In many cases of ventricular tachycardia, the heart sounds are split and of variable intensity, making this rhythm sound somewhat similar to that of atrial fibrillation. In classic ventricular tachycardia, the ectopic rhythm is fairly regular and produces occasional cannon A waves in the jugular pulse. In some patients, supraventricular tachycardia may be converted to sinus rhythm by ocular or carotid sinus massage. Sinus tachycardia does not slow permanently, but may slow transiently.

5. AV blocks (2° and 3°) usually produce distinct pauses or bradycardia. Second-degree AV block causes irregularity of the S_1-S_1 interval with a relatively normal or slow rate. There is no pulse deficit. It is difficult to distinguish 2° AV block from marked sinus arrhythmia or sinoatrial block. The ventricular escape rhythm of complete (3°) AV block produces a slow (30 to 50 beats/min) bounding pulse and S_1-S_1 rhythm. An escape rate of 80 to 100 beats/min is typically noted in affected cats. Hyperkinetic arterial pulses are present (which distinguish this from hyperkalemia secondary to Addison's disease in which the pulse is very thready) and cannon A waves. Independent soft atrial (S_4) sounds may be heard. Bradycardia from AV block must be distinguished from sinus bradycardias caused by hyperkalemia, brain stem lesions, hypothermia, elevated CSF pressure (Cushing's reflex), sinus node disease, and drugs (digitalis, narcotics, acetylpromazine).

6. The diagnostic approach to auscultable cardiac rhythm disturbances includes the following steps (see section on cardiac arrhythmias for greater detail):

A. Obtain an up-to-date drug history.

B. Obtain a complete resting and a post-exercise rhythm strip and ECG.

C. Evaluate serum biochemistries, particularly electrolytes (Na, K, Cl, Ca) and serum T_4.

D. Search for causes of autonomic imbalance (e.g., neurologic deficits, obstructive pulmonary diseases).

E. Complete a cardiovascular evaluation, including physical and roentgenographic examination, blood pressure, and echocardiogram, if indicated.

7. Splitting of the heart sounds is present normally in some animals, but is abnormal when associated with ventricular conduction disturbances (bundle branch block) and dirofilariasis. Most "split" sounds are actually normal sounds coupled to systolic clicks (see the section on gallop rhythm that follows).

Cardiac Murmurs and Precordial Thrills

Definitions

1. A *cardiac murmur* is a prolonged vibration heard during a normally silent period of the cardiac cycle.[44] Cardiac murmurs are valuable physical findings and may lead the clinician to an anatomic cardiac diagnosis. Murmurs are described by their timing (systolic, diastolic, continuous), intensity (grades I to VI), point of maximal intensity (PMI), and configuration and quality (ejection or crescendo-decrescendo; regurgitant or plateau; blowing or decrescendo; "machinery"). Descriptive terms, such as "musical" and "harsh," are also used.

2. A *precordial thrill* is a palpable vibration that accompanies some murmurs. Often, the precordial thrill is palpated at the PMI and origin of the murmur. The palm is used to identify a thrill and the fingertips are used to localize the vibration source.

3. The clinician should locate the auscultatory cardiac valve area by examining the standing animal and carefully palpating for the left and right apical impulses. In general, proceeding cranially from the left apex, the valve sounds encountered are mitral, aortic, and pulmonic. The tricuspid valve area is located at the right hemithorax, slightly cranial to the mitral area (Fig. 9-2).

Types of Murmurs

1. Functional murmurs are heard frequently in small animals. They may be subdivided into two classes:
    A. Physiologic murmurs, or those related to altered physiologic state, including:
        1) Decreased blood viscosity (anemia and hypoproteinemia)
        2) Large stroke volume (athletic heart and bradycardia)
        3) Hyperkinetic circulation (fever, thyrotoxicosis, high sympathetic tone)
    B. Innocent murmurs, or those that cannot be attributed to heart disease or otherwise explained
2. Organic murmurs are caused by recognizable lesions of the heart and are important physical signs of heart disease.
    A. Organic murmurs are caused by both congenital and acquired heart diseases.
    B. Many organic murmurs sound alike, and their etiology must be distinguished by other physical or laboratory clues.
3. Important organic murmurs and their causes in animals include:
    A. Continuous murmurs secondary to PDA
    B. Systolic murmurs
        1) Ejection murmurs
            a) Pulmonary stenosis (PS)—subvalvular or valvular congenital lesion; relative PS caused by excessive right ventricular flow secondary to an atrial septal defect (ASD) or ventricular septal defect (VSD); pulmonary endocarditis (rare)
            b) Aortic stenosis—subaortic (most common), valvular, or supravalvular congenital lesion; dynamic muscular subvalvular stenosis caused by hypertrophic cardiomyopathy; aortic valvular endocarditis
        2) Plateau or regurgitant murmurs
            a) VSD
            b) Mitral valve insufficiency (MVI)

(or regurgitation)—congenital mitral dysplasia; degenerative thickening of the mitral valve (endocardiosis); mitral valvular endocarditis[22]; mitral insufficiency secondary to cardiomyopathies, hyperthyroid or hypertensive heart disease, or viral myocarditis; ruptured chorda tendineae, gross left ventricular (LV) dilation (e.g., from PDA)
            c) Tricuspid valve insufficiency (TVI)—etiologies similar to those of mitral insufficiency; also caused by heartworm disease, pulmonary stenosis, and pulmonary hypertension
    C. Diastolic murmurs (less common in small animals)
        1) Decrescendo murmurs
            a) Aortic insufficiency—secondary to congenital aortic disease, aortic endocarditis, or VSD (loss of aortic root support)
            b) Pulmonic insufficiency—secondary to congenital pulmonary valve disease; surgical correction of pulmonary stenosis; pulmonary endocarditis; heartworm disease (dilated main pulmonary trunk), pulmonary hypertension
        2) Diastolic flow murmurs
            a) Mitral stenosis (congenital or acquired)
            b) Relative mitral or tricuspid stenosis from excessive atrioventricular flow (ASD, VSD), severe AV valvular insufficiency

Clinical Diagnostic Approach[44]

1. Describe the cardiac murmur completely, including timing, PMI, configuration, intensity, quality, and radiation. Draw a picture of the murmur in relation to the heart sounds.
2. Examine the precordium, arterial and venous pulses, mucous membranes, and body cavities.
3. Form an initial assessment as to whether the murmur is functional or organic (Fig. 9-3).
    A. Functional murmurs are heard frequently in young animals (< 6 months of age). Typically, these murmurs are soft (< 3/6), heard best on the left side (aortic area), decrescendo or ejection in configuration, and unassociated with a precordial thrill. The second heart sound is obvious and normal. Functional murmurs often are high-

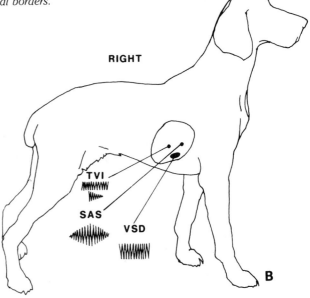

Figure 9-2. *Phonocardiographic configurations of various cardiac murmurs as recorded at the usual points of maximal murmur intensity. (A) View of left hemithorax. MVI, mitral valve insufficiency; SAS, subaortic stenosis; AS, valvular aortic stenosis; PDA, patent ductus arteriosus; PS, pulmonary stenosis. (B) View of the right hemithorax. TVI, tricuspid valve insufficiency; VSD, ventricular septal defect. Note: MVI is often loudest at the point of the left apical impulse. In the cat, many murmurs are loudest at the sternal borders.*

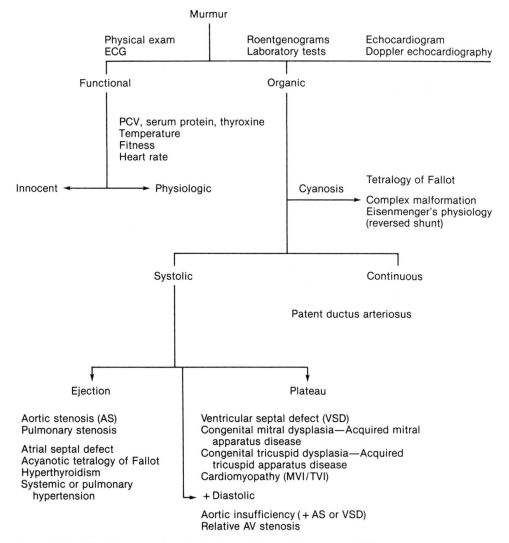

Figure 9-3. *Clinical approach to the patient with a cardiac murmur.* ECG, *electrocardiogram;* PCV, *packed cell volume;* MVI, *mitral valve insufficiency;* TVI, *tricuspid valve insufficiency;* AV, *atrioventricular*

pitched and musical, and change intensity with changes in body position or heart rate. They usually do not radiate over the thorax.

B. Physiologic outflow murmurs are expected in anemic, febrile, or bradycardiac patients, and in cats with hyperthyroidism.

C. Murmurs that are atypical of those described above as functional murmurs, and those associated with cyanosis, abnormal precordial palpation, pathologic pulses, or clinical signs, warrant further study.

4. Organic murmurs are evaluated by noting the signalment, completing the physical examination and laboratory evaluation, and answering the following questions:

A. What is the timing of the murmur?

B. When the animal is standing, where is the murmur heard best? Is there a precordial thrill?

C. What is the configuration, quality, and intensity of the murmur?

D. Do abnormalities in the arterial or venous pulses suggest a left ventricular or right ventricular lesion or a shunt?

E. Is there cyanosis? Ascites? Pulmonary edema? Pleural effusion?

F. Does precordial palpation suggest either right or left ventricular hypertrophy?

G. What are the results of history, physical examination, and ancillary tests?

1) Consider the age, species, and breed. The most common causes of organic murmurs in the mature cat are cardiomyopathy, hyperthyroidism, and hypertension associated with chronic renal disease. Young animals are more likely than older animals to have congenital defects. Mature, small breed dogs often develop mitral and tricuspid valve insufficiency. Giant breed dogs usually develop MVI or TVI from dilated cardiomyopathy. A diastolic murmur in a dog with fever and a hyperkinetic pulse is almost always caused by aortic endocarditis.

2) Taking into account the animal's age, is anemia or polycythemia evident from the CBC?

3) Does the ECG suggest left or right ventricular or atrial enlargement?

4) Does the thoracic roentgenogram reveal:

a) Left or right ventricular enlargement?

b) Enlargement of the great vessels (aorta, pulmonary trunk)?

c) Pulmonary venous or caudal vena cava engorgement?

d) Pulmonary overcirculation or undercirculation?

5) Is there azotemia or elevated T_4 levels?

5. The clinician can make valuable assumptions after considering the following:

A. If cyanosis and polycythemia are noted, a congenital right-to-left shunt, such as occurs with tetralogy of Fallot, is likely. These important findings are usually lacking with other lesions (Tables 9-3 and 9-4). Exceptions to this rule occur when there is florid pulmonary edema, extensive pleural effusion, or shock secondary to heart failure. These conditions lead to ventilation–perfusion mismatches in the lung, and they predispose the patient to cyanosis. Low-output, shock-like states, such as those caused by cardiomyopathy, also result in cyanosis if there is peripheral vasoconstriction and avid extraction of arterial oxygen by underperfused tissues.

B. An ECG, radiographs, and an echocardiogram should be performed to determine whether the lesion primarily affects the right or left ventricle.

1) Aortic stenosis, PDA, aortic insufficiency, and mitral insufficiency primarily result in signs of left-sided disease.

2) Pulmonary stenosis, tetralogy of Fallot, dirofilariasis, tricuspid insufficiency, pulmonary hypertension, and atrial ASDs result in signs related to right ventricular disease.

3) VSD, hyperthyroidism, and cardiomyopathies usually cause signs of left-sided or biventricular disease.

C. The clinician should determine whether the lungs are overcirculated or undercirculated, and whether there is evidence of right or left ventricular failure.

1) Overcirculation is expected in left-to-right shunts.

2) Undercirculation is expected in right-to-left shunts, pulmonary stenosis, congenital TVI, and failure secondary to low output.

3) Pulmonary venous congestion and caudal vena cava engorgement typify left and right ventricular failure, respectively.

6. This integrative approach is particularly valuable for young animals with congenital heart disease. For example, the diagnosis of PDA is usually straightforward because the auscultatory diagnosis is substantiated by other findings. Typical features include a left basilar continuous thrill, a prominent left apical cardiac impulse, ECG evidence of left or right ventricular enlargement, and roentgenographic signs of generalized cardiomeg-

Table 9-3. Clinical findings in acquired nonvalvular heart disease

Lesion	Pulse	Precordium	Cardiac Auscultation	Electrocardiogram	Thoracic Roentgenograms	Other Features
Pericardial disease (effusion) Cardiac neoplasia	N, ↓, or changing	↓ LAp	Muffled heartsounds	↓ voltages, ST-T elevation or depression, electrical alternans	Globoid silhouette, pleural effusion, distended veins, arrhythmias	German shepherds, brachycephalic breeds, venous distention-pulsation, hepatomegaly, ascites common, elevated CVP, positive pericardiocentesis*
Dirofilariasis	V	↑ RAp	V, TVI, PA flow murmur, split or loud S_2	N or RVH	↑ RA, RV, VC, MPA and lobar PA, lung density	Jugular pulsations, pulmonary adventitial sounds, positive microfilaria or ELISA test, eosinophilia
Canine dilated cardiomyopathy (congestive = dilated form)	N to ↓	V	Atrial fibrillation, V murmur, AV insufficiency, gallop	Atrial fibrillation, sinus rhythm—LAE, LVD; ST-T rhythm, PVC	V, generalized cardiomegaly; congestive heart failure changes	Giant to large breeds, dyspnea, ascites, ↓ serum proteins*
Feline cardiomyopathy Dilated form	↓	↓ LAp	V murmur, AV insufficiency, gallop rhythm	LAE, LVD, conduction disturbances: arrhythmias, bradycardia	Generalized cardiomegaly, congestive heart failure, small aorta (↓ output) pleural effusion	Hypothermia, pallor, cyanosis, dyspnea, aortic thromboembolism, prerenal azotemia, secondary to taurine deficiency*
Hypertrophic form	N to ↓	↑ LAp	V murmur, AV insufficiency, subaortic stenosis, gallop rhythm	LAE, LVH, conduction disturbances, arrhythmias	↑ LA, LV ("Valentine heart") apex shift to right, pulmonary edema	Aortic thromboembolism, dyspnea*
Hyperthyroid heart disease	↑	↑	Systolic murmurs, gallop rhythm, tachycardia	↑ Voltages, premature complexes	Cardiomegaly, dilated aorta	Palpable thyroid nodule, weight loss, anxiety, elevated thyroxine level

* Doppler echocardiography can define abnormal anatomy, cardiac contraction, and abnormal blood flow and associated lesion (e.g., tumor, thrombus, effusion).

Key: N, normal; ↑, increased or prominent; ↓, decreased; R, right; L, left; Ap, apex; RA, right atrium; RV, right ventricle; CVP, central venous pressure; AV, atrioventricular; LAE, left atrial enlargement; LA, left atrium; LV, left ventricle; LVD, left ventricular dilation; RAE, right atrial enlargement; RVH, right ventricular hypertrophy; LAD, left axis deviation; MPA, main pulmonary artery; PA, pulmonary artery; VC, vena cava; V, variable; PVC, premature ventricular contractions.

Table 9-4. **Clinical findings with common valvular and congenital heart diseases**

Lesion	Typical Breeds	Arterial Pulse	Venous Pulse	Pre-cordium	Timing	Cardiac Murmur Point of Maximal Intensity	Configuration
Mitral valve insufficiency (MVI)	Acquired—small breeds; congenital—Great Danes, German shepherds, bull terriers	N to ↓	N	↑ LAp	Systolic	LAp	Plateau, decrescendo
Tricuspid valve insufficiency (TVI)	Acquired—small breeds; congenital—large breeds, male retriever breeds	N to ↓	N to ↑	↑ RAp	Systolic	RAp	Plateau, decrescendo
Ventricular septal defect (VSD)	None in dogs; common in cats	N	N	Systolic	V	Right sternal border	Plateau, decrescendo
Pulmonary stenosis (PS)	Beagle, terriers, Chihuahua, bulldog, schnauzer	N to ↓	N to ↑	↑ RAp	Systolic	LB	Ejection
Atrial septal defect (ASD)	Unusual isolated lesion; boxer, Doberman	N	N to ↑	↑ RAp	Systolic	LB	Ejection
Tetralogy of Fallot	Keeshond, English bulldog	N to ↓	N to ↑	↑ RAp	Systolic	LB	Ejection
Aortic stenosis (AS)	Newfoundland, boxer, German shepherd, golden retriever, rottweiler	↓	N	↑ LAp	Systolic	LB, RB, or subaortic	Ejection
Patent ductus arteriosus	Poodles, Pomeranians, collies, German shepherds (female > male)	↑	N to ↑	↑ LAp	Continuous	LB (high)	Machinery
Aortic insufficiency	—	↑	N	↑ LAp	Diastolic	LB and LAp	Decrescendo

* Doppler echocardiography can document anatomical lesions and abnormal blood flow.

Key: *N*, normal; ↑, increased; ↓, decreased; *R*, right; *L*, left; *Ap*, apex/apical impulse; *B*, base; *RA*, right atrium; *RV*, right ventricle; *LA*, left atrium; *LV*, left ventricle; *AV*, atrioventricular; *LAE*, left atrial enlargement; *LVD*, left ventricular dilatation; *LVH*, left ventricular hypertrophy; *RAE*, right atrial enlargement; *RVH*, right ventricular hypertrophy; *LAD*, left axis deviation; *MPA*, main pulmonary artery; *Circ*, pulmonary circulation; *PV*, pulmonary vein; *VC*, vena cava; *V*, variable.

aly with dilation of the great arteries and pulmonary overcirculation. This approach is emphasized in Tables 9-3 and 9-4.

7. Although unavailable in most practices except by referral, echocardiography is an excellent means of diagnosing the causes of cardiac murmurs.[66] When combined with Doppler echocardiography, abnormal blood flow can be detected. Thus, anatomical and flow disturbances can be detected noninvasively.

Electrocardiographic Findings	*Thoracic Roentgenograms*									*Other Features*
	RA	*RV*	*LA*	*LV*	*Aorta*	*MPA*	*Circ*	*PV*	*VC*	
LAE, LVD	N	N	↑	↑	N	N	N	↑	N	Acquired often with tricuspid insufficiency; secondary murmur in cardiomyopathy, shunts, AS, and endocardial cushion defect
RAE, RVH (especially with congenital disease or pulmonary hypertension)	↑	↑	N	N	N	N	(N,↓)	N	↑	Acquired with heartworm disease and caval syndrome, congenital right heart disease, pulmonary hypertension, and cardiomyopathy
Variable; ± LAE, ± LVD; cats: LVD + RVH	V	N↑	N↑	N↑	N	N↑	↑	N,↑	N	May be murmur of relative PS. In cats, it is part of endocardial cushion defect (+ ASD and cleft AV valve).
RAE + RVH	↑	↑	N	N	N	↑	↓	N	↑	Displacement of apex to left may mimic LVH, secondary TVI
RAE + RVH	↑	↑	N↑	N	N	N↑	↑	N	N↑	Split S$_2$; murmur of relative PS; occurs as part of complete endocardial cushion defect
RVH, dogs; RVH or LAD, cats	N	↑	N↓	N↓	N↑	N↑	↓	N	V	With hypoplastic pulmonary artery and polycythemia, murmur may be absent. Cyanosis is worse with exercise. Abnormal (cranial) aortic position
N or LAE + LVH; ST-T depression; ventricular arrhythmias	N	N↑	N↑	N↑	↑	N	N	↑	N	Syncope common
LAE + LVD; ± RVH (precordial) deep Q waves (Lead II)	N	↑	↑	↑	↑	↑	↑	↑	N	Secondary MVI and atrial fibrillation in advanced cases
LVD	N	N	N↑	↑	N↑	N	N	N↑	N	Occurs in endocarditis, subaortic VSD, and congenital AS; concurrent systolic murmur is common.

Gallop Rhythm

Definition

1. A gallop rhythm is produced when extra diastolic sounds are auscultated. The rapid sequence of the first, second, and diastolic sound is similar to the cadence of a galloping horse.

2. By definition, gallop rhythms are diastolic sounds that can be classified according to the following categories (Fig. 9-4):

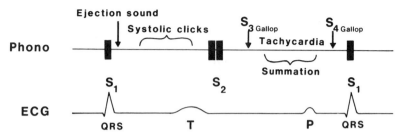

Figure 9-4. *Timing of gallops and other transient sounds. Abnormal cardiovascular transient sounds are timed relative to the first (S_1) and second (S_2) heart sounds. Following activation of the ventricles, S_1 is heard. The two components of S_2 (aortic and pulmonic) indicate the end of ventricular systole. Ejection sounds, such as those that occur with valvular pulmonary stenosis and pulmonary hypertension, are heard immediately following S_1. Systolic clicks can be auscultated throughout systole. They usually indicate mitral valve disease. Ventricular (S_3) gallops, atrial (S_4) gallops, and summation gallops ($S_3 + S_4$) are diastolic sounds that indicate ventricular decompensation or stiffness.*

A. Ventricular gallops (S_3), right or left ventricle in origin

    B. Atrial gallops (S_4)

    C. Summation gallops (S_{3-4})

3. Gallop rhythms are not audible in normal small animals. Since gallops may be present before overt signs of heart failure, they are valuable diagnostic clues and may lead to an early diagnosis of heart disease.

4. In simple terms, gallop rhythms indicate ventricular dysfunction; they are labile, being dependent on heart rate, myocardial compensation, and therapy.

5. Because most small animals have rapid heart rates, it is often difficult to distinguish S_3 from S_4 gallops without the benefit of phonocardiography.

Basic Principles

1. Gallop rhythms are particularly significant in the following types of patients:

    A. Animals with cardiomyopathies without obvious heart murmurs may have gallop rhythms. For example, it is common to auscultate a loud gallop in an otherwise asymptomatic cat. The patient may subsequently manifest roentgenographic evidence of cardiomyopathy, hyperthyroidism, or systemic hypertension.

    B. Animals with chronic valvular, myocardial, or congenital disease often develop loud gallops coincident with heart failure. These extra sounds are labile, and their disappearance may herald a favorable response to therapy.

2. Some etiologic generalizations are possible:

    A. S_3 gallops are common in failing, dilated ventricles, and are associated with congestive (dilated) cardiomyopathies and chronic volume overloads, as in AV valve insufficiency or left-to-right shunts.

    B. S_4 gallops usually indicate that an atrium is contracting against a thickened or stiff ventricle; therefore, these sounds are heard frequently in hypertrophic cardiomyopathy or with pressure overloads, as occurs in semilunar valve stenosis or chronic hypertension.

Clinical Diagnostic Approach

1. True gallops must be distinguished from other extra sounds, particularly systolic clicks and ejection sounds (see Fig. 9-4).

    A. Nonejection, left apical, systolic clicks occur commonly in small animals and probably indicate congenital (cats) or acquired (dogs) mitral apparatus disease. They may be associated with systolic murmurs of mitral valve insufficiency. They are easily distinguished from gallops by their timing and frequency (clicks are high-pitched). They usually coincide with the left apical cardiac impulse and the systolic peripheral arterial pulse. They wax and wane with ventilation.

B. Ejection sounds are less common, high-pitched, early systolic sounds that are associated most frequently with a stenotic pulmonary valve or dilated pulmonary trunk.

2. Gallops are sounds of lower frequency, and are most apparent when auscultated with the bell of the stethoscope. They also wax and wane with ventilation. An apical gallop usually involves S_3, whereas a basilar location is more likely related to an S_4.

3. In uncertain cases, such as cats with tachycardia, proper characterization of the timing of the extra sound requires phonocardiography.

4. Occasionally, pericardial knocks are auscultated. These are closely timed with S_3, but indicate a constrictive pericardial disease. (Pericardial effusion, if present, may generate a friction rub and can dampen the intensity of the heart sounds.)

5. There is no particular treatment for gallop rhythms because they are secondary manifestations of a specific disorder of the heart.

6. The practice of routine prophylactic drug therapy to prevent the development of heart failure in animals with gallop rhythms but no other signs of disease should be considered empirical unless other studies indicate significant heart disease.

7. An echocardiogram is valuable for identifying cardiomyopathy or hypertrophy of the ventricle. In cats, aspirin may be indicated if there is atrial dilation.

8. Arterial blood pressure should be measured to rule out hypertensive heart disease. Antihypertensive drug therapy is indicated in animals with systemic hypertension.

Cyanosis

Definition

1. Cynaosis, a bluish color of the mucous membranes, nail beds, and skin, usually indicates the presence of at least 5 g/dL of reduced hemoglobin (Fig. 9-5).

2. Cyanosis is classified as follows:
   A. Central from arterial hypoxemia (low

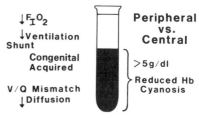

Figure 9-5. *Mechanisms of cyanosis. Cyanosis indicates arterial oxygen desaturation. Cyanotic patients generally have greater than 5 g/dL of reduced hemoglobin (Hb). This imparts a bluish tint to the mucous membranes. Causes of cyanosis include decreased inspired oxygen concentration (F_IO_2), hypoventilation, congenital right-to-left cardiac shunts, acquired pulmonary shunts, mismatching of ventilation and perfusion in the lung (V/Q), and possibly, a diffusion barrier.*

partial pressure of O_2 [PaO_2] within the blood), caused by pulmonary or cardiovascular disease

   B. Peripheral from tissue hypoxia (low tissue levels of O_2 but normal PaO_2), caused by poor circulation, hypoxemia, or altered hemoglobin states

   1) Central cyanosis is caused by congenital heart disease with right-to-left shunting (e.g., tetralogy of Fallot) or by pulmonary disease. Pulmonary disorders include:
      a) Major airway obstruction
      b) Obstructive lower airway disease, asthma
      c) Alveolar disease
         i. Pneumonia
         ii. Pulmonary edema
         iii. Atelectasis
      d) Restrictive disease, fibrosis, and pleural space disease
      e) Pulmonary embolism
      f) Decreased inspired oxygen concentration ($\downarrow$ FiO$_2$)

   2) Peripheral cyanosis is caused by abnormal circulation secondary to arterial obstruction, cold exposure, shock, or low-output heart failure (e.g., dilated cardiomyopathy). Altered hemoglobin states produce cyanosis by changing the affinity of hemoglobin for oxygen. These disorders include methemoglobinemia and sulfhemoglobinemia. A leftward shift of the oxyhemoglobin dissociation curve increases the binding of oxygen to hemoglobin and prevents its release to the tissues. Metabolic alkalosis and decreased body temperatures are examples of disorders that shift the curve to the left.

Clinical Diagnostic Approach

1. Explore the history and examine the patient carefully for signs of heart disease, pulmonary disease, or chemical or drug exposure (e.g., nitrites, phenacetin).

2. If cyanosis is localized to a limb, examine the regional arterial pulses.

3. Determine arterial blood gas values. Hypoxemia ($PaO_2 < 60$ mmHg) indicates central cyanosis caused by heart or pulmonary disease.

4. If the blood appears brown and does not turn red after shaking with air, congenital or acquired methemoglobinemia is likely. Rule out polycythemia vera or polycythemia that is secondary to right-to-left shunts. Anemia does not cause cyanosis.

5. Examine a chest roentgenogram for cardiopulmonary disease or pulmonary vascular disease.

6. Doppler echocardiography or contrast echocardiography, with saline injections in the venous system, can outline right-to-left intracardiac shunts.

7. Cardiac catheterization may be needed to rule out congenital heart disease.

8. Mass spectroscopy is used to confirm a diagnosis of methemoglobinemia.

9. Lung scans or angiography may document pulmonary embolism.

Pulmonary Adventitious Sounds

Definitions

1. Normal breath sounds are caused by air flowing through the major conducting and peripheral airways. Tracheal, bronchial, vesicular, and bronchovesicular sounds are normally auscultated over the trachea, hilus, and lung fields. Absence of these normal sounds usually indicates pulmonary atelectasis, effusion, a space-occupying mass, pneumothorax, or a pleural space disorder. Accentuation

of these sounds is common in a variety of pulmonary disorders, including pneumonia and some cases of consolidation, and dorsal to areas of pleural effusion.

2. Obstructive pulmonary sounds are particularly common in animals. A snoring inspiratory sound (stertor) is common with redundant soft palate. Stridor, a high-pitched inspiratory wheeze, is a sign of laryngeal obstruction or paralysis. The dog with collapsing trachea has loud tracheal and bronchial sounds punctuated by a "snapping" sound and honking cough. Compression of major bronchi leads to loud bronchial sounds with dyspnea and wheezing. The point of maximal intensity of the obstructive sound generally indicates its origin.

3. Continuous adventitious sounds include low-pitched (sonorous) rhonchi and high-pitched wheezing (sibilant rhonchi). These sounds indicate accumulation of secretions (as in bronchitis and bronchopneumonia) or airway narrowing (as in asthma). They occur most frequently during expiration.

4. Pulmonary crackles (rales) are discontinuous sounds that presumably indicate small airway closure, pulmonary fluid, or fibrosis. These sounds are often heard best ventrally when the animal is forced to breathe deeply. The clinical distinction between "wet" and "dry" crackles is very difficult to make, and often results in inappropriate use of diuretics in some dogs with fibrosis or bronchitis. In fact, loud, coarse crackles are more common in animals with bronchitis and fibrosis than in those with pulmonary edema.

5. Auscultation of abnormal lung sounds should alert the clinician to the probable location and type of pulmonary disease. Adventitious sounds are an indication for thoracic roentgenograms and other cardiorespiratory tests (see section on cough). Obstructive sounds may prompt endoscopic evaluation.

Arterial Thromboembolism

Definition

1. When a thrombus travels from its point of formation to lodge elsewhere in the circulation, the occlusion is termed a *thromboembo-lism*. Systemic arterial thromboembolism is uncommon in small animal medicine; it occurs most frequently in the cardiomyopathic cat. Although the overall incidence of arterial thromboembolism is low, there are particular situations in which the disorder occurs:

    A. Aortic embolism associated with feline or (rarely) canine cardiomyopathy

    B. Arterial or pulmonary embolism associated with hypoalbuminemia and hypercoagulable states, such as renal amyloidosis, glomerular disease, Cushing's disease, chronic pericarditis, and chronic nonmobile patients

    C. Embolism secondary to DIC or immune-mediated hemolytic conditions

    D. Pulmonary embolism associated with dirofilariasis or its treatment

    E. Septic or bland (sterile) embolism secondary to disruption of a heart valve vegetation

    F. Embolism caused by a missile (e.g., bullet or pellet)

    G. Fat embolism secondary to bone trauma

    H. Air embolism secondary to roentgenographic procedures

    I. Trauma

    J. Aberrant dirofilariasis (systemic artery)

    K. Neoplastic embolization

2. The signs of arterial embolism are proportional to the location and duration of the obstruction, and the presence or absence of arterial collateral circulation.

3. The origin of arterial emboli is not always obvious. In cardiomyopathy, the presumed origin of the clot is the left atrium.

4. Abnormal vascular dynamics are related both to the physical obstruction and the presence of vasoactive chemicals produced by the clot, which result in secondary constriction of collateral vessels.

5. The end result and clinical signs of complete arterial occlusion are related to degeneration and necrosis of the tissues supplied by that vessel. Additional abnormalities in the case of pulmonary embolism are associated with sudden obstruction of ventricular out-flow, leading to dyspnea, shock, and heart failure.

Clinical Diagnostic Approach

1. Arterial embolism is suspected when there is a sudden cessation of organ or tissue function related to clinical signs of hypoperfusion.

    A. Aortic emboli usually lodge in the iliac arterial bifurcation or in a femoral artery of its branches. Typical signs include sudden paresis, loss of motor and sensory limb function, muscle pain and contracture, lack of peripheral arterial pulsations with pallor and coolness of the distal extremity, lack of bleeding, and loss of segmental spinal reflexes (lower motor neuron).

    B. The classic triad of acute pulmonary embolism includes an increased heart rate, respiratory rate, and body temperature (if ischemic necrosis is present). The animal frequently exhibits acute respiratory distress. If the obstruction is complete, acute right ventricular failure, shock, and death can ensue. Pleural effusion may be evident.

    C. Arterial embolism of other organs is difficult to diagnose, but is suspected in cases of peracute neurologic deficit, colic, or biochemical disorders (e.g., acute oliguric renal failure, acute hypoparathyroidism, or acute hypoadrenocorticism).

    D. Other causes of arterial obstruction, including atherosclerotic disease from hypothyroidism or primary hypolipidemia, hyperviscosity of blood, trauma, and neoplasia, may mimic signs of arterial embolism.

2. The clinician must maintain a high level of suspicion to diagnose embolism of visceral or nervous tissues.

3. Depending on the clinical presentation and knowledge of current patient problems, the following tests are appropriate:

    A. In arterial embolism of the limbs, the diagnosis is usually made by physical examination.

    B. A tentative diagnosis of major pulmonary embolism is made when peracute dyspnea is associated with typical clinical signs and clinical laboratory evidence of the previously mentioned disorders. Laboratory evaluations of importance include blood microfilaria or heartworm ELISA test, chest roentgenogram (increased lung densities and pulmonary artery hypervascularity), arterial blood gas, serum protein and albumin, clotting profile, PCV, serum lipid profile, and serum T_3, T_4 levels.

C. Angiography may be necessary to delineate arterial obstruction, particularly in deep vascular occlusions. Radioisotope scans, when available, may also assist in the diagnosis.

D. Vascular occlusion of the nervous system is diagnosed on the basis of the history, neuroroentgenography, and exclusion of other considerations (see Chapter 17).

Treatment

1. Surgical removal of a thrombus is optimal; however, it is seldom feasible in animals. Irreversible tissue damage usually occurs within a few hours. The cardiovascular and pulmonary status must be considered before subjecting a patient to general anesthesia.

2. Mechanical removal of arterial emboli using balloon (Fogarty) catheters, enzymatic fibrinolytic therapy, and tissue plasminogen activator have been attempted experimentally.[81] These treatments also hold some promise in clinical veterinary practice.

3. Acute iliac thrombosis may be managed with:

A. Analgesics or sedatives (low doses)

B. Surgery, if the clot is proximal to the renal arteries (follow the serum BUN)

C. Sodium heparin to prevent the extension of the clot

D. Antiplatelet drugs, such as aspirin

E. Vasodilator drugs, such as promazine-derivative tranquilizers, to increase collateral circulation

F. Supportive care of the limb

G. Tissue plasminogen activator

4. Acute pulmonary embolism is treated with:

A. Mild sedation

B. Oxygen therapy

C. Corticosteroids

D. Bronchodilators

E. Rest

F. Diuretics (furosemide), which are sometimes helpful in embolization following heartworm therapy or sudden death of a filarial parasite

G. Heparin for non-heartworm–related pulmonary embolism

Extravascular Fluid Accumulation

Definition

1. Accumulation of fluid outside of the vascular space is a common problem associated with cardiopulmonary disease. Common disorders include subcutaneous edema, pleural effusion,[11] ascites,[20] pericardial effusion,[83,92] and pulmonary edema.[46,96] These problems are not specific for cardiac or respiratory diseases; however, they are frequently associated with disease of these systems.

2. Subcutaneous edema is diagnosed on the basis of physical examination, discussed below.

3. Physical examination reveals signs suggestive of pulmonary edema, pleural effusion, ascites, and pericardial effusion. These disorders are substantiated and qualified by roentgenographic, ultrasonographic, and laboratory analysis. Physical, chemical, and cytologic analysis of the fluids is germane to the evaluation of extravascular fluid accumulation. For this reason, these four problems are discussed later in this chapter. Differential considerations for pericardial effusion are also listed.

4. It should be emphasized that the physical examination, although vital for the detection of these problems, is not the endpoint of diagnostic evaluation. For example, dogs with dyspnea, cyanosis, and crackles may have either congestive heart failure or chronic bronchitis. The definitive diagnosis is not possible until all available information has been analyzed.

Subcutaneous Edema

1. Subcutaneous edema is attributable to increases in extracellular, extravascular water and solute localized in the subcutaneous tissues. The characteristic physical feature of advanced subcutaneous edema is swelling with pitting: the persistent deformation of the tissue following release of digital pressure.

2. Subcutaneous edema results from elevated venous pressure, as in heart failure, arteriovenous fistula, or venous thrombosis; from lymphatic obstruction, as in cancer; from reduced plasma oncotic pressure, which is usually the result of hypoalbuminemia; or from increased permeability of small vessel walls, as occurs in hypersensitivity reactions or vasculitis (Fig. 9-6); and in iatrogenic diseases associated with extravasation of fluids or perivascular injection of chemotherapeutic drugs.

3. Subcutaneous edema is an unusual feature of heart disease in small animals.

4. In this discussion, generalized or bilaterally symmetrical edema is explained. Localized edema, commonly associated with trauma, AV fistulas, hypersensitivity, insect bites, constricting bands, or localized neoplasms, is not discussed here. A list of common causes of generalized or symmetrical subcutaneous edema follows.

A. Heart failure or elevated venous pressure secondary to:

1) Pericardial disease

2) Right heart lesions (pulmonary stenosis, dirofilariasis, right atrial obstruction or tumor)

3) Dilated cardiomyopathy

4) Cardiac arrhythmia

5) Fluid overload

B. Hypoproteinemia secondary to:

1) Renal loss (amyloidosis, glomerular disease)

2) Protein-losing (gastro-) enteropathy

3) Liver disease

4) Cutaneous protein loss from disseminated skin disease or crush injury

5) Vasculitis

6) Nutritional disorders

C. Venous or lymphatic obstruction secondary to:

1) Mediastinal or pelvic neoplasm

2) Other tumors or mass lesions

3) Vena caval thrombosis

4) Metastatic or lymphoreticular cancer

D. Altered vascular or lymphatic permeability (e.g., vasculitis, trauma, transfusion reaction)

E. Lymphatic dysplasia or aplasia (congenital)

F. Myxedema from hypothyroidism

G. Ehrlichiosis (advanced cases)/Rocky Mountain spotted fever (vasculitis)

Clinical Diagnostic Approach

1. The physical examination must be thorough. The clinician should search for objec-

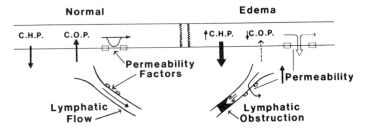

Figure 9-6. *Mechanisms of subcutaneous edema and pulmonary edema. (Left) The factors responsible for normal microcirculatory fluid dynamics are shown. CHP, capillary hydrostatic pressure; COP, capillary oncotic pressure. Permeability factors include normal capillary membranes and normal lymphatic wall integrity. (Right) Increased CHP (as occurs with congestive heart failure), decreased COP (as occurs with hypoalbuminemia), lymphatic obstruction (as occurs with neoplasia), and increased permeability (as occurs with immunologic injury) disrupt normal fluid movement and result in positive pressure within the interstitial space. This leads to demonstrable edema.*

tive signs of venous hypertension such as heart disease, jugular venous or superficial venous distention, and palpable masses, or evidence of active inflammation or immune disease (e.g., thrombocytopenia) that might suggest a permeability mechanism for the edema.

2. Obtain a thoracic roentgenogram and possibly an echocardiogram to evaluate heart size, rule out a mediastinal mass, and diagnose heart failure, pericardial disease, or a cardiac tumor.

3. Obtain abdominal and pelvic roentgenograms if the edema is limited to the rear limbs or if renal or hepatic disease is a primary consideration. Evaluate these for intraabdominal masses and abnormal size and shape of the kidneys, liver, and prostate. Follow this examination with ultrasonography if available.

4. Obtain routine laboratory tests, including:

A. CBC and serum albumin

B. Urine protein (interpret in light of specific gravity and sediment and the urine protein/creatine ratio).

C. Serum cholesterol (elevated in nephrotic syndrome)

D. Immunologic testing or vessel biopsy if an autoimmune disorder leading to immune vasculitis is suspected (poorly defined in animals)

E. Echocardiogram if heart failure, pericarditis, or a heart-base or cardiac tumor is suspected

Treatment

1. Therapy for subcutaneous edema is directed at the underlying etiology.

2. Furosemide may result in symptomatic relief, but is associated with the typical side effects and other disadvantages of diuretic therapy, such as reduced cardiac filling.

3. Provide soft bedding to prevent decubital ulcers.

4. If all other causes of subcutaneous edema are ruled out, the use of immunosuppressive doses of glucocorticosteroids may be beneficial if the underlying disorder is increased vessel permeability from vasculitis.

5. Tetracycline is used in suspected cases of rickettsial-induced vasculitis.

Congestive Heart Failure

Definition

1. *Heart failure* is a state of circulatory dysfunction characterized by normal or elevated venous pressures and reduced cardiac output relative to exercise needs.[19,39,56,57,59,82,83,92,95,96] Clinical signs of heart failure are related to:

A. Circulatory venous congestion causing pulmonary edema, ascites, pleural effusion, subcutaneous edema, hepatosplenomegaly, or pericardial effusion.

B. Low arterial output causing depression, weakness, syncope, azotemia, pallor, hypothermia, and cardiac arrhythmias

2. The causes of heart failure can be arbitrarily classified as follows:

A. Endocardial diseases

1) Chronic myxomatous valvular heart disease in dogs (endocardiosis)

2) Bacterial endocarditis

3) Congenital endocardial fibroelastosis

4) Congenital valve malformation

B. Myocardial diseases

1) Myocardial disease, degeneration, or failure secondary to another disorder (e.g., taurine deficiency, drugs, parvovirus, trypanosomiasis, Lyme disease, hypothyroidism, carnitine deficiency)

2) Primary myocardial diseases (idiopathic cardiomyopathies)

a) Feline cardiomyopathies

b) Canine cardiomyopathies

3) Acute myocardial infarction (rare)

C. Pericardial diseases

1) Constrictive pericardial diseases

2) Cardiac tamponade (effusions) (e.g., idiopathic hemorrhagic pericardial effusion in the dog)

3) Cardiac or pericardial neoplasia (e.g., hemangiosarcoma, lymphosarcoma, aortic body tumor, ectopic thyroid carcinoma, mesothelioma)

D. Congenital heart disease

1) Intracardiac and extracardiac

shunts (PDA, ASD, VSD, endocardial cushion defect)

    2) Semilunar valvular stenosis (aortic and pulmonic stenosis)

    3) Abnormal development of the tricuspid and mitral valves (dysplasia)

  E. Cardiac arrhythmias

  F. Cor pulmonale

    1) Dirofilariasis

    2) Other causes of cor pulmonale (e.g., pulmonary embolus, primary pulmonary hypertension)

  G. Miscellaneous causes

    1) Peripheral arteriovenous fistula

    2) Thyrotoxicosis (e.g., thyroid neoplasia)

    3) Chronic anemia

  3. A search for objective signs of heart disease is imperative. Dyspnea, cyanosis, and crackles are not specific for heart failure, and the clinician must substantiate a diagnosis before attributing any clinical sign to cardiovascular dysfunction. As illustrated throughout this chapter, there are no objective historical signs of heart disease. All historical problems have alternative diagnoses. On the other hand, certain physical and laboratory findings are highly suggestive of heart disease. These include:

  A. Loud cardiac murmur and precordial thrill

  B. Gallop rhythm

  C. Arrhythmia and concurrent pulse deficits

  D. Abnormal ECG or echocardiogram

  E. Roentgenographic evidence of cardiomegaly or heart failure

  F. Measurable increase in venous pressure

The absence of any of these findings makes a diagnosis of heart failure untenable.

Clinical Diagnostic Approach

  1. Obtain a history, including previous therapy and clinical response, complete the physical examination, and evaluate an ECG and thoracic roentgenograms. Microfilaria tests, heartworm ELISA, and routine hematologic studies are obtained as needed.

  2. Other studies, including echocardiography, Doppler studies, measurement of vascular pressures, angiocardiography, cardiac catheterization, phonocardiography, and pericardiocentesis may be indicated in select cases. Physiochemical and cytologic analysis of pleural or ascitic fluid should be performed.

  3. Most disorders leading to heart failure are accompanied by a heart murmur arrhythmia, or a gallop rhythm. The approach to the patient with a heart murmur has already been described in the earlier section on cardiac murmurs and precordial thrills. However, there are situations in which significant heart failure is present without obvious heart murmur. Important causes of heart failure with absent or variable cardiac murmur include:

  A. Heartworm disease (dirofilariasis)

  B. Pericardial disase

  C. Myocardial disease—*Note:* Often, a gallop rhythm or cardiac arrhythmia is evident. In myocardial disease, it is common for the murmur associated with AV valve insufficiency to wax and wane, coincident with dilatation of the ventricles. After digitalization or diuretic therapy, these murmurs may not be evident, only to recur with severe heart failure.

  4. Thoracic roentgenography, ECG, and echocardiography are keys to the diagnosis of heart failure in dogs without murmurs. Significant abnormalities are usually detected by these methods.

  5. Common clinical findings in small animal patients with heart failure from various causes are described in Tables 9-3 and 9-4.

The underlying cause of heart failure can usually be determined through analysis of all of the test results. Salient features distinguishing the different causes of heart failure are listed in the tables and references.

Treatment

  1. The medical management of heart failure has been described in detail elsewhere.[19,39,56,57,59,82,92]

2. Treatment for heart failure may be divided into specific and symptomatic treatment.

A. Specific treatment is predicated on establishment of the correct diagnosis. Examples of specific therapy include surgical ligation of PDA, valvulotomy for pulmonary stenosis, taurine administration in cats with dilated cardiomyopathy,[82] pericardectomy for pericardial constriction, and chemotherapy for dirofilariasis or cardiac arrhythmias.

B. Symptomatic therapy is directed toward abnormalities that cause clinical signs of heart failure. These include pulmonary edema, pleural effusion, ascites, and decreased cardiac output. Since many cardiac disorders, including chronic valvular and myocardial disease, are not amenable to specific treatment, heart failure secondary to these problems must be managed symptomatically.

    1) The principles underlying symptomatic therapy for heart failure include:

      a) Reduction of activity, and decreased psychic and thermal stress

      b) Sedation when required

      c) Improvement of gas exchange
        i. Oxygen
        ii. Ethyl alcohol nebulization
        iii. Aminophylline for bronchodilatation

      d) Reduction of capillary pressure
        i. Furosemide or thiazide diuretics
        ii. Vasodilator therapy (nitroglycerine, captopril, enalapril)
        iii. Positive inotropic agents

      e) Increase in cardiac output
        i. Digitalis glycosides
        ii. Catecholamines (dobutamine and dopamine)
        iii. Amrinone, milrinone
        iv. Vasodilator therapy (hydralazine, prazosin, captopril, enalapril)

      f) Antiarrhythmic therapy

      g) Aspiration of pleural or pericardial effusions

      h) Aspiration of large peritoneal effusion

Cardiopulmonary Arrest

Definition

1. *Cardiopulmonary arrest* (CPA) is a sudden, unexpected cessation of circulation and ventilation.

2. CPA occurs in many clinical settings, including anesthesia and surgery, trauma, metabolic disorders, pulmonary disease, and heart disease. The ability to resuscitate and maintain a patient is proportionate to the preparedness and skill of the clinician and the underlying cause and duration of the CPA.

3. CPA is recognized by the lack of
    A. Consciousness
    B. Ventilation
    C. Pulse and blood pressure
    D. Heartbeat
    E. Circulation or bleeding
    F. Pupillary light reflexes (PLRs)

4. The clinician must initiate immediate resuscitative measures before irreversible CNS damage occurs or the patient dies. The principles of management are outlined in Figure 9-7 and include:[36,48]
    A. Establishing an airway (*A*)
    B. Breathing for the animal (*B*)
    C. Restoring circulation (*C*)
    D. Administering drugs or defibrillation shocks (*D*)
    E. Evaluating the ECG to guide therapy (*E*)

Treatment

1. Verify the CPA by physical examination.

2. Establish an airway with a cuffed endotracheal tube.
    A. Use positive pressure ventilation.
    B. Use 100% oxygen.
    C. Ventilate 12 to 16 times/min.
    D. Do not overinflate the lungs because this leads to pneumomediastinum and decreased venous return.

3. If there is no heartbeat, begin external cardiopulmonary massage.
    A. Compress the chest 80 to 120 times/min.

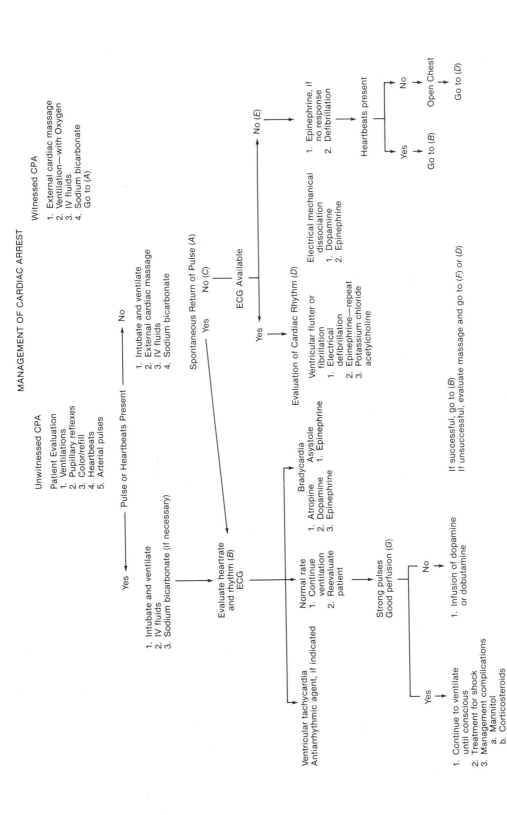

Figure 9-7. *Management of cardiopulmonary arrest (CPA). Essential steps in the management of cardiopulmonary arrest are indicated. ECG, electrocardiograms.*

B. Coordinate with ventilation.

1) Ratio of 5 to 6 massages to 1 ventilation (team)

2) Ratio of 15 massages to 2 ventilations (alone)

C. Abdominal counterpulsation or wrapping may increase the effectiveness of CPR.

D. Open chest massage is indicated in some cases.

4. Establish an intravenous line; administer large doses of isotonic fluids to increase venous return (unless there is lung edema).

5. Administer sodium bicarbonate IV.

6. If an ECG is available, determine the rhythm and provide appropriate therapy.

A. For asystole, administer epinephrine by the intravenous or the intratracheal route or by intracardiac (IC) injection into the left ventricle.

B. For ventricular fibrillation, electrical defibrillation is applied. Energy levels are dependent on the size of the animal and on the positioning of the paddles internally or externally.

C. Electrical-mechanical dissociation (normal ECG without contraction) is managed by inotropic drugs, including dopamine hydrochloride and epinephrine.

7. If an ECG is not available, administer epinephrine. If this is unsuccessful, follow it with defibrillation and consider opening the chest.

A. Direct visualization of the heart generally permits the identification of the cardiac rhythm.

B. Appropriate drugs can then be given IC.

8. If sinus rhythm is restored, the circulation is supported with a dopamine infusion, and other agents are administered as needed.

A. Antiarrhythmic drugs (e.g., procainamide or lidocaine)

B. Bicarbonate for metabolic acidosis

C. Positive inotropic-chronotropic drugs (dopamine is both)

D. Mannitol for cerebral edema

E. Glucocorticoids (dexamethasone, prednisolone)

F. Supportive care and monitoring

9. Occassionally, respiratory failure occurs in patients that maintain normal cardiovascular status.

A. Mechanisms include central and peripheral failure (exhaustion), trauma, and severe lung disease.

1) Central failure occurs with CNS disease or with drug overdose (narcotics, barbituates, anesthetics).

2) Peripheral failure secondary to chronic dyspnea, neuromuscular blockade (aminoglycosides), myasthenia gravis, polyradiculoneuritis, cervical spinal cord disease, botulism, and tetanus have been reported.

3) Severe pulmonary parenchymal disease as with intrapulmonary hemorrhage, pneumonia, embolic disease, and acute respiratory distress syndrome (shock lung), leads to respiratory failure.

4) Chest trauma can cause respiratory failure.

B. Patients in respiratory failure usually exhibit marked tachypnea and hypoxemia ($PaO_2 < 60$ torr). Cyanosis is prominent in most patients, and many are hypercapnic.

C. Management principles include the following (consult the references for more detailed therapy[36,48]):

1) Mechanical ventilation of apneic patients (by tracheotomy if needed)

2) Administration of oxygen

3) Clearance of airways

4) Treatment of shock, cardiac arrhythmias, or anemia

5) Treatment of the underlying etiology

6) Correction of acid–base and electrolyte imbalances

7) Maintenance of proper ventilation and patient nursing care

Other Disorders Associated with Heart Disease

Hepatosplenomegaly

1. Severe right ventricular failure results in palpable enlargement of the liver (and sometimes the spleen) secondary to congestion of these organs.

2. Congestion and hypoperfusion of the liver also result in laboratory abnormalities, including elevations in liver enzymes and elevated serum bile acids.

3. Constrictive pericarditis, cardiac tamponade, heart-base tumors, and obstructive right atrial tumors can cause dramatic hepato-megaly that may direct the clinician away from the underlying etiology of venous obstruction. In most cases, there is jugular venous distention (except in intracardiac or caudal vena caval obstruction).

4. Evaluation of the patient with an enlarged liver is discussed in Chapter 11.

Persistent Fever

1. Fever is a nonspecific sign associated with numerous disorders. Animals with persistent fever occasionally are found to have infective endocarditis.[22] This differential diagnosis should be considered in any animal with persistent or recurrent fevers.

2. Intravenous therapy and protracted immunosuppressive therapy (steroids) predispose animals to infective endocarditis.

3. Endocarditis should be considered in patients with "new" or rapidly changing murmurs. The presence of a new holosystolic murmur or a decrescendo diastolic murmur related to aortic insufficiency should alert the clinician to probable vegetative endocarditis. Remember, however, that fever is a common cause of physiologic systolic murmurs, and many animals with early endocarditis do not have murmurs.

4. The diagnosis of bacterial endocarditis is confirmed by isolating the infectious agent from the blood. Echocardiography can detect valvular vegetations.

5. Treatment of bacterial endocarditis includes long-term administration of bactericidal antibiotics, management of attendant heart failure or arrhythmias, and monitoring for signs of secondary arterial embolization.

Roentgenographic, Electrocardiographic, and Laboratory Problems

Cardiomegaly

Definition

1. Cardiomegaly is a frequent finding on inspection of thoracic roentgenograms.[62,88,89]

The clinical significance of this problem is evident only after a careful review of the following:

    A. Technical quality of the x-ray films

    B. History and physical examination findings

    C. Thoracic roentgenograms, analyzed for:

        1) Cardiac rotation and apex displacement

        2) Species and breed variability

        3) Size of individual chambers

        4) Size of the aorta and main pulmonary artery

        5) Pulmonary undercirculation or overcirculation

        6) Pulmonary venous or systemic venous congestion

        7) Intrapulmonary or peribronchial disease

        8) Intrapleural disease

        9) Obstructive large airway (tracheo-bronchial) disease

        10) Thoracic restrictive disease (e.g., in obesity)

    D. Laboratory and ancillary data, such as an ECG, heartworm test, and tracheal aspiration cytology

    E. An echocardiogram

2. Often, cardiomegaly is of little clinical significance. For example, moderate right ventricular enlargement is common in dogs with long-standing chronic lung disease, yet secondary right ventricular failure is rare.

3. Do not overinterpret x-ray films. For instance, underexposure leads to abnormally dense lungs. Pure right ventricular enlargement usually displaces the apex to the left, mimicking left ventricular enlargement. Inability to expand the chest (e.g., as a result of lung fibrosis or obesity) causes the heart to appear relatively larger.

4. Integration of roentgenographic and clinical findings has already been emphasized. Typical roentgenographic abnormalities are described in Tables 9-2 and 9-3.

Etiology

1. When right atrial and ventricular enlargement predominate, consider (Fig. 9-8):

    A. Pulmonary stenosis

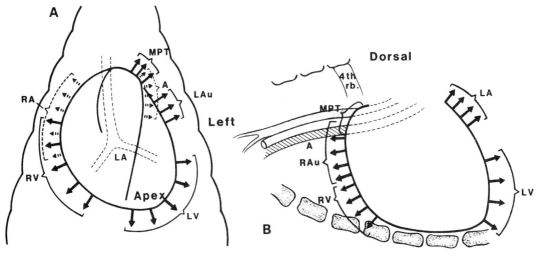

Figure 9-8.   *Cardiomegaly associated with various cardiac lesions in the dog. The typical patterns of cardiomegaly are shown for the dorsoventral (A) and lateral (B) thoracic roentgenograms. Pure right ventricular enlargement typically results in shifting of the apex dorsally and to the left. Enlargement of the left atrium leads to separation and compression of the mainstem bronchi. MPT, main pulmonary trunk; A, aorta; LAu, left auricle; LV, left ventricle; LA, left atrium; RV, right ventricle; RA, right atrium; RAu, right auricle. (The trachea and mainstem bronchi are indicated by the dashed lines in the center of the heart.)*

Assessment of the pulmonary circulation can be accomplished through analysis of the pulmonary arteries and veins supplying the cranial lung lobes. In normal animals, the pulmonary artery (shaded) and pulmonary vein (cross-hatched) are approximately equal in diameter and constitute approximately 75% of the diameter of the fourth rib. The bronchus lies between the two vessels. The MPT in the cat does not extend to the outer border of the cardiac silhouette.

    B. Tetralogy of Fallot
    C. Tricuspid dysplasia or insufficiency
    D. ASD
    E. Dirofilariasis
    F. Cor pulmonale
    G. Reversed congenital shunts (Eisenmenger's physiology)
    H. Pulmonary hypertension
  2. When left atrial and ventricular enlargement predominate, consider:
    A. PDA
    B. Mitral dysplasia or insufficiency
    C. Aortic insufficiency (AS)
    D. Mitral stenosis (rare)
    E. Anemia (chronic)
  3. Causes of biventricular enlargement include:

    A. VSD
    B. Endocardial cushion defect
    C. Bilateral AV valve insufficiency
    D. Cardiomyopathy
    E. Pericardial disease (apparent cardiomegaly)
    F. Hyperthyroidism
    G. Chronic left ventricular disease with pulmonary hypertension

Enlargement of the Great Vessels

  1. Causes of enlarged aorta include:
    A. PDA
    B. Aortic stenosis
    C. Tetralogy of Fallot (malpositioned)
    D. Pulmonary atresia

2. Causes of enlarged main pulmonary artery include:

    A. PS

    B. Dirofilariasis

    C. Left-to-right shunts

        1) PDA

        2) ASD

        3) VSD

    D. Pulmonary hypertension

Abnormal Pulmonary Circulation

1. Causes of undercirculation

    A. Tetralogy of Fallot

    B. Right-to-left shunt (e.g., reverse PDA)

    C. PS

    D. Tricuspid dysplasia

    E. Addison's disease

    F. Shock

    G. Hypovolemia from other causes

2. Causes of increased vascularity (arteries and veins) or pulmonary overcirculation

    A. ASD

    B. VSD

    C. PDA

    D. Endocardial cushion defect

    E. Anemia

    F. Hyperthyroidism

    G. AV fistula

    H. Biventricular congestive heart failure (CHF) with secondary pulmonary hypertension (cat)

    I. Fluid overinfusion

3. Causes of increased pulmonary arterial diameter

    A. Heartworm disease

    B. Pulmonary embolism

    C. Pulmonary vascular disease

    D. Reversed shunts (Eisenmenger's physiology)

    E. Causes of overcirculation (listed above)

4. Causes of increased pulmonary venous diameter

    A. Left-sided CHF

    B. Mitral stenosis

    C. Cor triatriatum

    D. Veno-occlusive disease

    E. Left-atrial mass

Increased Pulmonary Densities

Definitions

1. The correct interpretation of increased pulmonary densities noted on thoracic roentgenograms is important in the management of cardiopulmonary disease. The clinician must remember, however, that the lung only responds to injury in a limited number of ways. Consequently, the alterations in pulmonary roentgenographic patterns can be similar for different disorders.

2. As an initial measure, the clinician must decide whether the decreased or increased densities are within the lung parenchyma, the mediastinum, or the pleural space. There are few common causes of increased lucency, but these include: overexposure; asthma; gas trapping from bronchial disease; emphysema, as with bronchial hypoplasia; bullous lung lesions; and pneumothorax. Most lesions lead to increased radiodensity.

    A. Lesions within the pleural space silhouette the heart, diaphragm, and great vessels; blunt the costophrenic angles; cause a scalloped appearance of increased density on the lateral roentgenogram; and retract the lung lobes, separating the interlobar fissures.

    B. Widening of the mediastinum is nonspecific because it may be caused by fat, mass lesions, a dilated esophagus, or fluid accumulation. Often, roentgenographic contrast procedures (e.g., a barium swallow test) are needed to further define the cause of a widened mediastinum. Other tests, including ultrasonography, venography, aspiration cytology, or biopsy, may be necessary to diagnose tumors, abscesses, lymphadenopathy, fluid, mediastinitis, and cysts.

    C. Increased pulmonary parenchymal densities are defined based on number, size, location, and roentgenographic pattern. Patterns of intrapulmonary parenchymal disease include the following.[88,89]

        1) In alveolar disease, air brochograms, masking of the cardiac borders, and nondistinct, coalescing margins of increased pulmonary density are evident.

        2) Peribronchial densities cause demarcation of the walls of larger airways.

These often appear as air-filled "doughnuts" when viewed on end.

    3) Interstitial densities involve changes of the supporting tissues of the lung. The interstitial pattern may be a diffuse increase in linear density that obscures blood vessels, or a nodular lesion with distinct borders.

    3. The clinician must be very familiar with the roentgenographic appearance of many cardiopulmonary disorders. It is useful, for example, to know that cardiogenic pulmonary edema in the dog usually results in perihilar densities, whereas noncardiogenic pulmonary edema is frequently evident (and worse) in the peripheral zones. Similarly, bacterial bronchopneumonia usually involves the cranial, middle, and ventral pulmonary zones, whereas viral or mycotic pneumonia causes diffuse interstitial densities.

    4. The following list includes some of the underlying disorders associated with abnormal pulmonary densities, as described by Suter and Lord.[88,89]

    5. Since pulmonary densities are generally associated with respiratory symptoms, the clinical work-up pertinent to abnormal pulmonary densities is described in the earlier sections on cough and respiratory distress.

Causes of Increased Pulmonary Density[11]*

Alveolar density
    Pulmonary edema
    Pulmonary hemorrhage
    Bronchopneumonia
    Aspiration
    Atelectasis
    Alveolar microlithiasis
    Granulomatous disease
    Lungworms
    Pulmonary embolism
    Dirofilariasis
    Lung lobe torsion
    Eosinophilic pneumonitis
    Bronchial-alveolar cell carcinoma

    Lipid pneumonia (aspiration)
    Pulmonary lymphosarcoma
Diffuse Interstitial Density
    Interstitial edema
    Interstitial hemorrhage
    Interstitial pneumonia
    Dirofilariasis
    Lungworms
    Granulomatous diseases
    Pulmonary fibrosis
    Some neoplasms (e.g., lymphosarcoma)
    Artifacts (expiratory film; obesity)
    Cushing's disease
Nodular Interstitial Density
    Granulomatous disease (e.g., fungal or immunologic in origin)
    Primary and metastatic neoplasms
    Lungworms
    Dirofilariasis
    Pulmonary abscess
    Pulmonary cyst
    Pulmonary hematoma
    Broncholithiasis
    Disseminated alveolar microlithiasis
    Calcified hematomas and granulomas
    Bronchiectasis filled with fluid
    Artifact (end-on vessels)
    Artifact (nipples, thoracic wall lesions)
Peribronchial density
    Bronchitis (chronic)
    Bronchiectasis
    Dirofilariasis
    Cushing's disease
    Age-related changes
    Pneumonia

Pleural Effusion

Definition

    1. *Pleural effusion*, the accumulation of fluid within the pleural space, is a common sign of cardiopulmonary and thoracic disease. Pleural effusion is a sign that results from the many possible causes listed below.[9,11,14,15,26–28,29,31,42,43,45,55,64,72,74,80,98,100]

    2. Most cases of pleural effusion involve increased production of fluid secondary to transudative or exudative processes. Cytologic analysis of a pleural effusion is imperative in order to discern the underlying cause.[29]

---

* This material is summarized from tables originally published by Suter and Lord (see references). It should be obvious from this information that mixed patterns of pulmonary roentgenographic density are common. The clinician must always interpret thoracic roentgenograms in light of clinical and other laboratory findings.

3. Based on physical and chemical characteristics and cytologic evaluation, the causes pleural effusion can be subdivided as shown in the list that follows.[11,29,74]

4. The cytologic classification of an effusion varies depending on the mechanism of fluid production. For example, tumors may cause bleeding, lymphatic obstruction, or necrosis with inflammation.

Causes of Pleural Effusion

Transudates

CHF (generally biventricular)
Pericardial disease
Hypoalbuminemia
    Liver disease (ascites also has to be
      evident)
    Protein-losing enteropathy
    Renal disease
    Glomerulonephritis
    Amyloidosis
Other sources of protein loss
Overinfusion of IV fluids
Lymphatic dysplasia or ectasia

Modified Transudates and Obstructive Effusions

CHF or pericardial disease
Neoplastic obstruction
Long-standing transudation
Atelectasis
Diaphragmatic hernia
Lung lobe torsion
Postthoracotomy or chest drainage
Pulmonary embolus
Lymphatic obstruction or dilation

Chylous Effusions

Ruptured thoracic duct
Lymphatic dysplasia (dilation)
Chronic CHF (cardiomyopathy, pericardial
    disease)
Trauma
Lymphatic obstruction (neoplasia)
Pericardial disease/heart-base tumors
Thoracic neoplasia

Inflammatory Effusions (Exudative)

Bacterial infection (idiopathic) pyothorax
    Anaerobic
    Aerobic

Extension of infection from
    Trachea, bronchi, lung
    Esophagus
    Thoracic wall
    Penetrating foreign body
Sterile inflammatory effusions
    Previous infection
    Steatitis
    Surgery or chest drain
    Trauma
    Diaphragmatic hernia
    Pleuritis
    Pancreatitis
Pyogranulomatous effusion
    FIP

Neoplastic Effusions

Inflammatory
Obstructive
Hemorrhagic
Tumor cells may or may not be detected.

Hemorrhagic Effusions

Trauma
Coagulopathy
Lung lobe torsion
Neoplasia

Clinical Diagnostic Approach

1. Pleural effusions can be small, detectable only by roentgenography or ultrasonography, or they may be large, resulting in dramatic clinical signs. Tachypnea, distress, cyanosis, open-mouthed breathing, muffling of heart and lung sounds, and orthopnea are the clinical signs of pleural effusion. Dyspneic patients should undergo immediate thoracocentesis as a therapeutic and diagnostic procedure. Stable patients first undergo roentgenography to determine the optimal site for thoracocentesis. Dorsoventral roentgenograms should be substituted for ventrodorsal views, because struggling may initiate respiratory arrest.

2. Complete a thorough physical examination to detect abnormalities that may be associated with pleural effusion. For instance, cardiac murmurs, gallops, arrhythmias, or jugular venous distention suggest an underlying cardiovascular disorder. In a cat, active chorioretinitis suggests an underlying viral cause, such as FeLV-related disease or FIP. The detection of mammary tumors is suggestive of metastatic neoplasia with pleural involvement. Unilateral heart sounds may indicate a diaphragmatic hernia. A noncompressible cranial chest in cats is associated with thymic lymphosarcoma and concurrent pleural effusion.

3. Obtain roentgenograms to determine the presence and extent of fluid accumulation; any underlying cardiac, mediastinal, or pulmonary lesions; and the optimal site for thoracocentesis. Drain large effusions bilaterally and as completely as possible to permit visualization of the thoracic viscera and to allow more complete cardiac auscultation.

4. Perform thoracocentesis. Fluid is cultured (aerobic and anaerobic tests in the case of inflammatory exudate); analyzed for specific gravity, protein concentration, LDH values, and white blood cell (WBC) count (per mm^3); and centrifuged for sediment analysis, as described by Creighton and Wilkins.[29,74] Consultation with an experienced clinical pathologist is recommended because reactive mesothelial cells appear to be neoplastic to the uninformed. Categorize the effusion and seek an underlying etiology. Often, roentgenograms and fluid analysis will provide the diagnosis.

5. Collect blood and urine. Of particular importance in patients with transudates are determinations of serum protein, albumin/globulin (A/G) ratio, urine protein concentration, and hematologic evidence of hemorrhage or inflammation. Compare serum to effusate triglycerides and cholesterol[43] if chylothorax is suspected. Chyle is high in triglycerides. Liver function tests, ultrasonography, and abdominal roentgenograms are helpful in evaluating the animal for liver disease when there is concurrent ascites.

6. An ECG and echocardiogram are useful if you suspect cardiovascular disease. As a general rule, pleural effusion is most common in cats with biventricular CHF (e.g., cardiomyopathy) and in dogs with pericardial disease, atrial fibrillation, and severe pulmonic stenosis, but is uncommon in animals with heartworm disease or chronic valvular disease when there is sinus rhythm.

7. Determination of central venous pressure (CVP) may help rule out pericardial disease[83] (see the section on elevated venous pressure that follows).

8. Blood tests for FeLV and FIP serum titers may be useful.

9. If the mediastinum is widened and a mass is suspected, request thoracic ultrasonography and/or employ fine-needle aspiration biopsy and cytology to check for lymphosarcoma or thymoma.[10,11,74]

10. Lymphangiography is useful in the diagnosis of lymphatic disorders and chylothorax.[15,42,45,64,100] Thoracotomy is necessary for diagnosis in some cases. Lung lobe torsion, diaphragmatic hernia, constrictive pericardium, thymoma, esophageal lesions, solitary primary tumors, chylothorax, and other disorders may require surgical treatment. Diagnosis is substantiated at the time of surgery.

Treatment

1. The causes of pleural effusion are so diverse that a definitive diagnosis is needed for successful management of most cases.[9,11,29,72,74]

2. Thoracocentesis is indicated in life-threatening pleural effusion from any cause. Chest drainage tubes or surgery may be needed for management of pyothorax[9]; alternatively, pleurovenous shunting may be useful for chylothorax.[15,42,43,45,64,100]

3. Transudate and modified transudates usually decrease in volume if the underlying disorder (e.g., heart failure, hypoproteinemia) is treated.

4. Treatment of FIP- or FeLV-associated lymphosarcoma is attempted in some cases.[19,29]

5. Whole blood transfusion, vitamin K_1, or fresh plasma or platelet transfusions may be indicated in the management of pleural hemorrhage. Autotransfusion does occur from the pleural space, and can be used with blood obtained by chest drainage in certain cases.

6. As previously noted, surgery may be curative.

7. Other modes of therapy should be directed at the primary disorder.

8. Pleurodesis is a method of last resort for controlling pleural effusion.[14]

Pulmonary Edema

Definition

1. Pulmonary edema refers to the accumulation of abnormal quantities of liquid and solute in the lung. Edema can accumulate in the pulmonary connective tissue (interstitial edema) or in the alveoli and terminal airspaces (alveolar edema).[46,96]

2. Pulmonary edema is a common cause of the increased interstitial and alveolar pulmonary densities seen on thoracic roentgenograms.

3. Alveolar edema usually results in clinical abnormalities, including dyspnea, cyanosis, pulmonary crackles, coughing, and hypoxemia.

4. Pulmonary edema can occur secondary to many disorders, including both cardiogenic and noncardiogenic causes. As indicated in Figure 9-9, the forces responsible for normal fluid movement in the terminal lung unit may be summarized as follows:

A. Capillary hydrostatic pressure—Increases can result in pulmonary edema.

B. Pulmonary capillary oncotic pressure—Decreases can result in pulmonary edema.

C. Lymphatic flow—Obstruction of pulmonary lymphatic flow may lead to pulmonary edema.

D. Pulmonary alveolar-capillary membrane permeability—Increases in permeability lead to pulmonary edema of high protein content.

E. Other factors play a role in pulmonary circulatory dynamics.

5. Table 9-5 lists the various causes of pulmonary edema in small animal patients.

Clinical Diagnostic Approach

1. Previous information included in the earlier section on cough and respiratory distress is germane to the clinical approach to pulmonary edema.

2. The medical history may provide important clues to the cause of pulmonary edema. Explore the possibilities of advancing heart failure, aspiration of gastric contents, trauma, electric shock, near-drowning, overinfusion of fluids, and adverse reactions to drugs or insect bites.

3. The physical examination should be identical to that described earlier in the section on respiratory distress.

4. Obtain thoracic roentgenograms. The distinction between cardiogenic and noncardiogenic pulmonary edema is significant. Cardiac edema is usually observed with left

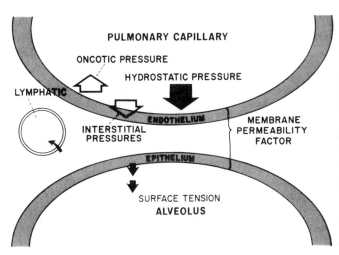

Figure 9-9. *Mechanisms of pulmonary edema. Pulmonary edema can result from increased capillary hydrostatic pressure, decreased plasma oncotic pressure, lymphatic obstruction, or altered capillary endothelial-alveolar epithelial membrane permeability. See text for a description of the common causes of these changes. (Bonagura JD: Pulmonary edema. In Kirk RW (ed): Current Veterinary Therapy VII, p. 245. Philadelphia, WB Saunders, 1980)*

Table 9-5. **Causes of pulmonary edema**

Mechanism or Etiology	Comments
Increased pulmonary capillary pressure	
Cardiogenic	Multiple causes of left ventricular failure
Noncardiogenic	
Pulmonary veno-occlusive disease	Not well described in animals
Overinfusion of crystalloid fluids or blood	
Decreased plasma oncotic pressure (hypoproteinemia)	Usually requires an additional mechanism
Hepatic disease	Inadequate protein synthesis
Renal disease	Protein loss secondary to glomerulonephritis or amyloidosis
Protein-losing enteropathies	Caused by lymphangiectasia, or inflammatory/neoplastic bowel disease
Nutritional disorders	
Altered alveolar-capillary permeability	
Infectious pulmonary disease	Protein content of edema very high
"Toxic" damage to membrane	
Inhaled toxins	Smoke inhalation, aspiration of gastric contents
Circulating exogenous toxins	Snake venom, alphanaphthyl thiourea (ANTU), paraquat, endotoxins, monocrotaline
Circulating endogenous toxins	Uremia, pancreatitis, vasoactive substances released from thrombosis or shock
Drowning and near-drowning	Direct flooding of alveolus with secondary atelectasis and edema related to tonicity of water (fresh vs. salt) and damage to membrane
Disseminated intravascular coagulation (e.g., secondary to heat stroke)	Microembolic damage of capillary endothelial membrane
Immunologic reactions and anaphylaxis	Drug and blood transfusion reactions
Shock and nonpulmonary trauma	"Shock lung;" noncardiogenic pulmonary edema possibly related to release of chemicals or tissue components into the circulation
Pulmonary contusion	
Aspiration of gastric contents	Increased mortality if pH < 2.5
Oxygen toxicity	$> 100\%$ O_2 for 24–48 h
Lymphatic insufficiency	From neoplastic infiltration
Mixed or undetermined causes	
Neurogenic	Seizure disorders, head trauma, electrical shock through brain stem
Electrocution and cardioversion	
Drug-induced (?)	? ketamine HCl, anesthetic agents
Rapid removal of pleural fluid associated with reduction of diaphragmatic hernia	Expands atelectatic lung, favors pulmonary capillary ultrafiltration, and alters surface tension

From Bonagura JD: Pulmonary edema. In Kirk RW (ed): Current Veterinary Therapy VII. Philadelphia, WB Saunders, 1980 atrial enlargement, pulmonary venous (and possibly arterial) distention, and a perihilar (often right > left-sided), caudal distribution. Fulminant edema or CHF in cats may lead to diffuse or predominantly right caudal alveolar lung infiltration. Noncardiac edema is often generalized, and often peripheral in location. Right-sided cardiac enlargement with prominent lobar arteries may be observed. Analysis of thoracic roentgenograms, in conjunction with history, physical examination, and electrocardiographic findings, usually permits the identification of cardiogenic edema.

5. Obtain an ECG and echocardiogram.

6. Analyze arterial blood gases, if they are available. This analysis permits more accurate assessment of ventilation and diffusion capacity of the lung.

7. Elevated capillary pulmonary wedge pressures indicate untreated cardiogenic pulmonary edema.

Treatment

1. General therapeutic measures
   A. Reduction of activity by cage rest
   B. Sedation
2. Measures to improve gas exchange
   A. Oxygen therapy[39]
   B. Bronchodilator therapy[76]
   C. Endotracheal suction, if needed
   D. Ventilator therapy[72,78]
3. Measures to reduce pulmonary capillary pressure
   A. Administration of furosemide
   B. Positive inotropic agents (digitalis glycosides, dobutamine hydrochloride) if congestive heart failure exists
   C. Control of cardiac arrhythmias, if present
   D. Vasodilator therapy (nitroglycerine ointment, sodium nitroprusside, hydralazine, enalopril, captopril) if cardiogenic edema is noted
4. Other therapy
   A. High-dose, short-term, corticosteroid therapy may be useful in treating some causes of permeability pulmonary edema.
   B. See the earlier section on therapy, included under the heading of Congestive

Heart Failure, for information concerning management of CHF.

Cardiac Arrhythmias

Definitions

1. The normal sequence of electrical activation of the heart (Fig. 9-10) begins in the sinoatrial (SA) node, and subsequently spreads to:
   A. Atrial and special internodal (SA to AV) pathways
   B. AV node, bundle of His, and bundle branches
   C. Specialized ventricular conduction pathways (bundle branches, fascicles, Purkinje network)
   D. Ventricular myocardium
2. Electrocardiographic analogues
   A. P wave (atrial depolarization)
   B. PR (Q) interval (time for spread of impulse from SA node, through AV node, to onset of ventricular activation)
   C. QRS (ventricular depolarization)
   D. ST-T (ventricular repolarization)
3. Normal rhythms in the dog and cat are sinus rhythm and sinus arrhythmia (less common in cats).[35,93] Sinus rhythm causes regular activation of the heart with normal P waves and (if electrical conduction is normal) normal intervals and QRS-T configuration. Sinus arrhythmia is characterized by irregular impulse formation. The irregularity is cyclic, gradual, and often related to phases of ventilation (Fig. 9-11). Because sinus arrhythmia is vagally mediated, there can be cyclic changes in the P wave configuration ("wandering atrial pacemaker") and PR interval. These alterations are normal variants and should not be confused with atrial premature complexes. In some dogs, particularly puppies, 2° AV block is normal.

4. A cardiac arrhythmia is an abnormality of impulse formation (secondary to increased automaticity of reentry) or impulse conduction (Table 9-6). Examples of the former are atrial, junctional, and ventricular premature impulses. Conduction disturbances include atrial standstill and AV blocks.

(text continues)

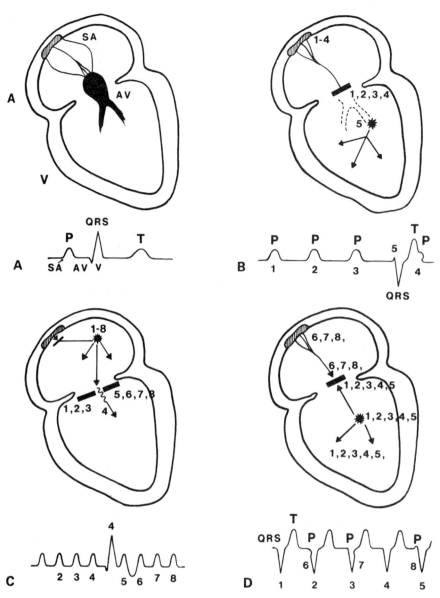

Figure 9-10. *Mechanisms of atrioventricular dissociation. (A) The normal atrioventricular conduction pathways are shown. The impulse is initiated in the sinoatrial (SA) node, spreads through internodal pathways to the atrioventricular (AV) node and then enters the ventricles through the bundle branches. (B) Complete AV block as a result of anatomic dissociation of the atria and ventricles. Sinus node impulses result in atrial activation (1–4), but all impulses are blocked in the AV nodal region. The ventricle is activated by a ventricular escape focus (5). (C) Physiologic AV block as a result of AV nodal refractoriness to rapid impulse information in the atria. The atria are activated by an ectopic atrial pacemaker (atrial tachycardia) or circuit movement (atrial flutter). Most atrial impulses arrive at the AV node when the node is refractory owing to partial conduction of previous impulses (concealed conduction). Most impulses are blocked (1–3, 5–8), with only an occasional impulse (4) being conducted to the ventricles. This type of dissociation is a normal response of the AV node to rapid atrial activation. (An additional P wave occurs simultaneously with QRS,*

Table 9-6. **Clinical associations of common arrhythmias**

Rhythm	*Clinical Association(s)*
Sinus rhythms	
Sinus rhythm	Normal, but can be associated with other disorders of impulse formation or conduction
Sinus arrhythmia	Normal; secondary to vagotonia; less common in cats
Sinus bradycardia	High vagal tone; increased CSF pressure; head trauma; brain stem lesions; hyperkalemia; hypothermia; low-output heart failure; drugs; hypothyroidism
Sinus tachycardia	High sympathetic tone; anticholinergic drugs; pain, excitement, fright; fever; hypothermia; hypotension; hypovolemia; hyperthyroidism; chocolate toxicosis
Supraventricular ectopic rhythms	
Atrial and AV junctional premature depolarizations (= impulses, "beats," complexes)	Chronic myocardial disease, particularly valvular insufficiency, congenital heart disease, cardiomyopathy; hypoxia; chronic pulmonary disease; digitalis intoxication; drugs; "toxemia"
Supraventricular (atrial and AV junctional) tachycardia	Same for atrial and AV junctional premature depolarizations; accessory AV pathways; electrocution; electrolyte disorder
Junctional escapes or escape rhythm	A secondary rhythm, the result of normal protective mechanisms; SA block or arrest; sinus bradycardia; AV block
Atrial dysrhythmias	
Atrial flutter or fibrillation	Atrial disease; chronic AV valvular insufficiency; cardiomyopathy; long-standing congenital heart disease
Atrial standstill	Hyperkalemia (Addison's disase, urinary obstruction); persistent atrial standstill as part of a generalized muscular dystrophy or myocarditis
AV blocks	
First-degree	Vagotonia; digitalis; xylazine; AV nodal disase; doxorubicin; cardiomyopathy
Second-degree	Same as for first-degree; also normal in some dogs; high-grade ($> 3 : 1$ QRS) block usually indicative of AV junctional disease
Third-degree (complete)	AV nodal disease; infarcts; endocarditis; replacment with connective tissue; neoplasia; cardiomyopathy; senile degeneration
Ventricular ectopia	
Ventricular escapes or escape rhythm	Same as for junctional escapes
Ventricular extrasystoles, accelerated (enhanced) ventricular rhythm, and ventricular tachycardia	Hypokalemia; hypoxia; autonomic imbalance; myocardial ischemia and hypoxia; heart failure; cardiomyopathy; endomyocarditis; trauma; neoplasia; pyometra; gastric dilatation/torsion; pancreatitis; acidosis; pulmonary disease; drugs and anesthetics; organic heart disease

Key: *CSF,* cerebrospinal fluid; *AV,* atrioventricular; *SA,* sinoatrial

---

but is omitted for purposes of clarity). (D) AV dissociation secondary to ventricular tachycardia. An ectopic ventricular focus rapidly activates the ventricle, resulting in abnormal QRS-T complexes (1–5). Sinoatrial impulses are blocked (6, 7, 8) owing to interference in the AV junctional region. The primary abnormality is increased ventricular automaticity.

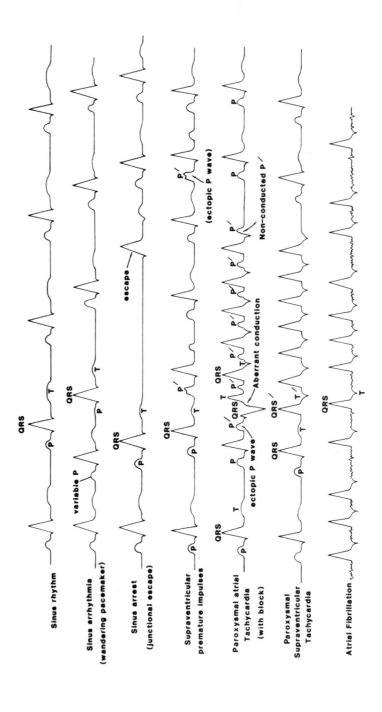

Sinus rhythm

Sinus arrhythmia
(wandering pacemaker)

Sinus arrest
(junctional escape)

Supraventricular
premature impulses

Paroxysmal atrial
Tachycardia
(with block)

Paroxysmal
Supraventricular
Tachycardia

Atrial Fibrillation

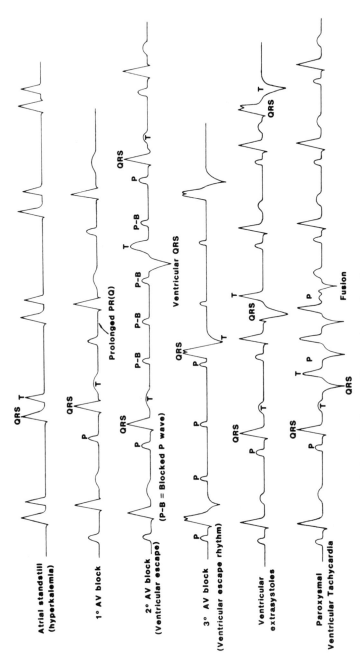

Figure 9-11. *Common cardiac rhythm disturbances. See text for explanation.*

A. Arrhythmias arise when there is either an absence of impulse formation or usurpation of the pacemaker role by an ectopic pacemaker focus or as a result of circuit movement of the impulse (reentry). In sinoatrial arrest, the normal pacemaker stops. In ventricular tachycardia, the SA node is normal but cannot drive the ventricles owing to the presence of an ectopic, dominating ventricular pacemaker (see Fig. 9-10).

B. Conduction blocks can be of primary clinical significance; for example, complete AV block often causes syncope. Other conduction disturbances, such as the bundle branch and fascicular blocks, do not cause clinical signs, yet they may indicate significant myocardial disease.

C. Abnormalities in the P wave or QRS complex occur also as a result of cardiac chamber enlargement. These changes do not indicate primary electrical problems.

Clinical Diagnostic Approach

1. Rhythm disturbances may be recognized by careful analysis of the ECG. The clinician, by identifying certain problems noted on the ECG, can correctly interpret most electrocardiographic studies. To this end, some of the ECG abnormalities that are associated frequently with cardiac arrhythmias are:

A. Abnormal ventricular rate
B. Irregular QRS (R-R) or P-P intervals
C. Lack of distinct P waves
D. More or fewer P waves than QRS-T complexes
E. Lack of consistent P to QRS-T relationship
F. Abnormality of P wave or QRS-T configuration or duration, or both
G. Abnormal P-R or Q-T interval
2. When any of these problems are noted, a long ECG rhythm strip is studied. The clinician examines the record for:

A. Repetitive patterns or cycles
B. Gradual changes versus abrupt changes
C. Relative rates and intervals of the atrial (P) and ventricular (QRS) complexes
D. The possibility of ventricular fusion, cardiomegaly, bundle branch block, or aberrant ventricular conduction whenever abnormal QRS-T complexes are detected
E. The predominant or underlying rhythm

3. The following discussion concentrates on the diagnosis of common dysrhythmias based on the detection of the aforementioned problems. It is assumed that the reader is familiar with the ECG features of common rhythm disturbances, which are described in detail in other texts.[35,93] Most of these disorders are diagrammed in Figure 9-11. Common ECG/clinicopathologic correlations are listed in Table 9-6, and the usual mode of treatment for each disturbance is set forth in Tables 9-7 and 9-8. As treatment of cardiac arrhythmias must be individualized according to the patient and the clinical situation, the idea of a "cookbook" approach to therapy for rhythm disorders is discouraged. Before embarking on antiarrhythmic treatment, the clinician must define and determine the clinical importance of the disturbance and be familiar with relevant pharmacologic principles. This is imperative if patients are receiving a regimen involving multiple drugs.

Abnormal Ventricular Rate

1. The normal ventricular rate for dogs varies from 60 to 180/min; smaller breeds have higher heart rates. In cats, the ventricular rate is usually between 160 and 240/min.

2. Decreased ventricular rate (bradycardia) is associated with:

A. Sinus bradycardia
B. Sinus arrest or sinus block with escape rhythm (AV junctional or ventricular)
C. AV blocks, with or without escape rhythms
D. Hyperkalemia, leading to sinus bradycardia, sinoventricular rhythm, or SA block. Secondary idiojunctional or idioventricular escape rhythms can result.
E. Persistent atrial standstill with escape rhythm

3. Increased ventricular rate (tachycardia) is associated with:

A. Sinus tachycardia
B. Atrial, junctional, or supraventricular tachycardia (paroxysmal or nonparoxysmal)
C. Atrial flutter and fibrillation
D. Ventricular tachycardia

Table 9-7. **Initial treatment of cardiac arrhythmias**

Arrhythmia	First	Second	Third
Supraventricular			
Sinus bradycardia	Atropine	Dopamine	Epinephrine
Premature atrial depolarizations	Digitalis	Propanolol	Diltiazem
Atrial tachycardia*	Vagal maneuver	Digitalis	Calcium channel blocker
Atrial fibrillation† or flutter	Digitalis	Diltiazem	Propanolol
Atrioventricular			
Junctional tachycardia*	Vagal maneuver	Digitalis (unless a cause)	Propranolol or quinidine
High-grade 2° and 3° heart block	Atropine	Dopamine	Pacemaker (transvenous)
Ventricular			
Extrasystoles	Lidocaine	Procainamide	Propranolol
secondary to digitalis	Lidocaine	Phenytoin	Potassium chloride
Ventricular tachycardia			

* Atrial and junctional (supraventricular) reentrant tachycardias are best treated with verapamil or digoxin if there is concurrent congestive heart failure (CHF).

† Acute atrial tachyarrhythmias that are not associated with CHF can be treated with quinidine.

Table 9-8. **Treatment of chronic cardiac arrhythmias**

Arrhythmia	First	Second	Third
Supraventricular			
Sick sinus syndrome (sinoatrial arrest)	Pacemaker	—	—
Premature atrial depolarizations	Digitalis	Propranolol**	Diltiazem
Atrial tachycardia	Digitalis	Propranolol	Diltiazem
Atrial fibrillation or flutter	Digitalis	Diltiazem	Propranolol
Atrioventricular (AV)			
Junctional tachycardia	Digitalis	Propranolol	Quinidine
Complete (3°) AV block	Pacemaker		
Ventricular*			
Ventricular extrasystoles	Procainamide, Quinidine, Tocainide, Mexiletine, beta-blocker		
Paroxysmal ventricular tachycardia	Procainamide, Quinidine, Tocainide, Mexiletine, beta-blocker		
Ventricular tachycardia	Procainamide, Quinidine, Tocainide, Mexiletine, beta-blocker		

* Choice of drug depends on experience during acute management, concomitant drug therapy, and myocardial function.

** Or other beta-blocker.

Irregular P-P or R-R Intervals

1. Associated with abnormal pacemaker activity

    A. Sinus arrhythmia (normal)

    B. Premature atrial, junctional, or ventricular complexes

    C. Sinus arrest

2. Irregular AV conduction secondary to:

    A. AV block (slow or normal heart rate)

    B. Atrial fibrillation or atrial flutter

    C. Atrial tachycardia with physiologic AV block

Absence of P Waves

1. Associated with abnormal atrial activity
   A. Sinus arrest or SA block
   B. Atrial fibrillation (if waves) or atrial flutter (F waves)
   C. Atrial standstill
      1) Hyperkalemia
      2) Persistent atrial standstill
2. Superimposition of QRS on P waves ("buried P waves")
   A. AV junctional rhythm with simultaneous retrograde atrial and anterograde ventricular activation
   B. AV dissociation from junctional or ventricular tachycardia
3. Inapparent or isoelectric P waves in a particular ECG lead (common in cats)
4. Sinus tachycardia (P waves superimposed on T waves)

More or Fewer P Waves Than QRS-T Complexes

1. More P waves
   A. AV block (see Fig. 9-10*B*)
   B. Atrial tachycardia with physiologic AV block (see Fig. 9-10*C*)
   C. Atrial premature impulses nonconducted to ventricles
2. Fewer P waves
   A. Sinus arrest with escape rhythm (absent retrograde conduction)
   B. AV junctional or ventricular tachycardia

Lack of P to QRS-T Relationship

1. When P waves are not associated with QRS-T complexes, there is either altered AV conduction, ectopic junctional or ventricular rhythm, or both (see Fig. 9-10).
   A. In primary AV conduction disorders, atrial impulses may be blocked, thus preventing them from reaching the ventricles. Some P waves are not associated with QRS-T complexes, and escape complexes are not associated with P waves. Second-degree AV block is an example. The ventricular rate is typically slow.
   B. Ectopic rhythms originating in the junction or ventricle can cause the AV junction to depolarize prematurely, preventing

anterograde conduction of sinus impulses. If the ectopic focus does not depolarize the atria in retrograde fashion, the result is AV dissociation (see Fig. 9-10*D*). The atria (driven by the sinus mode) and the ventricles (discharged by the ectopic impulse) are never related during the period of rhythm disturbance. Thus, the P waves and QRS-T complexes are unrelated except by chance. This is found with digitalis toxicosis.
   C. Dissociation of P and QRS-T complexes is often short-lived, particularly if the sinus node is able to capture the ventricle and dominate the ectopic focus (see Fig. 9-11).
2. Supraventricular ectopia may lead to isolated P waves that are not associated with QRS-T complexes. This results from physiologic refractoriness of the AV node, which is unable to conduct some premature impulses (see Fig. 9-10*C*). The ventricular rate is normal to increased, and the atrial rate is rapid, often greater than 300/min.

Abnormal P-QRS-T Configuration

1. An abnormal configuration of the P-QRS-T complex results from abnormal activation of the atria or ventricles. Ectopia, conduction disturbances, and cardiomegaly lead to abnormal complexes.
2. Abnormal P waves result from:
   A. Atrial or junctional ectopia (usually associated with a normal QRS-T complex)
   B. Atrial enlargement
      1) P-mitrale (widened, often notched P waves associated with left atrial enlargement or right atrial conduction delay)
      2) P-pulmonale (peaked, often widened P waves associated with either right or left atrial enlargement)
3. Abnormal QRS complexes result from:
   A. Ventricular ectopia
   B. Bundle branch or fascicular block
      1) Right bundle branch block results in widened complexes and right axis deviation (terminal ventricular activation in leads I and aV$_F$ is primarily negative), as shown in Figure 9-12.
      2) Left anterior fascicular block results in left axis deviation (terminal ventric-

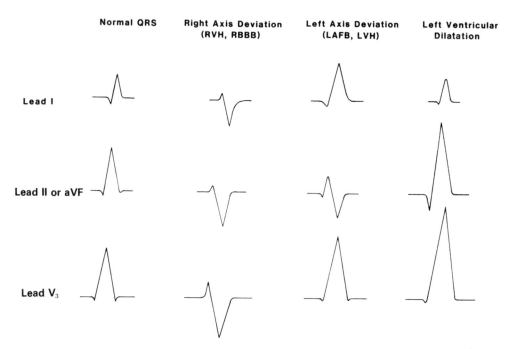

| Normal QRS | Right Axis Deviation (RVH, RBBB) | Left Axis Deviation (LAFB, LVH) | Left Ventricular Dilatation |

Lead I

Lead II or aVF

Lead V₃

Figure 9-12. *Electrocardiographic (ECG) configurations associated with heart disease. Typical configurations of the QRS complexes in various ECG leads associated with cardiomegaly or conduction disturbances are demonstrated. Right ventricular hypertrophy (RVH) and right bundle branch block (RBBB) result in a right axis deviation with typical S waves in leads I, aV$_F$, and V$_3$. Left ventricular concentric hypertrophy (LVH) and (possibly) left anterior fascicular block (LAFB) lead to a left axis deviation with R waves of increased amplitude in leads I and V$_3$ and with terminal negative forces in aV$_F$. Left ventricular dilatation (with hypertrophy) typically causes a normal frontal axis with R waves of increased voltage in leads II and aV$_F$*

ular activation in leads I and aV$_L$ is positive, whereas in aV$_F$, it is negative).

3) Left bundle branch block results in normal or left axis deviation with widened QRS complexes.

4) Abnormal QRS complexes lead to widened, abnormal T waves (secondary T wave changes). The resultant QRS-T complex may be misinterpreted as ventricular in origin.

5) Transient or phasic aberrant ventricular conduction secondary to bundle branch block can complicate supraventricular ectopia and atrial fibrillation (see Fig. 9-11)

C. Cardiomegaly (see Fig. 9-12)

1) Right ventricular hypertrophy leads to right axis deviation and prominent S waves in leads I, II, aV$_F$, and V$_3$.

2) Left ventricular hypertrophy leads to increased voltages in leads II and aV$_F$, and sometimes in lead I.

3) Secondary T wave changes are common.

4. The ST-T segment is frequently abnormal. Changes can be primary repolarization abnormalities or alterations that are secondary to abnormal depolarization. Hyperkalemia, for example, leads to primary repolarization changes, whereas the large, widened T wave that follows a ventricular extrasystole is secondary to abnormal ventricular activation. Prominent causes of ST-T changes include:

A. Left ventricular hypertrophy (covering, slurring, depression)

B. Myocardial ischemia (elevation or depression)

C. Pericarditis (elevation)

D. Hypoxia and hyperkalemia (negative or positive peaking, or tenting)

E. Digitalis (hammocking, depression)

F. Miscellaneous causes of nonspecific ST-T changes

    1) Electrolytes (K, Ca)

    2) Exercise

    3) Sympathetic tone

    4) Anesthetics

    5) Hypothermia

Abnormal PR and Q-T Intervals

1. Abnormal PR(Q) interval

A. The shortened PR interval results from ventricular preexcitation or, more commonly, from AV dissociation.

    1) Ventricular rhythm with fusion (see Fig. 9-11)

    2) Unrelated, coincidental (unconducted) P waves

    3) Preexcitation

        a) Wolff-Parkinson-White syndrome

        b) Lown-Ganong-Levine

B. A prolonged PR(Q) interval is diagnostic for 1° AV block secondary to:

    1) Vagotonia

    2) Digitalis or other drugs (beta-blockers, calcium channel blockers, xylazine, doxorubicin, procainamide, quinidine)

    3) AV nodal disease

    4) Physiologic refractoriness or concealed conduction

2. The Q-T interval varies inversely with the heart rate and should be corrected for instantaneous R-R interval. Hyperkalemia and hypercalcemia can shorten the Q-T interval; hypocalcemia and hypothermia may prolong it.

Treatment

1. Treatment of cardiac arrhythmias must be individualized according to the patient and the clinical circumstances.[16,18,35,70,71,85–87,93,97] In some situations, arrhythmias are important clues to underlying disorders, but require no treatment. In other cases, such as in complete AV block, multifocal ventricular tachy-cardia, or atrial standstill, the arrhythmia requires prompt management.

2. Important management considerations

A. Hemodynamic state—Hypotension, oliguria, weakness, and syncope are indications for therapy.

B. Electrolyte status—Hypokalemia in particular predisposes the animal to arrhythmias and can render them refractory to therapy.

C. Ventricular rate—In dogs, ventricular tachycardia with rates exceeding 140/min is particularly likely to cause hypotension.

D. Multifocal ventricular rhythms and ectopic QRS on the previous T wave (R on T) indicate vulnerability to ventricular fibrillation and should be treated promptly.

E. Left ventricular function—Decreased myocardial function, as in patients with cardiomyopathy, is an indication to control concurrent cardiac arrhythmias.

F. Anesthetized patients are less tolerant of arrhythmias.

3. Life-threatening arrhythmias are managed initially by IV therapy. For example, postoperative canine patients with ventricular tachycardia receive (in the order given):

A. IV lidocaine or procainamide bolus(es)

B. Constant-rate IV infusion of the drug

C. IM and oral maintenance antiarrhythmic drugs

4. The usual treatment of acute and chronic cardiac arrhythmias in the dog is outlined in Tables 9-6 and 9-7. The clinician should be cognizant of recent developments in antiarrhythmic therapy; many new drugs are being tested and are available for use. For example, verapamil may be highly effective therapy for acute supraventricular tachycardia.

5. Combination therapy (e.g., procainamide plus a beta-blocker) may be required. Choose drugs from separate classes. For example, Lidocaine (class 1B) and procainamide (1A) may be used together.

Elevated Venous Pressure

Definition

1. The venous pressure is an important determinant of venous return and ventricular filling.

A. The systemic venous pressure is estimated by assessing jugular venous distention and pulsation relative to the level of the right atrium, and is measured by placing a catheter into an intrathoracic vein or the right atrium. This CVP reflects the right ventricular filling pressure.

B. The left ventricular filling pressure cannot be accurately estimated from the CVP, but must be assessed by insertion of a catheter into the pulmonary artery. The catheter is advanced until it is wedged into a peripheral arterial branch. At this point, the pulmonary capillary wedge (PCW) pressure (a correlate of left atrial pressure) is recorded.

2. Venous pressure is not routinely measured in clinical practice. However, its determination can be of value in establishing certain diagnoses.

A. Pericardial effusion/constriction
B. Right atrial tumors
C. Cardiomyopathy
D. Cardiogenic versus noncardiogenic pulmonary edema
E. Left ventricular failure versus bronchitis with compensated heart disease

3. Most patients with untreated right-sided CHF have elevated CVP (> 12 cm H_2O). This finding is helpful when a diagnosis is not obvious, or is confused by concomitant disease.

A. Pericardial constriction can be difficult to detect; however, high venous pressure supports the diagnosis.

B. Obstruction to venous inflow, as might occur with right atrial tumors, may elevate the CVP.

C. Cardiomyopathy leads to increased venous pressure.

D. Unlike edema from increased capillary permeability, pulmonary edema from overinfusion of fluids or from heart failure is associated with elevated PCW pressure.[6]

E. Dogs with compensated valvular disease often have concomitant chronic bronchitis and pulmonary fibrosis. The clinical signs resemble symptomatic left ventricular failure. Measurement of PCW pressure may illustrate the primary problem.

4. Venous pressures must be interpreted as part of the patient's data base, not as absolute determinants of heart failure.

5. Intrapleural disease, mediastinal masses, and positive pressure ventilation may lead to increased CVP.

Other Laboratory Problems

1. Microfilaremia is usually associated with *Dirofilaria immitus* infection, although a considerable percentage of dogs have occult heartworm disease.

A. In dogs with clinical, hematologic, and roentgenographic features of dirofilariasis, a negative microfilaria test with positive heartworm antigen ELISA test is highly suggestive of heartworm disease.

B. The clinician should measure and examine filaria to distinguish *D. immitus* (width > 5.8 μm) from *Dipetalonema reconditum* (width < 5.8 μm).

C. Ivermectin, levamisole, dithiazanine iodide (Dizan), organophosphates, milbemycin, and diethylcarbamazine citrate (DEC) may clear the blood of microfilaria and may affect blood examination results.

2. Positive blood cultures should alert the clinician to the consideration of bacterial endocarditis.

3. Abnormalities of the hemogram (CBC) occur in cardiopulmonary disease.

A. Polycythemia is common in right-to-left shunts and severe chronic pulmonary disease.

B. Nucleated red blood cells (RBCs) may be present in acute pulmonary edema or severe respiratory disease. Hemangiosarcoma is associated with circulating nucleated RBCs.

C. Eosinophilia, basophilia, and monocytosis and hyperglobulinemia are common in dirofilariasis, lungworm infection, and allergic pulmonary disease.

D. Plasma protein is often low (5 to 6 g/dL) in dogs with dilated cardiomyopathy. The mechanism for this is unclear.

4. Heart disease frequently leads to mild elevations of liver enzymes and serum bile acids. Presumably, this is related to altered hepatic circulation, congestion, and hypoxia.

5. Prerenal azotemia is common in severe heart failure or in chronic heart failure treated with diuretics. Patients not receiving diuretics and with otherwise normal kidneys will concentrate their urine. Often, a moderate number of hyaline or finely granular casts will be detected in animals with acute heart failure.

6. Hypoxemia (a decrease in arterial PO_2) indicates arterial desaturation. It is frequently associated with cyanosis, as previously described.

References

1. Adams WM, Withrow SJ, Walshaw R, et al: Radiotherapy of malignant nasal tumors in 67 dogs. J Am Vet Med Assoc 191: 311–315, 1987

2. Allsion N, Willard MD, Bentinck-Smith J, et al: Nasal rhinosporidiosis in two dogs. J Am Vet Med Assoc 188: 869, 1986

3. Amis TC, Hager D, Dungworth DL, et al: Congenital bronchial cartilage hypoplasia with lobar hyperinflation (congenital lobar emphysema) in an adult pekingese. J Am Anim Hosp Assoc 23: 321–329, 1987

4. Amis TC, Haskins SC: Respiratory failure. Semin Vet Med Surg 1: 261–275, 1986

5. Anderson GI: Pulmonary cavitary lesions in the dog: A review of seven cases. J Am Anim Hosp Assoc 23: 89–94, 1987

6. Armstrong PJ: Hemoptysis. In Ford RB (ed): Clinical Signs and Diagnosis in Small Animal Practice. New York, Churchill Livingstone, 1988

7. Aron DN, Crowe DT: Upper airway obstruction: General principles and selected conditions in the dog and cat. Vet Clin North Am (Small Anim Pract) 15: 891–917, 1985

8. Barr FJ, Gibbs C, Brown PJ: The radiological features of primary lung tumors in the dog: A review of thirty-six cases. J Small Anim Pract 27: 493–505, 1986

9. Bauer T: Pyothorax. In Kirk RW (ed): Current Veterinary Therapy IX. Philadelphia, WB Saunders, 1986

10. Bauer TG: Diagnostic approach to cardiopulmonary disorders. In Kirk RW (ed): Current Veterinary Therapy X. Philadelphia, WB Saunders, 1989

11. Berkwitt L, Berzon JL: Pleural cavity diseases. In Morgan RV (ed): Handbook of Small Animal Practice. New York, Churchill Livingstone, 1988

12. Biller DS, Myer CM: Case examples demonstrating the clinical utility of obtaining both right and left lateral thoracic radiographs in small animals. J Am Anim Hosp Assoc 23: 381–386, 1987

13. Birchard SJ: A simplified method for rhinotomy and temporary rhinostomy in dogs and cats. J Am Anim Hosp Assoc 24: 69–72, 1988

14. Birchard SJ, Fossman TW, Gallagher L: Pleurodesis. In Kirk RW (ed): Current Veterinary Therapy X. Philadelphia, WB Saunders, 1989

15. Birchard SJ, Smeak DD, Fossum TW: Results of thoracic duct ligation in dogs with chylothorax. J Am Vet Med Assoc 193: 68–71, 1988

16. Bonagura JD: Therapy of atrial arrhythmias. In Kirk RW (ed): Current Veterinary Therapy X. Philadelphia, WB Saunders, 1989

17. Bonagura JD, Hamlin RL, Gaber C: Chronic respiratory disease in the dog. In Kirk RW (ed): Current Veterinary Therapy X. Philadelphia, WB Saunders, 1989

18. Bonagura JD, Muir WW: Antiarrhythmic therapy. In Tilley LP (ed): Essentials of Canine and Feline Electrocardiography, 2nd ed. Philadelphia, Lea and Febiger, 1985

19. Bonagura JD, Muir WW: Vasodilator therapy. In Kirk RW (ed): Current Veterinary Therapy IX. Philadelphia, WB Saunders, 1986

20. Bunch SE: Abdominal effusion. In Ford RB (ed): Clinical Signs and Diagnosis in Small Animal Practice. New York, Churchill Livingstone, 1988

21. Burgener DC, Clocombe RF, Zerbe CA: Lymphoplasmacytic rhinitis in five dogs. J Am Anim Hosp Assoc 23: 565–568, 1987

22. Calvert CA: Endocarditis and bacteremia. In Fox PR (ed): Canine and Feline Cardiology. New York, Churchill Livingstone, 1988

23. Calvert CA, Mahaffey MB, Lappin MR, et al: Pulmonary and disseminated eosinophilic granulomatosis in dogs. J Am Anim Hosp Assoc 24: 311–320, 1988

24. Calvert CA, Rawlings CA: Pulmonary manifestations of heartworm disease. Vet Clin North Am 15: 991–1009, 1985

25. Calvert CA, Rawlings CA: Therapy of canine heartworm disease. In Kirk RW (ed): Current Veterinary Therapy IX. Philadelphia, WB Saunders, 1986

26. Carothers M, Couto CG: Respiratory neoplasia. In Kirk RW (ed): Current Veterinary Therapy X. Philadelphia, WB Saunders, 1989

27. Carpenter JL, Myers AM, Conner MW, et al: Tuberculosis in five basset hounds. J Am Vet Med Assoc 192: 1563–1568, 1988

28. Crawford M, Robertson S, Miller R: Pulmonary complications of Cushing's syndrome: Metastatic mineralization in a dog with high dose chronic corticosteroid therapy. J Am Anim Hosp Assoc 23: 85–87, 1987

29. Creighton SR, Wilkins RJ: Pleural effusions. In Kirk RW (ed): Current Veterinary Therapy VII. Philadelphia, WB Saunders, 1980

30. Creighton SR, Wilkins RJ: Transtracheal aspiration biopsy: Technique and cytologic evaluation. J Am Anim Hosp Assoc 10: 219, 1974

31. Crystal RG, Bitterman PB, Rennard SI, et al: Interstitial lung diseases of unknown cause. N Engl J Med 310: 154–166 and 235–244, 1984

32. Dillon AR, Pechman RD, Spano JS, et al: Results of ancillary tests for respiratory disease in normal dogs. J Small Anim Pract 24: 533, 1983

33. Dobbie GR, Darke PGG, Head KW: Intrabronchial foreign bodies in dogs. J Small Anim Pract 27: 227, 1986

34. Easley JR, Meuten DJ, Levy MG, et al: Nasal rhinosporidiosis in the dog. Vet Pathol 23: 50, 1986

35. Edwards NJ: Bolton's Handbook of Canine and Feline Electrocardiography, 2nd ed. Philadelphia, WB Saunders, 1987

36. Evans AT: Cardiopulmonary resuscitation. In Fox PR (ed): Canine and Feline Cardiology. New York, Churchill Livingstone, 1988

37. Evinger JV, Kazacos KR, Cantwell HD: Ivermectin for treatment of nasal capillariasis in a dog. J Am Vet Med Assoc 186: 174, 1985

38. Fingland RB, Dehoff WD, Birchard SJ: Surgical management of cervical and thoracic tracheal collapse in dogs using extraluminal spiral prostheses: Result in seven cases. J Am Anim Hosp Assoc 23: 173, 1987

39. Fitzpatrick RK, Crowe DT: Nasal oxygen administration in dogs and cats: Experimental and clinical investigations. J Am Anim Hosp Assoc 22: 293, 1986

40. Ford RB: Sneezing and nasal discharge. In Ford RB (ed): Clinical Signs and Diagnosis in Small Animal Practice. New York, Churchill Livingstone, 1988.

41. Ford RB, Roudebush P: Chronic cough. In Ford RB (ed): Clinical Signs and Diagnosis in Small Animal Practice. New York, Churchill, Livingstone, 1988

42. Fossum TW, Birchard SJ, Arnold PA: Mesenteric lymphography and ligation of the thoracic duct in a cat with chylothorax. J Am Vet Med Assoc 187: 1036, 1985

43. Fossum TW, Jacobs RM, Birchard SJ: Evaluation of cholesterol and triglyceride concentrations in differentiating chylous and nonchylous pleural effusions in dogs and cats. J Am Vet Med Assoc 188: 49, 1986

44. Gompf RE: Heart murmur. In Ford RB (ed): Clinical Signs and Diagnosis in Small Animal Practice. New York, Churchill Livingstone, 1988

45. Harpster NK: Chylothorax. In Kirk RW (ed): Current Veterinary Therapy IX. Philadelphia, WB Saunders, 1986

46. Harpster NK: Pulmonary edema. In Kirk RW (ed): Current Veterinary Therapy X. Philadelphia, WB Saunders, 1989

47. Harvey CE: Tracheotomy and tracheostomy. In Kirk RW (ed): Current Veterinary Therapy IX. Philadelphia, WB Saunders, 1986

48. Haskins SC: Cardiopulmonary resuscitation. In Kirk RW (ed): Current Veterinary Therapy X. Philadelphia, WB Saunders, 1989

49. Haskins SC: Physical therapeutics for respiratory disease. Semin Vet Med Surg [Small Anim] 1: 276, 1986

50. Hendricks JC, O'Brien JA: Tracheal collapse in two cats. J Am Vet Med Assoc 187: 418, 1985

51. Herrtage ME, Clarke DD: Congenital lobar emphysema in two dogs. J Small Anim Pract 26: 453, 1985

52. Hirsh SC: Bacteriology of the lower respiratory tract. In Kirk RW (ed): Current Veterinary Therapy IX. Philadelphia, WB Saunders, 1986

53. Hoffmann WE, Wellman ML: Tracheobronchial cytology. In Kirk RW (ed): Current Veterinary Therapy IX. Philadelphia, WB Saunders, 1986

54. Hribernik T: Respiratory distress or difficulty. In Ford RB (ed): Clinical Signs and

Diagnosis in Small Animal Practice. New York, Churchill Livingstone, 1988

55. Jay SJ: Diagnostic procedures for pleural disease. Ann Chest Med 6: 33, 1985

56. Keene BW: Canine cardiomyopathy. In Kirk RW (ed): Current Veterinary Therapy X. Philadelphia, WB Saunders, 1989

57. Keene BW: Cardiovascular drugs. In Bonagura JD (ed): Cardiology—Contemporary Issues in Small Animal Practice. New York, Churchill Livingstone, 1987

58. Kirkpatrick CE, Megella C: Use of ivermectin in treatment of aelurostrongylus abstrusus and toxocara cati infections in a cat. J Am Vet Med Assoc 190: 1309, 1987

59. Kittleson MD: Management of heart failure: Concepts, therapeutic strategies, and drug pharmacology. In Fox PR (ed): Canine and Feline Cardiology. New York, Churchill Livingstone, 1988

60. Kraman SS: Lung sounds for the clinician. Arch Intern Med 146: 1411, 1986

61. Krotje LJ, McAllister HA, Engwall MJA, et al: Chronic obstructive pulmonary disease in a dog. J Am Vet Med Assoc 191: 1427, 1987

62. Lord PR: Radiologic examination. In Fox PR (ed): Canine and Feline Cardiology. New York, Churchill Livingstone, 1988

63. Love S, Barr A, Lucke VM, et al: A catheter technique for biopsy of dogs with chronic nasal disease. J Small Anim Pract 28: 417, 1987

64. Martin RA, Barber DL, Richards LS, et al: A technique for direct lymphangiography of the thoracic duct system in the cat. Vet Radiol 29: 116, 1988

65. McKiernan BC: Bronchoscopy in the small animal patient. In Kirk RW (ed): Current Veterinary Therapy X. Philadelphia, WB Saunders, 1989

66. Moise NS: Echocardiography. In Fox PR (ed): Canine and Feline Cardiology. New York, Churchill Livingstone, 1988

67. Moise NS, Spaulding GL: Feline bronchial asthma: Pathogenesis, pathophysiology, diagnostics, and therapeutic considerations. Compend Contin Educ Vet 3: 1091, 1981

68. Morrison WB, Wilsman NJ, Fox LE, et al: Primary ciliary dyskinesia in the dog. J Vet Intern Med 1: 67, 1987

69. Moses BL, Spaulding GL: Chronic bronchial disease of the cat. Vet Clin North Am [Small Anim Pract] 15: 929, 1985

70. Muir WW: Beta-blocking therapy in dogs and cats. In Kirk RW (ed): Current Veterinary Therapy IX. Philadelphia, WB Saunders, 1986

71. Muir WW, Sams RA: Pharmacology and pharmacokinetics of antiarrhythmic drugs. In Fox PR (ed): Canine and Feline Cardiology. New York, Churchill Livingstone, 1988

72. Murtaugh RJ, Spaulding GL: Initial management of respiratory emergencies. In Kirk RW (ed): Current Veterinary Therapy X. Philadelphia, WB Saunders, 1989

73. Neer TM, Waldron DR, Miller RI: Eosinophilic pulmonary granulomatosis in two dogs and literature review. J Am Anim Hosp Assoc 22: 593, 1986

74. Noone KE: Pleural effusions and diseases of the pleura. Vet Clin North Am [Small Anim Pract] 15: 1069, 1985

75. O'Brien JA, Buchanan JW, Kelly DF: Tracheal collapse in the dog. Vet Radiol 7: 12, 1966

76. Papich MG: Current concepts in pulmonary pharmacology. Semin Vet Med Surg [Small Anim] 1: 289, 1986

77. Parker NR, Binnington AG: Nasopharyngeal polyps in cats: Three case reports and a review of the literature. J Am Anim Hosp Assoc 21: 473, 1985

78. Pascoe PJ: Short-term ventilatory support. In Kirk RW (ed): Current Veterinary Therapy IX. Philadelphia, WB Saunders, 1986

79. Pearson GR, Lane JG, Holt PE, et al: Chondromatous hamartomas of the respiratory tract in the dog. J Small Anim Pract 28: 705, 1987

80. Phillips L, Schaer M: Idiopathic pleural effusion in a dog. J Am Vet Med Assoc 192: 788, 1988

81. Pion PD, Kittleson MD: Therapy of feline aortic thromboembolism. In Kirk RW (ed): Current Veterinary Therapy X. Philadelphia, WB Saunders, 1989

82. Pion PD, Kittleson MD, Rogers QR, et al: Cardiomyopathy in the cat and its relation to taurine deficiency. In Kirk RW (ed): Current Veterinary Therapy X. Philadelphia, WB Saunders, 1989

83. Reed JR: Pericardial diseases of the dog and cat. In Bonagura JD (ed): Cardiology—

Contemporary Issues in Small Animal Practice. New York, Churchill Livingstone, 1987

84. Saik JE, Toll SL, Diters RW, et al: Canine and feline laryngeal neoplasia. A 10-year survey. J Am Anim Hosp Assoc 22: 359, 1986

85. Schollmeyer M: Pacemaker therapy. In Fox PR (ed): Canine and Feline Cardiology. New York, Churchill Livingstone, 1988

86. Sisson DD: Bradyarrhythmias and cardiac pacing. In Kirk RW (ed): Current Veterinary Therapy X. Philadelphia, WB Saunders, 1989

87. Sisson DD: Clinical management of cardiac arrhythmias in the dog and cat. In Fox PR (ed): Canine and Feline Cardiology. New York, Churchill Livingstone, 1988

88. Suter PF: Thoracic Radiography. Wettswil, Switzerland, PF Suter, 1984

89. Suter PF, Lord PF: Radiographic differentiation of disseminated pulmonary parenchymal diseases in dogs and cats. Vet Clin North Am 4: 687, 1974

90. Tams TR: Aspiration pneumonia and complications of inhalation of smoke and toxic gases. Vet Clin North Am 15: 971, 1985

91. Tams TR: Pneumonia. In Kirk RW (ed): Current Veterinary Therapy X. Philadelphia, WB Saunders, 1986

92. Thomas WP: Pericardial disease. In Kirk RW (ed): Current Veterinary Therapy IX. Philadelphia, WB Saunders, 1986

93. Tilley LP: Essentials of canine and feline electrocardiography, 2nd ed. Philadelphia, Lea and Febiger, 1985

94. Venker-van Haagen AJ: Laryngeal diseases of dogs and cats. In Kirk RW (ed): Current Veterinary Therapy IX. Philadelphia, WB Saunders, 1986

95. Ware WA, Bonagura JD: Cardiovascular problems. In Bonagura JD (ed): Cardiology—Contemporary Issues in Small Animal Practice. New York, Churchill Livingstone, 1987

96. Ware WA, Bonagura JD: Pulmonary edema. In Fox PR (ed): Canine and Feline Cardiology. New York, Churchill Livingstone, 1988

97. Ware WA, Hamlin RL: Therapy of ventricular arrhythmias. In Kirk RW (ed): Current Veterinary Therapy X. Philadelphia, WB Saunders, 1989

98. Weiss RC, Scott FW: Feline infectious peritonitis. In Kirk RW (ed): Current Veterinary Therapy VII. Philadelphia, WB Saunders, 1980

99. Wheeldon EB, Pirie HM, Fisher EW, et al: Chronic respiratory disease in the dog. J Small Anim Pract 18: L229, 1977

100. Willauer CC, Brexnock EM: Pleurovenous shunting technique for treatment of chylothorax in three dogs. J Am Vet Med Assoc 191: 1106, 1987

101. Withrow SJ: Diagnostic and therapeutic nasal flush in small animals. J Am Anim Hosp Assoc 13: 704, 1977

CHAPTER TEN

Gastrointestinal Diseases

Donna S. Dimski and Robert G. Sherding

This chapter provides an overview of the diagnostic approaches to problems affecting the alimentary tract and abdomen. The following clinical problems are addressed:

Oral ulcers and stomatitis
Oral mass lesions
Dysphagia
Regurgitation
Vomiting
Diarrhea
Constipation
Abdominal pain
Abdominal effusion

Although guidelines for therapy are suggested, the reader is encouraged to consult with more specific references for further therapeutic recommendations. Suggested readings are provided.

Oral Ulcers and Stomatitis

Oral ulceration or stomatitis occurs when the balance between the normal flora and mucosal defenses of the oral cavity is altered. Common causes of oral disease include decreased mucosal defenses, immunosuppression, and overgrowth of pathogenic organisms.

Etiology

The common causes of oral ulceration and stomatitis in dogs and cats are listed in Table 10-1 and can be grouped as follows:

1. Decreased mucosal defense barrier—Physical abrasion, erosion, or ulceration of the mucosa may allow overgrowth of normal flora or the establishment of pathogenic flora in the oral cavity. Breakdown of the mucosa occurs with trauma, foreign bodies, viral infections, caustic chemical injury or heavy metal toxicity, immune-mediated diseases, and uremia. Dental disease may also allow an overgrowth of oral microbes.

2. Immunosuppression—Immunosuppression secondary to viral diseases, systemic diseases, or immunosuppressive therapy may permit an overgrowth of normal or pathogenic flora in the oral cavity. Examples include feline leukemia virus (FeLV) and feline immunodeficiency virus (FIV).

History and Physical Findings

1. An adequate history to evaluate the chronicity of the problem and involvement of other body systems is needed to rule out acute viral diseases (for example, feline calicivirus or herpesvirus).

2. Animals with oral disease often exhibit pain or difficulty prehending food when eating. Hypersalivation and halitosis may also be noted.

3. The oral cavity should be examined thoroughly for the presence of foreign bodies, mass lesions, lacerations, ulcers, bullae, or burns. The examiner should look under the tongue (especially in cats) for string foreign bodies. Sedation or anesthesia may be needed for a thorough examination.

Table 10-1. **Causes, diagnosis, and treatment of oral ulceration and stomatitis**

Causes	Basis for Diagnosis	Mode of Treatment
Infectious		
Feline calicivirus Feline herpesvirus	Associated evidence of fever and oculonasal discharge	Symptomatic therapy for upper respiratory infection (URI)
Feline leukemia virus (FeLV) Feline immunodeficiency virus (FIV)	ELISA tests for FeLV and FIV	Oral and systemic antimicrobial agents to manage immunosuppression
Ulcerative necrotizing stomatitis (fusobacterium, spirochetes) Nocardia stomatitis Secondary periodontitis Candida stomatitis	Cytology of ulcerated mucosa, bacterial and fungal cultures	Dental prophylaxis, cleansing of oral cavity, systemic antibiotics
Physical and chemical		
Oral foreign body (e.g., grass burrs)	Oral examination	Removal of foreign body, cleansing of oral cavity
Caustic substances (e.g., lye, acids) Thermal or electrical burns Trauma Ingestion of heavy metals (e.g., thallium)	History of exposure, oral examination	Cleansing of oral cavity, supportive care
Immune-mediated		
Pemphigus vulgaris Bullous pemphigoid Systemic lupus erythematosus (SLE)	Physical and oral examination, immunofluorescent studies of biopsy samples, ANA testing, lupus erythematosus	Immunosuppressive therapy, as indicated
Systemic diseases		
Renal failure	Serum biochemical studies	Treatment of renal failure
Immunosuppression	Tests of immune function	Oral and systemic antimicrobials
Other causes		
Feline plasma cell gingivitis/pharyngitis	Oral examination histopathologic studies	Immunosuppressives, antibiotics
Eosinophilic granuloma complex	Oral examination histopathologic studies	Glucocorticoids, progestational drugs, surgery

4. A thorough dental examination should be performed to rule out tooth root abscesses, periodontal disease, or other dental problems.

5. If immune-mediated disease is suspected, other mucocutaneous junctions should be examined for lesions.

6. Submandibular lymphadenopathy is often present in animals with chronic oral disease.

Diagnostic Approach

1. Laboratory findings

A. Mycotic cultures and impression smear cytology to detect fungal infection

B. Enzyme-linked immunosorbent assay (ELISA) to detect FeLV and FIV in cats

C. Evaluation of renal function to detect renal failure

D. Biopsy of oral lesions, including any chronic ulcerative disease or proliferative lesion, for routine histopathologic examination as well as immunofluorescent examination to detect immune-mediated disease

2. Radiographic findings

A. Evaluation of skull radiographs to diagnose invasive neoplastic diseases involving the oral cavity

B. Radiographs of the teeth and tooth roots to diagnose dental disease

Therapeutic Approach

1. Traumatic oral injuries and acute viral diseases are usually self-limiting and do not require specific treatment.

2. If oral disease is secondary, diagnosis and treatment of the underlying cause is necessary. For example, animals with periodontal disease should have appropriate dentistry performed, and animals with uremic stomatitis should be treated for renal failure.

3. Dietary support is very important. Depending on the severity and degree of pain, this may range from feeding soft food to bypassing the oral cavity via nasogastric tube feeding.

4. Cleansing of the oral cavity may facilitate the healing of many oral diseases.

A. Saline solution (0.9%)

B. Dilute chlorhexidine solution

C. Gly-Oxide (10% carbamide peroxide in anhydrous glycerol)

D. Sodium bicarbonate solution

5. Antibiotics may be indicated in primary or secondary oral infections. Penicillins and metronidazole are good choices for oral bacterial pathogens.

6. Long-term anti-inflammatory or immunosuppressive therapy may be needed for immune-mediated or idiopathic forms of stomatitis.

Oral Mass Lesions

Etiology

1. Non-neoplastic

A. Eosinophilic granuloma complex

B. Feline plasma cell gingivitis-pharyngitis

C. Gingival hyperplasia

D. Salivary mucocele

2. Benign neoplastic masses

A. Papillomatosis

B. Epulis

C. Odontogenic tumors

3. Malignant neoplastic masses

A. Squamous cell carcinoma

B. Malignant melanoma

C. Fibrosarcoma

History and Physical Findings

1. Oral mass lesions will commonly cause hypersalivation, halitosis, and difficulty in eating. Occasionally, pet owners will notice the mass lesion within their pet's mouth.

2. A thorough oral examination is needed to diagnose the presence of mass lesions. Mass lesions may be located anywhere within the oral cavity, including the lips, gingiva, sublingual area, oropharynx, and palatine tonsils.

3. Examination of the submandibular lymph nodes may reveal enlargement (secondary to metastatic disease or reaction to chronic oral inflammation).

Diagnostic Approach

1. Biopsy examination of any mass lesion of the oral cavity should be performed for histopathologic diagnosis.

2. Fine-needle aspiration of the oral lesion or of enlarged submandibular lymph nodes may be helpful in diagnosing some types of mass lesions.

Therapeutic Approach

1. Appropriate treatment of oral mass lesions depends on the cause; therefore, diagnosis is essential.

2. Many oral mass lesions are treated surgically. Salivary mucoceles require excision of the associated salivary gland and duct to prevent recurrence. Neoplastic masses may be removed surgically with wide margins. Occasionally, radical excision via partial mandibulectomy or maxillectomy may be required.

3. Adjunctive therapy may be required for some neoplastic diseases or the oral cavity, depending on tumor type. Chemotherapy, radiation therapy, and hyperthermia may be recommended by a veterinary oncologist after a diagnosis has been established.

4. Some oral mass lesions are treated medically. Immunosuppressive doses of corticosteroids or other agents are used to treat feline plasma cell gingivitis/pharyngitis and eosinophilic granuloma complex.

Dysphagia

1. *Dysphagia* is a difficulty or inability to prehend, chew, or swallow food or water. It implies structural or functional disease of the oral cavity or pharynx. Dysphagia is often accompanied by hypersalivation.

2. Dysphagia may be caused by diseases of the oral cavity (as discussed previously), or it may occur secondary to neuromuscular disease or mechanical obstruction to swallowing.

Etiology

1. Oral or pharyngeal foreign body

2. Oral or pharyngeal neoplasia

3. Pharyngeal or retropharyngeal abscess/cellulitis

4. Immune-mediated masticatory myositis (see Chapter 17)

5. Cricopharyngeal achalasia

6. Mandibular neurapraxia (idiopathic cranial nerve V paralysis) (see Chapter 17)

7. Rabies

History and Physical Findings

1. Rabies should always be considered in the evaluation of dysphagia, and a thorough vaccination and exposure history should be obtained.

2. Animals with a pharyngeal or retropharyngeal abscess or cellulitis often exhibit pain when the mouth is opened.

3. Animals with masticatory myositis may initially present with swollen, painful masticatory muscles; however, later in the disease, the muscles may fibrose and the animal may be unable to open the mouth widely.

4. Dogs with mandibular neurapraxia have a "dropped jaw" and are unable to close the mouth.

5. Animals with cricopharyngeal achalasia make repeated attempts to swallow, and regurgitation of undigested food occurs soon after eating. Aspiration pneumonia may occur secondary to regurgitation of food. Cachexia is common because of the chronic nature of the disease.

6. A thorough oral and pharyngeal examination should be performed. This may require anesthesia or sedation.

Diagnostic Approach

1. Laboratory findings

   A. A leukogram may reveal inflammatory changes in animals with a pharyngeal or retropharyngeal abscess/cellulitis.

   B. Elevated muscle enzyme levels (creatine phosphokinase, aspartine aminotransferase) may accompany masticatory myositis.

2. Radiographic findings

   A. Aspiration pneumonia may be seen with cricopharyngeal achalasia.

   B. A barium swallow study with fluoroscopy may be needed to confirm a diagnosis of cricopharyngeal achalasia.

3. Other findings

   A. Electromyography may indicate masticatory myositis or mandibular neurapraxia.

   B. Masticatory muscle biopsy confirms and characterizes myositis.

Therapeutic Approach

1. Maintenance of food intake is essential.

2. Surgical intervention may be necessary for abscesses, cricopharyngeal achalasia, or pharyngeal polyps or neoplasia. Pharyngeal foreign bodies may require anesthesia for extraction.

3. Immunosuppressive therapy with corticosteroids or other immunosuppressants is required for immune-mediated masticatory myositis.

4. Mandibular neurapraxia usually resolves within weeks if supportive alimentation is maintained.

Regurgitation

Regurgitation is the passive expulsion of a food bolus from the pharynx or esophagus. It involves only the gag reflex, with retrograde movement of food out of the oral cavity.

Etiology

Regurgitation is a sign of esophageal disease (Table 10-2). Megaesophagus is dilatation of the esophagus. Although primary or secondary causes of megaesophagus are common causes of regurgitation, other diseases of the esophagus that affect motility without resulting in obvious esophageal dilatation must also be considered.

History and Physical Findings

1. It is essential to differentiate between regurgitation and vomiting in obtaining a history, as the diagnostic approaches to and causes of each are different. Regurgitation occurs abruptly, without warning, and the preparatory events that characterize vomiting, such as hypersalivation, retching, and abdominal contractions, are absent.
2. The signalment may be helpful in identifying a cause. Idiopathic megaesophagus is most common in German shepherd dogs, Great Danes, and Irish setters. Persistent right aortic arch (PRAA) is usually recognized in young dogs shortly after weaning, and occurs most commonly in young German shepherds.
3. A history of ingestion of caustics or recent anesthesia may suggest esophagitis.
4. A travel history to the Southern United States could suggest *Spirocerca lupi* infection.
5. Horner's syndrome, or dyspnea (pleural effusion) associated with a noncompressible cranial thorax (in cats), may suggest a mediastinal mass causing esophageal obstruction.
6. Systemic signs, such as weakness, muscle atrophy, muscle pain, neurologic deficits,

or poor hair coat and obesity, may suggest a diagnosis of secondary megaesophagus.
7. Because aspiration pneumonia may occur secondary to regurgitation, a thorough auscultation of the chest for abnormal lung sounds should be performed.

Diagnostic Approach

1. Laboratory findings
  A. Leukocytosis suggests an inflammatory esophageal disease or the presence of aspiration pneumonia.
  B. Elevated muscle enzyme levels (creatine phosphokinase) may be associated with megaesophagus caused by polymyositis.
  C. Evaluation of blood lead concentration, serum acetylcholine receptor antibody titer, thyroid function, and adrenal function may be indicated in animals with megaesophagus.
  D. Fecal flotation may be performed to evalute the animal for *Spirocerca lupi* infection.
2. Radiographic findings
  A. Plain thoracic radiographs are often diagnostic of megaesophagus, PRAA, radiopaque esophageal foreign body, or external esophageal compression by a mediastinal mass. In PRAA, the esophageal dilatation occurs cranial to the base of the heart. Thoracic radiographs should also be evaluated for evidence of aspiration pneumonia.
  B. The most common sites of esophageal foreign bodies are the thoracic inlet, the base of the heart, and the diaphragmatic hiatus.
  C. Contrast studies are necessary if plain radiographs are not diagnostic. They are useful in the diagnosis of radiolucent esophageal foreign bodies, intraluminal esophageal masses, gastroesophageal intussusception, and esophageal strictures. Barium studies should be avoided if esophageal perforation is a possibility.
  D. Fluoroscopic studies are necessary to evaluate esophageal motility.
3. Endoscopy provides the greatest diagnostic information for intraluminal esophageal disease. Endoscopy is useful in visualizing strictures, foreign bodies, masses, gastro-

Table 10-2. **Causes, diagnosis, and treatment of regurgitation**

Causes	Basis for Diagnosis	Mode of Treatment
Megaesophagus	Thoracic radiography Esophageal contrast radiography	Management of feeding Mangement of pneumonia
Idiopathic	Rule out secondary causes	
Secondary		
Polymyositis	Elevated serum levels of muscle enzymes Involvement of other muscles	Immunosuppressive therapy
Myasthenia gravis	Tensilon test, acetylcholine receptor antibodies	Edrophonium chloride therapy
Lead poisoning	Elevated blood lead levels	EDTA therapy

Hypothyroidism	Thyroid-stimulating hormone
	  (TSH) stimulation test
		Thyroid hormone replacement
		  therapy

Systemic lupus erythematosus
  (SLE)
	ANA, lupus erythematosus (LE)
	  prep
	Other evidence of immunologic
	  disease
		Immunosuppressive therapy

Canine distemper	History of distemper Vaccination history	Management of feeding
Feline dysautonomia	Other autonomic dysfunction Origin in United Kingdom	Management of feeding
Hypoadrenocorticism	ACTH stimulation test	Mineralocorticoid supplementation
Persistent right aortic arch	History Esophageal contrast radiography	Corrective surgery
Esophagitis		
Gastroesophageal reflux	History of recent anesthesia Esophageal contrast fluoroscopy Esophageal endoscopy	Cimetidine, metoclopramide
Hiatal hernia	Esophageal/gastric contrast radiography	Surgical correction
Esophageal foreign body	Thoracic radiography Esophageal contrast radiography	Foreign body removal Treatment of reflux
Other esophageal disorders		
Extraluminal obstruction (masses)	Thoracic radiography	Surgical correction
Neoplasia	Thoracic radiography Esophageal contrast radiography Esophageal endoscopy	Surgical correction Adjunctive chemotherapy
Spirocerca lupi granuloma or neoplasia	Thoracic radiography Esophageal contrast radiography Fecal flotation	Surgical correction
Laceration	History of trauma or foreign body ingestion Esophageal contrast radiography Esophageal endoscopy	Medical management, as for reflux Surgical correction
Stricture	Esophageal contrast radiography Esophageal endoscopy	Breakdown of stricture (bougienage or balloon dilation) Prednisone
Gastroesophageal intussusception	Thoracic radiography Esophageal contrast radiography Esophageal endoscopy	Treatment of shock Surgical correction

esophageal intussusception, and lesions affecting the esophageal mucosa. Endoscopic biopsies may be performed to diagnose intraluminal mass lesions or esophagitis.

Therapeutic Approach

1. Idiopathic megaesophagus is managed by feeding the affected animal small, frequent meals of a blended gruel in an elevated position, and maintaining the animal in an erect posture for 10 to 15 minutes after feeding.
2. PRAA is managed surgically by ligation and separation of the ligamentum arteriosum via thoracotomy. The dilated portion of the esophagus may never regain normal motility, thus necessitating upright feeding.
3. Esophageal foreign bodies are managed by using a rigid endoscope to retrieve the foreign body through the mouth or advance it into the stomach. Endoscopic removal may not be possible if the foreign body is firmly lodged in the mucosa; in such cases, surgery is required. Gastrotomy may be useful in reaching a distal esophageal foreign body. Esophagotomy frequently results in severe stricture formation, and should be avoided if possible.
4. Esophagitis should be treated with drugs that decrease gastric acidity (antacids, cimetidine) and metoclopramide to increase the tone of the gastroesophageal junction. If the esophageal wall is damaged, antibiotics should be administered to decrease the risk of infection, and anti-inflammatory doses of corticosteroids may be given to reduce stricture formation. Severe stricture formation may be treated with esophageal bougienage or balloon dilation techniques.
5. Gastroesophageal intussusception is treated by reduction of the intussusception and gastropexy via laparotomy. Hiatal hernia is also treated by gastropexy.

Vomiting

Vomiting is a reflex act that results in the forceful expulsion of gastric contents through the oral cavity. The major clinical significance of vomiting lies in the recognition of the numerous primary diseases associated with vomiting. Whatever its cause, protracted vomiting can have serious metabolic consequences, the most important of which are sodium and potassium depletion, dehydration, and either metabolic acidosis or hypochloremic metabolic alkalosis.

Vomiting occurs whenever there is stimulation of the vomiting center in the medulla. The stimulation may be direct (e.g., elevated CSF pressure, CNS inflammation), secondary to stimulation of the chemoreceptor trigger zone (e.g., as a result of drugs, uremia, acidosis, bacterial endotoxins, vestibular input), or secondary to stimulation of peripheral receptors (vagal and sympathetic fibers) located in the gastrointestinal tract, liver, pancreas, peritoneum, urinary tract, and heart.

Etiology

1. The causes of vomiting can be grouped into primary gastrointestinal causes and secondary metabolic aberrations that result in vomiting. The major causes of vomiting and the appropriate diagnostic and therapeutic approaches for each of those causes are listed in Table 10-3.
2. Often, vomiting is a sign of an acute and transient illness or nonspecific gastrointestinal upset. In such cases, supportive care for 24 to 48 hours will result in resolution of signs without determination of a definitive diagnosis.
3. Many ingested toxins or drugs can result in acute vomiting (Table 10-4).

History and Physical Findings

1. A thorough history should be obtained, including vaccination status, parasite control, diet, exposure to other animals, and potential exposure to drugs, toxins, or foreign bodies.
2. A historical review of other body systems should be evaluated to determine whether a metabolic cause for vomiting exists. Pertinent findings may include polyuria/polydipsia, weight loss, fever, recent estrus, and the like.
3. A history of the timing of the vomiting may be helpful. Proximal obstructive gastrointestinal (GI) diseases usually result in vomit-

Table 10-3. **Causes, diagnosis, and treatment for vomiting**

Causes	Basis for Diagnosis	Mode of Treatment
Primary gastrointestinal causes		
Infectious		
Viral		
Feline panleukopenia	Signs and history	Supportive care
Canine distemper	Signs and history	Supportive care
Canine parvovirus	Fecal viral antigen test (Hemagglutination, ELISA) Leukopenia, fever History	Supportive care
Canine coronavirus	Signs and history	Supportive care
Infectious canine hepatitis	Signs and history	Supportive care
Bacterial or rickettsial		
Leptospirosis	Serum titers Urine dark field microscopy Compatible renal and hepatic disease	Penicillin, streptomycin
Salmonellosis	Culture	Systemic antibiotics
Salmon poisoning	History of salmon ingestion Fecal examination for fluke eggs Lymphadenopathy, fever	Tetracycline
Parasitic		
Intestinal nematodes	Fecal flotation	Anthelmintics
Physaloptera species	Fecal flotation Visualization of parasite in vomitus or by endoscopy	Pyrantel pamoate
Ollulanus tricuspis (cats only)	Microscopic identification of parasite larvae in vomitus	Pyrantel pamoate
Inflammatory		
Dietary indiscretion	Compatible history	Supportive care
Gastric ulceration	Blood in vomitus Fecal occult blood Endoscopy	Cimetidine Sucralfate Supportive care
Gastric neoplasm	Barium contrast GI radiography Endoscopy and biopsy	Surgical excision Adjunctive chemotherapy
Mast cell tumor (MCT)	Identification of MCT anywhere in body	Surgical removal of MCT Cimetidine Antihistamines Prednisone
Severe liver disease	Identification of liver disease (see Chapter 11) Vomiting of blood Fecal occult blood	Treatment of liver disease Cimetidine or ranitidine
Uremic gastritis	Identification of renal failure (see Chapter 12)	Treatment of renal failure Cimetidine
Gastrinoma (Zollinger-Ellison syndrome)	Elevated serum gastrin levels Identification of pancreatic nodule	Removal of pancreatic tumor Cimetidine
Hemorrhagic gastroenteritis	Compatible history Hemoconcentration	Supportive care

(*continued*)

Table 10-3. (Continued)

Causes	Basis for Diagnosis	Mode of Treatment
Primary gastrointestinal causes		
Inflammatory		
Inflammatory bowel disease	(See Table 10-7)	(See Table 10-7)
Mechanical obstruction		
Pyloric stenosis or pylorospasm	Barium GI contrast radiography	Surgical correction
Hypertrophic gastritis	Barium GI contrast radiography	Surgical correction
GI foreign body	Abdominal radiography Barium GI contrast radiography	Endoscopic or surgical removal
Gastric dilatation/volvulus complex	Abdominal radiography	Surgical correction Shock therapy
Intussusception/intestinal volvulus	Abdominal radiography Abdominal ultrasonography Barium GI contrast radiography	Surgical correction
GI neoplasm	Abdominal radiography Barium GI contrast radiography Endoscopy and biopsy	Surgical excision Adjunctive chemotherapy
Functional obstruction		
Gastric emptying disorder	Compatible history Barium GI contrast radiography	Metoclopramide
Paralytic ileus	Compatible history	Metoclopramide
Metabolic diseases		
Liver disease (see Chapter 11)	Laboratory evaluation	Treatment of liver disease
Uremia (see Chapter 12)		
Primary renal failure	Laboratory evaluation	Treatment of renal failure
Postrenal obstruction	Identification of obstruction	Removal of obstruction Fluid therapy
Diabetic ketoacidosis (see Chapter 25)	Laboratory evaluation	Treatment of ketoacidosis
Hypoadrenocorticism (see Chapter 14)	Laboratory evaluation	Mineralocorticoid supplementation
Pyometra (see Chapter 13)	Compatible history and physical examination CBC Abdominal radiography	Ovariohysterectomy
Neurologic Disease (see Chapter 17)		

Elevated intracranial pressure
    Head trauma
    Brain tumor
    Hydrocephalus
	Neurologic evaluation	Treatment of underlying disorder(s)

Cerebellar or vestibular disorders	Neurologic evaluation	Treatment of underlying disorder(s) Antiemetics

Table 10-4. *Toxins and drugs associated with vomiting*

Heavy metals
  Lead
  Mercuric chloride
  Arsenic
  Thallium
  Copper sulfate

Pesticides
  Organophosphates
  Alpha-naphthylurea (ANTU)
  Fluoroacetate
  Zinc phosphamide

Solvents
  Ethylene glycol
  Isopropanol
  Methanol
  Acetone
  Benzene
  Nitrobenzene
  Phenol

Miscellaneous toxins
  Ethanol
  Hexachlorophene
  Oxalates

Therapeutic drugs
  Apomorphine
  Ipecac
  Morphine
  Digitalis glycosides
  Ammonium chloride
  Salicylates
  Lincomycin
  Erythromycin
  Tetracyclines
  Chloramphenicol
  Nitrofurantoin
  Mebendazole
  Antineoplastic agents

ing sooner after eating than do obstructions that are lower in the GI tract.

4. The character of the vomitus may allow identification of a disease process. Vomitus with the appearance of coffee grounds suggests gastric ulceration. Ascarids or other parasites may be seen in the vomitus, as may small portions of gastric foreign bodies. Bile-tinged vomitus, or the presence of undigested food in vomitus six to eight hours after eating, suggest a gastric emptying disorder.

5. A thorough physical examination should be performed. Often, animals with metabolic causes for vomiting will exhibit abnormalities on physical examination that are unrelated to the GI tract. In addition, an evaluation of hydration, attitude, and general condition is necessary for appropriate decisions to be made regarding fluid therapy, hospitalization, and the need for medical versus surgical intervention.

6. Abdominal palpation may reveal a cause for vomiting. Foreign bodies, intussusception, abdominal tumors, enlarged mesenteric lymph nodes, enlarged uterus, and thickened bowel loops may be found. Abdominal pain may also be elicited.

Diagnostic Approach

1. Laboratory findings

  A. A CBC is helpful in assessing the hydration status of the patient and the severity of the inflammatory response. In hemorrhagic gastroenteritis (HGE), the packed cell volume (PCV) is dramatically elevated, whereas the total plasma protein (TPP) is often normal. In dehydration secondary to hypovolemia, both the PCV and TPP are elevated. In acute feline panleukopenia and canine parvovirus infections, a profound leukopenia is observed. Leukocytosis may be seen with inflammatory causes of vomiting.

  B. Determination of serum amylase and lipase concentrations may be useful in the diagnosis of canine pancreatitis, but they are of limited value in the assessment of feline pancreatitis.

  C. Serum electrolyte, BUN, creatinine, and glucose determinations, as well as liver function tests, are useful in the diagnosis of metabolic causes of vomiting (hypoadreno-corticism, renal failure, diabetic ketoacidosis, liver disease).

  D. Prolonged vomiting secondary to any cause leads to dehydration, electrolyte depletion, and derangement of acid–base balance. Serum electrolytes and blood gas determinations allow the identification of these imbalances so that proper treatment may be instituted.

  E. Fecal examination may be needed to diagnose endoparasitism. Most helminth eggs are found by fecal flotation; however, the eggs of *Nanophyetus salmincola*, the fluke that transmits the etiologic agent of salmon poisoning, are found by fecal sedimentation. The larvae of the gastric nematode *Ollulanus tricuspis* are identified by direct microscopic examination of the vomitus.

2. Radiographic findings

A. Plain abdominal radiographs may detect radiopaque foreign bodies, pyometra, abdominal masses, GI obstructive gas patterns, peritonitis, and abdominal fluid accumulation.

B. Contrast studies are indicated if plain films and supportive laboratory studies are not diagnostic. If GI perforation is suspected, iodinated contrast materials may be preferred over barium administration.

3. Endoscopy may be used to visualize and obtain biopsy specimens from the gastric and duodenal mucosa. This technique is useful in the diagnosis of gastric ulceration, gastric mass lesions, gastric foreign body, and inflammatory diseases of the stomach and duodenum.

Therapeutic Approach

1. Vomiting is a clinical sign and not a diagnosis. The clinician must make a conscientious effort to discover the primary disease process responsible for vomiting prior to instituting therapy. The goal of therapy is the elimination of the disease process.

2. Obstructive diseases involving the GI tract are usually emergencies, requiring immediate surgical intervention. Surgery (or endoscopy) may also be performed for removal of gastric foreign bodies.

3. Fluid, electrolyte, and acid–base derangements should be treated on the basis of previously obtained laboratory findings. If these laboratory values are unavailable, the fluid of choice for rehydration of the vomiting animal is 0.9% sodium chloride supplemented with potassium.

4. In patients with a history of recent onset of vomiting, normal physical examination, and no major laboratory abnormalities, conservative symptomatic therapy may be instituted.

A. Food intake should be restricted for 24 hours. Small amounts of water or ice may be given. After 24 hours, a bland diet, such as Prescription Diet i/d® (Hill's Pet Products), low-fat cottage cheese, boiled chicken, or boiled hamburger and rice, may be given in small amounts for one to two days. If the patient does not respond, further diagnostic tests are warranted.

B. Antiemetic drugs are occasionally useful. Recommended antiemetics include phenothiazine tranquilizers (e.g., chlorpromazine, prochlorperazine), metoclopramide, and adsorbents (e.g., Kaopectate, Pepto-Bismol). Anticholinergic drugs (e.g., atropine) are not recommended because of their side effects and lack of efficacy.

Diarrhea

Diarrhea results from excessive fecal water content and is the most important clinical sign of intestinal disease in the dog and cat. It is characterized by an abnormal increase in the frequency, fluidity, or volume of feces. The pathogenesis involves derangement of transmucosal water and solute fluxes caused by abnormal digestion, absorption, secretion, permeability, or motility. Most intestinal disorders cause diarrhea by a complex integration of the following pathophysiologic mechanisms.

1. Osmotic diarrhea—the osmotic retention of water in the lumen by osmotically active substances that are malabsorbed as a result of:

A. Maldigestion caused by exocrine pancreatic insufficiency (EPI)

B. Primary intestinal malabsorption caused by diffuse mucosal lesions, such as inflammatory, neoplastic, or villous atrophy disorders

2. Secretory diarrhea—the active secretion or inhibition of ion absorption, independent of malabsorption of ingesta or changes in mucosal permeability

3. Permeability diarrhea—the loss of intestinal water and solute secondary to the passive leakage of interstitial fluid and outpouring of blood, mucus, or protein (exudation) from sites of mucosal damage

4. Motility derangements

    A. Abnormally reduced peristalsis (hypomotility), which promotes stasis and bacterial overgrowth within the small intestine

    B. Disturbance of contact time between luminal contents and mucosa resulting from accelerated intestinal transit (hypermotility)

    C. Premature emptying of the colon associated with colonic inflammation or "irritability"

In addition to this mechanistic classification, diarrhea may be categorized by temporal (acute versus chronic), anatomic (small bowel versus large bowel), functional (maldigestion versus malabsorption), and etiologic or histopathologic classification schemes (Table 10-5). These categorizations correspond to the sequential steps used for ap-

proaching the diagnosis of diarrheal diseases in a logical manner.

Etiology and General Approach to Management

Acute Diarrhea

The etiologic origins of diarrhea are numerous and diverse. Acute diarrhea is common, and is characterized as diarrhea of abrupt or recent onset and short duration. Many of the disorders that cause acute diarrhea are self-limiting or easily resolved, typified by simple dietary indiscretion or uncomplicated intestinal parasitism; however, others are fulminant and life-threatening, as typified by parvoviral enteritis or acute hemorrhagic gastroenteritis (Table 10-6).

Table 10-5. **Classification schemes used to categorize diarrhea and the corresponding sequential steps for diagnosis**

Classification Schemes	Sequential Steps for Diagnosis
Temporal Acute diarrhea Chronic diarrhea	**Step 1** Historical characterization of the duration of the problem. (Many cases of acute diarrhea are self-limiting or resolved in this stage and do not require further evaluation.) Rule out dietary causes, intoxications, parasitism, infectious enteritides, and systemic disorders
Anatomic Small bowel diarrhea (small intestine, pancreas) Large bowel diarrhea (cecum, colon, rectum) Diarrhea secondary to nonenteric disease (kidney, liver, adrenal, thyroid, etc.)	**Step 2** Anatomic localization of the process to the small or large bowel using history, physical examination, fecal characteristics, and preliminary results of laboratory tests Identification of nonenteric causes using a data base of routine laboratory tests (e.g., serum chemistries, urinalysis, CBC, T_4 levels)

Functional
Normal assimilation
Malassimilation
  Maldigestion (pancreatic)
  Malabsorption (intestinal)
Diarrhea accompanied by protein-losing enteropathy
	Step 3
	Functional characterization (in chronic small bowel diarrhea) to identify malassimilation (steatorrhea) and then to differentiate maldigestion (serum trypsin-like immunoreactivity [TLI] or N-benzoyl-L-tyrosyl-*p*-aminobenzoic acid [BT-PABA] test) from malabsorption (xylose absorption test)
	Identification and evaluation of hypoproteinemia

Etiologic	**Step 4** Establishment of a definitive etiologic or histopathologic diagnosis through an extended data base consisting of more sophisticated laboratory tests, radiographs, endoscopic biopsies, biochemical tests, or therapeutic trials

Table 10-6. **Diagnosis and treatment of acute diarrhea**

Causes	Basis for Diagnosis	Mode of Treatment
Dietary Abrupt dietary changes Overfeeding Indiscretion—"garbage" ingestion; ingestion of abrasive or indigestible material Food hypersensitivity or intolerance	History; response to dietary modification	Restricted diet
Drug- and Toxin-induced Anti-inflammatory drugs—steroidal, nonsteroidal Antimicrobials Parasiticides—anthelmintics, dithiazanine Antineoplastic agents Heavy metals—e.g., lead, aresenic, thallium Insecticides—e.g., organophosphates	History of exposure	Eliminate exposure to the offending drug or toxin

Parasitic
Helminths
  Ascarids
  Hookworms
  Whipworms
  Strongyloides
  Others (cestodes, trematodes, Trichinella, etc.)
Protozoa
  Coccidia—Isospora, Cryptosporidia
  Giardia
  Others (Pentatrichomonas, Entamoeba, Balantidium)
	Fecal examinations	Specific anthelmintics and antiprotozoal drugs

Viral Parvovirus Coronavirus Rotavirus Astrovirus Others (canine distemper, feline infectious peritonitis, feline leukemia virus)	Clinical signs; demonstration of virus in feces by electron microscopy or ELISA; serologic results	Supportive therapy (fluid therapy; control of secondary bacterial complications)
Bacterial Salmonella species Campylobacter jejuni Yersinia enterocolitica *Bacillus piliformis* Others (*Escherichia coli,* Clostridium species)	Specialized fecal cultures	Specific antibiotics
Rickettsial Salmon poisoning disease	Clinical signs; endemic habitat; fecal examination for fluke eggs; lymph node cytologic studies	Tetracycline

(continued)

Table 10-6. (*Continued*)

Causes	Basis for Diagnosis	Mode of Treatment
Idiopathic Hemorrhagic gastroenteritis	Clinical signs; hematocrit	Supportive therapy (fluid therapy); antibiotics
Obstructive Intestinal foreign body Intussusception Intestinal volvulus	Abdominal palpation; barium contrast GI radiography	Surgery
Extraintestinal Renal failure Hepatic disease Hypoadrenocorticism Acute pancreatitis	Serum biochemistry determinations and organ function tests	Various treatments to control the underlying extraintestinal disorder

From Sherding RG: Diseases of the small bowel. In Ettinger SJ (ed): Textbook of Veterinary Internal Medicine, 3rd ed. Philadelphia, WB Saunders, 1989

Management of acute diarrhea is based on rehydration therapy and dietary restriction. Symptomatic therapy with antidiarrheal agents may also be a consideration (see the section on Therapeutic Approach that follows). In many cases of mild or nonspecific acute diarrhea, resolution occurs spontaneously within a day or two without any treatment except for restriction of food intake. Because the treatment of acute diarrhea is mainly supportive and nonspecific, many animals can be managed without determination of a definitive diagnosis. The exception to this is when infectious agents may be involved (see Table 10-6); in this situation, it is important to identify enteropathogens for which specific treatment (e.g., antibiotics) is available.

Chronic Diarrhea

Diarrhea is generally categorized as chronic, rather than acute, if within three to four weeks it has not resolved or responded to symptomatic therapy, or if there is a pattern of episodic recurrence. This time frame usually excludes most cases of dietary indiscretion, intoxication, and viral enteritis.

Management of chronic diarrhea is based on diagnosis of the underlying disorder, rather than symptomatic treatment. Specific intervention or treatment is often necessary,

requiring a specific diagnosis or histopathologic characterization. The first step in diagnosis is to classify the diarrhea as primarily small bowel or large bowel in origin (see the section on History and Physical Examination that follows). The causes of chronic small and large bowel diarrhea and the appropriate means of diagnosis and therapy for each are presented in Tables 10-7 and 10-8.

History and Physical Findings

History

Animals with intestinal disease most often present to the veterinarian because of diarrhea or because of concern over other abnormalities that may accompany diarrhea, such as anorexia, vomiting, inactivity, weakness, or weight loss. The history is especially helpful in localizing the disease process to the small or large bowel. It also may indicate extraintestinal causes of diarrhea (such as renal failure, hypoadrenocorticism, or hyperthyroidism) or identify important predisposing factors, such as breed, diet, environmental stress, exposure to infectious agents or parasites, and drug or toxin exposures. The following historical aspects of the diarrhea may be diagnostically useful:

Table 10-7. **Diagnosis and treatment of diseases of the small intestine**

Disorder	Basis for Diagnosis	Mode of Treatment
Exocrine pancreatic insufficiency	Fecal stains; serum trypsin assay; N-benzoyl-L-tyrosyl-*p*-aminobenzoic acid (BT-PABA) test	Enzyme replacement
Chronic inflammatory small bowel disease		
Eosinophilic enteritis	Eosinophilia; biopsy	Prednisolone
Lymphocytic-plasmacytic enteritis	Biopsy	Lamb and rice diet; prednisolone (also, tylosin, metronidazole, azathioprine)
Immunoproliferative enteropathy of basenjis	Serum protein electrophoresis; biopsy	Diet; prednisolone; antibiotics
Granulomatous enteritis	Radiography; biopsy	Prednisolone (± azathioprine, ± metronidazole); surgical resection
Lymphangiectasia	Hypoproteinemia; hypocholesterolemia; lymphopenia; biopsy	Fat-restricted diet (medium chain triglycerides added); prednisolone
Villous atrophy		
Wheat-sensitive enteropathy	Response to wheat-free diet; biopsy	Wheat-free (gluten-free) diet
Idiopathic	Biopsy	Diet; prednisolone; antibiotics (±)
Histoplasmosis	Serology; cytology; biopsy	Amphotericin B: ketoconazole
Pythiosis	Biopsy	Surgical excision ± ketoconazole
Lymphosarcoma	Biopsy	Chemotherapy (antineoplastic drugs)
Bacterial overgrowth syndrome	Culture of intestinal aspirate; serum B_{12}/folate; response to antibiotics	Antibiotics (tetracycline, tylosin, metronidazole, etc.)
Giardiasis	Fecal examination; response to parasiticides	Metronidazole or quinacrine
Lactase deficiency	Response to lactose-free diet	Elimination of milk from diet

From Sherding RG. Chronic diarrhea. In Ford RB (ed): Clinical Signs and Diagnosis in Small Animal Practice. New York, Churchill Livingstone, 1988, by permission

Mode of onset (abrupt versus gradual)
Duration (acute versus chronic)
Clinical course (intermittent versus continuous; progressiveness)
Correlation with diet (food intolerances, dietary indiscretions)
Correlation with medication usage (drug side effects)
Response to previous treatment (e.g., prescribed diets, antibiotics, anthelmintics, corticosteroids)

Association with other signs (e.g., weight loss, vomiting, or dyschezia)

Small Bowel Versus Large Bowel Diarrhea

The medical history should also include the characteristics of the patient's feces (frequency, volume, consistency, color, odor, and composition) in order to localize the disease process to either the small or large bowel (Table 10-9). This distinction is an

Table 10-8. **Diagnosis and treatment of diseases of the large intestine**

Disorder	Basis for Diagnosis	Mode of Treatment
Chronic colitis Lymphocytic-plasmacytic (L-P) Histiocytic Eosinophilic	Colonoscopy; colon biopsy	Lamb and rice diet (L-P colitis); sulfasalazine, prednisolone, metronidazole
Abrasive colitis	Dietary history; inspection of feces	Elimination of dietary indiscretions
Whipworm colitis	Fecal flotation; colonoscopy; response to fenbendazole	Anthelmintics (fenbendazole)
Protozoan colitis Amebiasis Balantidiasis Trichomoniasis	Saline fecal smears	Metronidazole
Histoplasma colitis	Fecal cytology; colon biopsy; serology; culture	Amphotericin B, ketoconazole
Salmonella colitis	Culture	Antibiotics (e.g., trimethoprim-sulfa)
Campylobacter colitis	Culture	Antibiotics (e.g., erythromycin)
Protothecal colitis	Colon biopsy	None
Rectocolonic polyps	Digital palpation; barium enema	Surgical excision
Colonic adenocarcinoma	Colonoscopy; barium enema	Surgical resection
Colonic lymphosarcoma	Colon biopsy	Chemotherapy (antineoplastic drugs)
Cecal inversion	Barium enema; colonoscopy	Cecectomy
Functional diarrhea ("irritable colon")	History and diagnostic work-up that excludes all other diseases	Diet; diphenoxylate, anticholinergics, tranquilizers

From Sherding RG. Chronic diarrhea. In Ford RB (ed): Clinical Signs and Diagnosis in Small Animal Practice. New York, Churchill Livingstone, 1988, by permission

Table 10-9. **Clinical differentiation between small bowel and large bowel diarrhea**

Clinical Sign	Small Bowel	Large Bowel
Fecal volume	Markedly increased daily output (large quantity of bulky or watery feces with each defecation)	Normal or slightly increased daily output (small quantities with each defecation)
Frequency of defecation	Normal, or slightly increased	Very frequent
Urgency or tenesmus	Rare	Common
Mucus in feces	Rare	Common
Blood in feces	Dark black (digested)	Red (fresh)
Steatorrhea (malassimilation)	May be present	Absent
Weight loss and emaciation	May be present	Rare
Flatulence	May be present	Absent
Vomiting	Occasional	Occasional

important one because it determines the direction of subsequent diagnostic evaluations in animals with chronic, unresponsive diarrhea. Diffuse disease may produce concurrent small and large bowel signs.

1. Chronic small bowel diarrhea
   A. Characteristics—voluminous, malodorous, unformed or liquid diarrhea with minimal mucus and an absence of fresh blood; often accompanied by loss of body weight
   B. Diagnostic overview
      1) Rule out dietary causes (food trials, hypoallergenic diets).
      2) Rule out giardiasis (fecal examination; metronidazole therapeutic trial).
      3) Perform function tests to differentiate EPI from primary intestinal disease and to identify protein-losing enteropathy.
      4) Perform endoscopic small bowel biopsy to assess mucosal lesions.
2. Chronic large bowel diarrhea
   A. Characteristics—urgency and frequent attempts to defecate with passage of small quantities of bloody mucoid diarrhea
   B. Diagnostic overview
      1) Rule out dietary causes (food trials, hypoallergenic diets).
      2) Rule out trichuriasis (fecal examination; fenbendazole therapeutic trial).
      3) Perform tests to rule out invasive enteropathogens.
      4) Perform colonoscopic biopsy to assess colonic mucosal lesions.

Physical Examination

A complete physical examination may reveal important clues about the severity, nature, and cause(s) of intestinal disease (Table 10-10). An effort should be made to identify any underlying systemic disease that may be a cause or consequence of diarrhea. Significant physical findings may include:

Fever, weight loss, malnutrition, dehydration, weakness, or depression
Pallor (GI blood loss) or effusions/edema (enteric plasma protein loss)
Palpable thyroid nodules (feline hyperthyroidism)

Abnormalities noted on palpation of the liver
Abnormalities noted on palpation of the intestinal loops (masses, thickenings, distention, aggregation, pain, or associated lymphadenopathy)
Abnormalities noted on digital palpation of the rectum (foreign objects, masses, strictures, mucosal irregularities, abnormal fecal material)

Diagnostic Approach

The reader is referred to Table 10-5 for an overview of the sequential steps involved in the diagnosis of diarrhea. Specific diagnostic modalities are discussed in this section. Please refer to Tables 10-6 through 10-8 for applications of these modalities to specific diseases. An overview of the various diagnostic findings in categories of chronic diarrhea may be found in Table 10-11.

Routine Hematologic and Blood Chemistry Studies

1. Hematologic findings and their implications in diarrhea
   A. Eosinophilia—parasitism, eosinophilic enteritis, hypoadrenocorticism
   B. Neutrophilia—infectious or inflammatory disease
   C. Neutropenia—parvovirus, endotoxemia, or overwhelming sepsis (e.g., peritonitis from bowel perforation)
   D. Monocytosis—chronic or granulomatous inflammation (e.g., mycosis)
   E. Lymphopenia—intestinal lymphangiectasia
   F. Anemia—enteric blood loss or depressed erythropoiesis (e.g., chronic inflammation, malnutrition)
   G. Elevated hematocrit—hemoconcentration from intestinal fluid loss
   H. RBC microcytosis—chronic GI blood loss (iron deficiency)
   I. RBC macrocytosis—nutritional deficiencies (rare), feline hyperthyroidism, or FeLV
2. Biochemical findings and their implications in diarrhea

Table 10-10. **Clinical significance of abnormal physical findings associated with intestinal disease**

Physical Findings	Potential Clinical Associations
General physical examination	
Dehydration	Diarrheal fluid loss
Depression/weakness	Electrolyte imbalance; severe debilitation
Emaciation/malnutrition	Chronic malabsorption; protein-losing enteropathy
Dull, unthrifty haircoat	Malabsorption of fatty acids, protein, and vitamins
Fever	Infection; transmural inflammatory bowel disease; lymphosarcoma
Edema, ascites, pleural effusion	Protein-losing enteropathy
Pallor (anemia)	GI blood loss, anemia or chronic illness or inflammation
Intestinal palpation	
Masses	Foreign body; neoplasia; granuloma
Thickened loops	Infiltration (inflammatory, neoplastic)
"Sausage loop"	Intussusception
Aggregated loops	Linear intestinal foreign body; peritoneal adhesions
Pain	Inflammation; obstruction; ischemia
Gas or fluid distention	Obstruction; ileus
Mesenteric lymphadenopathy	Inflammation; infection; neoplasia
Rectal palpation	
Masses	Polyp; granuloma; neoplasia
Circumferential narrowing	Stricture; spasm; neoplasia
Coarse mucosal texture	Colitis; neoplasia

From Sherding RG. Chronic diarrhea. In Ford RB (ed): Clinical Signs and Diagnosis in Small Animal Practice. New York, Churchill Livingstone, 1988, by permission

A. Panhypoproteinemia—protein-losing enteropathy

B. Hyperglobulinemia—basenji enteropathy

C. Azotemia—dehydration, primary renal failure

D. Hyperkalemia/hyponatremia—hypoadrenocorticism, trichuriasis

E. Hypocalcemia—hypoalbuminemia, lymphangiectasia

F. Hypocholesterolemia—lymphangiectasia, liver disease

G. Elevated serum liver enzymes, bile acids—liver disease

H. Elevated serum thyroxine (T_4) levels —feline hyperthyroidism

Fecal Examination

Fecal examinations are an important aspect of the diagnostic approach to diarrhea. They may involve gross inspection (see previous section on Large Bowel Versus Small Bowel Diarrhea), examination for parasites, microscopic examination, quantitative fecal collection and analysis, chemical determinations, and cultures (Table 10-12). An examination of feces for parasites should be part of the data

Table 10-11. **Typical findings and diagnostic criteria in various categories of chronic diarrhea**

Easily or rapidly diagnosed diarrhea

1. Dietary diarrhea (food hypersensitivity, dietary indiscretion) is usually self-limiting with dietary restriction or trial feeding of a controlled diet.
2. Drug-induced diarrhea resolves with dosage reduction or discontinuation of the drug.
3. Parasitic diarrhea is diagnosed by identification of ova, larvae, or trophozoites in the feces and by the animal's response to parasiticidal drugs.
4. Nonenteric causes of diarrhea, such as liver disease, renal failure (increased BUN and creatinine), or hypoadrenocorticism (hyperkalemia and hyponatremia), are often identified by serum biochemistry profiles and urinalysis.
5. Thyroid palpation and measurement of serum thyroxine (T_4) levels will indicate the presence of hyperthyroid-related diarrhea in aged cats.

Exocrine pancreatic insufficiency

1. Severe steatorrhea (positive Sudan stain for unsplit fat, excessive quantitative fecal fat excretion)
2. Amylorrhea (positive iodine stain for undigested starch)
3. Lack of plasma turbidity after oral fat load (corrected with enzymes)
4. Normal xylose absorption (unless there is secondary mucosal injury or bacterial overgrowth)
5. Abnormal oral bentiromide (BT-PABA) digestion test
6. Very low serum trypsin-like immunoreactivity assay
7. Responsive to oral pancreatic enzyme therapy

Intestinal malabsorption

1. Steatorrhea (positive Sudan stain for split fat, increased quantitative fecal fat excretion)
2. Flat xylose absorption curve
3. Normal pancreatic function tests
4. Nonspecific infiltrative lesions of the bowel wall detected on barium upper GI radiography (in some cases)
5. Abnormal serum levels of folate and vitamin B_{12} (in some cases)
6. Decreased brush border enzyme activities (measured by specialized assays)
7. Histopathologic lesions detected on biopsy of small intestine
8. Response to therapeutic trials: d/d Prescription Diet® (lymphocytic-plasmacytic enterocolitis); metronidazole (occult giardiasis); tetracycline (bacterial overgrowth)

Protein-losing enteropathies

1. Panhypoproteinemia, including hypoalbuminemia and hypogammaglobulinemia (hyperglobulinemia in lymphoproliferative enteropathy of basenjis)
2. Steatorrhea and abnormal xylose absorption may be noted, but are inconsistent findings
3. Lymphopenia
4. Hypocholesterolemia
5. Hypocalcemia
6. Transudative or chylous body cavity effusion
7. Characteristic lesions found on biopsy of the small bowel

Large bowel disease

1. Fecal examinations may yield positive results for:
   Ingested foreign material (abrasive colitis)
   Parasitic ova (whipworm colitis)
   Protozoal trophozites (colitis secondary to Entamoeba, Balantidium, etc.)
   Campylobacter-like organisms
   Leukocytes (exudative colitis)
2. Responsive to whipcidal drugs (e.g., fenbendazole) in cases of occult, non–egg-producing trichuriasis
3. Fecal cultures may be positive for specific bacterial enteropathogens, especially when fecal leukocytes are present (Salmonella, Campylobacter).
4. Cecocolonic lesions may be delineated by barium enema radiography.
5. Colonic lesions may be identified by colonoscopic examination and biopsy.

Table 10-12. *Fecal examinations used for diagnosis of intestinal disease*

Examination/Procedure	Diagnostic Significance
Gross inspection	
Volume (bulk)	Small *v* large bowel diarrhea
Consistency, color, odor	Small *v* large bowel diarrhea
Composition	Blood, mucus, foreign matter
Examinations for parasites	
Visual inspection	Tapeworm proglottids
Flotation (conventional—e.g., sodium nitrate)	Nematode and cestode ova
Zinc sulfate centrifugation-flotation	Giardia and coccidia cysts
Sheather's sugar centrifugation-flotation	Cryptosporidium cysts
Saline suspension	Protozoan trophozoites
Sedimentation/Baermann	Strongyloides larvae
Microscopic examination	
Sudan preparation	Fat (steatorrhea)
Iodine preparation	Starch (amylorrhea)
Cytologic preparation	Leukocytes, infectious agents
Quantitative 24-hour fecal collection	
Quantitative fecal fat analysis	Malassimilation
Fecal weight (daily fecal output)	Malassimilation
Chemical determinations	
Fat content	Steatorrhea—malassimilation
Water content	Correlated with fecal weight
Nitrogen content	Azotorrhea—malassimilation
Electrolytes	Osmotic *v* secretory diarrhea
Osmolality	Osmotic *v* secretory diarrhea
pH	Carbohydrate malassimilation
Occult blood test	GI bleeding
Proteolytic (trypsin) activity	Pancreatic insufficiency
Alpha$_1$-antitrypsin	Protein-losing enteropathy
Toxin assays	*Clostridia difficile* infection
Cultures	
Bacterial	Salmonella, Campylobacter, Yersinia, etc.
Fungal	Histoplasmosis, etc.

From Sherding RG. Chronic diarrhea. In Ford RB (ed): Clinical Signs and Diagnosis in Small Animal Practice. New York, Churchill Livingstone, 1988, by permission

base for all animals with diarrhea; for those with chronic, unresponsive diarrhea, the data base should be expanded to include microscopic examination of stained fecal smears for fat, starch, and leukocytes. If circumstances suggest infection, fecal culture for specific enteropathogenic bacteria (e.g., Salmonella, Campylobacter) is warranted.

Tests of Digestive and Absorptive Function

In dogs, once simple dietary, parasitic, or infectious causes for chronic diarrhea have been ruled out, diagnostic efforts should then be directed toward determining the presence or absence of EPI. An attempt to characterize intestinal malabsorption should then be made. This is accomplished through tests that evaluate digestive and absorptive function.

1. Fecal microscopy—preliminary in-office screening procedure involving the examination of Sudan- and iodine-stained fecal smears for steatorrhea and amylorrhea

A. Direct Sudan stain—detects excessive undigested fat (neutral, unsplit), which appears as numerous, large, refractile orange droplets, indicating steatorrhea of pancreatic maldigestion

B. Indirect Sudan stain—the addition of acetic acid and heating render fatty acids (split fat) stainable as well; thus, the presence of numerous droplets in fecal specimen that tests negative on direct Sudan stain suggests steatorrhea caused by malabsorption of fatty acids.

C. Lugol's iodine stain—detects undigested starch as blue-black granules, suggesting amylorrhea secondary to pancreatic maldigestion

2. Serum trypsin-like immunoreactivity (TLI) test

A. The TLI test is a highly specific and sensitive assay requiring a single fasted serum sample; thus, it is the test of choice for confirmation of EPI

B. Normal dogs have a TLI of 5 to 35 μg/L, whereas dogs with EPI generally have values of less than 2.5 μg/L.

3. Oral bentiromide (BT-PABA) digestion test

A. The N-benzoyl-L-tyrosyl-*p*-aminobenzoic acid (BT-PABA) test is a fairly reliable test for confirming EPI in dogs, but it is not as easy to perform as the TLI test.

B. The bentiromide test substrate, a chymotrypsin-labile peptide, is administered orally, after which serum samples are taken at 60 and 90 minutes and assayed for PABA. Dogs with EPI, because they secrete very little chymotrypsin, develop a negligible rise in plasma PABA levels.

C. The test is not reliable in the cat.

4. Xylose absorption test

A. The xylose absorption test is the standard test for evaluating canine intestinal absorptive function; however, it is relatively insensitive and does not help distinguish between the numerous small intestinal diseases capable of causing malabsorption.

B. In normal dogs, following oral administration of xylose (0.5 g/kg as a 5% to 10% solution), plasma xylose concentrations peak at greater than 60 mg/dL 60 to 120 minutes after administration.

C. Intestinal malabsorption is indicated by an abnormally low plasma xylose level.

D. This test is unreliable in the cat.

5. Measurement of serum folate and vitamin B_{12}

A. Serum levels of folate and vitamin B_{12} (cobalamin) reflect intestinal absorptive function and the status of intestinal flora.

B. Serum folate levels (normally 3.5 to 11.0 μg/L) depend on the absorptive function of the jejunum, whereas serum levels of vitamin B_{12} (normally 300 to 700 ng/L) depend on absorption in the ileum. Thus, serum folate may be decreased in enteropathies that affect the proximal small intestine, serum vitamin B_{12} may be decreased in enteropathies that affect the distal small intestine, and the levels of both vitamins may be decreased in diseases that cause diffuse intestinal malabsorption. In small intestinal bacterial overgrowth, serum folate levels may actually be increased owing to synthesis of folate by the overgrown bacteria, whereas vitamin B_{12} may be decreased because bacteria can utilize or bind the vitamin, making it unavailable for absorption.

6. Diagnosis of small intestinal bacterial overgrowth

A. An overproliferation of bacterial flora within the proximal small intestine, usually the result of stasis ("stagnant loop"), has been recognized as a cause of small bowel diarrhea, but is difficult to document. Confirmation requires quantitative aerobic and anaerobic culture of intestinal contents obtained by duodenal intubation or aspiration. This is impractical for routine clinical application.

B. Indirect criteria for the diagnosis of bacterial overgrowth include increased serum folate levels, decreased serum vitamin B_{12} levels, and response to certain antibiotics (e.g., oxytetracycline, tylosin, metranidazole, or chloramphenicol).

Gastrointestinal Radiography and Ultrasonography

1. Upper GI barium contrast radiography should be considered when other tests fail to determine the cause of small bowel diarrhea. The study may help to detect obstructive lesions, stagnant loops, and neoplastic or inflammatory lesions that cause an irregular mucosal pattern.

2. Barium enema radiography is helpful in selected cases of large bowel diarrhea for evaluating the colon and cecum for intussusceptions, neoplasms, polyps, strictures, and inflammatory lesions. Colonoscopy is generally preferred over barium enema for evaluating the colon.

3. Abdominal ultrasonography can be useful for defining intestinal and other abdominal masses, for evaluating the pancreas for tumors and abscesses, and for detecting evidence of biliary tract disease.

Gastrointestinal Endoscopy

1. Upper GI endoscopy—duodenoscopy with a flexible fiberoptic endoscope can be performed in the anesthetized animal for visual examination of the duodenum, duodenal aspiration (for quantitative bacterial culture or detection of Giardia), and mucosal biopsy.

2. Colonoscopy—definitive diagnosis of many large bowel diseases, especially colitis, is made by colonoscopic examination and biopsy.

Intestinal Biopsy

1. Most chronic small and large bowel diarrhea cases in which EPI and extraintestinal, dietary, parasitic, and infectious causes have been excluded require mucosal biopsy for definitive diagnosis or accurate characterization.

2. The least invasive and, in many cases, preferred method for procurement of biopsy material is endoscopy; if this is unavailable, laparotomy should be considered.

Diagnosis by Response to Therapy

A therapeutic drug or dietary trial may be used as an empirical approach to diagnosis when supported by adequate clinical information.

1. Trial-and-error test diets may be employed to determine dietary hypersensitivity, as in the restriction of wheat and other gluten-containing grains in Irish setters with wheat-sensitive enteropathy and the use of a hypoallergenic diet, such as lamb and rice, in lymphocytic-plasmacytic enteritis.

2. Response to antibacterial therapy may be a useful indicator of small intestinal bacterial overgrowth.

3. Occult parasitic infections involving Giardia or whipworms may be excluded by response to metronidazole or fenbendazole, respectively.

Therapeutic Approach

Acute Diarrhea

Acute diarrhea is frequently self-limiting and resolves without treatment; however, dietary, supportive, and symptomatic therapy is beneficial in many cases. In severe cases, rehydration therapy can be life-saving.

1. Diet

A. The initial goal in acute diarrhea is to put the GI tract to rest by restricting food intake for at least 24 hours.

B. When feeding is resumed, bland, low-fat foods are fed in small amounts at frequent intervals. Examples of appropriate foods include boiled rice, potatoes, or pasta (as carbohydrate sources) combined with boiled, skinless chicken; yogurt; or low-fat cottage cheese (as protein sources). Ready-made prescription diets can also be used.

C. Once the diarrhea has been resolved for 48 hours, the animal can gradually be reintroduced to its regular diet.

2. Fluid therapy

A. In severe, acute diarrhea, such as occurs with parvoviral enteritis, intestinal fluid loss may lead to serious dehydration, shock, and death. Fluid and electrolyte replacement therapy is, therefore, essential.

B. Parenteral methods of fluid therapy are preferred in most cases; however, oral glucose-electrolyte solutions (Entrolyte, Beecham) are available for counterbalancing intestinal fluid losses in cases of mild diarrhea.

3. Antidiarrheal drugs

A. Symptomatic treatment of diarrhea depends upon drugs that modify motility and fluid secretion/absorption, or drugs that act locally within the lumen as protectants/adsorbents.

B. In most cases, these drugs are reserved for short-term use, usually for periods of less than five to seven days.

1) Opiate and opioid narcotic analgesic drugs—probably the most effective all-purpose antidiarrheal agents

a) They inhibit intestinal fluid loss through modification of mucosal fluid and electrolyte transport.

b) They impede bowel transit by stimulating nonpropulsive contractions (segmentation) and decreasing propulsive motility (peristalsis), thereby allowing more contact time for absorption.

c) Examples include paregoric, diphenoxylate (Lomotil), and loperamide (Imodium).

2) Anticholinergic/antispasmotic drugs

a) They, too, inhibit fluid loss, presumably through an antisecretory effect.

b) They cause a generalized suppression of gut motility that may potentiate ileus; however, their antispasmodic action may be most beneficial in controlling the urgency and discomfort of colitis.

c) Examples include atropine, isopropamide (Darbid), aminopentamide (Centrine), propantheline (Pro-Banthine), and dicyclomine (Bentyl).

3) Prostaglandin-inhibiting drugs

a) They have an anti-inflammatory/antisecretory action.

b) They may be used for intraluminal delivery of antiprostaglandin to the proximal GI tract (bismuth subsalicylate [Pepto-Bismol]).

c) They may be used for intraluminal delivery of antiprostaglandin to the lower GI tract or colon (sulfasalazine [Azulfidine] or 5-aminosalicyclic acid).

d) Systemic prostaglandin inhibitors (nonsteroidal anti-inflammatory drugs) should be avoided because they tend to cause gastric ulceration.

4) Chlorpromazine—possible antisecretory effects

5) Protectant/adsorbent drugs

a) Some oral agents work in the lumen to adsorb injurious bacteria and toxins and to provide a protective coating on inflamed mucosal surfaces.

b) The efficacy of these drugs remains unproven. Large doses are often required, and the drugs may be difficult to administer.

c) Examples include kaolin-pectin, bismuth, activated charcoal, and barium.

4. Antibiotics

A. Antibiotics should not be used routinely as empirical therapy in cases of uncomplicated diarrhea of undetermined cause because of their adverse effects on normal intestinal flora and their tendency to promote resistant strains of bacteria.

B. Antibiotics are indicated when specific bacterial or rickettsial enteropathogens, such as Salmonella or Campylobacter, are suspected causes.

C. Antibiotics are also appropriate in conditions associated with severe mucosal damage and a high risk of secondary sepsis or endotoxemia, such as in parvoviral enteritis or hemorrhagic gastroenteritis. Thus, reasonable indications for antibacterial therapy in the animal with acute GI disease include bloody diarrhea, fever, leukocytosis, leukopenia, fecal leukocytes, and signs of shock.

Chronic Diarrhea

Chronic diarrhea does not usually resolve spontaneously or in response to symptomatic antidiarrheal agents. Specific intervention or treatment is desirable and requires a specific diagnosis (see Tables 10-7 and 10-8). As adjunctive therapy, however, dietary modification may be beneficial in the animal with chronic diarrhea.

1. Chronic small bowel diarrhea

A. In the dog, the diet should be highly digestible, consisting of 80% carbohydrates (such as rice); it should provide adequate amounts (15% to 20%) of high-biologic-quality protein derived from one or two food sources (such as skinless chicken, lean lamb, yogurt, or low-fat cottage cheese); and it should contain a minimum of fat, lactose, and additives.

B. In cats, being true carnivores, a high-protein, moderate-fat, low-carbohydrate diet is more appropriate.

C. Daily food intake should be divided into three or four small meals to avoid overloading digestive/absorptive capacity.

D. Supplementation of the diet with vitamins, minerals, medium-chain triglycerides, or pancreatic enzymes should be considered.

2. Chronic large bowel diarrhea

A. A meat-based diet, such as lamb and rice, is suitable.

B. In dogs, supplementation of the diet with crude fiber, such as cellulose, hemicellulose, or pectin, seems to have a normalizing effect on colonic motor function.

Constipation and Dyschezia

Definitions

1. *Constipation* is a clinical sign characterized by absent, infrequent, or difficult defecation associated with retention of feces within the colon and rectum. When feces are retained for a prolonged period of time, the mucosa continues to absorb water from the fecal mass, which gradually results in impacted feces that become progressively harder and drier.

2. *Obstipation* is a condition of intractable constipation in which the colon and rectum become so impacted with excessively hard feces that defecation cannot occur.

3. *Dyschezia* is a clinical sign characterized by difficult or painful evacuation of feces from the rectum, and is usually associated

with lesions in or near the anal region. Dyschezia often leads to fecal retention and constipation.

4. *Tenesmus* is a clinical sign characterized by straining to defecate, usually ineffectively or painfully; thus, it usually accompanies dyschezia.

5. *Megacolon* is a disorder (not a sign) in which the colon becomes markedly dilated and hypomotile, usually irreversibly so. It is one of the important causes of chronic constipation/obstipation, especially in cats.

Etiology

Underlying causes or predisposing factors for constipation, listed in Table 10-13, include ingested foreign material, environmental factors, painful defecation, colonic obstruction, neuromuscular diseases, fluid and electrolyte disturbances, and drug-related effects.

1. Ingested foreign material, such as indigestible fibrous material (especially hair in cats from their grooming behavior) or abrasives (especially bones in dogs), may become incorporated into the fecal mass, resulting in the formation of hard fecal impactions that are difficult or painful to evacuate from the colon.

2. Environmental factors that are not conducive to defecation or that vary from the daily routine to which the animal is accustomed may cause the animal to inhibit the urge to defecate, leading to constipation. For example, this may occur when an animal is kept in strange surroundings, such as in a kennel or veterinary hospital, or when a cat's litter box is too dirty.

3. Painful defecation caused by anorectal diseases (e.g., anal sacculitis, perianal fistulas) or orthopedic disorders that limit positioning for defecation (e.g., disorders affecting the pelvis, spine, or hips) will often result in voluntary inhibition of defecation and lead to constipation.

4. Rectocolonic obstruction, which mechanically impedes the passage of feces, may result from intraluminal causes, such as foreign bodies or stenosing neoplastic or inflammatory lesions, or from extraluminal causes,

Table 10-13. **Classification and causes of constipation**

Category	Cause
Dietary	Ingested foreign material mixed with feces (hair, bones, kitty litter, plant material)
Environmental/psychological	Dirty litter box Inadequate exercise Hospitalization Change in habitat or daily routine

Painful defecation	Anorectal disorders
	  Anal sac impaction/abscess
	  Anorectal stricture, tumor, or foreign body
	  Perianal fistula
	  Perianal bite wound cellulitis/abscess
	  Pseudocoprostasis
	Orthopedic disorders
	  Spinal disease or injury
	  Injuries of the pelvis, hip joints, or pelvic limbs

Colonic obstruction	Extraluminal
	  Prostatic hypertrophy or tumor; prostatitis
	  Paraprostatic cyst
	  Pelvic fracture (malunion)
	  Pelvic collapse secondary to nutritional bone disease
	  Perianal tumor
	  Pseudocoprostasis
	Intraluminal
	  Rectocolonic stricture, tumor, or foreign body
	  Rectal diverticulum or perineal hernia

Neuromuscular disease	Lumbosacral spinal cord disease, deformity (Manx cats), or injury (e.g., intervertebral disk disease) Bilateral pelvic nerve injury Dysautonomia (Key-Gaskell syndrome) Hypothyroidism Idiopathic megacolon (?)
Fluid and electrolyte abnormalities	Dehydration Hypokalemia Hypercalcemia (hyperparathyroidism)
Drug-induced	Anticholinergics Opiates/opioids Diuretics Antihistamines Aluminum hydroxide Barium sulfate

such as prostatic enlargement, paraprostatic cysts, compressive pelvic fractures, anorectal masses, or pseudocoprostasis (feces matted to the hair of the perianal area).

5. Neuromuscular disorders may lead to constipation by interfering with colonic inner-vation or smooth muscle function or the ability of the animal to assume the normal defecation stance. For example, this may occur in association with disease or injury of the lumbosacral spinal cord, spinal deformity (as occurs in Manx cats), endocrine disease (hypothyroidism), or dysautonomia, a progressively fatal autonomic polyneuropathy of young cats. When innervation of the anus is also impaired, fecal incontinence may be an associated clinical sign. The pathogenesis of idiopathic megacolon is poorly characterized, but probably involves a primary or secondary neuromuscular dysfunction of the colon.

6. Fluid and electrolyte disorders may predispose an animal to constipation, particularly in the case of dehydration, which can cause the feces to become excessively dry and hard, and in hypokalemia or hypercalcemia, either of which can affect colonic smooth muscle function.

7. Drug-induced constipation may be a side effect of motility-modifying drugs (anticholinergics, opiates, opioids), antihistamines, barium sulfate, aluminum hydroxide, or diuretics.

Clinical Signs

1. Constipated animals are usually presented for failure to defecate over a period of days. The owner may notice tenesmus or frequent attempts to defecate with little or no passage of feces.

2. Dyschezia usually indicates anorectal disease. The animal first may cry out as it attempts to defecate, usually with straining (tenesmus) during the attempt. Then, it may cease the effort, walk around anxiously, and repeatedly try again.

3. Mucosal irritation caused by impacted feces may provoke a secretion of fluid and mucus which bypasses the retained fecal mass and is expelled paradoxically as diarrhea during attempts to defecate.

4. Other signs may include anorexia, lethargy, vomiting, dehydration, and a hunched-up appearance caused by abdominal discomfort.

5. Constipation tends to be a recurrent problem in many animals.

Diagnostic Approach

1. The history should identify dietary, environmental, behavioral, psychological, and medication-related factors or predispositions.

2. Physical examination

A. Abdominal palpation generally reveals a colon distended with hard feces.

B. Digital anorectal examination should be performed to detect painful or obstructive lesions of the anorectum.

C. A neurologic examination (see Chapter 17) should be performed to identify any underlying neurologic causes of constipation.

D. The rear limbs, coxofemoral joints, pelvis, and lumbosacral spine should be examined for orthopedic problems that could cause either difficulty in maneuvering into the defecation stance or painful defecation.

E. In cats with constipation secondary to dysautonomia (Key-Gaskell syndrome), additional manifestations of progressive autonomic failure that may be seen include urinary/fecal incontinence, megaesophagus, bradycardia, mydriasis, decreased lacrimation, and prolapse of the nictitating membranes (see Chapter 17).

3. Serum biochemical profile, urinalysis, and CBC

A. These tests should be performed in animals with recurrent constipation or with signs indicating the potential for underlying systemic disease that could cause constipation secondary to dehydration or electrolyte disturbances.

B. These parameters should also be evaluated in severely constipated/obstipated animals, especially those that are vomiting or markedly depressed, in order to detect the metabolic consequences of prolonged fecal retention (e.g., fluid and electrolyte imbalances, endotoxemia, azotemia, etc.) and to guide supportive treatment.

4. Serum T_4 levels should be measured in dogs with recurrent constipation and other signs compatible with hypothyroidism.

5. Abdominal radiography

A. Confirms the extent of colonic impaction with densely packed feces

B. Identifies the extreme dilatation of the colon that indicates megacolon

C. Identifies radio-opaque foreign material (e.g., bone chips) in the retained feces that would indicate a dietary cause of constipation.

D. Identifies pelvic, coxofemoral, or

spinal lesions that may predispose an animal to constipation

E. Identifies underlying prostatic enlargement that may be the cause of constipation

6. Barium enema contrast radiography or colonoscopy may be performed after removal of retained feces to evaluate the lumen of the colon when intraluminal obstructive lesions are suspected.

7. Myelographic and electrodiagnostic evaluation of the lumbosacral spinal cord and spinal nerves (see Chapter 17) should be considered in selected patients when impaired anorectal innervation is suspected.

Therapeutic Approach

1. Evacuation of impacted feces from the colon using enemas and/or manual extraction of retained feces is the initial treatment for constipation. Phosphate enemas must never be used in cats or small dogs because they result in dangerous hypernatremia, hyperosmolality, hyperphosphatemia, and hypocalcemia.

2. Any accompanying dehydration or electrolyte imbalances that may complicate severe constipation/obstipation should be corrected.

3. Underlying causes of constipation (identified in Table 10-13) should be eliminated or controlled.

4. Laxative therapy and dietary adjustments are used as follow-up therapy aimed at preventing recurrences (Table 10-14).

5. Subtotal colectomy is the treatment of choice for severe, recurrent constipation/obstipation or megacolon that is unresponsive to medical management.

Abdominal Pain

Abdominal pain is caused by stretching or distention of the peritoneum or visceral organs, or by peritoneal irritation secondary to chemical or septic material (as in peritonitis). In general, the severity of abdominal pain in acute disorders correlates with the severity of the underlying process. Therefore, the finding of abdominal pain indicates a need for further diagnostic evaluation.

Table 10-14. **Treatment of constipation*,†**

Enemas

Tap water (± soap)
Isotonic saline solution (± soap)
Dioctyl sodium sulfosuccinate
Mineral oil
Sodium phosphate‡
Bisacodyl

Rectal suppositories

Glycerin
Dioctyl sodium sulfosuccinate
Bisacodyl

Bulk-forming laxatives

Canned pumpkin
Coarse bran
Psyllium

Lubricant laxatives

White petrolatum
Mineral oil

Emollient laxatives

Dioctyl sodium sulfosuccinate
Dioctyl calcium sulfosuccinate

Saline laxatives

Magnesium hydroxide

Osmotic laxatives

Lactose
Lactulose
Polyethylene glycol and electrolytes§

Stimulant laxatives

Bisacodyl
Castor oil§

* Ancillary treatment measures include regular grooming to prevent ingestion of loose hair (especially in cats); prevention of ingestion of abrasive foreign materials; provision of fresh drinking water; provision of clean litter for cats; and a program of regular exercise.

† For severe recurrent or refractory cases, subtotal colectomy may be necessary.

‡ Should not be used in cats or small dogs.

§ Used mainly to prepare the colon for radiography or endoscopy.

Etiology

1. Abdominal pain may be caused by disorders of several body systems of the abdominal cavity (Table 10-15).

2. Because many causes are surgical emergencies, rapid identification of the cause of abdominal pain is essential.

Table 10-15. **Causes, diagnosis, and treatment of abdominal pain**

Causes	Basis for Diagnosis	Mode of Treatment
Gastrointestinal		
Inflammatory		
Hemorrhagic gastroenteritis	Clinical signs CBC (hemoconcentration)	Supportive care (fluids, antibiotics)
Feline panleukopenia	Clinical signs CBC (leukopenia)	Supportive care (fluids, antibiotics)
Canine parvovirus	Clinical signs CBC (leukopenia)	Supportive care (fluids, antibiotics)
Obstructive		
Foreign body	Abdominal palpation Abdominal radiography Barium GI contrast radiography	Surgical or endoscopic removal
Gastric dilatation/volvulus complex	Abdominal palpation Abdominal radiography	Gastric decompression Surgical correction
Intussusception	Abdominal palpation Abdominal radiography Barium GI contrast radiography	Surgical correction
Intestinal volvulus	Abdominal palpation Abdominal radiography	Surgical correction
Neoplasia	Abdominal palpation Abdominal radiography Surgical biopsy	Surgical excision Adjunctive chemotherapy
Traumatic (gastric or intestinal rupture)	Abdominal radiography Abdominocentesis	Surgical correction
Urogenital		
Inflammatory or infectious		
Acute renal failure	Compatible history Laboratory evaluation (see Chapter 12)	Fluid therapy (See Chapter 22)
Acute pyelonephritis	Laboratory evaluation (see Chapter 12) Urine culture	Antibiotic therapy (see Chapter 12)
Ruptured pyometra	Compatible history Laboratory evaluation Abdominal radiography	Surgical correction
Acute prostatitis	Physical examination Urine or prostatic wash culture	Antibiotic therapy Castration
Traumatic		
Renal trauma	History of trauma	Supportive care
Ruptured bladder	History of trauma Hematuria Palpation of bladder Laboratory evaluation Contrast cystogram	Surgical correction
Ruptured ureter	Excretory urogram	Surgical correction

(*continued*)

Table 10-15. *(Continued)*

Causes	Basis for Diagnosis	Mode of Treatment
Urogenital		
Obstructive		
Ureteral obstruction	Excretory urogram	Surgical correction
Urethral obstruction	Bladder palpation	Urethral catheterization
	Contrast cystogram	Surgical correction
Splenic		
Traumatic rupture	History of trauma	Splenectomy
	Abdominocentesis	
Torsion of splenic pedicle	Abdominal radiography	Splenectomy
	Identification of hemoglobinuria	
	Palpation of spleen	
Rupture of splenic neoplasm	Palpation of spleen	Splenectomy
	Abdominal ultrasonography	
	Abdominocentesis	
Peritoneal		
Chemical peritonitis		
Acute pancreatitis	Serum amylase and lipase	Supportive care
	Diagnostic imaging (radiography, ultrasonography)	
Early gastric rupture	Abdominal radiography	Surgical correction
	Abdominocentesis	
Ruptured urinary tract	Serum creatinine	Surgical correction
	Excretory urogram	
	Abdominocentesis	
Ruptured biliary system	Abdominocentesis	Surgical correction
Hemoperitoneum	Abdominocentesis	Correction of underlying disorder
Septic peritonitis		
Ruptured GI tract	Abdominocentesis	Surgical correction
	Laparotomy	
Ruptured abscess	Abdominocentesis	Surgical correction
	Laparotomy	
Ruptured pyometra	Compatible history	Surgical correction
	Abdominal radiography	

History and Physical Findings

1. If vomiting or diarrhea are part of the history, obstructive and inflammatory diseases of the GI tract and pancreatitis should be considered.

2. A history of trauma suggests the possibility of a ruptured abdominal organ.

3. Abdominal auscultation may reveal a lack of sounds, suggesting ileus, or high-pitched sounds that have an increased frequency, suggesting mechanical obstruction.

4. Careful palpation of the abdomen is essential. In addition to pain, palpation may reveal abnormal masses, organomegaly, an air-filled tympanic stomach, or distention of bowel loops. In addition, abdominal fluid may be detected by ballotment.

5. An attempt should be made to localize the site of abdominal pain. Pancreatitis results in pain in the cranioventral abdomen. Renal pain is usually localized to the paralumbar region. Intestinal pain is often difficult to localize. Peritonitis and gastric dilatation/volvulus cause generalized abdominal pain.

6. The presence of fever suggests inflammatory or infectious cause for the abdominal pain.

7. Clinical signs of shock indicate a serious problem (intestinal obstruction, gastric dilatation/volvulus complex, ruptured abdominal organ, fulminant acute pancreatitis, etc.).

Diagnostic Approach

1. Laboratory findings

A. The CBC is useful in judging the severity of the disorder. A degenerative left shift indicates a grave process (e.g., ruptured viscus). Hemoconcentration or hypovolemia may also be seen.

B. Serum amylase and lipase concentrations are used to diagnose pancreatitis.

C. Azotemia may be present as a result of dehydration (prerenal) or rupture of the urinary tract (postrenal) (see Chapter 12). A urinalysis (including specific gravity measurements) may be useful in distinguishing between these two conditions.

D. Abdominocentesis or diagnostic peritoneal lavage may be necessary to obtain samples for bacterial culture and cytologic examination.

2. Radiographic findings

A. Plain abdominal films may reveal GI obstruction, gastric dilatation/volvulus, organomegaly, or abdominal effusion, thereby facilitating establishment of a diagnosis.

B. Contrast studies of the GI tract may be required if plain films are not diagnostic. Barium tests should be avoided if GI perforation is possible.

3. Exploratory laparotomy may be the most expedient diagnostic approach in cases of "acute abdomen."

Therapeutic Approach

1. Stabilization of the patient frequently involves treatment for hypovolemic or endotoxic shock, including aggressive fluid therapy.

2. Surgical intervention is often imperative, so early diagnosis is of utmost importance.

Abdominal Effusion

Abdominal distention may be caused by organomegaly, hernias of the abdominal wall, or the accumulation of fluid within the peritoneal cavity. Fluid within the peritoneal cavity can be ascites (serous fluid), hemorrhage, or exudate.

Etiology

1. The accumulation of fluid within the abdominal cavity can be a result of active bleeding, exudation, or changes in vascular hydrostatic pressure or intravascular colloid osmotic pressure (Table 10-16).

2. If exudate and hemorrhage are ruled out based on examination of abdominal fluid, an evaluation of cardiac, renal, hepatic, and gastrointestinal function is warranted.

History and Physical Findings

1. A history of polyuria/polydipsia suggests the possibility of renal or liver disease.

2. A history of chronic diarrhea suggests protein-losing enteropathy.

3. A history of coughing, exercise intolerance, or lack of a heartworm prevention program may suggest a cardiogenic cause for ascites. The presence of muffled heart sounds, jugular vein distention, or abnormal cardiac auscultation indicate cardiogenic ascites (see Chapter 9).

4. Abdominal palpation should be performed to evaluate the animal for abdominal pain and organomegaly, as may be associated with exudative and hemorrhagic abdominal effusions.

Table 10-16. **Causes of and diagnostic tests for abdominal effusion**

Causes	Diagnostic Tests
Ascites—transudate with hypoalbuminemia	

Nephrotic syndrome
  Glomerulonephritis
  Renal amyloidosis
	Urinalysis
	Urine protein: creatinine ratio
	Renal biopsy

Protein-losing enteropathy
  Lymphangiectasia
  Intestinal lymphosarcoma
  Histoplasmosis
  Inflammatory bowel disease
	Panhypoproteinemia
	Intestinal biopsy

Liver disease Cirrhosis	Serum bile acids Liver biopsy
Ascites—modified transudate	
Liver disease	Serum bile acids Liver biopsy

Right-sided congestive heart failure
  Dirofilariasis
  Pericardial disease
  Cardiomyopathy
	Microfilaria test
	Occult heartworm test
	Thoracic radiography
	Echocardiography
	ECG

Abdominal neoplasm	Abdominal radiography Abdominal ultrasonography Laparotomy
Chylous or pseudochylous effusion	Triglyceride and cholesterol determinations on effusion Abdominal lymphangiography
Exudate	

Nonseptic inflammatory
  Bile peritonitis secondary to ruptured
    biliary system
  Urine peritonitis secondary to
    ruptured urinary system
  Peritonitis secondary to pancreatitis
  Early gastric rupture
  Feline infectious peritonitis
	Cytology of exudate
	Creatinine analysis of exudate
	Laboratory evaluation
	Laparotomy

Septic inflammatory
  Bacterial or mycotic peritonitis
  Ruptured abscess
  Ruptured pyometra
  Ruptured GI tract
	Cytology of exudate
	Cultures of exudate
	Laparotomy

Hemorrhage	

Traumatic splenic rupture
Ruptured splenic hemangiosarcoma
Coagulopathy
  Secondary to warfarin intoxication
  Secondary to disseminated
    intravascular coagulopathy
  Secondary to congenital coagulopathy
	Cytology of exudate
	Hemostasis evaluation
	Laparotomy

Diagnostic Approach

1. Laboratory findings

A. A CBC is useful in identifying inflammatory causes, which are usually associated with exudative effusions.

B. Serum albumin levels should be evaluated. Hypoalbuminemia is associated with nephrotic syndrome, protein-losing enteropathies, and liver disease. A decrease in both albumin and globulin suggests GI protein loss.

C. Abdominocentesis should be undertaken to determine the type of abdominal effusion. Cytologic evaluation and bacterial culture may be performed on the sample. Transudates are associated with nephrotic syndrome and protein-losing enteropathies, and modified transudates are associated with liver and cardiac diseases. Rupture of the biliary tract will cause a yellow- to green-stained modified transudate. Chylous effusions are lactescent in nature. Biochemical evaluation of the effusion may aid in diagnosis, as in creatinine determinations to diagnose uroabdomen.

D. A urinalysis will reveal proteinuria in patients with nephrotic syndrome. Hemoglobinuria may be seen in dogs with postcaval syndrome of heartworm disease (see Chapter 9).

2. Radiographic findings

A. Abdominal radiographs are often useful in differentiating abdominal effusion from other causes of abdominal enlargement, but they cannot distinguish the cause of effusion in most cases.

B. Thoracic radiographs are helpful if a cardiovascular cause for ascites is suspected.

3. Ultrasonographic findings

A. Ultrasonography is helpful in evaluating organs that cannot be visualized by radiographic means in patients with abdominal effusion.

B. The size and architecture of the liver, kidneys, and spleen, as well as the presence of abdominal masses, can be determined.

C. Cardiac ultrasonography can usually identify pericardial disease or other cardiac abnormalities.

Therapeutic Approach

1. Appropriate treatment is contingent upon establishing a definitive diagnosis.

2. Surgery is imperative in the management of a ruptured viscus or spleen.

3. Ascites may need to be treated symptomatically once a diagnosis is made. A low-sodium diet, diuretics, and angiotensin-converting enzyme inhibitors (e.g., captopril) are all used in the management of ascites. Therapeutic abdominocentesis should be reserved only for patients with severe respiratory compromise.

Suggested Readings

Burrows CF: Constipation. In Kirk RW (ed): Current Veterinary Therapy IX, p 904. Philadelphia, WB Saunders, 1986

Johnson SE: Diseases of the esophagus. In Sherding RW (ed): The Cat: Diseases and Management, p 907. New York, Churchill Livingston, 1988

Johnson SE: Medical emergencies of the digestive tract and abdomen. In Sherding RG (ed): Medical Emergencies, p 213. New York, Churchill Livingstone, 1985

Leib MS: Megaesophagus in the dog. In Kirk RW (ed): Current Veterinary Therapy IX, p 848. Philadelphia, WB Saunders, 1986

McKeever PJ: Stomatitis. In Kirk RW (ed): Current Veterinary Therapy IX, p 846. Philadelphia, WB Saunders, 1986

Sams DI, Harvey CE: Oral and dental diseases. In Sherding RW (ed): The Cat: Diseases and Management, p 875. New York, Churchill Livingstone, 1988

Sherding RG: Chronic diarrhea. In Ford RB (ed): Clinical Signs and Diagnosis in Small Animal Practice, p 473. New York, Churchill Livingstone, 1988

Sherding RG: Diseases of the intestines. In Sherding RW (ed): The Cat: Diseases and Management, p 995. New York, Churchill Livingstone, 1988

Sherding RG: Diseases of the small bowel. In Ettinger SJ (ed): Textbook of Veterinary Internal Medicine, 3rd ed, p 1323. Philadelphia, WB Saunders, 1989.

Twedt DC, Tams TR: Diseases of the stomach. In Sherding RW (ed): The Cat: Diseases and Management, p 929. New York, Churchill Livingstone, 1988

Twedt DC, Wingfield WE: Diseases of the stomach. In Ettinger SJ (ed): Textbook of Veterinary Internal Medicine, 2nd ed, p 1233. Philadelphia, WB Saunders, 1983

CHAPTER ELEVEN

Liver Failure

William A. Rogers

Liver failure is a difficult subject because the liver performs so many complex metabolic and excretory functions, any of which may fail in a patient with liver disease. It is necessary to simplify the subject of hepatic failure (at the risk of oversimplification) to allow "quick reference" to this disease process. The reader is reminded that liver diseases without failure are not included in this discussion.

Consequences of Liver Failure

Table 11-1 lists important clinical concepts in patients with acute or chronic liver failure.

1. Hepatoencephalopathy develops as a result of the failure of the liver to remove toxic factors, such as ammonia, from portal vein blood or to process nutrients in portal blood. This inability to process portal blood represents parenchymal failure, portacaval shunting, or both. Consequences may include amino acid imbalance or abnormal fatty acid metabolism.

2. The result is a metabolic encephalopathy (hepatoencephalopathy) associated with a variety of neurologic signs, including grand mal seizure, coma, and aggressive behavior. These signs are usually episodic, and depend on the rise or fall in the blood level of "hepatotoxins" normally cleared by the healthy liver.

3. The liver is the metabolic center of the body, and intermediary metabolism is impaired when it fails. Stunted growth, lack of energy, and weight loss are common. Hypoglycemia is a result of depleted glycogen stores or impaired gluconeogenesis in the face of decreased energy intake secondary to anorexia. Protein metabolism is severely deranged. The resultant hypoalbuminemia and decreased plasma oncotic pressure cause edema or ascites. The transport function of albumin and other carrier proteins, such as transferrin, ceruloplasmin, and haptoglobin, is reduced. Malnutrition and portcaval shunting rob the liver of important and hepatotrophic nutrients, causing further liver malfunction and atrophy.

4. Coagulopathies in patients with liver failure may result from lack of clotting factors, inability to clear fibrinolytic factors, disseminated intravascular coagulopathy (DIC), or thrombocytopenia. Because blood is a rich source of ammonia, a major complication is gastrointestinal hemorrhage, which may be followed by fatal encephalopathy.

5. Nearly all drugs undergo biotransformation by the liver, so that patients with liver failure do not metabolize drugs in a predictable way. A history of prolonged recovery from anesthesia is common. Caution should be used when selecting drugs and drug dosages for patients with liver failure.

6. Increased vascular resistance to portal blood flow may lead to portal venous hypertension. The consequences of portal hypertension include ascites, formation of portacaval shunt vessels, and possibly, extravasation of protein into the gut. The latter would contribute to hypoalbuminemia and worsen ascites.

Table 11-1. **Liver failure**

Major Consequences	Clinical Manifestation
Hepatoencephalopathy	Dementia Personality change Seizures Coma Anorexia Polydipsia
Impaired metabolic activity	Hypoglycemia Hypoproteinemia Weight loss Low BUN—polydipsia
Clotting disturbances	Gastrointestinal bleeding Prolonged bleeding time Petechial hemorrhage
Altered drug metabolism	Exaggerated response to drugs Prolonged bleeding time
Portal hypertension	Ascites Protein-losing enteropathy Gastrointestinal bleeding
Impaired bilirubin excretion	Icterus Bilirubinuria

7. Liver failure may cause icterus, but an absence of icteric membranes does not rule out liver failure. Dogs (especially males) have an increased ability to excrete bilirubin in urine compared to cats or human beings; thus they may become jaundiced less readily than similarly affected cats or human beings.

Medical History and Physical Exam

A complete physical examination and history taking are imperative. Special note should be made of the following:

1. Exposure to drugs or environmental chemical toxins. Drugs suspected of hepatotoxicity include primidone, phenytoin, mebendazole, oxybendazole, and mitotane (OP ddd), but the list is probably longer than currently appreciated. Corticosteroid drugs cause hepatopathy, but not liver failure. Nevertheless, steroid therapy may cause marked increases in serum liver enzyme values, thus confusing the interpretation of the liver profile.

2. A history of gastrointestinal bleeding or bilirubinuria may be elicited by asking the owners for a description of feces and urine characteristics.

3. Age, sex, and breed factors may influence the practitioner's clinical suspicion of a given liver disease. For example, female Doberman pinscher dogs with liver failure are most likely to have a characteristic chronic active hepatitis. Congenital portacaval shunting is more likely to occur in young dogs than in older dogs.

4. On physical examination, body condition should be noted as an indicator of chronicity, and precipitous weight loss in obese cats should be considered indicative of feline hepatic lipidosis. Palpate the liver carefully for size, consistency, and surface contour. In cases of cirrhosis and portacaval shunt, the liver is small. Neoplasia and acute hepatitis may cause hepatomegaly with increased turgidity and tenderness. The liver surface is irregular and nodular in cirrhotic animals and in some animals with hepatic neoplasia.

5. Examine the mucous membranes for jaundice.

6. Perform a neurologic examination, including a subjective evaluation of the state of mentation.

Diagnostic Approach

1. All patients suspected of having liver disease should undergo liver profile testing (see Table 11-2). Most chemistry profiles include tests that make up an adequate liver profile. Select a competent laboratory with quality control. A liver profile should include serum glutamic-pyruvic transaminase (SGPT/ALT), serum alkaline phosphatase (SAP), bilirubin, glucose, total protein, and albumin determinations. Determinations of serum gamma glutamyl transpeptidase (SGGT) and lactic dehydrogenase (LDH) are often added.

2. Urinalysis is performed to detect significant bilirubinuria.

3. An activated coagulation time (ACT; normal <125 sec in dogs and <65 sec in cats) or a clotting profile (one-stage prothrombin time [OSPT], activated partial thromboplas-

min time [APTT], platelet count) should be performed to assess risk of bleeding and to prepare for liver biopsy.

4. Abdominal radiographs should be obtained to assess liver size.

5. The van den Bergh test adds little diagnostic information.

6. Dogs with marked increases in SAP levels and near-normal values for other liver profile tests are often found to have undergone enzyme induction as a result of corticosteroid drugs, cortisol (in Cushings' syndrome), or other drugs (e.g., anticonvulsants). Glucocorticoid-induced hepatopathy does not cause liver failure.

7. An abnormal liver profile with a predominance of increased SAP and bilirubin levels or significant bilirubinuria usually indicates liver disease that is secondary to cholestasis, as occurs in biliary cirrhosis.

8. Marked increases in SGPT values often indicate acute or active liver necrosis, as occurs in toxin- or drug-induced hepatitis.

9. Marked increases in SAP levels in cats occurs most commonly with feline hepatic lipidosis. All increased SAP values in cats should be investigated, as the SAP level is not as volatile in cats as in dogs.

Table 11-2. **Normal laboratory values in liver failure***

Test Name	Range of Normal Values	
	Dog	*Cat*
SGPT	15–85 IU/L	30–80 IU/L
Serum alkaline phosphatase	0.0–105 IU/L	10–60 IU/L
Serum gamma glutamyl transpeptidase	1.0–11.0 IU/L	0.0–2.0 IU/L
Bilirubin	0.0–0.4 mg/dL	0.0–0.5 mg/dL
Glucose	75–120 mg/dL	70–135 mg/dL
Total protein	5.2–6.9 gm/dL	5.7–8.0 gm/dL
Albumin	2.7–4.2 gm/dL	2.7–3.9 gm/dL
BUN	6–28 mg/dL	15–35 mg/dL
Ammonia-fasting	10–74 μg/dL	Same
Ammonia tolerance test	>3× the fasting value	Same
Total serum bile acid	<5 μM/L	<5 μM/L
Two-hour postprandial bile acid	<10× the fasting value	Same
BSP dye excretion	<5% retention/30 min	Same
Activated coagulation time	<125 sec	<65 sec

* These values should be checked against the normal values established by the laboratory in which the tests are performed.

10. Hypoglycemia, hypoalbuminemia, and low BUN levels may indicate parenchymal liver failure, as in severe hepatic necrosis, cirrhosis, or portacaval shunts with hepatic atrophy.

11. Other useful parameters to test in patients with liver failure include:

A. Blood ammonia. Increased values indicate an inability to clear portal blood of ammonia, and correlate with the presence of hepatoencephalopathy. These values may be used to monitor the effectiveness of therapy for hepatic coma or encephalopathy. The test is performed after the patient has fasted for 12 hours. An ammonium chloride tolerance test to challenge hepatic function can be done in selected animals whose test results are borderline.

B. Total serum bile acid. Similar in rationale to the determination of blood ammonia levels, total serum bile acid tests are also performed after a period of fasting. A competent laboratory with a technique that has been validated in dogs, cats, or both should be used. A preprandial and postprandial test, similar to the ammonium chloride tolerance test, can be done. The bile acid level indicates contamination of systemic blood by portal blood. It is a good measure of portacaval shunting.

C. Bromsulphalein (BSP) dye excretion test. The indications and usefulness of this test are extremely limited. Its value is supplanted by that of blood ammonia or total serum bile acid assays.

D. Liver biopsy. A liver biopsy should be performed in cases of liver disease in which the etiology cannot be determined by noninvasive means. Liver biopsy should be avoided in dogs with bleeding tendencies, microhepatica, predictable steroid hepatopathy, congenital portacaval shunts, and biliary disease detectable by ultrasonography or radiologic studies. Liver biopsy should usually be obtained by percutaneous Menghini needle aspiration, preferably under ultrasonographic guidance. If the clinician lacks experience in liver biopsy, the patient should be referred to a specialist with such expertise.

E. Ultrasonography of the liver. Ultrasonography is a new and exciting diagnostic aid in animals with liver failure. Experience is a prerequisite to avoid interpretation errors. The biliary tree is easily imaged, and the parenchyma may be assessed by the degree of echogenicity and structural organization. Portacaval shunt vessels can be imaged. Needle biopsy can be guided by ultrasonography for increased safety. Postbiopsy ultrasonographic examination can detect hemorrhage. Unless the clinician has considerable experience in ultrasonography, the patient should be referred to a competent ultrasonographer for examination.

F. Portal vein angiography. Angiography may be used to detect portacaval shunts and to plan surgical correction of portacaval shunts. Arterial angiography has largely been replaced by splenoportography, mesenteric vein angiography, or both. Splenoportograms are easily obtained with ultrasonographic guidance of a needle into the spleen, followed by intrasplenic induction of contrast medium. Mesenteric venography is performed by injecting a mesenteric vein, isolated at laparotomy with contrast medium; it is the more invasive of the two tests.

G. Ammonium chloride tolerance test. When the fasting value is normal, administer 100 mg/kg of ammonium chloride orally. Repeat a blood ammonia assay in 30 minutes.

Etiologic Considerations

As the clinician attempts to establish an accurate diagnosis, consideration should also be given the potential causes of and predisposing factors underlying liver failure. Etiologic and prognostic factors relating to this condition are summarized in the following list. In addition, the clinician should consider the first five disorders listed in Table 11-3 in all cases of liver failure.

Causes of Liver Failure in Dogs and Cats

Congenital Portacaval Shunt
- Breeds most often affected—miniature schnauzer, Yorkshire terrier, Doberman pinscher
- Usually, but not always, affects young animals, often causing stunted growth

Table 11-3. **Treatment of liver failure**

Condition	Therapy	Dosage/Dietary Regimen
1. Hepatoencephalopathy	Lactulose	0.5 mL/kg orally, q8h, or as retention enema Retention enema: 15 mg/kg
	Glucose	2.5–5.0% in intravenous (IV) fluids
	Cleansing enema	To effect (removal of colon blood)
	Diet—acute cases	Carbohydrates (e.g., rice, potatoes, pastas)
	Diet—chronic cases	Low-salt/low-protein (e.g., dairy products, vegetables, k/d Prescription diet)
2. Hypoglycemia	Glucose	5% IV to maintain normoglycemia
3. Metabolic alkalosis/hypokalemia	Potassium	See Chapters 24 and 25
4. Hypoalbuminemia	Plasma	Slow IV administration, to effect
5. Disseminated intravascular coagulopathy	Heparin	150 U/kg subcutaneously (SC) q6h, to effect
6. Hepatitis	Prednisone Azathioprine D-penicillamine	1–2 mg/kg orally or IV 2 mg/kg orally 10–15 mg/kg orally, 30 min before meals
7. Fibrosis	Colchicine	Experimental antifibrotic; 0.03 mg/kg/day orally
	D-penicillamine	10–15 mg/kg orally, 30 min before meals
8. Copper accumulation	D-penicillamine	10–15 mg/kg orally, 30 min before meals
	Diet	Low-copper foods

- Hepatoencephalopathy is a major feature
- Polydipsia is common
- Ptyalism is a diagnostic clue in cats
- Ammonium biurate crystalluria and urolithiasis are common
- Treatment: Consider referral to a clinic capable of performing surgical correction
- Prognosis: Good, if successful surgery is accomplished; otherwise, it is poor, but medical therapy may be successful

Chronic Active Hepatitis (CAH) or Chronic Active Liver Disease (CALD)
- May be drug-induced (e.g., primidone, phenytoin, mebendazole, and others)
- Doberman pinscher is predisposed to developing these conditions (possibly inherited)
- Often idiopathic
- Occurs most commonly in middle-aged, female dogs
- Not well described in cats
- May lead to cirrhosis
- Treatment: see items 1 through 8 of Table 11-3
- Prognosis: Poor, as liver failure is already present; however, the prognosis may be fair when detected early

Acute Hepatic Necrosis
- Usually idiopathic

- Viral (e.g., infectious canine hepatitis)
- Acute toxic hepatitis
- Drug-induced
- Environmental toxins
- Endotoxin
- Treatment: Consider mannitol for animals exhibiting cerebral edema. The role of steroids remains controversial
- Prognosis: Poor

Feline Hepatic Lipidosis
- Obese cats with acute, severe weight loss
- Anorexia
- Icterus
- Delayed gastric emptying and vomiting
- Hepatomegaly
- Treatment: Nutrition is a main factor. Provide enteral hyperalimentation if necessary. In the author's experience, administration of choline (250 mg/day) has proven helpful
- Prognosis: Poor (approximately 50% survival rate)

Copper-associated Hepatitis
- Breeds most often affected: Bedlington terrier, West Highland white terrier
- Treatment: See items 1 through 4 and 8 of Table 11-3
- Prognosis: Guarded when liver failure is present; good when diagnosed and treated early

Cirrhosis
- Occurs most commonly in female dogs
- Active (end stage of CAH) versus inactive
- End result of chronic biliary obstruction
- Often idiopathic—end stage of many liver diseases
- Treatment: See items 1 through 5 and 7 of Table 11-3. In animals with active cirrhosis, see item 6
- Prognosis: Grave

Primary Liver Tumors
- Hepatoma
  —Those animals affected often have hypoglycemia
  —Treatment: None effective
  —Prognosis: Grave

Infections
- Leptospirosis
  —Usually caused by *Leptospira icterohaemorrhagiae*
  —Occurs most commonly in rural areas and in male dogs
  —Conduct serologic tests or blood culture and consider public health importance
  —Treatment: Intramuscular (IM) procaine penicillin G, 40,000 U/kg q12h, for leptospiremic phase
  —Follow-up is warranted to eliminate carrier state
- Infectious canine hepatitis
  —Rare incidence as a result of the effectiveness of vaccination; included because it is a known cause of CALD, which can lead to cirrhosis
- Histoplasmosis
  —Treatment: Amphotercin B, 0.25 to 0.50 mg/dL intravenously (IV) 3 days/week to a total dose of 2.5 to 5.0 mg/dL and oral ketoconazole, 10 mg/kg daily for 60 days
  —Prognosis: Fair
- Feline infectious diseases with liver failure
  —Toxoplasmosis
  —Feline leukemia virus
  —Feline infectious peritonitis
  —Treatment and prognosis: Currently, there is no known effective treatment for these diseases. Consequently, they are associated with a grave prognosis

The prognosis in liver failure should not be estimated by the degree of hepatic encephalopathy or the degree of increase in serum liver enzyme levels, as these two factors may not reflect the severity of hepatic parenchymal damage, malfunction, or capability for regeneration.

General Treatment Methods

Treatment of liver failure is directed at maintaining life until the liver can recover, and preserving hepatic function in chronic cases. Control of hepatoencephalopathy is of key importance. The treatment of ascites is intentionally ignored, as its presence is not usually detrimental and vigorous treatment with diuretics can worsen hepatoencephalopathy and cause hypokalemia or dehydration. Amino acid administration to correct plasma amino acid imbalances should be routine therapy in the near future.

CHAPTER TWELVE

Renal Failure

Dennis J. Chew and Stephen P. DiBartola

···

Definitions

1. The term *renal disease* denotes the presence of a pathologic process within the kidney.

A. There is no specified amount of nephron damage.

B. Renal disease may be present without renal failure if extensive nephron damage has not occurred.

2. The term *renal failure* applies when the kidneys are no longer able to maintain the conservation, excretion, and endocrine functions required of them.

A. The results are retention of nitrogenous solutes; derangement of fluid, electrolyte, and acid–base balance; and other extrarenal manifestations.

B. Renal failure occurs when glomerular filtration is reduced by 75% or more.

C. This reduction may be temporary or permanent.

3. *Azotemia* refers to increased concentrations of nitrogenous solutes (urea, nitrogen, and creatinine) in the plasma. The BUN and serum creatinine concentrations do not increase above normal until more than 75% of the glomeruli are not filtering. Clinical signs associated with azotemia may or may not be apparent.

4. The constellation of clinical signs and biochemical abnormalities resulting from renal failure is called *uremia*.

5. The finding of renal failure refers to a level of organ function without regard to a specific disease (Figures 12-1 and 12-2). It does not specify whether it is:

A. Prerenal, postrenal, or primary (intrinsic)

B. Acute or chronic

C. Reversible or irreversible

D. Progressive or nonprogressive

6. The magnitude of azotemia (increased BUN or serum creatinine levels) does not differentiate between prerenal, primary renal, and postrenal azotemia.

7. The magnitude of azotemia does not help differentiate acute from chronic renal failure, nor reversible from irreversible renal failure.

8. *Chronic interstitial nephritis* (CIN) is a histopathologic term used to describe the generalized fibrosis of renal interstitial tissue accompanied by a mononuclear inflammatory cell infiltrate and loss of functioning nephrons. The glomeruli are relatively unaffected by the pathologic process. No specific etiology is implied. Rather, the term is a description of the histologic appearance of the kidneys of many dogs and cats with chronic renal failure.

9. *End-stage renal disease* is a term used to describe the end result of all inflammatory, degenerative, and ischemic renal diseases that are generalized, progressive, and irreversible. End-stage renal disease has a variety of causes.

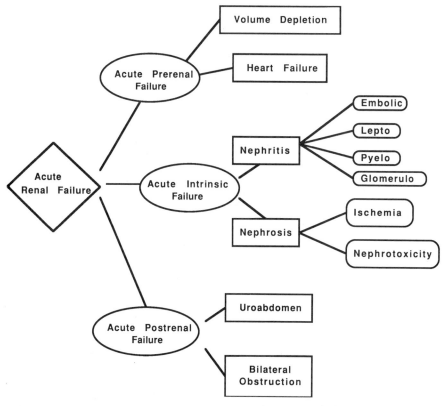

Figure 12-1. *Potential causes for acute azotemia (renal failure)*

Prerenal Failure

1. Azotemia is the result of decreased renal perfusion.

2. The kidneys are normal initially, but cannot excrete nitrogenous waste adequately because of decreased hydrostatic pressure within glomeruli.

3. Decreased renal perfusion may result from decreased cardiac output and decreased vascular volume secondary to:

    A. Cardiac failure

    B. Shock or hypovolemia

    C. Severe dehydration

    D. Hyponatremia (hypoadrenocorticism)

    E. Hypoalbuminemia

4. It is important to recognize these prerenal factors because their influence on azotemia may be readily reversible.

5. Sustained, uncorrected renal hypoperfusion may result in primary renal parenchymal damage.

6. Prerenal factors frequently coexist with primary renal and postrenal disease.

7. In certain phases of disease, it may be difficult to determine how much of the problem is prerenal and how much is actually caused by renal parenchymal disease. This differentiation will be discussed later.

8. Prerenal azotemia usually is characterized by physiologic oliguria.

    A. Decreased renal perfusion is monitored within the kidney and in peripheral baroreceptors; it results in increased renal conservation of salt and water from the glomerular filtrate.

    B. High urine specific gravity (sp gr >1.030) or high urine osmolality is expected

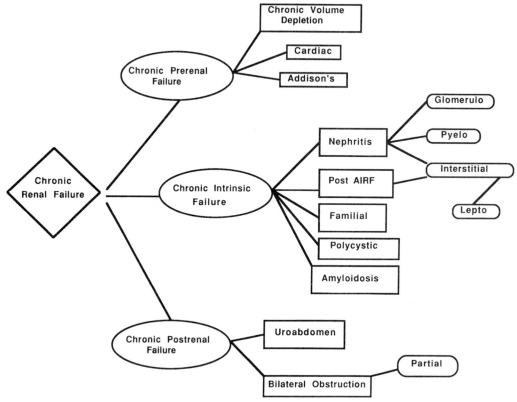

Figure 12-2.   *Potential causes for chronic azotemia (renal failure)*

in samples obtained prior to fluid or diuretic therapy.

C. Low urinary sodium concentration (<20 mEq/L), as advocated to document dehydration in humans, is unreliable for use in dogs.

D. Low fractional excretion of sodium may help document prerenal azotemia.

$$FE_{Na} = U_{Na}/S_{Na} \div U_{CR}/S_{CR} \times 100\%$$

The normal value is less than 1%.

E. A BUN-to-creatinine ratio of greater than 25:1 as a result of enhanced reabsorption of urea at low tubular flow rates may occur.

F. Urinalysis is normal. A few hyaline casts may be seen owing to the concentration of urinary mucoprotein.

G. Rehydration with intravenous (IV) fluids should lead to increased urine volume and improved renal function (↓ BUN and creatinine). If oliguria or poor renal function persists (↑ BUN and creatinine), suspect primary renal failure.

9. Treatment involves reestablishing vascular volume and improving cardiac output if the azotemia is purely prerenal. (See sections on Postrenal and Primary Renal Failure for treatment if these components are also present.)

Postrenal Failure

1. Postrenal azotemia is the result of interference with excretion of urine from the body secondary to:

    A. Obstruction

    B. Uroabdomen

2. The kidneys initially are normal morphologically and are capable of normal function.

A. Obstruction results in increased renal tubular pressure, a force opposing glomerular filtration rate (GFR), with subsequent retention of nitrogenous waste.

B. Uroabdomen results in azotemia secondary to recycling of nitrogenous waste across the semipermeable peritoneal membranes.

3. Obstruction may occur anywhere from the renal pelvis to the urethra, but (assuming two normal kidneys prior to the obstruction) both kidneys must be involved in order for azotemia to develop.

A. Obstruction may be acute or chronic, partial or complete.

B. Primary renal disease or failure may result from the obstruction, depending on its extent and duration.

4. Causes of obstruction

A. Calculi

B. Neoplasia

C. Prostatic disease

D. Neurologic disease (e.g., bladder atony)

E. Congenital ureterocele

F. Bladder or urethral entrapment (e.g., by a hernia)

G. Intravesical foreign body or blood clots

H. Ureteral obstruction from a severely thickened bladder wall

5. Rupture of the urinary conduit (kidney, renal pelvis, ureter, bladder, or urethra) may result from the following:

A. Trauma

1) Blunt abdominal (e.g., from a vehicle or kick)

2) Penetrating (e.g., from a knife or bullet wound)

3) Iatrogenic

a) Improper urinary catheterization technique

b) Accidental surgical rent

c) Improper cystotomy closure or breakdown of closure

B. Rupture secondary to severe obstruction (e.g., ruptured bladder in a cat with urethral obstruction or ruptured ureter secondary to longstanding erosive ureteral calculus)

C. Breakdown of friable neoplastic tissue

6. Diagnosis of postrenal azotemia (obstructive)

A. Variable degrees of oliguria or polyuria may be seen, depending on the location, severity, and chronicity of the obstruction.

B. The initial specific gravity may be either increased or decreased.

C. Urinalysis findings may reflect the underlying disorder (e.g., hematuria, pyuria, proteinuria, bacteriuria).

D. Physical examination may disclose the site of obstruction.

1) Turgid bladder from urinary retention

2) Visible crystalline material at the urethral tip of male cats

3) Palpable urethral calculi distal to the os penis or in the perineal or pelvic urethra

4) Cystic calculi

5) Renal enlargement

6) Abdominal mass

E. Abdominal imaging

1) Plain abdominal or perineal radiographs

2) Contrast urethrocystography

3) Excretory urography (intravenous pyelography [IVP])

4) Abdominal ultrasonography

F. The combination of a thorough physical examination and pertinent radiographic studies localize the obstruction.

G. Treatment consists of:

1) Relieving the obstruction (e.g., urinary catheterization for urethral obstruction, surgical repair of a bladder entrapped in a hernia)

2) Proper fluid therapy to maintain vascular volume and minimize prerenal azotemia.

7. Diagnosis of postrenal azotemia (urinary rent)

A. A ruptured bladder is the most common type of urinary rent.

B. A significant volume of urine may still be voided in animals with a ruptured bladder.

C. Physical examination

1) Pain near the site of rupture is often elicited.

2) Abdominal fluid may be palpable, especially after IV fluid therapy.

3) A small urinary bladder may be palpable in animals with bladder rupture. The bladder may fail to fill following IV fluid therapy because fluid continues to leak into the abdomen.

D. Return of substantial fluid volume following urethral catheterization does not exclude rupture of the bladder or urethra. On occasion, the catheter may pass through the tear into the abdomen, retrieving accumulating abdominal fluid.

E. Abdominocentesis in suspected cases of uroabdomen may be helpful in confirming the diagnosis.

1) Retrieval of fluid from the abdominal tap does not prove conclusively that the fluid is urine.

2) Chemical tests of the fluid add greater certainty that the fluid is urine, or that it is urine modified by equilibration in the peritoneal cavity.

a) Fluid and serum urea nitrogen measurements may demonstrate a gradient such that the suspect fluid urea nitrogen concentration is higher than the serum urea nitrogen concentration, if indeed the suspect fluid is urine. However, this comparison does not always demonstrate a marked gradient, because urea rapidly equilibrates between urine in the abdomen across the peritoneal membranes and into plasma. Dipstick methods for urea concentration (Azostix) may provide the same information regarding suspect fluid and serum urea nitrogen concentration if a large difference in the two color reactions can be demonstrated.

b) Measurement of the creatinine concentration of the suspect fluid and serum is the chemical determination of choice. A large concentration gradient is most likely in using creatinine concentrations, because creatinine is a larger molecule and does not readily equilibrate across the peritoneum.

F. Injection of air through a urethral catheter may allow the clinician to hear a hissing sound as air leaves the bladder tear. Inability to distend the bladder adequately may occur if the tear is in the bladder.

G. Injection of methylene blue through a urethral catheter may be useful to document a tear of the urethra or bladder. Abdominocentesis performed after this injection will yield blue fluid.

H. Radiography is required to localize the site of urinary rupture.

1) Positive contrast cystography is the procedure of choice in bladder rupture.

2) Pneumocystography may demonstrate the bladder tear, but it is difficult to detect in most cases.

3) Excretory urography (IVP) is necessary to demonstrate the lack of integrity in renal or ureteral anatomy.

8. To treat urinary rupture, presurgical radiographic studies are performed to localize the tear and to assess the amount of damage.

A. Urethra

1) Use of an indwelling urethral catheter as a stent for seven days may suffice if the tear is small.

2) Primary closure is required if the tear is large.

B. Bladder—primary closure after debridement

C. Ureter—largely depends on location of tear (proximal or distal)

D. Kidney

1) Pelvic tears usually cannot be closed, and nephrectomy is often required.

2) Partial nephrectomy may be possible if leakage is occurring from one pole of the kidney.

Primary (Intrinsic) Renal Failure

1. Azotemia is the result of disease within the renal parenchyma that causes loss of nephron function. GFR may be reduced for a variety of reasons:

A. Decreased number of nephrons and their replacement with nonfunctional tissue

B. Decreased function of remaining nephrons

1) Glomerular permeability change

2) Intrarenal hydronephrosis

3) Intrarenal blood maldistribution

2. Some prerenal component of the azotemia (dehydration from vomiting or hypodipsia) usually accompanies primary renal azotemia.

3. Dilute urine (sp gr <1.030) and azotemia (increased BUN and creatinine concentration) indicate primary renal failure as the cause of the azotemia.

A. Dilute urine and azotemia may coexist without primary renal failure if nonrenal factors interrupt the urinary concentrating mechanism. (For example, severe dehydration in a patient with diabetes insipidus may result in azotemia and dilute urine, yet no lesions will be found in the kidney.)

B. Rarely, concentrated urine (sp gr >1.030) and azotemia may coexist in a patient with primary renal failure, most notably in animals with early glomerular disease and relatively maintained tubular function (glomerulotubular imbalance).

C. Concentrated urine and azotemia occur commonly in subtotally nephrectomized experimental cats, yet dilute urine occurs most often in cats with clinical renal failure.

4. Azotemia from primary renal failure fails to respond rapidly and completely to fluid therapy, although a partial improvement in renal function tests (decreased BUN and creatinine levels) may occur as prerenal factors are corrected.

5. After deciding that the failure is attributable to primary renal involvement, the predominant anatomic site of injury (vascular, glomerular, tubular, interstitial, or a combination) remains to be determined.

A. There exists a functional interdependence of the units of the nephron.

B. Injury at the level of the glomerulus eventually influences units supplied by postglomerular capillaries.

C. Interstitial diseases are not isolated derangements of the interstitial tissue, but commonly affect tubules and glomeruli adversely, just as tubular injury may initiate interstitial changes.

D. Thus, a disease process that is primarily active in one particular anatomic area may progress to involve other functional areas.

6. The diagnostic approach should be directed toward differentiating acute from chronic disorders and reversible from irreversible processes.

A. The prognosis may be greatly affected by these decisions, suggesting either euthanasia or further treatment.

B. These decisions are based on radiographic findings (especially kidney size), serial biochemical studies, hematology, urinalysis, and the patient's response to therapy. Renal biopsy is also of value in selected patients.

Acute Intrinsic Renal Failure

Acute intrinsic renal failure (AIRF) is a syndrome characterized by an abrupt deterioration of renal function with retention of nitrogenous compounds and loss of ability to regulate solute and water balance. The etiology of AIRF is varied, but nephrotoxins are most important, followed by renal ischemia and nephritis. Sudden recognition of azotemia does not necessarily mean that it developed recently, as some animals (with chronic renal failure) tolerate azotemia for long periods.

1. Urine volume

A. There is no characteristic urine volume in dogs or cats with AIRF.

1) Older definitions required the presence of oliguria.

B. Anuria is uncommon unless severe cortical necrosis has occurred.

C. Severe oliguria can occur following ethylene glycol poisoning.

D. Nonoliguria typifies aminoglycoside nephrotoxicity.

E. Severe oliguria parallels the degree of tubular injury (the more severe the tubular injury, the greater the likelihood of oliguria).

F. An alteration in urine volume is neither sensitive nor specific for the diagnosis of AIRF.

2. AIRF can be caused by nephritis or nephrosis, but nephrosis is more common.

3. Phases of primary AIRF (Figure 12-3)

A. Induction (latent, incipient)

1) This phase extends from exposure to a toxin, infectious agent, or ischemic epi-

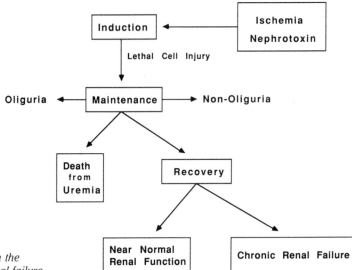

Figure 12-3. *Potential phases in the development of acute intrinsic renal failure*

sode until the development of intrarenal lesions.

    B. Maintenance (well-established, fixed)

        1) In this phase, a critical mass of intrarenal lesions has been achieved, so that simple removal of the inciting cause will not result in immediate improvement in renal function.

        2) Fluid therapy also does not cause renal function to be regained immediately.

        3) This phase may last 7 to 21 days, or longer, if renal insult is severe.

    C. Recovery

        1) GFR, BUN, and serum creatinine levels can return to near normal if adequate intrarenal healing occurs.

        2) Chronic renal failure can occur if healing is by fibrosis.

        3) A period of months may ensue before complete recovery occurs.

Nephritis

  1. Leptospirosis*
  2. Pyelonephritis (more often associated with chronic renal failure)

  3. Glomerulonephritis (more often associated with chronic renal failure)

    A. Systemic lupus erythematosus (SLE)
    B. Heartworms
    C. Pyometra
    D. Endocarditis
    E. Feline leukemia virus (FeLV)
    F. Borreliosis
    G. Rocky Mountain spotted fever
    H. Idiopathic disease

  4. Viral nephritis (Usually, renal disease is only a small part of systemic illness.)

    A. Canine distemper virus
    B. Infectious canine hepatitis
    C. Herpesvirus

Nephrosis

  1. Disease within the kidney characterized by degenerative or necrotic tubular lesions
  2. Synonyms include acute tubular necrosis (ATN), acute tubular insufficiency, and lower-nephron nephrosis.

  3. Nephrosis

    A. Nephrotoxins*
    B. Hypoperfusion (ischemia)*
    C. Thrombosis
    D. Pigments (myoglobin or hemoglobin)

  4. AIRF associated with nephrotoxins

A. Glycols*
    1) Ethylene glycol
    2) Diethylene glycol
B. Antimicrobials*
    1) Aminoglycosides*
    2) Amphotericin B*
    3) Cephaloridine
    4) Sulfonamides
    5) Tetracyclines
    6) Polymyxin B
    7) Colistin
C. Chemotherapeutic agents used in the treatment of cancer
    1) Cisplatin
    2) High-dose methotrexate
    3) High-dose doxorubricin
    4) High-dose cyclophosphamide
    5) Mithramycin
    6) Streptozotocin
D. Hypercalcemia/hypercalciuria
    1) Humoral hypercalcemia of malignancy
        a) Most commonly causes chronic renal failure
    2) Hypervitaminosis D (iatrogenic, new-generation rodenticide*)
E. Heavy metals
    1) Arsenic
    2) Mercury
    3) Thallium
    4) Cadmium
F. Hydrocarbons
    1) Methanol
    2) Carbon tetrachloride (solvent)
    3) Toluene (solvent)
    4) Chlordane (insecticide)
    5) Paraquat (herbicide)
G. Intravenous radiocontrast agents
H. Fluorinated inhalational anesthetics
    1) Methoxyflurane/enflurane
I. Miscellaneous
    1) Thiacetarsamide (organic arsenical)
    2) Cyclosporin
    3) Elemental phosphorus (rodenticide)
    4) EDTA
    5) Mushroom poisoning
    6) Mycotoxins
    7) Hemoglobinuria/myoglobinuria

* Most common cause

    8) Snake bite/bee sting (may involve significant hypoperfusion also)
J. Nephrotoxic nephropathy results in tubular lesions predominantly affecting the proximal tubule, with a tendency to preserve the integrity of the tubular basement membranes.
5. AIRF associated with renal ischemia (hypoperfusion)
    A. Intravascular volume depletion*
        1) Dehydration (vomiting, diarrhea, sequestration, hypodipsia)*
        2) Blood loss
        3) Hypoalbuminemia
        4) Trauma
        5) Hypoadrenocorticism
    B. Altered renal and systemic vascular resistance
        1) Renal vasoconstriction*
            a) Catecholamines (epinephrine, norepinephrine)
            b) Sympathetic nervous stimulation
            c) Vasopressin
            d) Angiotensin II
            e) Hypercalcemia
            f) Amphotericin B
            g) Hypothermia
            h) Myoglobinuria/hemoglobinuria
        2) Systemic vasodilatation
            a) Arteriolar vasodilator treatment
            b) Anaphylaxis
            c) Inhalational anesthesia
            d) Sepsis
            e) Heatstroke
    C. Interference with renal autoregulation during hypotension
        1) Nonsteroidal anti-inflammatory drugs* (e.g., aspirin, indomethacin, ibuprofen, banamine)
            a) Inhibition of renal prostaglandin synthesis
    D. Decreased cardiac output
        1) Congestive heart failure
        2) Low output without overt failure
            a) Pericardial disease
            b) Arrhythmias
            c) Following cardiac arrest
    E. Renal hypoperfusion may result in an ischemic nephropathy associated with patchy anatomic areas of tubular necrosis or degen-

eration, and with a tendency to disrupt the integrity of the tubular basement membranes.

6. The mechanisms for reduced GFR, renal blood flow, oliguria, or diuresis in AIRF have been studied in experimental nephrosis, although these mechanisms may also be operative in nephritis. Renal ischemia and nephrotoxins share the common end point of lethal renal tubular cell injury when severe. The precise contribution of each possible mechanism to the induction or maintenance of AIRF in clinical nephrosis is presently unknown. Mechanisms may be different during the induction phase than in the maintenance phase of AIRF.

7. Mechanisms that may contribute to decreased GFR and/or oliguria

A. Vasoconstriction of preglomerular blood vessels

1) "Vasomotor" nephropathy

B. Tubular backleak

C. Tubular obstruction

1) Intraluminal casts

2) Extraluminal compression from swelling or infiltrates

D. Decreased permeability of glomerular capillary wall

8. Conversion from oliguria to diuresis or increased GFR may be expected to occur when resolution of vasoconstriction, tubular backflow, tubular obstruction, and decreased glomerular permeability take place.

A. Diuresis is aided by:

1) Solute diuresis induced by solute that accumulated during the oliguric phase

2) Sodium wasting secondary to decreased proximal tubular reabsorption of sodium

3) Insensitivity of collecting tubules to antidiuretic hormone

4) Overzealous administration of fluids during the oliguric phase (overhydration)

Diagnosis

1. Diagnosis of AIRF and its differentiation from chronic renal failure (CRF) is of paramount importance because AIRF is a potentially treatable, reversible disease, whereas CRF is not.

2. In most cases, the animal will be evaluated by the veterinarian during the maintenance phase. Common findings include:

A. A serum creatinine at least 50% to 100% greater than previously measured values, despite correction of prerenal factors

B. A progressive increase in serum creatinine and BUN concentrations (early), despite fluid therapy

3. There is no single test or finding that can confirm a diagnosis of AIRF.

History and Physical Findings

1. Abrupt onset of clinical signs of uremia (can also occur with acute decompensation of CRF)

2. No long-standing history of polyuria or polydipsia

3. Questioning of the owner may elicit the precipitating cause, such as trauma, blood loss, anesthesia and surgery, or exposure to nephrotoxins, such as antibiotics, ethylene glycol (did the owner recently change a car's radiator fluid?), or amphotericin B.

4. Hypothermia (98°F to 100°F) is often seen in AIRF; it is not seen in CRF unless the affected patient is terminal.

5. Normal to increased renal size is noted on palpation and radiography. (Kidneys are small to normal in size in CRF.)

A. Renal pain may be elicited upon palpation.

6. Dehydration, oral ulcers, gastrointestinal bleeding, and necrosis of the tongue tip may be signs of uremia, but are not specific for AIRF.

7. Absence of anemia early in the course of the disease (A normochromic, normocytic anemia is a frequent finding in CRF.)

Laboratory Findings

1. Increased BUN and serum creatinine concentrations

2. Increased PO_4 and decreased Ca^{++} concentrations

3. Increased serum potassium concentration, which may be life threatening

A. Most likely if the animal is oliguric, or if severe metabolic acidosis is also present

4. Low urine specific gravity and osmolality

5. Fractional urinary sodium excretion greater than 1%

6. Urine sediment: ± RBCs, WBCs, tubular epithelial cells, cellular casts, coarsely granular casts

7. Blood gases: decreased pH, decreased HCO_3^-, mildly decreased P_{CO_2}

    A. Metabolic acidosis with mild respiratory compensation

    B. The metabolic acidosis in CRF is usually very mild, whereas in AIRF, it may be severe.

8. If AIRF is attributable to pyelonephritis, bacteria and WBC casts may be found.

9. If it is the result of ethylene glycol poisoning, there may be:

    A. Severe metabolic acidosis

    B. Increased anion gap

    C. Increased osmolar gap

    D. Increased ethylene glycol or metabolites in serum (based on positive results of an in-house test kit for ethylene glycol)

        1) Test yields positive results if it is performed within 12 to 24 hours of ingestion.

Renal Biopsy

1. May be needed to differentiate between AIRF and CRF

2. May provide prognostic information

    A. Extent of tubular cell damage

    B. Status of basement membranes (needed for repair of tubules)

    C. Extent of healing by fibrosis

    D. Extent of mineralization

    E. Evaluation of underlying renal disease prior to AIRF

Chronic Intrinsic Renal Failure

1. Chronic real failure is characterized by the slowly progressive development of irreversible renal lesions and loss of renal function. Systemic arterial hypertension is common in dogs with CRF and probably also in cats.

    A. It is not a specific diagnosis, but rather the end point of a variety of disease processes, including generalized vascular, glomerular, interstitial, and tubular processes (see Figure 12-2 and section on Causes, below).

    B. The natural history in dogs and cats with untreated clinical CRF is not well-documented, but clinical experience indicates that it is progressive.

    C. The rate of progression is variable, but can be estimated by serial evaluation of serum creatinine concentrations in an individual animal.

    D. Clinical signs and history will reflect the loss of the conservation, excretion, metabolism, and endocrine functions of the kidneys.

2. Why do animals with CRF develop progressive loss of renal function and renal lesions (sometimes called the "inexorable progression of CRF")?

    A. It is not known for certain.

    B. The original cause for renal injury may still be present and ongoing.

    C. The original cause for the renal injury may no longer be present, yet progressive renal injury continues.

        1) A critical mass of nephron loss appears to be necessary before self-perpetuating mechanisms continue to destroy the remaining viable renal tissue.

            a) An excess of 75% to 80% loss of nephron mass may be necessary for this to occur.

            b) The greater the loss of functional nephron mass, the greater the degree of self-perpetuating injury to the remaining "healthy" renal tissue.

    D. The so-called adaptive response of the remaining viable nephrons following substantial injury and loss of function to other units may actually contribute to their eventual injury. Renal hypertrophy of function results in "super nephrons."

        1) Intraglomerular hypertension (hyperfiltration)

            a) Increased single nephron GFR

            b) Increased glomerular plasma flow

            c) Increased transglomerular capillary hydraulic pressure

        2) Increased tubular metabolism

3) Increased tubular cell ammo-niagenesis
  E. Mineralization of renal tissue
    1) Related to phosphate retention
    2) Influenced by the magnitude of the calcium × phosphorus product
  F. Systemic arterial hypertension
  G. Intrarenal coagulation
  H. Immune-mediated mechanisms

Etiology

1. Idiopathic CIN is most common.
2. Pyelonephritis
3. Amyloidosis
  A. Idiopathic—most common
  B. Secondary
  C. Familial in Abyssinian cats and Shar Pei dogs
4. Glomerulonephritis
  A. Idiopathic type is most common.
  B. Infectious—canine
    1) Adenovirus 1
    2) Ehrlichiosis
    3) Brucellosis
    4) Leishmaniasis
    5) Bacterial endocarditis
    6) Pyometra
    7) Dirofilariasis
    8) Borreliosis?
    9) Rocky Mountain spotted fever?
  C. Infectious—feline
    1) Feline leukemia virus (FeLV)
    2) Feline infectious peritonitis (FIP)
    3) Polyarthritis (mycoplasma gatae)
    4) Feline immunodeficiency virus?
  D. Inflammatory
    1) Pancreatitis
    2) SLE
  E. Neoplastic
    1) Lymphosarcoma
    2) Hemolymphatic neoplasia
    3) Mastocytoma
    4) Others
  F. Familial
    1) Doberman pinscher?
    2) Glomerulonephritis in sibling cats
5. Familial renal disease
  A. Lhasa apso
  B. Shih Tzu
  C. Norwegian elkhound
  D. Cocker spaniel

E. Doberman pinscher
F. Samoyed
G. Standard poodle
H. Soft-coated wheaten terrier
I. Golden retriever
6. Polycystic kidneys
  A. Acquired
  B. Congenital
  C. Familial in Persian cats
7. Resolution of AIRF by fibrosis
8. Hypercalcemia in dogs (rare in cats)
9. Bilateral renal neoplasia (e.g., renal lymphosarcoma in cats)
10. Bilateral hydronephrosis
11. Pyogranulomatous nephritis
  A. FIP
  B. Fungal
12. Renal occlusive vascular disease (uncommon in dogs and cats)
13. Leptospirosis (uncommon in dogs; rare to nonexistent in cats)

Stages of Development

1. Diminished renal reserve (up to 50% loss of functioning nephrons)
  A. No azotemia
  B. Concentrating ability remains
  C. Well-preserved excretory function
2. Renal insufficiency (50% to 75% loss of functioning nephrons)
  A. Azotemia absent or mild
  B. Impaired concentrating ability
  C. Stress may precipitate overt renal failure.
3. Renal failure (>75% loss of functioning nephrons)
  A. Moderate to severe azotemia
  B. Impaired concentrating ability
  C. Variable loss of diluting ability
  D. Hyperphosphatemia
  E. Metabolic acidosis
  F. Nonregenerative anemia
  G. Extrarenal manifestations of uremia (e.g., uremic gastroenteritis)

Differentiation Between Chronic Renal Failure and Acute Intrinsic Renal Failure

1. May be clinically difficult
2. Differentiation is important because AIRF

is potentially reversible and treatable, but CRF is not.

A. Renal size is small to normal in CRF, but normal to large in AIRF.

B. A history of previous polyuria and polydipsia is often present in CRF, but absent in AIRF.

    1) Oliguria following rehydration suggests AIRF, or terminal CRF.

C. Anemia is often detected in animals with CRF, but not in those with AIRF.

D. Hypothermia is occasionally detected in patients with AIRF, but not in those with CRF unless they are terminal.

E. Hyperkalemia suggests AIRF (of primary parenchymal or postrenal cause), or terminal CRF with oliguria.

Diagnosis

1. Historical findings

    A. Polyuria or polydipsia

        1) May be first abnormality noted by owner

        2) Nocturia

        3) Some owners may think the animal is incontinent because it urinates in the house although it never did so in the past.

    B. If the owner fails to detect polyuria/polydipsia, signs of uremia may be the first signs detected.

2. Azotemia (increased BUN and serum creatinine)

3. Dilute urine (sp gr <1.030, and usually <1.017)

4. Urinalysis

    A. Inactive sediment

    B. Proteinuria if underlying glomerulopathy is present

        1) The urine protein to urine creatinine ratio ($U_P : U_{CR}$) may be helpful in evaluating proteinuria that is thought to arise from renal loss.

        a) Highly concentrated urine can result in increased concentration of urinary protein when 24-hour excretion of protein is normal.

        b) Very dilute urine can result in low concentrations of urinary protein when 24-hour excretion of protein is increased.

        c) The effect of urine concentration or dilution is minimized when urinary protein and creatinine are compared.

        d) Urinary protein is measured by Coumassie Brilliant Blue (CBB) or trichloroacetic acid Ponceau-S (TCA-PS) methods that detect both albumin and globulin.

        e) Normal $U_P : U_{CR}$ is less than 1 for both dogs and cats.

        f) Glomerulonephritis, renal amyloidosis, and CIN usually result in $U_P : U_{CR}$ of greater than 1.

        g) One large study of dogs showed a median $U_P : U_{CR}$ of 5.73 (0.4 to 34.39) for glomerulonephritis, 22.50 (11.17 to 46.65) for amyloidosis, and 2.89 (1.51 to 10.52) for CIN.*

        h) The large overlap in U_P to U_{CR} ratios shown above indicates that increased values cannot be used to identify the renal disease responsible for the increased protein loss.

        i) Urine samples with obvious hematuria or pyuria usually exhibit an increased $U_P : U_{CR}$ that may not be indicative of glomerulopathy.

    C. Bacteriuria may or may not be observed in pyelonephritis.

5. Kidneys may be small (<2.5 × L_2 in length for dogs; <2 × L_2 for cats).

6. Nonregenerative anemia

7. Normal to low serum K^+ concentration (except in the case of extremely advanced CRF, in which hyperkalemia may be seen)

8. Mild to moderate metabolic acidosis

9. Hyperphosphatemia

10. Low, normal, or, rarely, increased serum calcium concentration

Treatment of Intrinsic (Primary) Renal Failure

1. Rarely is the exact type of intrinsic renal failure known at the time therapy must be started. Consequently, therapy and further diagnostic studies must continue simultaneously.

---

* Center SA, Wilkinson E, Smith CA, Lewis RM: 24-hour urine protein/creatinine ratio in dogs with protein-losing nephropathies. J Am Vet Med Assoc 187(8): 820–824, 1985

2. In all cases of presumptive primary renal failure, one must:

A. Correct existing dehydration within 6 to 8 hours using physiologic crystalloid solutions, as continuing renal hypoperfusion could be detrimental.

B. Provide maintenance fluids, considering the possible wide range of urine output.

C. Provide contemporary loss fluids as calculated from estimates of losses via vomiting or diarrhea.

D. Correct severe electrolyte or acid–base disturbances.

E. Rule out urinary obstruction by radiographic examination.

    1) Relieve any existing obstruction by medical or surgical methods.

F. Rule out urinary tract infection by urine culture.

    1) Initiate a regimen of non-nephrotoxic antibiotics if infection is present.

G. Rule out hypercalcemia as a possible cause of renal failure (see Chapter 25).

H. Perform serial measurements to evaluate the patient.

    1) Body weight b.i.d. to t.i.d. initially

    2) Packed cell volume and total solids (PCV/TS) b.i.d., then s.i.d. later

    3) Skin turgor and other clinical monitors of hydration

    4) BUN and serum creatinine concentrations to detect deterioration or improvement of renal function

    5) Serum electrolyte concentrations (Na, K, Cl) during severe diuresis or oliguria to monitor effects of therapy, particularly in terms of hyperkalemia and hypokalemia

3. In cases of primary renal failure, the clinician must determine whether it is polyuric or oliguric in nature. Evaluation of urine volume is made by an assessment of historical and physical findings, metabolism cage collections, or measured urine output through an indwelling urinary catheter. Normal urine volume production for dogs and cats is 0.5 to 1.0 mL/lb/h.

4. In oliguric intrinsic renal failure, the patient must be monitored for retention of water and electrolytes.

A. Hyperkalemia frequently accompanies azotemia in this type of renal failure.

B. Hyperphosphatemia, hypocalcemia, and metabolic acidosis also may be seen.

C. During oliguria, meticulous attention must be directed to the volume and type of fluid administered in order to avoid iatrogenic overhydration and hypernatremia.

    1) Overhydration may appear as subcutaneous edema, pulmonary edema, or congestive heart failure.

    2) The ideal fluid for administration during this period would not contain potassium (e.g., 0.9% saline, 2.5% dextrose in 0.45% saline).

    3) Fluids that are low in sodium are helpful in avoiding hypernatremia. Patients with severe reductions in GFR that receive sodium-rich fluids frequently develop hypernatremia.

5. Polyuric renal failure is characterized primarily by losses of water and electrolytes. Serum potassium concentrations usually are normal to low, in contrast to those in the oliguric state. Other biochemical measurements are similar to those found in oliguric renal failure. Animals with severely decreased GFR may exhibit polyuria and hyperkalemia, however.

6. In renal failure, the oral and subcutaneous routes of fluid administration are not satisfactory for the initial phase of management. The azotemic animal may be vomiting, and its gastrointestinal absorption of water and electrolytes may be unreliable. Subcutaneous absorption of fluids also may be unreliable, particularly if moderate or severe dehydration exists. Also, it is difficult to administer large volumes of fluid by this route. Consequently, the IV route is essential during initial treatment.

7. Fluid therapy in the dog and cat with primary renal failure ideally allows the patient to remain alive long enough so that repair of renal tissue and hypertrophy of function in the remaining viable nephrons results in improved renal function. With fluid therapy, the aim is to ensure adequate renal perfusion by maintaining peripheral plasma volume. Frequently, fluid therapy can be continued until a definitive diagnosis is made. Intravenous fluid therapy also offers the clinician an avenue for intensive diuresis of the patient with primary renal failure so that azotemia is reduced.

8. Control of vomiting

A. Circulating uremic toxins may stimulate the chemoreceptor trigger zone.

B. Gastrointestinal uremic ulceration may stimulate reflex vomiting.

C. Gastric hyperacidity, which is often encountered in uremia, should be reduced. This often is successful in reducing the severity or frequency of vomiting.

    1) Cimetidine (Tagamet)

        a) 10 mg/kg IV initially, followed by 5 mg/kg IV b.i.d. to t.i.d.

        b) Can be administered orally when vomiting stops

    2) Ranitidine, 2 to 4 mg/kg b.i.d.

D. Central control of vomiting may be helpful when cimetidine alone is not successful.

    1) Chlorpromazine (Thorazine), 0.5 mg/kg

    2) Prochlorperazine (Compazine), 1.0 mg/kg

    3) Trimethobenzamide (Tigan), 3.0 mg/kg

    4) Metoclopramide (Reglan), 0.2 to 0.4 mg/kg t.i.d. to q.i.d.

E. Gastrointestinal coating agents for ulcerations

    1) Kaolin-Pectin

        a) 1 mL/kg t.i.d. to q.i.d. orally

    2) Sucralfate

        b) 1 tablet/25 kg t.i.d. to q.i.d.

F. No food for at least 24 to 48 hours during therapy; also consider restriction of oral water intake if vomiting is severe.

9. Severe uremic oral ulcers, stomatitis, and tongue-tip necrosis

A. Topical lidocaine (Xylocaine viscous)

B. Glycerine and hydrogen peroxide mouthwash (Gly-Oxide)

Acute Renal Failure

1. *Primum non nocere* (first, do no harm).

A. The primary aim of therapy in AIRF is to minimize alterations in the patient's internal milieu and give the kidneys an opportunity to repair themselves.

B. The renal lesion itself is not amenable to therapy.

C. Try to maintain proper fluid, electrolyte, and acid–base balance during the phases of AIRF.

2. Meticulous attention to detail in fluid volume administration is necessary to provide optimal hydration and to avoid overhydration if oliguria persists. Overhydration may occur in animals without oliguria because their ability to excrete a water load also may be severely impaired.

A. Replace dehydration, contemporary fluid loss, and maintenance fluid volumes by IV administration.

    1) If oliguria persists, an additional IV fluid volume equal to 3% to 5% of body weight may be justified.

        a) This much dehydration may be misjudged easily owing to the inaccuracy of clinical estimations of dehydration.

3. If the additional volume expansion does not result in diuresis, attempt to increase urine production by administering diuretics.

A. Rehydration must be completed before administration of diuretics.

B. The goal of intensive diuresis is to increase the turnover of body water, electrolyte, and metabolic waste products.

C. Diuresis will result in loss of substances that have accumulated in the uremic environment, causing many of the signs of uremia.

D. In certain instances, glomerular filtration actually increases during diuresis; in other cases, an increase in urine production is not accompanied by increased glomerular filtration.

E. An increase in urine volume should not be equated with improved renal function. In some cases, it is not possible to increase urine flow.

F. The efficacy of diuretic therapy in AIRF has not yet been established, but most clinicians use them anyway.

4. Osmotic diuresis

A. Osmotic diuresis with 10% or 20% dextrose in water has been effected at a dosage of 10 to 30 mL/lb IV. The salutary effect of dextrose solutions does not appear to be as good as that of mannitol, furosemide, or dopamine, however.

1) To create hyperglycemia, the dextrose solution is administered at a rate of 2 to 10 mL/min for the first 10 to 15 minutes. This is followed by administration at a rate of 1 to 5 mL/min. After this dose has been given, a polyionic solution, such as lactated Ringer's solution, is administered IV to prevent dehydration and excessive depletion of electrolytes. This treatment is repeated two or three times daily as needed.

2) During attempts to produce diuresis, careful attention must be directed toward body weight, glucosuria, urine output, and changes in BUN or serum creatinine concentrations. After a normally hydrated body weight has been established as a baseline, this weight should be kept constant throughout the administration of the osmotic diuretics. Progressive weight loss during attempts at diuresis indicates dehydration, whereas progressive weight gain indicates overhydration. The appearance of glucosuria indicates that appropriate hyperglycemia has been achieved. Urine output should approach 1 to 3 mL/min if this procedure has been successful in initiating diuresis. If the urine volume remains inadequate, further attempts at osmotic diuresis are not warranted.

B. Use mannitol as an alternative osmotic agent at an initial dose of 0.25 to 0.50 g/kg of body weight as a 20% to 25% solution administered IV over a period of 3 to 5 minutes to initiate diuresis.

1) Expect diuresis within 20 to 30 minutes.

2) The concerns about dextrose apply to mannitol, except that there is no practical way to measure the appearance of mannitol in the urine.

3) To maintain diuresis, administer 2 to 5 mL/min of a 5% to 10% solution of mannitol IV.

a) Mannitol may also be diluted in lactated Ringer's solution to supply necessary fluids.

b) Do not exceed a total mannitol dose of 2 g/kg/d.

4) Mannitol may be superior to dextrose in initiating diuresis in cases of acute renal failure in which cellular swelling is important in the maintenance of oliguria or reductions in glomerular filtration.

a) Dextrose equilibrates with the intracellular and the extracellular spaces, but mannitol stays within the extracellular compartment and, consequently, may have a more dramatic effect in reversing cellular swelling.

5. Furosemide and ethacrynic acid are natriuretic agents that may promote diuresis when dextrose and mannitol have failed to do so. These drugs also may be used initially, in place of dextrose or mannitol.

1) Administer furosemide at a dose of 1 to 2 mg/lb IV.

2) Expect a diuresis within 5 to 15 minutes that may last as long as two hours.

3) Furosemide may be given every eight hours to maintain diuresis.

4) If diuresis does not occur within 30 minutes, double the dosage of furosemide and administer it again IV.

6. Dopamine alone or in combination with furosemide may be successful in promoting diuresis when other treatments have failed.

A. It is more difficult to use in practice because it must be administered in accurate amounts by constant infusion to avoid adverse effects.

B. Dosage: 2 to 10 μg/kg/min.

1) A dosage of 1 to 3 μg/kg/min usually is tried initially.

2) If this is unsuccessful, increase the dosage, or add furosemide (Lasix), 1 mg/kg/h.

3) Use an ECG to monitor the animal for development of tachyarrhythmias, which can be fatal.

7. If intensive diuresis with osmotic and natriuretic agents fails, consider other measures to sustain life, such as peritoneal dialysis or hemodialysis in selected dogs and cats with potentially reversible renal disease.

8. If diuresis is established by administration of diuretics or spontaneous renal repair, continue to direct meticulous attention to fluid therapy, as tendencies toward dehydration, hyponatremia, and hypokalemia will develop and may last for weeks.

9. The aim of nutritional therapy is to reduce protein catabolism, which serves as a source of nitrogenous solutes, phosphorus, potassium, and hydrogen ions, and to promote anabolism.

A. Glucose supplementation of IV fluids to provide nonprotein calories in an attempt to spare protein is unsuccessful in all but the smallest of patients.

B. Anabolic steroids

C. Maintain a low-quantity, high-quality protein intake while the animal remains severely azotemic, if oral alimentation is possible. (See the section on dietary management of chronic renal failure, below, for further details.)

D. Consider enteral or parenteral nutrition in selected cases.

10. Management of hyperkalemia

    A. Acute

        1) Administer sodium bicarbonate

            a) 1 to 2 mEq/kg; repeat after 15 to 30 minutes, if necessary

            b) Monitor the patient with ECG (see Chapter 25).

    B. Subacute or chronic

        1) Sodium polystyrene sulfonate (Kayexylate) per rectum 25 to 50 g t.i.d. to dogs.

        2) Peritoneal dialysis

11. Management of metabolic acidosis

    A. Administer sodium bicarbonate as needed to maintain bicarbonate serum levels >15 mEq/L.

    B. Do not be overzealous with alkali therapy.

        1) Sodium retention

        2) Seizures or tetany

12. Management of infections

    A. Acutely uremic patients have an increased susceptibility to infection. Infection is a leading cause of mortality from AIRF in humans, and can also occur in dogs and cats.

    B. Pneumonia may result from prolonged recumbency.

    C. Urinary tract infections (UTIs)

        1) The damaged kidney is increasingly susceptible to infection.

        2) Prolonged use of indwelling urinary catheters is a source of sepsis. The clinician must weigh the high risk of UTI against the need to monitor urine output.

    D. Intravenous catheters are a potential source of thrombophlebitis, septicemia, and bacteremia.

    E. Administer non-nephrotoxic antibiotics as infections emerge.

        1) Adjust the dosage or time interval if the drug is eliminated by the kidneys.

13. Dialysis should be considered if azotemia is progressive and symptomatic despite aggressive fluid and diuretic therapy, or if intractable metabolic acidosis, hyperkalemia, or overhydration develop.

    A. Dialysis is of greatest benefit to animals with reversible AIRF.

    B. It is not recommended if the uremia is caused by chronic renal failure.

    C. Hemodialysis is possible in medium- to large-sized dogs, but not practical.

    D. Peritoneal dialysis is feasible in practice or at referral centers owing to the development of the column-disc catheter, but even in these settings, it can have disadvantages.

        1) Expensive

        2) Many complications

             a) Hypoalbuminemia

             b) Catheter obstruction

             c) Peritonitis

             d) Subcutaneous edema

             e) Electrolyte disturbances

        3) Special expertise needed

    E. Patient well-being is improved by dialysis while awaiting definitive diagnosis and potential renal healing.

Prognosis in AIRF

1. Guarded to poor if the animal is in the maintenance phase with severe uremic signs, regardless of cause

2. Poor to grave if the animal is in the maintenance phase as a result of ethylene glycol nephrotoxicity

3. Grave if severe oliguria persists despite treatment during the maintenance phase, regardless of cause

4. Death during initial treatment often is attributable to hyperkalemia, metabolic acidosis, or overhydration.

5. Death from uremia or infections often occurs before renal lesions have an opportunity to heal.

6. The prognosis following treatment with dialysis is unknown.

Chronic Renal Failure

1. Animals that are acutely decompensated require IV fluid therapy to reestablish hydration, as previously discussed in the section on Treatment of Intrinsic (Primary) Renal Failure.

A. Fluid requirements are greater than those for normal animals because of polyuria.

B. If dehydration is severe, the animal initially may be oliguric.

C. Intensive diuresis, as described for AIRF, may be beneficial in improving renal function, reducing the severity of azotemia, decreasing the severity of uremic signs, and enabling the animal to survive without IV fluids.

2. Conservative medical management is started when the severity of uremic signs has decreased and oral intake of food and water is possible.

A. Maintain fluid, electrolyte, acid–base and caloric balance.

B. Reduce the magnitude of retained uremic solutes.

C. Minimize the effects of lost renal endocrine functions of the kidneys.

D. Stem the progressive loss of renal function and development of renal lesions that otherwise characterize CRF (controversial).

3. Maintain free access to water at all times.

A. Impairment of urinary concentrating ability leads to polyuria and a secondary compensatory polydipsia.

B. Dehydration and prerenal azotemia develop if the animal with CRF is not allowed adequate water intake.

C. Water deprivation and subsequent dehydration may precipitate a uremic crisis.

Dietary management

1. Introduction

A. Mainstay of conservative therapy

B. Many of the solutes retained in the plasma of uremic animals are by-products of protein catabolism.

C. Clinical signs frequently can be attributed directly or indirectly to these uremic toxins (e.g., vomiting, anorexia, depression, anemia, neurologic disease).

1) The severity of uremic signs may parallel the magnitude of BUN more than serum creatinine concentration.

2) Urea itself is not considered a major toxin, but other unmeasured toxic substances also may accumulate in proportion to the increase in BUN concentration.

D. Factors that may be controlled by dietary manipulation include the quantity and quality of:

1) Calories

2) Proteins and amino acids

3) Phosphorus

4) Sodium

5) Potassium

6) Lipids and fatty acids

7) Vitamins

E. The major goal of dietary therapy is to provide a reduced quantity of high-quality (high-biologic-value) protein while supplying enough carbohydrates and fats to serve as nonprotein calories.

1) Fewer uremic toxins should be generated if this is accomplished.

a) BUN will decrease, but serum creatinine concentration will not change.

2) It is essential that adequate nonprotein calories be provided at the time of protein intake; otherwise, the ingested protein or body tissue protein will be catabolized for energy.

3) Other beneficial effects of dietary protein restriction

a) Reduction in phosphorus intake

b) Reduction in acid by-products of protein catabolism

F. The sodium intake of animals with CRF may contribute to the development of systemic arterial hypertension and so may be important to consider when formulating a diet.

1) Salt supplementation is not routinely recommended.

2) Normal or reduced amounts of salt are recommended in the absence of a severe, salt-losing nephropathy.

3) Change the diet gradually over several weeks to a lower salt composition, as the CRF kidney adjusts slowly to this restriction; otherwise, dehydration and salt depletion could occur.

2. Potential benefits of dietary modification (protein, phosphorus, and sodium restriction)

   A. Patient well-being improves as the degree of nitrogenous waste retention is reduced. Higher quality and greater length of life may be achieved.

      1) Less vomiting

      2) Improved appetite

      3) Increased activity level

      4) Less severe anemia

   B. A reduction in the degree of polyuria and polydipsia because less solute is presented for urinary excretion (less breakdown of protein and less salt)

   C. Renal secondary hyperparathyroidism may be blunted following phosphorus restriction, and less soft tissue mineralization may occur.

   D. Less metabolic acidosis (less breakdown of protein)

   E. Systemic blood pressure may be decreased by sodium restriction.

   F. The inexorable progression of the underlying renal disease may be slowed or halted.

      1) Single nephron GFR may be reduced by decreased protein intake, and this may prevent glomerular sclerosis.

      2) Less renal mineralization and fibrosis may result from phosphorus restriction.

3. Potential deleterious effects of dietary modification (protein, phosphorus, and sodium restriction)

   A. Malnutrition from inadequate protein

      1) Weight loss or loss of lean muscle mass

      2) Lethargy

      3) Poor hair coat and skin

      4) Progressive anemia

      5) Hypoproteinemia

   B. Decreased GFR and renal blood flow from decreased protein intake may increase the concentration of nitrogenous substances in plasma.

   C. Salt depletion and hypovolemia may

occur if the sodium content of the diet is too low or too quickly changed.

4. Guidelines for dietary protein restriction

   A. Controversy persists as to when and to what extent protein restriction should be prescribed in animals with CRF.

   B. Unfortunately, the actual protein requirements of dogs or cats with CRF presently are unknown.

   C. There is some experimental evidence to suggest that protein requirements during uremia may be increased above normal.

   D. There is no evidence to suggest that high-protein feedings harm dogs or cats with normal kidneys.

   E. There is no evidence to suggest that early dietary protein restriction is prophylactic for the eventual development of primary renal failure in dogs and cats.

   F. Dietary protein restriction for the control of uremic signs is a well-established treatment regimen.

   G. A balance between the degree of protein restriction needed to ameliorate uremic signs and that needed to prevent malnutrition is desired.

   H. Homemade diets

      1) Egg protein is the standard source for the highest quality/biological value protein.

      2) Egg, muscle meats, fish, or cottage cheese can be used as primary protein sources.

         a) Recent experimental evidence from dogs with CRF suggests that egg-based protein-restricted diets may result in hyperchloremic metabolic acidosis when compared to diets based on animal and vegetable proteins.

      3) Calories can be supplied by a variety of carbohydrates and fats.

   I. Improving palatability of protein-restricted diets

      1) Warming in microwave oven

      2) Frying in oils

      3) Use of additives

         a) Bacon fat

         b) Meat drippings

         c) Clam juice or tuna juice for cats

   J. Dogs

1) Normal adult dogs require 1.25 to 1.75 g/kg/d of high-biologic-value protein.

2) Commercial dog foods provide approximately 5 to 7.5 g/kg/d of protein in dry or canned preparations.

3) Mild renal failure (serum creatinine <2.5 mg/dL in the hydrated state)

  a) No protein restriction or mild protein restriction

  b) Mild protein restriction may prepare the animal for more severe restriction later if disease progresses.

4) Moderate renal failure (serum creatinine of 2.5 to 5.0 mg/dL in the hydrated state)

  a) 2.5 to 4.0 g/kg/d of high-biologic-value protein

  b) Prescription Diets G/D® or K/D®*

  c) Homemade diets

5) Severe renal failure (serum creatinine >5.0 mg/dL)

  a) 1.5 t 2.5 g/kg/d of high-biologic-value protein

  b) Prescription Diet U/D®*

  c) Homemade diets

  K. Cats

1) Healthy cats require approximately three times more protein in their diet than do dogs.

2) In comparison to dogs, cats use more of their dietary protein for calories. Approximately 20% of a cat's calories are normally derived from protein sources.

3) Commercial cat foods provide approximately 6 to 7 g/kg/d of protein in dry or canned preparations.

4) A total of 3.3 to 3.7 g/kg/d is recommended as a regimen of moderate protein restriction for cats.

5) Feline K/D® supplies 20% protein and about 3.5 g/kg/d when fed to meet caloric needs.

6) Unfortunately, many cats will not eat a protein-restricted diet.

  L. If CRF is attributable to glomerulopathy and substantial proteinuria, additional protein should be provided based on the amount of protein lost in daily urine. Daily urine protein loss also can be estimated using the U_P/U_{CR} ratio.

1) $U_P : U_{CR} + (0.036) \div (0.05) =$ estimated 24-hour urinary protein loss in dogs when protein is measured by CBB

2) $U_P : U_{CR} - (0.006) \div (0.033) =$ estimated 24-hour urinary protein loss in dogs when protein is measured by TCA-PS

  M. If progressive weight loss, anemia, poor hair and skin condition, or loss of lean body muscle mass develop despite "adequate" control of nitrogenous waste products, gradually increase the protein and caloric content of the diet until weight gain is achieved or weight stabilizes.

  5. Calories

  A. For dogs, provide 70 to 110 cal/kg/d.

  B. For cats, provide 70 to 80 cal/kg/d.

  6. Vitamin supplementation

  A. Water-soluble vitamins are provided as supplements to the diets of dogs and cats with CRF as the ability of the kidney to conserve these vitamins during polyuria is unknown.

  B. Vitamin A should not be supplemented because it is normally excreted by the kidney.

  7. Phosphorus restriction and control of hyperphosphatemia

  A. Phosphorus restriction in rats, cats, dogs, and human beings with CRF may have beneficial effects on renal histopathology, renal function, and mortality, but results have been inconsistent.

  B. Phosphorus restriction may blunt renal secondary hyperparathyroidism.

  C. It may improve the conversion of vitamin D metabolites to calcitriol.

1) Increased phosphorus concentration inhibits the activity of 1-alpha-hydroxylase, which is necessary for conversion to calcitriol (1,25-dihydroxycholecalciferol).

  D. It may lessen the degree of soft tissue mineralization (including that within the kidney).

  E. Dietary phosphorus restriction and intestinal phosphorus binders are indicated in the presence of hyperphosphatemia.

  F. Dietary phosphorus restriction and intestinal phosphorus binders also may be

* Hills

indicated when the serum phosphorus level is normal.

1) Renal secondary hyperparathyroidism occurs early during the loss of renal mass (long before hyperphosphatemia is detectable). It is the increased serum concentration of parathyroid hormone (PTH) that initially maintains normal serum phosphorus and calcium concentrations, despite the loss of renal function.

G. Protein restriction alone may result in a decrease in serum phosphorus concentrations to normal levels in some instances.

H. In cases of a severe reduction in renal function, dietary restriction alone will be insufficient to return serum phosphorus concentrations to normal. In these instances, intestinal phosphorus binders will be needed.

I. Most commercially available phosphorus binders contain aluminum

1) Aluminum salts are good phosphorus binders, but aluminum accumulation and toxicity is a potential problem in animals with CRF.

a) Dosage: 10 to 30 mg/kg t.i.d. with meals (Phosphorus binders are much less effective in fasting patients.)

2) Aluminum hydroxide gel (Amphojel, AlternaGEL)

3) Aluminum carbonate gel (Basaljel)

J. Consider nonaluminum, calcium-containing compounds for chronic phosphorus restriction.

1) Do not use until the calcium × phosphorus product is less than 70.

2) Monitor the serum calcium concentration to detect development of hypercalcemia.

3) Administer calcium carbonate (Tums, Os-Cal), 30 mg/kg b.i.d. to t.i.d. with meals.

Medical Management

1. Management of acidosis

A. The metabolic acidosis associated with CRF often is mild owing to compensatory renal tubular ammonia excretion, respiratory hyperventilation, and bone buffering.

B. Treatment may not be necessary unless the patient is symptomatic.

C. Low, steady-state bicarbonate concentrations increase the animal's susceptibility to an acidotic crisis (e.g., diarrhea).

D. Chronic acidosis contributes to osteodystrophy as a result of the skeletal demineralization that is associated with bone buffering.

E. Sodium bicarbonate may be supplemented in the diet as needed to maintain a serum bicarbonate concentration exceeding 18 mEq/L.

1) Initially, 8 to 12 mg/kg of sodium bicarbonate t.i.d. is recommended.

F. Consider treating metabolic acidosis with calcium carbonate when additional calcium or intestinal phosphorus binding is desired.

1) Monitor serum calcium concentrations periodically to detect hypercalcemia.

G. As with AIRF, overzealous administration of alkali can result in tetany or seizures.

H. Early supplementation of sodium bicarbonate may slow the development of the tubulointerstitial lesions that are characteristic of CRF in experimental rats.

1) The underlying mechanism may be related to renal ammonia levels that are decreased during bicarbonate therapy.

2. Management of potassium homeostasis

A. Hyperkalemia usually is not a problem in CRF unless severe oliguria or metabolic acidosis occurs.

1) Emergency treatment may include sodium bicarbonate or calcium gluconate infusion, as described in the preceding section on the treatment of AIRF.

B. Hypokalemia is more common in CRF than is hyperkalemia.

1) Chronic hypokalemia can cause functional renal lesions (urinary concentrating defects and decreased GFR), structural intrarenal lesions, and chronic renal failure.

2) Chronic potassium depletion in cats apparently can result in chronic renal failure, but the exact mechanisms remain to be proven.

3) Cats with primary renal failure may have an exaggerated response in the excretion of urinary potassium such that the fractional urinary excretion of potassium is high at a time when serum potassium concentration is low. This same phenomenon occasionally has been observed in dogs with CRF.

    4) Oral potassium supplementation with potassium gluconate in dogs and cats with CRF and hypokalemia is indicated, but a sudden potassium load may not readily be excreted by the chronically failing kidney. (See Chapter 25 for further details regarding potassium supplementation.)

    5) Intravenous potassium supplementation may be required if hypokalemia and clinical signs are severe.

  3. Anabolic steroids

    A. Potential benefits include enhancement of erythropoiesis, increased appetite, increased anabolism (positive nitrogen balance), increased calcium deposition in bone, and increased delivery of oxygen to tissue from increased 2,3-diphosphoglyceric acid concentrations in RBCs.

    B. None of these potential beneficial effects have been validated in the dog or cat; consequently, some veterinary nephrologists do not advocate their use.

    C. Anabolic steroids have been used in an attempt to stimulate erythropoiesis in animals with nonregenerative anemia.

      1) A beneficial effect may require 1 to 3 months.

    D. Available products

      1) Methyltestosterone

      2) Stanozolol (Winstrol-V)

      3) Oxymetholone (Anadrol, Adroyd)

      4) Nandrolone decanoate (Deca-Durabolin)

        a) May be the anabolic steroid of choice for treatment of anemia

        b) Injectable only

          i. An oral preparation may become available, but requires much higher doses.*

        c) 1 to 5 mg/kg/week intramuscularly (IM); total dose not to exceed 200 mg

  4. Vitamin D and calcium supplementation

    A. Decreases in serum calcitriol and ionized calcium concentrations can occur as renal disease advances.

    B. Replacement therapy using vitamin D metabolites and calcium supplementation has not been used routinely in dogs and cats with CRF.

    C. Indications include severe fibrous osteodystrophy and symptomatic hypocalcemia.

    D. Initiate therapy only after serum phosphorus concentrations have been returned to normal; otherwise, there is risk of soft tissue mineralization.

    E. Rehydration and intestinal phosphorus binders may lower serum phosphorus concentration and subsequently increase serum calcium concentration.

      1) Based on mass law interaction

      2) Increased rate of conversion to calcitriol as serum phosphorus decreases

    F. Calcium-containing intestinal phosphorus binders (calcium carbonate) are indicated when hypocalcemia is present.

    G. Hypercalcemia is an undesirable side effect of vitamin D therapy and calcium supplementation. Serum calcium concentration should be measured periodically, and the dosage of calcitriol adjusted if necessary.

    H. Recent evidence suggests that calcitirol supplementation may blunt renal secondary hyperparathyroidism

      1) Calcitriol receptors are present in the parathyroid glands, and stimulation of these receptors may be necessary to decrease the synthesis and secretion of PTH, independent of the serum calcium concentration.

    I. Vitamin D supplementation

      1) Dihydrotachysterol (Hytakerol)

        a) Synthetic vitamin D derivative that does not require renal activation

        b) Dosage: 125 μg per dog three times per week

        c) May take weeks to attain maximal effect

        d) After discontinuation of treatment, it may take a week for the effects of the drug to abate.

      2) Calcitriol (1,25-dihydroxycholecalciferol; Rocaltrol)

        a) No activation required

        b) Short half-life (hours)

        c) Rapid onset of action

        d) A dosage of 0.25 μg per dog has been recommended three times per week.

          i. This dose may be excessive.

---

* Personal communication, Dr. Sharon Center

ii. Very small doses of calcitriol may be effective in reducing renal secondary hyperparathyroidism $(0.003 - 0.006 \ \mu g/kg/d)$.

3) Hypervitaminosis D and toxicity can occur in dogs in the absence of hypercalcemia.

5. Treatment of anemia

   A. Reduction of nitrogenous waste products with effective dietary therapy may prolong the life of existing erythrocytes and reduce suppression of bone marrow production of erythrocytes by uremia.

   B. Healing of gastrointestinal ulcers will reduce blood loss and allow anemia to stabilize or improve.

   C. The chronic nonregenerative anemia of CRF is largely attributable to the lack of the trophic effect of erythropoietin on bone marrow.

   1) Anabolic steroids may be helpful, but their efficacy has not been proven.

   2) Synthetic human erythropoietin recently has been marketed.

   a) Its use in dogs or cats presently is under investigation.

   i. It is expensive.

   D. Blood transfusions occasionally are needed, particularly when acute blood loss occurs because replacement with new RBCs by bone marrow is not adequate.

6. Treatment and prevention of chronic dehydration

   A. Some dogs and cats do not drink an adequate amount of fluid to maintain normal hydration.

   1) Add additional fluids to food.

   2) Force fluids orally with a syringe.

   3) Teach owners to administer subcutaneous fluids periodically at home (e.g., lactated Ringer's solution) when water intake is low, particularly when episodes of vomiting occur.

7. Hypertension

   A. Occurs commonly in dogs with chronic renal failure, but the need for its treatment remains to be proven.

   B. Difficult to document in practice

   1) Direct arterial puncture is the best method for detection.

   2) Doppler or oscillometric methods are less attractive because of difficulties in reproducing results.

   C. Clinical signs may include:

   1) No signs

   2) Ocular changes

   a) Blindness

   b) Retinal hemorrhages

   c) Retinal detachments

   3) Neurologic changes

   a) Seizures

   b) Fatigue/lethargy

   4) Epistaxis

   D. Consequences of systemic arterial hypertension

   1) Largely unknown in dogs and cats

   a) Left ventricular hypertrophy has been documented.

   2) End-organ damage may occur.

   3) Further renal damage may occur if the increased pressure is transmitted to the kidneys.

   E. Treatment should not be undertaken without a method to monitor blood pressure serially during therapy.

   1) Salt restriction (10 to 40 mg/kg/d)

   2) Diuretics (furosemide, chlorothiazide)

   3) Arterial vasodilators (e.g., prazosin)

   4) Calcium channel blockers (e.g., diltiazem, nifedipine)

   5) Converting enzyme inhibitors (e.g., captopril, enalapril)

   6) β blockers (propranolol)

   a) Avoid using with cimetidine

8. Avoidance of stress if at all possible

   A. The influence of stress is difficult to quantitate, but may contribute to dehydration as a result of inadequate intake of food and water.

   B. Perform procedures on an outpatient basis when feasible.

   C. Avoid surgery if possible.

   D. Administer fluids during all anesthetic procedures.

   1) Consider the use of diuretics during anesthesia also.

   E. Avoid the use of any nephrotoxic drugs.

   F. Avoid boarding the animal.

   1) Consider prophylactic subcutaneous fluids if boarding is essential.

9. Follow-up after release of the patient from the hospital

A. Initially, recheck the animal in one to two weeks, and monthly thereafter for the first three months.

1) Follow-up visits thereafter can be tailored to how well the individual animal is doing.

B. Determinations of body weight, estimation of lean muscle mass, PCV (packed cell volume), and serum albumin concentrations are helpful in the assessment of nutritional status.

C. BUN concentration

1) Helpful in assessing the degree of control of the uremic environment owing to protein restriction. However, it is no longer a very good tool with which to monitor renal function.

D. Serum creatinine concentration

1) Helpful in assessing the stability of the animal's renal function

E. Serum electrolyte concentrations

1) Phosphorus

a) Adequacy of dietary restriction and intestinal binders

2) Calcium

a) Adequacy of supplementation and vitamin D administration

3) Sodium, potassium, chloride

a) Adequacy of salt needs and fluid volume status

4) Bicarbonate

a) Adequacy of alkali replacement

10. Prognosis

A. The prognosis is poor as a result of the progressive nature of CRF.

B. The rate of progression of CRF can vary considerably among individual patients.

C. With conservative medical treatment, some uremic dogs and cats may survive 3 to 24 months or longer.

D. Findings suggestive of a poor prognosis

1) Severe nonregenerative anemia

2) Advanced renal osteodystrophy

3) Progressive increases in BUN and serum creatinine despite maintenance of hydration and conservative medical management

4) Progressive electrolyte and acid–base abnormalities

a) Hyperkalemia or hypokalemia

b) Hyperphosphatemia

c) Hypocalcemia or hypercalcemia

d) Hypernatremia or hyponatremia

e) Decreased serum bicarbonate concentration

5) Progressive weight loss

6) Severe end-stage lesions detected on renal biopsy

E. Approximate survival time may be predicted by plotting $1/S_{CR}$ on the ordinate versus time in months on the abscissa.

Suggested Readings

Allen TA: Management of advanced chronic renal failure. In Kirk RW (ed): Current Veterinary Therapy X—Small Animal Practice, pp 1195–1198. Philadelphia, WB Saunders, 1989

Allen TA, Jaenke RS, Fettman MJ: A technique for estimating progression of chronic renal failure in the dog. J Am Vet Med Assoc 190: 866–888, 1987

Chew DJ, DiBartola SP: Manual of Small Animal Nephrology and Urology. New York, Churchill Livingstone, 1986

Chew DJ, DiBartola SP: Pathophysiology and diagnosis of renal disease. In Ettinger SJ (ed): Textbook of Internal Medicine, 3rd ed. Philadelphia, WB Saunders, 1989

Fettman MJ: Feline kaliopenic polymyopathy/nephropathy syndrome. Vet Clin North Am [Small Anim Pract] 19(3): 415–432, 1989

Finco DR, Brown SA: Newer concepts and controversies on dietary management of renal failure. In Kirk RW (ed): Current Veterinary Therapy X—Small Animal Practice, pp 1198–1201. Philadelphia, WB Saunders, 1989

Polzin DJ, Osborne CA, Adams LD, O'Brien TD: Dietary management of canine and feline chronic renal failure. Vet Clin North Am [Small Anim Prac] 19(3): 539–560, 1989

CHAPTER THIRTEEN

Disorders of the Urogenital System

Ronald Lyman

Disorders of Urination

Difficult Urination and Bloody Urine

A routine problem in veterinary medicine centers on disorders causing dysuria (painful or difficult urination). Common presenting signs include stranguria (increased straining), pollakiuria (increased frequency of urination), or hematuria (urine with blood). Many acute cases are successfully treated with antibiotics without obtaining a specific diagnosis. The purpose of this section is to outline an approach for specific diagnosis and treatment of those animals requiring further work-up because of the chronicity of the disorder or specific associated clinical findings.

History

1. Pay special attention to the duration of the current episode, the number of past episodes, and the animal's prior response to therapy.
2. Ascertain the presence or absence of macroscopic hematuria.
3. Determine the ability to pass urine.

Physical Examination

Emphasize abdominal palpation, rectal palpation, and genital examination.

Clinicopathologic Examination

1. Obtain a urinalysis (UA) in all cases.
2. Obtain bacterial cultures of urine samples that have been collected aseptically by cystocentesis (preferably) or catheterization in cases in which the urine sediment may be contaminated by other genitourinary (GU) discharges (e.g., balanoposthitis).
3. Other clinicopathologic diagnostic techniques are discussed in the sections on specific disorders that follow.

Roentgenography

1. After the patient is thoroughly prepared by enemas, plain abdominal roentgenograms are performed in animals with chronic disorders and no specific historical or physical findings (e.g., bladder masses).
2. Special contrast studies (urethrocystography, intravenous pyelography [IVP], etc.) utilizing positive and double contrast techniques are often necessary.

Ultrasonography

Imaging via ultrasound may reveal mass effects, echogenic debris associated with infection, or calculi in the urinary tract.

Surgery

Consider diagnostic and therapeutic laparotomy or urethral surgery to observe the GU system and obtain tissue or cultures in selected cases.

Urinary Tract Infection (Bacterial)

1. Urinary tract infections (UTIs) may exist alone or in conjunction with other disorders causing dysuria.
2. Females are more commonly affected than males.
3. Congenital abnormalities, calculi, or previous urethral catherization predispose animals to this problem.

Clinical Recognition

1. The signs of UTI may be acute or chronic.
2. Stranguria, pollakiuria, or hematuria may be involved, or the infection may occur without signs.
3. Physical examination is usually unremarkable, although bloody urine may be expressed.
4. Urinalysis often reveals increased numbers of both RBCs and WBCs. Inflammation elevates the urine protein level, and the pH may be elevated in the presence of ureasplitting organisms. The presence of cellular casts is suggestive of renal involvement. Bacteria may be present in significant numbers.
5. Bacterial culture is usually positive (in the absence of concurrent antibiotic therapy). Quantitative cultures are recommended if cystocentesis is not used to collect the urine.) A bacterial count of 10^5 organisms/mL of urine is assumed to indicate infection.) Sensitivity to antibiotics should be determined in vitro. (Special culture techniques are required for mycoplasma or ureaplasma infections.)
6. Other diagnostic techniques are usually not employed unless indicated by specific physical findings or by chronically recurring bacterial infections.

Treatment

1. Administer appropriate antibiotics for at least two weeks.
2. Evaluate therapeutic effectiveness by means of a UA and culture one week after discontinuing antibiotics.
3. Chloramphenicol or tetracycline may be necessary to treat mycoplasma or ureaplasma infections.

Prognosis

1. Excellent, if the problem is acute.
2. If the problem is chronic, the prognosis is only fair. Evaluate the GU tract further; chronic, low-level antibiotics may be necessary in some cases.
3. Rare cases of fungal UTIs have been reported. The therapy and prognosis for such diseases is controversial at this time.

Dysuria with Urinary Tract Calculi

1. Dysuria with urinary tract calculi may occur in dogs or cats of any age. The most common site is the urinary bladder. Urethral, renal, and ureteral calculi occur also.
2. These calculi are commonly associated with UTIs (especially those caused by Staphylococcus).
3. Several different types of calculi exist. Examples include phosphate, urate, oxalate, silicate, and cystine. Combinations of these are possible.

Clinical Recognition

1. A chronic history of stranguria or hematuria is indicative of calculi.
2. Animals with a chronic history of UTI are at risk for the development of calculi (especially phosphate calculi).
3. Dalmations are predisposed to the development of urate calculi.
4. Animals with liver dysfunction or portosystemic vascular shunts may develop urate calculi.
5. Physical examination may disclose palpable cystic or urethral calculi.

6. Male dogs are predisposed to urethral obstruction from small calculi.

7. The UA is consistent with urinary tract inflammation. The sediment shows increased numbers of RBCs and bacteria (depending on the presence of infection). The presence of crystals in the sediment is not indicative of calculi.

8. Obstruction, chronic infection, or renal calculi may result in elevations of BUN, creatinine, and phosphorus levels in the serum. Potassium levels may be elevated in cases of obstruction.

9. Bacterial culture of the urine may be positive.

10. Plain abdominal or urethral roentgenograms (after enema preparation) demonstrate radio-opaque calculi in most cases. Some calculi (especially cystine and urate) are radiolucent and must be demonstrated by positive contrast studies or ultrasonographic imaging.

11. Perform calculi analysis when stones are obtained.

Treatment

1. Medical and surgical alternatives are available for calculi.

2. Propulsion of urethral calculi back into the bladder is necessary in cases of obstruction. Urethrostomy is necessary if calculi cannot be dislodged from the urethra. Treatment for obstructive renal failure may be necessary in these cases.

3. If calculi analysis reveals struvite stones, then medical management with prescription diet, canine S/D®* diet may be attempted. This diet is designed for use over a period of weeks to months, and should not be used indefinitely (or in growing animals). Calculi resorption should be monitored by monthly roentgenograms.

4. Surgical removal remains an important mode of therapy, and is often the only definitive means of allowing calculi analysis and deep calculi culture.

* Hills Products, Topeka, Kansas.

5. Treatment of concurrent bacterial infections is indicated.

6. The general principles of prophylaxis include induction of polyuria and polydipsia by the chronic administration of oral sodium chloride.

7. Oral administration of acetohydroxamic acid is advocated by some clinicians to inhibit struvite growth (although it is not intended for use in pregnant females or growing animals). The reader should consult this chapter's Suggested Readings for discussions of the various types of calculi and possible medical or adjunctive therapy.

Prognosis

1. Excellent for initial resolution of signs

2. Recurring calculi or UTIs are possible.

Feline Urologic Syndrome

1. Feline urologic syndrome (FUS) is a problem that affects both male and female cats.

2. The cause or causes are presently unknown, although many contributing factors have been postulated.

3. This subject is extremely controversial, especially with regard to etiology, therapy, and prevention.

Clinical Recognition

1. In the cat, FUS is characterized by hematuria, pollakiura and (sometimes) obstruction.

2. Males are at risk for obstruction, probably owing to the increased length and small diameter of their urethra. Females rarely develop obstruction.

3. The urethral obstruction is caused by formation of a proteinaceous crystalloid substance during inflammation. It cannot be predicted if a particular male will obstruct during an episode of FUS.

4. Obstruction is signaled either by a history of lethargy, anorexia, or vomiting, or by physical findings of dehydration, depression, and enlarged urinary bladder. Remember that a rupture of the urinary tract is possible in this syndrome.

5. Obstruction may lead to severe depression, postrenal azotemia, urinary tract rupture, acidosis, hyperkalemia, or acute renal failure; death may result from any of these complications.

6. The UA is characterized by a highly concentrated urine, hematuria, and minimal numbers of leukocytes. The pH is sometimes alkaline. Casts may be present if renal involvement has occurred secondary to an obstruction episode.

7. Urine cultures generally yield negative results (unless the animal has previously been catheterized).

8. Biochemical analysis may show acidosis, azotemia, or hyperkalemia if obstruction has occurred.

9. ECGs obtained during an acute episode of obstruction may reveal evidence of hyperkalemia (large T waves, conduction disturbances, bradycardia, etc.).

10. Other diagnostic techniques are rarely employed.

Treatment

1. The extent of therapy should be individualized in each case.

2. The basic procedures are as follows:

  A. Relieve obstructions if they occur.

  B. Maintain balanced fluid, electrolyte, and acid–base conditions.

  C. Educate the client about all possible consequences of this syndrome.

3. In the nonobstructed patient, the value of antibiotics, antispasmodics, and urinary acidifiers is questionable. All are often used empirically. The author believes that maintenance of adequate hydration with oral or parenteral fluids is beneficial.

4. Monitor the patient (especially if male) for possible obstruction.

5. Long-term stimulation of water intake by use of canned foods and the provision of fresh, free-choice water is recommended as such a regimen may be beneficial for animals afflicted with this problem.

6. Perineal urethrostomy prevents males

from obstructing during subsequent episodes in most cases.

7. Temporary use of a diet that causes struvite absorption (feline S/D®), followed by long-term use of a low-magnesium diet (C/D®) is advocated by some clinicians.

8. In the obstructed patient, the primary aim of therapy is to relieve the obstruction by passing a urinary catheter and flushing the bladder. Aseptic technique is very difficult to maintain, so consider the possibility that bacteria will be introduced and handle it appropriately by future cultures or prophylactic antibiotics.

9. Obstructed patients require prompt fluid management for postrenal azotemia and associated electrolyte abnormalities. (See Chapter 12 for a discussion of this management.)

10. Temporary indwelling catheters are sometimes necessary to maintain patency in a critical case or to monitor urine output.

11. Ruptured bladders require emergency laparotomy.

Prognosis

1. The acute prognosis varies from good to grave, depending upon the complicating factors.

2. Recurrence is common.

Dysuria Secondary to Previous Trauma

1. The most common cause of dysuria secondary to previous trauma is urethral stricture as a result of catheterization, calculi, or surgery.

2. Abnormal locations of the bladder may occur after blunt trauma (e.g., being hit by car).

Clinical Recognition

1. The most common sign is stranguria after the traumatic episode.

2. Physical examination may reveal the underlying problem (urethral stricture following perineal urethrostomy, abdominal hernia containing the bladder, etc.).

Treatment

1. Surgery to correct the anatomic abnormality is the treatment of choice.
2. Treatment of postrenal uremia may be necessary if the obstruction is severe.

Prognosis

The prognosis is excellent if a patent tract can be established.

Dysuria Secondary to Mass Lesions of the Urinary Tract

1. The most common mass lesions of the urinary tract involve neoplasia of the bladder or prostate.
2. Urethral masses, penile and vaginal tumors, and masses secondary to chronic infection occur less commonly. Foreign bodies are rare.

Clinical Recognition

1. Chronic hematuria is the most common sign.
2. Older animals with hematuria are at increased risk for neoplasia. Stranguria may occur with lower lesions (urethral, penile, etc.).
3. Physical examination may reveal genital masses (see section on Transmissible Venereal Tumor) or a thickened bladder wall.
4. The UA results are consistent with hemorrhage or inflammation.
5. Plain roentgenograms or contrast studies are most useful in outlining cystic or urethral filling defects, foreign bodies, and other abnormalities.
6. Ultrasonographic imaging may provide evidence for a pathologic mass.

Treatment

1. Surgical exploration and excisional biopsy represent definitive treatment.
2. Chemotherapy may be indicated in animals with neoplasia.

Prognosis

1. Excellent for foreign bodies
2. Fair for chronic inflammatory masses
3. Variable for neoplasia
   A. Excellent for transmissible venereal tumor
   B. Fair for leiomyoma (vaginal, cystic)
   C. Poor for transitional cell carcinoma of the bladder (the most common neoplasia of the urinary tract)

Prostatic Disease and Dysuria

1. In small animals, dysuria associated with prostatic disease is restricted to male dogs.
2. Stranguria or hematuria may occur, along with other signs of prostatic disease.
3. The reader is referred to the section of this chapter on prostatic disorders for a full discussion of this problem.

Drug-induced Dysuria

Clinical Recognition

1. Certain drugs have the potential to cause dysuria. The most notable drug causing dysuria is cyclophosphamide (Cytoxan), which is commonly used in oncologic and immunosuppressive therapy.
2. In a small percentage of dogs treated with cyclophosphamide, a sterile, hemorrhagic urinary tract inflammation results. Hematuria and stranguria are the predominant signs.
3. Urinary acidifiers have the potential to induce stranguria, especially if abrasions of the urethral or vaginal mucosa are present.
4. Appearance of clinical signs while a medication regimen is being continued is suggestive, but routine diagnostic techniques should, nonetheless, be employed to rule out more common causes.

Treatment

The drug in question should be withdrawn.

Prognosis

1. Guarded in the case of "Cytoxan-induced cystitis." Obtain a UA routinely while using this medication. Most cases regress following cessation of therapy, but some chronic cases persist.

2. Excellent in the case of acidifiers. Withdrawal of the drug ameliorates the signs.

Hematuria in Hemorrhagic Disorders

1. Disorders involving thrombocytes or the entire coagulation system may present with hematuria as a significant sign.

2. Physical examination and a routine workup should suggest a bleeding disorder (e.g., associated petechiae or hemorrhage elsewhere).

3. The reader is referred to Chapter 4 for a complete discussion of bleeding disorders.

Congenital Urinary Tract Anomalies

1. Signs referrable to congenital urinary tract anomalies may occur at any time in life.

2. The most common abnormalities include a complete or partially patent urachus, urachal cyst, cystic diverticulum, congenital penile anomalies, and congenital vaginal anomalies. Ectopic ureters are discussed under the heading of Incontinence.

Clinical Recognition

1. Clinical signs may occur as a direct result of the anomaly (persistent frenulum causing stranguria) or they may be attributable to UTI (patent urachus).

2. Physical examination may reveal the anatomic variation (as in a penile anomaly).

3. The UA may reflect urinary tract inflammation.

4. Plain or contrast roentgenography is most helpful in demonstrating anatomic abnormalities.

5. Many anomalies are found serendipitously during surgery for other causes (e.g., cystic calculi).

Treatment

1. Surgical correction of the anomaly, if possible, is advisable.

2. Secondary conditions, such as UTIs and calculi, should also be treated.

Dysuria from Miscellaneous Disorders of the External Genitalia and Urethra

1. Vaginal, penile, or preputial lesions may result in stranguria. Inflammation secondary to bacterial or fungal infection is the most common etiology. Self-mutilation exacerbates the signs. Young females commonly have a benign vaginitis before puberty.

2. Vulvovaginitis causes dysuria in the female. Obesity, dermatologic disease, and urinary incontinence are predisposing factors. Excessive skin folds may be seen in animals with this problem.

3. Granulomatous urethritis of unknown etiology occurs in female German shepherds.

Clinical Recognition

1. Physical examination usually reveals the cause of dysuria. Severe inflammation, with or without exudate, is seen.

2. Females with granulomatous urethritis may become obstructed.

3. Cytologic examination and bacterial or fungal culture of the genitalia provide evidence of the predominant organism involved in vaginitis or balanoposthitis.

4. Catheterization of the urethra is difficult in granulomatous urethritis. Biopsy of the urethra is indicated if this condition is suspected.

5. Perform a UA. Remember that voided samples may be contaminated by the external genitalia.

Treatment

1. Administer appropriate local and systemic antimicrobials for bacterial or fungal infections.

2. A temporary indwelling Foley catheter and anti-inflammatory doses of prednisolone are indicated for granulomatous urethritis.

3. Plastic surgery may correct the predisposing skin folds found in animals with vulvovaginitis.

Prognosis

1. Excellent for vulvovaginitis, although recurrences are likely
2. Excellent for vaginitis and balanoposthitis
3. Guarded to poor for granulomatous urethritis. Long-term, decremental doses of cortisone are necessary. Exacerbations are the rule.

Urinary Incontinence

Urinary incontinence is a difficult clinical problem to diagnose and manage. Current clinical definitions of incontinence are not standard. For the purposes of this discussion, incontinence is defined as the passage of urine without voluntary initiation. This condition is contrasted with stranguria, hematuria, pollakiuria, dysuria, and polyuria, which refer to alterations from the norm during willful micturition.

Work-up for Incontinence

1. Historical confirmation of incontinence is offered by a complaint of constant or very frequent passage of urine in an animal without evidence of willful micturition.
2. Straining or hematuria is uncommon in cases of urinary incontinence.
3. A common complaint is of a large wet area with urine odor where the animal sleeps.
4. Chronic vulvovaginitis in the female may be reported, with constant grooming of the genital region.
5. A history of rear limb weakness, pain, or self-mutilation is important. Frank vertebral trauma may be reported (e.g., hit by car).
6. Fecal incontinence may be reported in cases of neurogenic urinary incontinence.
7. A history of ovariohysterectomy is significant in a female with incontinence.
8. Physical examination often reveals malodorous, urine-scalded genital regions with a secondary chronic dermatitis.

9. Other physical findings are often unremarkable. Complete penile, preputial, and vaginal examinations are indicated.
10. Occasionally, congenital penile or vaginal anatomic anomalies may be found.
11. A complete neurologic examination is indicated, with emphasis on rear limb spinal reflexes, anal reflex and tone, and tail tone. Evaluate the paraspinal musculature for abnormal pain (hyperpathia).
12. Always obtain a UA for evidence of urinary tract inflammation.
13. Obtain plain roentgenograms of the abdomen, the surrounding skeletal structures, and the penile area in the male.
14. Imaging procedures to evaluate the GU tract may be necessary (IVP, urethrocystogram, double contrast study, ultrasonography, cystoscopy).
15. Electrodiagnostic studies such as electromyography (EMG), cystometrography, or other urodynamic studies, may be indicated in selected cases of neurogenic incontinence.
16. Magnetic resonance imaging (MRI) of the lumbosacral and caudal spine is indicated when EMG indicates an anatomic lesion in this area.
17. As always, response to therapy often offers a working diagnosis.

Neurogenic Urinary Incontinence

Lesions anywhere in the nervous system can cause loss of control over micturition, but signs of incontinence most commonly result from spinal cord or peripheral nerve (cauda equina) lesions. Occasional cases with lesions in unknown neuroanatomic locations (responsive to sympathomimetic drugs) do occur.

Clinical Recognition

1. Neurologic incontinence rarely presents as an isolated entity. Overt spinal cord disease (i.e., intervertebral disk disease or trauma) is often associated with incontinence.
2. Occasionally, vague signs of incontinence (both urinary and fecal) coexist with subtle gait abnormalities or apparent back

pain, suggesting that the lesion may exist in the cauda equina region of the spinal canal.

3. Physical examination is usually normal unless traumatic lesions are present.

4. Neurologic examination is abnormal and reflects the location of the lesion.

    A. Animals with lesions cranial to the L-4 spinal segment have upper motor (UMN) spinal reflexes to the rear limbs and sacral segments (anal reflex, perineal reflex). The spinal reflexes are present and possibly exaggerated.

    B. Lesions cranial to the S-1 spinal segment but caudal to the L-4 segment are associated with normal perianal and anal reflexes but depressed rear limb (patellar) reflexes.

    C. Animals with lesions involving the sacral segments (S-1, S-2) have absent or depressed anal reflexes and anal tone.

    D. Lesions involving the cauda equina are most often characterized by pain, with minimal to moderate changes in rear limb and anal reflexes. These lesions are often extradural and incomplete.

    E. Loss of perianal sensation indicates severe lesions causing neurologic urinary incontinence.

5. Animals with neurologically incontinent bladders are subject to other signs (dysuria, stranguria, hematuria) owing to their predisposition for UTIs.

6. Clinicopathologic tests are usually not helpful.

7. Roentgenograms may reveal skeletal abnormalities (e.g., intervertebral disk prolapse or vertebral fractures).

8. Electrodiagnostic studies (e.g., an EMG) may document neural involvement.

9. Magnetic resonance imaging (MRI) provides the most detailed information about actual compression of the cauda equina in the lumbosacral area (short of surgical exploration).

Treatment

1. In general, therapy for neurologic incontinence is based upon the supportive care of the bladder, as well as provisions for its emptying.

    A. Some UMN lesions (cranial to S1-S2)

are associated with abnormally hyperactive urethral sphincters and affected animals may resist reflex emptying or bladder expression. Intermittent catheterization may be necessary to remove residual urine.

    B. Some lower motor neuron (LMN) spinal lesions (S1-S2 segments affected) are characterized by detrusor muscle areflexia and poor sphincter tone, resulting in constant urine leakage. Intermittent catheterization or expression is still necessary.

    C. Unless the neurologic lesion is transient, UTI inevitably occurs and must be managed by appropriate cultures and antibiotics.

2. Occasionally, lesions of the cauda equina (vertebral canal stenosis, masses) can be managed by decompressive laminectomy.

3. A few cases have been managed by trigonal-colonic anastomosis.

4. Some cases of incontinence with a neurogenic cause may be managed by drug therapy. (See the discussion later in this chapter on functional failure of the bladder to store or empty urine adequately.)

5. Periurethral injection of Teflon® via cytoscopy has been used to improve continence in the canine.

Prognosis

Neurogenic urinary incontinence always carries a guarded prognosis. Unless a lesion is temporary (spinal cord contusion) or correctable (vertebral canal stenosis), minimal hope for resolution of the problem exists. A high incidence of UTIs results in cases managed by catheterization or trigonal-colonic anastomosis.

Nonneurogenic Urinary Incontinence

1. Nonneurogenic urinary incontinence encompasses a range of disorders from congenital anatomic anomalies to behavioral problems.

2. Specific diagnosis is a matter of exclusion of possibilities.

3. Empirical pharmacologic therapy is often the ultimate result of a work-up.

Behavioral or Psychogenic Urinary Incontinence

1. Young animals, hyperactive breeds, and animals with altered sensoria (e.g., dementia) are commonly involved. The loss of control often occurs during excitement.
2. All physical examinations and ancillary diagnostic test results are normal.
3. Neurologic examination may reveal signs that are compatible with cerebral disease.

Treatment

1. Young animals may outgrow the problem.
2. Other animals may be trained by specialists in behavior modification.
3. The cause of the cerebral signs may be treatable (e.g., administration of cortisone to decrease cerebral edema secondary to neoplasia).

Prognosis

1. Fair for young animals
2. Guarded for older animals or animals with CNS lesions

Congenital Lesions

1. Ectopic ureters are the most common congenital lesion.
2. Female dogs are most commonly affected.

Clinical Recognition

1. History is compatible with incontinence from a young age.
2. Physical examination is usually unremarkable except for the effects of the urine on the skin.
3. Occasionally, ureteral openings may be visualized in the vagina. Abnormal genital anatomy (pseudohermaphroditism) may be observed.
4. The most pertinent ancillary finding is positive contrast roentgenographic evidence of abnormal position and emptying of the ureter into the vagina or urethra. Some other possible anomalies are megaureter and hydronephrosis.

5. Occasionally, patent urachus may be observed in the dog and cat.

Treatment

1. In the case of ectopic ureter, employ urethral transplant to the bladder or heminephrectomy with ureterectomy.
2. Surgical extirpation of a patent urachus is indicated.

Prognosis
The prognosis for affected animals is good for future continence.

Iatrogenic Incontinence

This problem usually occurs after perineal urethrostomy in the cat, or after bladder surgery in the dog or cat.

Clinical Recognition

1. Onset of urinary incontinence postsurgically is suggestive.
2. Other examinations and ancillary studies are not contributory.

Treatment

"Tincture of time" may result in a functional return of the damaged sphincters or nerves.

Prognosis

1. Fair if acute
2. Poor if chronic

Estrogen-deficiency Incontinence

1. Estrogen-deficiency incontinence is primarily a problem affecting mature female dogs that have undergone ovariohysterectomy.
2. The incidence of occurrence is low, and the cause is not well understood.

Clinical Recognition

1. Development of incontinence in a spayed female dog is suggestive.
2. Physical examination, neurologic examination, and the results of ancillary diagnostic studies are usually normal.
3. Response to therapy is assumed to be diagnostic.

Treatment

1. Diethylstilbestrol (DES) at a total oral dose of 1 mg daily (for several days) is administered. Taper the dose to every third day, then every week until control is achieved. Lower doses (0.1 mg/dose) are often effective.

2. DES has been associated with bone marrow suppression, so forewarn the client and use the lowest effective dose.

3. Some clinicians prefer to use phenylpropanolamine (PPA) or ephedrine in an attempt to increase sphincter tone. These drugs may cause agitation or tachycardia. Concurrent cardiac disease is a relative contraindication.

4. Periurethral injection of Teflon® via cytoscopy has been used to improve continence in these cases in the canine.

5. Recent evidence suggests that estrogens cause increased sympathetic tone to the urethral sphincter. (This may actually represent a neurogenic incontinence.)

Prognosis

1. Excellent for continence

2. A slight possibility of bone marrow suppression exists with estrogen therapy. Death secondary to thrombocytopenic hemorrhage usually results from this complication of therapy.

Paradoxical Incontinence

Paradoxical incontinence is an occasional complication of urethral calculi or mass lesions, which may result in partial obstruction of urine outflow.

Clinical Recognition

1. Signs of incontinence usually are accompanied by signs of dysuria, hematuria, or stranguria.

2. Male dogs are most commonly affected.

3. Physical and neurologic examinations are often not contributory. Calculi may be palpable in the bladder or urethra. Catheterization may be difficult.

4. UA shows evidence of inflammation in some cases.

5. Plain roentgenograms or positive contrast studies demonstrate the calculus or obstructive mass lesion. Ultrasonographic imaging may reveal the lesion.

Treatment

1. Surgical removal of the lesion or urethrostomy proximal to the lesion is often curative.

2. Treat any urinary tract inflammation appropriately.

Prognosis

1. Good for continence if acute

2. Guarded if severe and chronic bladder distention has damaged the detrusor muscle

Incontinence Resulting from Functional Failure to Store Urine or Empty the Bladder Adequately

1. This category encompasses incontinence of multiple causes, including anatomic variables (e.g., "pelvic bladder"), neurologic causes ("reflex dyssynergia"), urge incontinence, and the like.

2. The reader is referred to the references at the conclusion of this chapter for a detailed discussion of the theory, diagnostic approach, and treatment of functional urinary incontinence.

Clinical Recognition

1. Signs of incontinence in these patients are related to an imbalance or incoordination of bladder muscle tone versus bladder sphincter tone.

2. Anatomic or pathologic disorders may be found in association with these problems (e.g., infections, prostatic disease).

3. Functional incontinence is suspected when the history, physical examination, UA, biochemical profiles, positive contrast roentgenograms, and/or empirical antibiotic therapy fail to define and correct the problem.

4. Special urodynamic studies, such as cystometography, may help to define functional urinary incontinence.

Treatment

1. Treatment is directed toward increasing or decreasing bladder contractility, or altering sphincter tone with pharmacologic agents. The following drugs and dosages are given for the canine:

    A. Phenylpropanolamine, an α-adrenergic agent to increase sphincter tone, 6.25 to 50 mg t.i.d. orally

    B. Phenoxybenzamine, an α-adrenergic blocker to decrease sphincter tone, 1 to 10 mg t.i.d. orally

    C. Ephedrine, a sympathomimetic agent to increase sphincter tone, 5 to 50 mg b.i.d. or t.i.d. orally

    D. Propantheline, an anticholinergic agent to decrease bladder muscle contraction, 5 to 15 mg t.i.d. orally

    E. Oxybutynin, an anticholinergic agent, 2 to 5 mg t.i.d. orally

    F. Bethanechol, a cholinergic agent to increase bladder muscle contraction, 2.5 to 10 mg subcutaneously (SQ) t.i.d.

    G. Diazepam, an internuncial neuron blocker, 0.5 to 10 mg t.i.d. orally (the lower dosage should be used in the feline), which may alter sphincter tone.

    H. All of these drugs should be used at the lowest dosage that can control incontinence.

    I. The reader should consult the suggested readings and a current *Physician's Desk Reference* to determine side effects and signs of overdose of these potent drugs.

2. Treatment of concurrent infections, intermittent catheterization, bladder expression, or the use of diapers may be necessary in many cases.

Prostatic Disorders

Disorders of the prostate gland cause a variety of clinical problems in the male dog. The cat does not possess a prostate as such. In this section, the general clinical signs of prostatic disease are discussed, followed by an outline of specific entities.

General Signs of Prostatic Disease

1. Dysuria, hematuria
2. Intermittent hemorrhage from the urethra
3. Fever
4. Tenesmus
5. Abdominal pain
6. "Ribbon" stools
7. Rear limb lameness (less common)
8. Rear limb edema secondary to lymphatic obstruction (less common)
9. Any one or several of these clinical signs may be present, and existing signs do not specify the nature of the prostatic disease.

Basic Principles for Evaluation of Prostatic Disease

1. Routine physical examination is indicated, with emphasis on rectal and abdominorectal palpation to assess the size, position, symmetry, and texture of the prostate.

2. Plain abdominal roentgenograms that include the entire caudal abdomen and vertebral bodies are useful. Preparation with enemas is very important before roentgenography. Thoracic roentgenograms may detect metastasis if neoplasia is present.

3. Urethrocystograms may be useful in documenting the position of the prostate or in outlining any large fistulous tracts or cysts.

4. Ultrasonographic imaging, computed tomography (CT scan), or MRI are useful in characterizing the type of lesion in a large prostate.

5. Prostatic washing by catheter or ejaculation are techniques available to obtain fluid for cytologic study, and bacterial culture and sensitivity.

6. Brucella serologic examination is indicated in cases of suspected inflammatory prostatic disease.

7. Biopsy by perineal fine-needle aspiration or laparotomy may be indicated to obtain a tissue diagnosis. Laparotomy is a more invasive technique, but it allows more reliable diagnosis and offers a chance for definitive therapy in cases of prostatic cysts or abscesses. (Castration may be performed under the same anesthesia.)

Benign Prostatic Hypertrophy

1. A common clinical entity that affects many mature males, with or without signs.
2. The disease has been associated with increased ratios of androgen to estrogen.

Clinical Recognition

1. Benign prostatic hypertrophy is usually an incidental finding on routine rectoabdominal palpation because it is rarely associated with severe signs.
2. The prostate is large, firm, symmetrical, and nonpainful.
3. Abdominal films reveal a symmetrically enlarged mass with no evidence of regional lymphadenopathy or bony metastasis.
4. Further diagnostic tests are usually unnecessary in the absence of clinical signs.

Treatment

1. If clinical signs are present, castration is the therapy of choice.
2. Use of estrogens is not recommended because of the possibility of inducing prostatic squamous metaplasia or bone marrow suppression. Three notable exceptions exist:
  A. Existing contraindications for surgery
  B. The value of the dog as a breeding animal
  C. Owner resistance to the surgery for personal or economic considerations
3. Ketoconazole administration blocks synthesis of testosterone and should be considered in the case of these exceptions.

Prognosis

1. Excellent if castration is performed
2. Temporary improvement should occur if estrogens are used. Temporary or long-term improvement may follow the use of ketoconazole.

Bacterial Prostatitis

1. Bacterial prostatitis (acute, chronic, abscessed) may present as an acute condition, or it may be a subclinical chronic entity.

2. The prostatic infection may be the underlying cause of chronic UTIs or infertility.

Clinical Recognition

1. Clinical signs often include fever, pain, and dysuria. Intermittent urethral hemorrhage also occurs.
2. Palpation reveals variable size and shape of the prostrate. If abscessed, fluctuant areas may be found. Palpation may induce pain or stimulate urethral discharge or hemorrhage.
3. The findings on plain roentgenograms vary, depending on the duration and extent of the problem. A large, fluid-density mass may represent an abscess. Local or diffuse loss of abdominal detail accompanies associated peritonitis (if present). Bony changes usually do not occur.
4. A urethrocystogram may show large fistulous tracts or fluid-filled cavities within the prostate.
5. Ultrasonography, CT scanning, or MRI may reveal abscess formation.
6. Cytologic studies reveal primarily a suppurative process that may be contaminated by hemorrhage. Culture and sensitivity often yield positive results if samples are taken before antibiotics are administered. Brucella serologic examination is recommended; positive results suggest the presence of this organism.
7. Biopsy is usually not performed.

Treatment

1. The presence of a large, fluid-filled abscess or cyst is an indication for abdominal exploration, biopsy, and surgical correction. Many procedures have been advocated, but this author recommends surgical extirpation of the abscess, prostatic drainage to the exterior by use of multiple Penrose drains, and a vigorous, long-term regimen of antibiotics selected on the basis of culture and sensitivity at surgery. Androgenic influence should be eliminated by concurrent castration. Avoid the use of estrogens because subsequent squamous metaplasia provides an ideal environment for chronic infection.
2. In the absence of an apparent abscess,

antibiotics, selected on the basis of culture and sensitivity of prostatic fluid, are indicated for at least one month. Castration is recommended if the problem is chronic (as discussed previously). Antibiotics that reach high levels in prostatic tissue include chloramphenicol, diaminopycimidine plus sulfonamides, erythromycin, tetracyclines, and cephalosporins.

3. Ketoconazole may be used in lieu of immediate castration for temporary reduction of testosterone production.

Prostatic Squamous Metaplasia

1. Prostatic squamous metaplasia occurs as a result of a decreased ratio of androgen to estrogen, with an excess in estrogens being the predominant cause.

2. This excess is usually attributable to:

A. Endogenous overproduction by a Sertoli cell neoplasm (occurring most commonly in retained testicles)

B. Previous estrogen therapy (iatrogenic)

3. Squamous metaplasia does not regress completely following the cessation of estrogen influence.

4. Squamous metaplasia provides an ideal environment for bacterial infection, so these two conditions often coexist.

Clinical Recognition

1. The concurrent presence of a Sertoli cell tumor or a history of previous estrogen therapy with clinical signs of prostatic diseases suggests the possibility of squamous metaplasia.

2. Rectal palpation usually reveals a large prostate that is symmetrical unless cysts or abscesses coexist.

3. Plain and contrast roentgenographic findings vary, depending on coexisting cysts or infection.

4. Cytologic studies may reveal increased numbers of squamous-type cells, or they may indicate an accompanying inflammatory process.

5. Biopsy is more reliable than cytologic examination (and is diagnostic for this condi-

tion). A shift toward squamous cell characteristics is noted in the prostatic parenchyma.

Treatment

1. Discontinue any further estrogen therapy, or remove the associated Sertoli cell tumor.

2. Castrate the animal to remove any androgenic influence.

3. Treat any associated cyst, infection, or abscess appropriately.

Prognosis

The prognosis associated with this condition is fair. Recovery from clinical signs is possible, but chronic infection may be a problem when associated with squamous metaplasia.

Prostatic Cyst

1. The origin of benign prostatic cysts is uncertain.

2. Clinical signs rarely develop until the cyst attains a large size, causing interference with local organ function (bowel, bladder, ureter).

Clinical Recognition

1. Tenesmus and dysuria do occur.

2. Physical examination usually reveals a huge caudal abdominal mass; it is often mistaken for a distended urinary bladder.

3. Plain roentgenograms commonly disclose the "double bladder sign," or what appears as two urinary bladders. The cyst is almost always dorsal to the bladder.

4. Emptying the bladder by catheterization and repeating the films should confirm the presence of the fluid-density mass. A urethrocystogram may reveal some contrast material entering the cyst by way of a tract, or it may simply serve to prove that the bladder is a separate structure from the cyst.

5. Ultrasonography, CT scanning, or MRI may define cystic borders.

6. Cytologic evaluation of the prostatic fluid is usually noncontributory, but helps to distinguish a cyst from an abscess.

Treatment

1. Treatment is effected by the same type of surgery as described for an abscess.
2. Culture and biopsy of the cyst are indicated at the time of surgery.

Prognosis

The long-term prognosis is good for complete recovery.

Prostatic Neoplasm

1. The most common tissue type is adenocarcinoma.
2. Older animals are generally affected.

Clinical Recognition

1. A chronic history of any or all of the signs of prostatic disease is usual, although rear limb edema and lameness are more suggestive of neoplasia than are the other prostatic problems.
2. Palpation reveals an irregular, large prostate that may be adhering to adjacent tissue. Pain is typically evident, and sublumbar lymph nodes may be enlarged.
3. Plain roentgenograms demonstrate an enlarged prostate. Sublumbar lymphadenopathy is often noted. A proliferative periosteal reaction in the caudal lumbar vertebrae is the hallmark of prostatic carcinoma with metastasis. Thoracic films may reveal multiple pulmonary metastatic nodules.
4. Ultrasonography, CT scanning, or MRI can define this lesion.
5. Cytologic study of the prostatic fluid may demonstrate clusters of immature neoplastic cells of epithelial derivation.
6. Perineal fine-needle aspiration or laparotomy confirms the diagnosis, if necessary.

Treatment

1. At the present time, no surgical or medical oncologic therapy results in an acceptable, long-term clinical result. Prostatectomy is indicated early in the course of the disease, but the disease is usually locally metastatic

by the time it is discovered. The persistent pain involved makes euthanasia an important consideration.
2. Ketoconazole to suppress testosterone production may be used as a palliative measure. Oncologists may be consulted for information on any new promising regimen.

Prognosis

At this time, the prognosis is routinely grave.

Summary

Prostatic problems indicate a need for aggressive diagnostic and therapeutic measures to prevent chronic diseases from developing. Rectal palpation during routine check-ups should be a part of all male canine physical examinations, as they allow early detection of prostatic disease.

Periparturient Disorders in the Female

Medical complications associated with pregnancy and parturition are occasional problems in the dog and rare problems in the cat. This section discusses these problems, with particular emphasis on dystocia, which is the most common of these clinical entities.

Dystocia

1. *Dystocia* is defined as abnormal or difficult parturition. It is more commonly encountered in the dog than in the cat, and the owner's lack of knowledge about normal periparturient behavior is a common reason for presentation of the animal for this complaint.
2. Routine physical examinations before breeding and prior to parturition often disclose potential problems and provide an opportunity for owner education.

Clinical Recognition

1. The breed and age of the animal are of prime importance. Past reproductive history, trauma, illnesses, and present environment all require inquiry. Note the breeding dates (if known). Ascertain owner experience with parturition in animals. Discuss the breeding value of the female, as well as future plans for the animal and her offspring.

2. Each clinical situation must be assessed individually; however, certain situations that suggest dystocia may be encountered.

A. Historical evidence indicating possible causes of dystocia (e.g., previous episodes of dystocia in the animal; previous trauma, especially to the pelvic region; current or recent illness; collapse; and muscular twitching or shaking)

B. Signs of active labor (contractions, panting) for more than one hour without delivery of offspring

C. Weak labor (infrequent contractions) for more than two hours without expulsion of offspring

D. Placental separation (dark green vaginal discharge) without signs of labor

E. More than a few hours between delivery of offspring, in which case, one must consider the possibility that all the offspring have been delivered

F. A deficit in the number of placentas passed relative to the number of offspring born

G. A calculated gestation period of greater than 68 to 70 days (in the dog or cat)

H. Abnormal vaginal discharge (purulent, foul smelling)

I. Evidence of fetal death

J. Evidence of maternal depression, weakness, or fever in lieu of contractions

3. Perform a physical examination with special emphasis on measurement of temperature, respiration and pulse rates, abdominal palpation, rectal palpation, and vaginal examination.

A. In the dog, body temperature usually drops to less than 100°F 24 hours prior to parturition.

B. Abnormal pelvic anatomy and mismatches between fetal head diameter and pelvic diameter can be appreciated on rectal examination.

C. Determine abnormal vaginal anatomy

and cervical relaxation by aseptic vaginal examination.

D. Determine the presence of a fetus in the birth canal or some abnormal presentation. (Remember that the "breech" or posterior presentation normally occurs about half the time in the dog and cat. A transverse presentation is abnormal.)

4. Ancillary diagnostic studies other than abdominal roentgenography or ultrasonography are rarely indicated in dystocia (unless complicated by some other systemic problem).

A. Determine fetal number, development, size, and positioning by the roentgenogram. The presence of gas around the fetuses suggests decomposition and possible infection.

B. Serum electrolyte studies may be indicated if hypocalcemia is suspected or if caesarian section is planned.

Disorders Associated with Dystocia in the Dog and Cat

Poor body condition with obesity
Inhibition of oxytocin release (psychogenic)
Senility
Uterine overstretching
Uterine prolapse
Myometrial defects or infection
Uterine torsion
Hypocalcemia, hypoglycemia
Ectopic pregnancy
Mismatch between fetal head diameter and pelvic size
Abnormal presentation (transverse)
Exhaustion secondary to lengthy parturition
Congenital anomalies of the birth canal
Fetal death
Inadequate fetal fluids

Treatment

1. The approach to treatment of dystocia depends upon the associated cause, future breeding considerations, the economic value of the mother and offspring, and personal preference.

2. A medical approach should be utilized when clinical and economic considerations indicate an attempt to preserve breeding potential and offspring life.

A. Document a clear birth canal and a dilated cervix by vaginal examination.

B. Attempt artificial lubrication and manual or instrument delivery if a fetus is palpated in the canal. Pull the fetus slightly dorsal until it reaches the pelvic brim. Then apply gentle traction ventrally and caudally.

C. "Feathering" the dorsal anterior vagina may help to stimulate uterine contractions.

D. Oxytocin, administered IM (3 to 5 U for the cat, 3 to 20 U for the dog), stimulates uterine contractions.

E. Ergonovine, administered IM (0.005 to 0.01 mg/lb), may be used in the dog to cause uterine contractions.

F. Administer 10% calcium gluconate solution (5 to 20 mL slowly, IV, until the desired effect is achieved) if hypocalcemia is known or suspected.

G. Administer 50% dextrose (1 mL/5 lb, IV) if hypoglycemia is known or suspected.

H. Repeat medical treatment every 30 minutes if initially unsuccessful. Place the female in a dark, quiet environment to allow evaluation of therapeutic efficacy.

3. Surgical therapy is indicated by clinical signs, time factors, economic considerations, or failure of medical therapy.

A. Inhalation anesthetics are most desirable. Isoflurane offers rapid recovery for mother and offspring.

B. Perform uterine culture and biopsy if a pathologic condition is suspected.

C. Consider ovariohysterectomy if future breeding is not desired. The females lactate despite ovariohysterectomy.

Prognosis

1. Offspring survival is always somewhat tenuous with dystocia. Death and injuries often occur.

2. Maternal prognosis is dependent upon the underlying condition and method of therapy.

3. Maintain close observation for periparturient disorders (e.g., retained placenta, uterine subinvolution).

Vaginal Discharges in the Postpartum Period

Postpartum Hemorrhage

1. Mild hemorrhagic vaginal discharge in a rapidly decreasing volume commonly persists for 7 to 14 days postpartum in the dog. A mild greenish tinge to the discharge is normal.

2. A hemorrhagic vaginal discharge is seldom noticed in the cat.

Clinical Recognition

1. A history of past episodes of hemorrhage or dystocia with instrument-assisted delivery may be obtained.

2. Inspect the vagina for lacerations.

3. Monitor mucous membrane color and refill, pulse rates, packed cell volume (PCV), and total protein in a severely hemorrhaging postpartum female.

4. Platelet estimates (by blood smear) or counts, and complete coagulation profiles are indicated in animals that fail to respond to conservative therapy. Consider hypocalcemia and evaluate serum calcium levels in these problem cases.

Treatment

1. Isotonic IV fluids provide volume replacement if necessary.

2. Ergonovine maleate (0.005 to 0.01 mg/lb IM once) has been used in the canine to promote uterine vasculature constriction.

3. Consider blood transfusion if bleeding continues. If a coagulopathy or platelet deficit (either numerical or functional) is suspected, choose whole fresh blood.

4. If present, hypocalcemia should be treated by slow IV administration of calcium gluconate or calcium chloride. The dosage is dependent on the magnitude of the exiting deficit, but a total dose of 5 to 25 mL of a 10% solution of either preparation is usually adequate.

5. Suture any vaginal lacerations.

6. Perform ovariohysterectomy if the problem persists.

Prognosis

Prognosis is good in terms of life, but variable in terms of future successful reproduction.

Retained Placenta

1. The retained placenta is primarily a problem in female dogs following an abnormal parturition.
2. Normally, these fetal membranes are expelled soon after delivery of the offspring.

Clinical Recognition

1. Make a direct count of offspring versus placentas passed.
2. A heavy, green-black, postpartum discharge that persists for more than two days is indicative of a retained placenta.
3. Depression, anorexia, dehydration, and fever may develop within a few days of parturition with retained placenta.
4. Abdominal palpation or vaginal examination may reveal a larger than expected uterus or fetal membranes at the cervix.
5. Abdominal roentgenograms or ultrasonographic imaging will demonstrate a large uterus.

Treatment

1. Oxytocin (3 to 10 U IM) and calcium gluconate (3 to 10 mL of a 10% solution IV) may stimulate further uterine contractions and expel the uterine contents if they are administered within hours of parturition.
2. Ergonovine maleate (0.005 to 0.10 mg/lb once), administered IM, has been advocated in the canine to stimulate uterine contractions.
3. Extra-abdominal message and instrumental delivery of placental membranes may be attempted using a gauze sponge on a forceps passed through the vagina to remove the retained tissue.
4. Abdominal exploratory examination and hysterotomy or ovariohysterotomy are indicated when other methods fail.

Prognosis

1. Good for life when recognized early
2. Guarded for future breeding because

uterine infections, subinvolution, or scarring may occur as sequelae.

Uterine Subinvolution

1. Uterine subinvolution is to be distinguished from subinvolution of the placental sites.
2. It results when normal posparturient uterine contractions fail to occur and the uterus is left full of fluid. It is hypothesized that the nursing offspring ingest a toxic factor from the milk in these cases.
3. The etiology is uncertain.

Clinical Recognition

1. The female shows no overt signs.
2. The offspring may be weak, depressed, and nursing poorly. Neonatal death may be a sign.
3. Physical examination of the female may demonstrate a palpably enlarged and fluctuant uterus. A slight serosanguineous vaginal discharge is often present (normal).
4. The body temperature of the female is usually normal (as compared to the fever caused by metritis or retained placenta).
5. Roentgenograms or ultrasonography will reveal a large uterus.
6. Brucella serologic tests are recommended in the dog.

Treatment

1. Handfeed offspring for 24 to 48 hours.
2. Infuse the uterus with an antibiotic solution administered through the vagina and cervix. (Use nitrofurazone solution; total dose of 3 to 10 mL)
3. Administration of ergonovine maleate (IM) is recommended in the dog (0.005 to 0.1 mg/lb once).
4. Administer broad-spectrum systemic antibiotics for two weeks.

Prognosis

1. Good for the life of the mother
2. Fair for the survival of the remaining offspring
3. Good for future breeding of the female

Subinvolution of the Placental Sites

1. Subinvolution of the placental sites is to be distinguished from subinvolution of the uterus as a whole.
2. The etiology is unknown.

Clinical Recognition

1. The female is normal in all respects except for a low-grade sanguineous vaginal discharge that persists for weeks after parturition.
2. The offspring are healthy.
3. The physical examination is normal except for the discharge.
4. Abdominal roentgenograms or ultrasonographic imaging demonstrates a small uterus. (The uterus is usually not seen roentgenographically.)
5. Brucella serologic testing yields negative results in the dog.
6. The results of hemostasis screening are normal.

Treatment

1. Spontaneous regression may occur.
2. Ergonovine maleate (0.005 to 0.01 mg/lb once) IM may cause the uterine vasculature to constrict.
3. Perform ovariohysterectomy if the problem is chronic and medical therapy fails.

Metritis

Overt bacterial uterine infection is most often recognized in association with dystocia, instrument-assisted delivery, retention of a fetus or placenta, or preexisting chronic endometritis.

Clinical Recognition

1. The female is usually febrile, anorexic, dehydrated, and oligogalactic. Offspring are often weak, depressed, or dying.
2. Physical examination reveals varying degrees of uterine discharge or an enlarged uterus.
3. Abdominal roentgenograms or ultrasonographic imaging may show an enlarged uterus or degenerating fetuses (if they were retained).

4. A leukocytosis with a left shift is common.
5. Brucella serologic testing yields positive results in the dog if this organism is involved.
6. Bacterial culture of the discharge may yield positive results.

Treatment

1. Initiate appropriate supportive fluid and electrolyte therapy.
2. Locally infused antibiotics (nitrofurazone solution, 3 to 10 mL by intrauterine administration), are recommended, followed by two weeks of systemic antibiotics.
3. Ergonovine maleate (0.005 to 0.10 mg/lb once) IM may be administered to expel uterine contents.
4. Tube feeding of the offspring is recommended.
5. Consider ovariohysterectomy if a poor response to medical therapy occurs, or if a canine female tests positive for Brucella.
6. Prostaglandins have been used experimentally to induce uterine contractions, but they are not presently approved for use in the dog or cat by the Food and Drug Administration (FDA). The recommended dosage is 100 to 250 μg/kg of prostaglandin F_2 alpha (nonsynthetic) administered SQ once daily for two days.

Prognosis

1. Good for the life of the mother
2. Fair for the life of the offspring
3. Guarded for future breeding potential

Pyometra (Cystic Endometrial Hyperplasia Complex)

1. Pyometra is considered under periparturient vaginal discharges, although it most commonly occurs in metestrus.
2. The causes involve abnormal interactions among the uterus, circulating hormones (estrogen, progesterone), and bacteria.
3. It occurs in the dog and cat.
4. Hormonal drugs used for contraception, or mismating, may be predisposing factors.
5. It may threaten life in several ways.
A. Absorption of toxins or bacteria into the circulation

B. Rupture of the uterus with frank peritonitis

C. Renal failure secondary to immune complex glomerulonephritis or prerenal factors

Clinical Recognition

1. Females may have a history of purulent vaginal discharge.
2. A history of polyuria, polydipsia, anorexia, or depression may be noted.
3. Physical examination may reveal various degrees of dehydration, abdominal distention, fever, vaginal discharge, and depression.
4. Abdominal roentgenograms are typically diagnostic of a huge, tubular, caudal, abdominal mass. Loss of abdominal detail may occur with a ruptured pyometra. (Ultrasonography may reveal a large uterus.)
5. Assess routine hematologic and biochemical profiles. Various degrees of azotemia may be detected. WBCs may be tremendously elevated (neutrophilic leukocytosis with a left shift), or there may be a degenerative left shift if the bone marrow is failing.
6. UA may reveal a failure to concentrate urine or a hyperproteinuria secondary to glomerular damage.

Treatment

1. Supportive fluid, antibiotic, and electrolyte therapy is indicated in all cases. The reader is referred to the discussion of renal failure for a more specific presentation of therapy (see Chapter 12).
2. Ovariohysterectomy is the treatment of choice in almost all cases, as it yields the most consistent results.
3. Medical management may be attempted in selected cases.
A. Owners may refuse surgery owing to valuable reproductive prospects in the female.
B. A serious contraindication to general anesthesia exists.
4. Medical management
A. Ensure the patency of the cervix. In selected cases, position a catheter by means of surgery or endoscopy.
B. Bacterial culture and sensitivity of the urine fluid are recommended.
C. Prostaglandin F_2 alpha (non-synthetic)

administered at 25 to 250 μg/kg SQ daily for 5 days, stimulates uterine evacuation in the canine. Point out to the owner that the drug is not approved for this use by the FDA. In addition, the drug causes severe side effects consisting of trembling, hyperpnea, vomiting, diarrhea, and excitement. The drug is used daily for three to five days until the uterus is judged to be normal by roentgenography or ultrasonography and the vaginal discharge ceases. Another course of treatment may be administered in two weeks if signs persist.
D. Administer concurrent broad-spectrum antibiotics and supportive fluid care.
5. If successful, breed the female immediately during the next estrus, and each estrus thereafter, ovariohysterectomy is recommended when further breeding is not desired.

Prognosis

1. Good if surgery is performed (provided serious renal damage or peritonitis have not occurred)
2. Guarded and uncertain if medical therapy is applied; experience with this therapy is limited

Miscellaneous Periparturient Disorders

Uterine Torsion

1. Uterine torsion develops late in pregnancy or is associated with pyometra.
2. The etiology is unknown.

Clinical Recognition

1. A history of impending parturition is usually obtained. Abdominal pain may be suspected.
2. Physical examination reveals a tubular abdominal mass or an extremely tense abdomen.
3. Other findings vary, depending on the duration of the condition or the presence of associated infection or rupture. Depression, dehydration, and shock may coexist.
4. Abdominal roentgenograms demonstrate the enlarged uterus; detail may be obscured by a homogeneous fluid density caused by uterine rupture or secondary ascites from venous occlusion.

Treatment

Abdominal exploration with ovariohysterectomy is recommended in all cases.

Prognosis

Prognosis is guarded for life, and future reproduction is not possible.

Prolapsed Uterus

A prolapsed uterus generally occurs during the act of parturition or as the result of assisted delivery with instruments. It has been reported to occur up to 48 hours postpartum in the feline.

Clinical Recognition

1. Physical examination is diagnostic. One or both uterus horns may be involved.
2. Inspect the animal carefully for evidence of lacerations, tissue necrosis, or self-mutilation.
3. This clinical entity is one differential diagnosis for vaginal mass.

Treatment

1. If fresh, the uterus should be flushed with sterile saline and replaced manually (laparotomy is usually necessary).
2. If necrotic, or if associated abdominal pathologic conditions are evident, perform ovariohysterectomy. Consider ovariohysterectomy as a primary mode of therapy in females of other than breeding quality.
3. Administer systemic antibiotics for two to four weeks.

Prognosis

The prognosis is good for life, but poor for future reproduction.

Uterine Rupture

1. Uterine rupture most commonly occurs with pyometra.
2. Other causes are traumatic (late pregnancy or an assisted delivery).

Clinical Recognition

1. A history of a late pregnancy or recent parturition is often elicited.

2. Vaginal discharge, polydipsia, or polyuria may occur if pyometra is involved.
3. The animal is usually depressed, and may have abdominal pain. Evidence of extrauterine fluid or masses may be found on palpation.
4. Abdominal roentgenograms confirm the presence of free abdominal fluid or fetuses.
5. Abdominal paracentesis and cytologic studies demonstrate the nature of the fluid, which varies from a modified transudate to a frankly suppurative exudate (depending on the presence of pyometra).

Treatment

1. Provide immediate supportive care (IV fluids), followed by abdominal exploratory and ovariohysterectomy.
2. Provide surgical treatment for peritonitis by lavage and drainage, and obtain a bacterial culture of the abdomen.
3. Initiate broad-spectrum antibiotics pending culture and sensitivity results.
4. Monitor renal function and electrolyte balance closely following surgery.

Prognosis

1. Guarded for life
2. Future breeding is impossible if ovariohysterectomy is performed.

Eclampsia (Periparturient Hypocalcemia)

1. Eclampsia is most common in toy breeds, although it has been reported in larger dogs and in cats.
2. It may occur before, during, or after parturition.
3. The signs result from a decreased availability of calcium to the female's neuromuscular system, owing to a preferential demand for its use in milk production.
4. Poor nutrition is commonly associated with eclampsia.

Clinical Recognition

1. Weakness, followed by muscle tremors, hyperpnea, and even generalized convulsions, may develop.
2. Body temperature is often elevated.

3. Muscle fasciculations may be noted on physical examination.

4. The serum calcium level is usually low. In some cases, the animal will respond to appropriate therapy, but will have normal serum calcium levels.

5. Pupillary light reflexes may be depressed.

Treatment

1. Slow IV infusion of 10% calcium gluconate or calcium chloride (3 to 30 mL), administered to effect, usually brings about a rapid response.

2. Auscultate the heart or perform an ECG during calcium therapy. Dysrhythmias or progressive bradycardia are indications for slowing or discontinuing calcium therapy.

3. Hypoglycemia may coexist, so a trial dose (2 to 20 mL) of 50% dextrose IV may be necessary if the calcium preparations are not effective.

4. When clinical signs abate administer 5 to 15 mL of calcium gluconate SQ.

5. Maintain the female on 0.5 to 2 g of oral calcium lactate daily, and 5,000 to 10,000 IU of oral vitamin D daily.

6. If the problem recurs during the same lactation, discontinue nursing and handfeed the offspring.

7. The effectiveness of corticosteroids in the treatment of this problem is controversial.

Prognosis

1. Excellent for recovery

2. The problem often recurs during subsequent lactations unless proper nutritional balance is accomplished.

Mastitis

1. Mastitis occurs most often in unsanitary environmental conditions.

2. Consider metritis as a potential concurrent problem.

Clinical Recognition

1. The female is febrile and depressed.

2. Offspring may be weak or dying.

3 Physical examination reveals an inflamed gland or glands, and an abnormal discharge from the involved teats.

4. A bacterial culture and sensitivity from the milk is strongly positive.

5. Other diagnostic techniques are usually unnecessary.

Treatment

1. Handfeed offspring during the acute course of the disease.

2. Select broad-spectrum systemic antibiotics pending sensitivity results.

3. Applying hot packs to the affected gland(s) provides pain relief and facilitates drainage.

Prognosis

1. Excellent for recovery and future breeding potential

2. Good for the life of the offspring, if detected early

Galactostasis

1. Galactostasis represents nonseptic mastitis.

2. It may occur in the dog or cat.

Clinical Recognition

1. The female has swollen, painful, mammary glands but normal-appearing milk.

2. Body temperature is normal.

3. Cytologic studies and cultures of the milk yield no evidence of bacterial infection.

Treatment

1. Apply hot soaks to the glands.

2. Administer nonsteroidal anti-inflammatory drugs.

3. Encourage suckling.

Prognosis

The prognosis is excellent for both the female and the offspring.

Agalactia or Oligogalactia

The causes of failure to produce milk in adequate quantities have not been investigated in the dog or cat.

Clinical Recognition

Physical examination reveals little or no expressible milk in the mammary glands. Offspring are weak or dying.

Treatment

1. Ensure an adequate nutritional intake for the female.
2. Feed offspring with commercial milk replacers if necessary.
3. Oxytocin therapy (3 to 10 U IM once) may be attempted.

Prognosis

Prognosis is fair for the survival of the offspring.

Postparturient Aggression

The etiology of postparturient aggression is uncertain.

Clinical Recognition

The female attacks or kills her offspring.

Treatment

1. Administer low doses of promazine derivatives or diazepam.
2. Remove the offspring from the mother and handfeed, or place them with a "foster mother."

Prognosis

This phenomenon may recur during subsequent pregnancies. Affected females are of questionable breeding stock.

Miscellaneous Genitourinary Problems

Urethral Prolapse

1. This problem is unusual in the male dog or cat, and rare in females.
2. Excessive licking, urinary tract infections or obstructions usually are associated problems.

Clinical Recognition

1. The everted urethral mucosa will be obvious on physical examination.

Treatment

1. If the mucosa appears viable and reducible, it may be held in place by a temporary suture with or without a concurrent catheter.
2. If the mucosa is judged inviable, resection and mucosal anastomosis is necessary.
3. Investigate any possible underlying cause such as calculi or U.T.I.

Prognosis

Good, but may recur, castration may control problem cases in males

Inguinal/Inguinalscotal Hernias

1. This problem is more common in canines than felines, and affects females more than males.
2. Severity is dependent upon the contents of the hernia.

Clinical Recognition

1. An inguinal mass is palpable, or scrotal enlargement is palpable in the male. The inguinal ring may be palpable at the base of the mass.
2. Radiographs or ultrasound may reveal abdominal structures within the hernia.
3. Contrast studies of the gastrointestinal tract or urinary tract may reveal obstructions in these systems.

Treatment

1. Reduction of the hernia and repair of the abdominal wall is necessary.
2. Intestinal anastomosis or genito-urinary tract surgery may be necessary if damage has occurred to vital structures.
3. Neutering should be considered due to the possible hereditary basis for this disorder.

Prognosis

1. Good results are expected unless necrosis of intestines or urinary tract structures has occurred.

2. Chronic inguinoscrotal hernia may have resulted in testicular atrophy on the affected side.

Testicular Torsion

1. This problem is unusual in the dog and rare in the cat.

2. Undescended testicles with tumors are the most likely to torse.

Clinical Recognition

1. Acute pain, lethargy, and slow, stiff gait are common historical complaints.

2. The abdomen or scrotum may be enlarged and/or painful to palpation.

3. Signs associated with excessive or abnormal hormonal production may be concurrent.

4. Radiographs or ultrasound may reveal the mass effect.

Therapy

Castration (Bilateral if cryptorchid) is indicated.

Prognosis

The outcome is usually dependent on the presence or absence of a concurrent tumor and its sequellae.

Priapism

1. This problem is persistent engorgement of the penis without sexual stimulation.

2. It is usually secondary to CNS lesions.

Therapy

Protect and lubricate the exposed penis while attempting to isolate and resolve the underlying etiology.

Prognosis

The outcome is dependent on the extent of damage to the penis, and resolution of the neurosurgical problem.

Paraphimosis

1. This problem is an engorged penis which will not retract into the prepuce.

2. Trauma (coital or non-coital), infections, tumors, or circumferential constriction of the penis by hair or foreign body represent the major causes.

Therapy

1. Lubrication of the penis, and resolution of the etiology are necessary.

2. An indwelling urinary catheter, surgical release of the prepuce, or debridement/amputation of the penis itself may become necessary.

Prognosis

Prognosis is dependent on the extent of damage to the penis and urethra.

Phimosis

Clinical Recognition

A rare condition in which the prepucial opening is too small for the release of an engorged penis. This will be observed during breeding attempts.

Therapy

Surgical enlargement of the prepucial opening

Prognosis

The prognosis is usually good.

Testicular Tumors

Clinical Recognition

1. Testicular tumors may be recognized by scrotal or abdominal palpation, or by the secondary conditions caused by altered hormonal concentrations in some cases.

2. In scrotal palpation, if one testicle is firm and the other is soft, the firm testicle is suspect for a tumor.

3. Males with feminine characteristics, prostatic disease, or signs of bone marrow suppression should be closely evaluated for possible testicular tumors.

4. Abdominal roentgenograms and ultrasonography may reveal retained testicular tumors (most often Sertoli cell types).

5. Serum estrogen or testosterone levels may be grossly altered (use control values).

6. Testicular biopsy may be necessary.

Therapy

1. Ultimate treatment is by orchiectomy.

2. Fresh whole blood transfusion may be necessary prior to surgery if anemia and thrombocytopenia are present.

Prognosis

1. Outcome is dependent on histopathologic cell type.

2. Prognosis in males with bone marrow suppression (associated with sertoli cell type) is guarded to grave. Most often the bone marrow will not naturally return to function.

Pseudocyesis (False Pregnancy)

1. Pseudocyesis is a routine clinical problem in the dog, but it rarely occurs in the cat.

2. The pathogenesis is presently uncertain.

3. The problem tends to recur in individual females.

Clinical Recognition

1. Mammary gland development and behavioral changes characteristic of a pregnant female occur two to three months after estrus in a female that has not been bred or has not been fertilized successfully.

2. The female may build a "nest" or adopt an inanimate object and treat it as her offspring.

3. Physical examination and roentgenograms fail to demonstrate pregnancy.

Treatment

1. Therapy is generally not recommended because most females gradually return to diestrual behavior.

2. If treatment is desired, administer oral mibolerone, 25 μg/lb once daily, for five consecutive days. (This androgenic steroid is not presently approved for this purpose by the FDA.)

3. Ovariohysterectomy provides a more permanent solution.

Prognosis

1. Good for resolution of the problem, with or without treatment

2. Excellent for a recurring problem

3. There is no definitive evidence of a predisposition to other reproductive problems as a result of pseudocyesis.

Vaginal Masses

1. Vaginal masses primarily occur in dogs and are uncommon in cats.

2. The differential diagnoses include transmissible venereal tumor (TVT) in the canine, other neoplasia, vaginal hyperplasia, and uterine prolapse.

Work-up of a Vaginal Mass

1. History and physical examination usually afford a diagnosis.

2. Biopsy or impression smear cytologic examination provides a definitive diagnosis in questionable cases or in cases of suspected neoplasia.

Transmissible Venereal Tumor (TVT)

1. Restricted to the dog (female and male)

2. May occur in other body locations (mouth, nose, penis)

3. Transmission occurs by cellular implantation during sexual activities.

Clinical Recognition

1. The history usually involves an adult animal of breeding age that has been allowed to breed indiscriminately.
2. The mass may occur anywhere in the vagina or on the vulva.
3. The mass is generally friable and fresh-colored, and it may hemorrhage.
4. Biopsy or impression smears reveal the typical "round cell" morphology of a TVT, with highly monomorphic nuclei and basophilic cytoplasm.
5. Metastasis (local or systemic) is rarely recognized.

Treatment

1. These tumors regress spontaneously in experimental cases.
2. Surgical excision may be necessary if hemorrhage secondary to excoriation or self-mutilation of the mass is a problem.
3. Chemotherapy with vincristine usually eliminates the tumor in less than six treatments.
4. Radiation therapy has been employed in some cases.

Prognosis

The prognosis is excellent for recovery and future reproductive potential.

Vaginal Hyperplasia

1. This problem usually occurs during proestrus or estrus in the dog. Cats are not affected.
2. The cause is thought to be the influence of estrogen on vaginal cells.

Clinical Recognition

1. The history may reveal previous occurrences.
2. A mass from the floor of the vagina is noted on physical examination.
3. Cytology reveals normal cornifying epithelial cells.

Treatment

1. Attempt conservative medical management (keeping the mass clean and lubricated until diestrus). The mass should regress spontaneously.
2. Perform surgical excision of the mass if it is excessively large or necrotic.
3. Ovariohysterectomy prevents recurrences.

Prognosis

1. Excellent for regression
2. Future episodes are possible during subsequent estrual periods.

Uterine Prolapse

See the previous section on Periparturient Disorders in the Female for a discussion of this entity.

Mismating (Pregnancy Termination)

1. Mismating is a problem encountered primarily in the dog.
2. Methods of clinical management are controversial, subject to undesirable side effects, and not approved by the FDA.

Clinical Recognition

1. Exposure to breeding is reported by the owner.
2. Vaginal smears should be examined to confirm estrus in acute mismatings if estrogen use is considered.
3. Late pregnancy is diagnosed by physical examination, ultrasound, or roentgenograms.

Treatment

1. Administer 22 μg/kg of estradiol cyclopentaneopropionate (ECP) IM once (total should not exceed 1.0 mg) for early pregnancy termination in the dog.
2. Administer 0.25 mg of ECP IM (total dose) for early termination in the feline.
3. Late termination in the dog (day 30 to 50)
   A. Ovariohysterectomy is recommended.

B. Administer prostaglandin F_2, prostaglandin F_2 alpha (non-synthetic), 25 to 50 μg/kg b.i.d. IM for nine days.

C. Administer prostaglandin F_2, prostaglandin F_2 alpha (non-synthetic), 500 to 1,000 μg/kg daily for two days.

4. Late termination in the cat (day 40 to 50)
A. Ovariohysterectomy is recommended.

5. After the sixth week of gestation, administration of 20 to 30 g/kg of bromocriptine twice daily for four days is effective in most bitches.

6. Monitor the animal with ultrasonographic examinations.

Prognosis

1. All of the treatments listed are effective, but ovariohysterectomy is the most reliable.

2. Side effects of the estrogens include possible induction of pyometra, bone marrow suppression, and persistence of estrus.

3. Side effects of the prostaglandins include severe gastrointestinal (GI) signs, uncontrolled muscular activity, and even sudden death.

4. Bromocriptine may cause transient vomiting or nausea.

Neonatal Weakness or Death

1. Neonatal weakness or death is handled primarily by preventive medicine and good husbandry techniques.

2. A specific diagnosis is often difficult to establish.

3. The mortality rate from birth to weaning is normally 10% to 30% in the dog and cat.

4. An environmental history and close examination of the mother are necessary.

Common Problems Associated with Neonatal Weakness or Death

Abnormal or traumatic birth
Congenital defects
Purposeful or accidental trauma by the mother
Neonatal viruses (herpes virus, feline infectious peritonitis [FIP], feline leukemia virus [FeLV], feline immunodeficiency virus [FIV], coronavirus, parvovirus, canine distemper)
Neonatal placental infections (Brucella, Staphylococcus)
Hypoglycemia
Unfavorable environmental temperature
Gastrointestinal parasites
Lactation failure
Undetermined causes

Clinical Recognition

1. Physical examination reveals weak or dying offspring. Signs are nonspecific in most cases.

2. Examination of the mother may reveal underlying causes, such as agalactia, mastitis, metritis, or uterine subinvolution.

3. Investigate the possibility of heavy parasite loads (i.e., hookworms in the first litter of a female dog).

4. Perform a thorough necropsy on dead offspring, and submit tissue for histopathologic examination.

5. Investigate any suspicious or chronic historical problems with available serologic or virologic studies.

Treatment

1. Supportive care of the offspring is accomplished by:
A. Incubation at 90°F to 100°F
B. Tube feeding several times daily with commercial milk replacers (following manufacturer's instructions)
C. Subcutaneous fluids if necessary
D. Intramedullary blood transfusions if necessary

2. Treat underlying problems in the mother, if present (e.g., mastitis, metritis).

3. Use oral or parenteral antibiotics empirically. Do not choose tetracyclines or aminoglycosides.

4. Employ intensive preventative medicine prior to future pregnancies.

Prognosis

1. For the affected offspring, prognosis is guarded to poor.

2. Prognosis for the other offspring is dependent on etiology.

Spontaneous Abortion

1. Spontaneous abortion occurs uncommonly in the dog and cat. The list below indicates associated causes.

2. Remember that unwitnessed abortion or fetal resorption is possible; this may explain problems otherwise considered as failure to conceive.

Clinical Recognition

1. Abortion most often presents as a primary client complaint.

2. A routine history and physical examination may indicate an obvious maternal cause for the abortion (e.g., trauma, uterine infection).

3. Plain abdominal roentgenograms are indicated to determine the state of the uterus or the presence of other fetuses.

4. Perform screening serologic tests for infectious diseases associated with abortion (Brucella, Toxoplasma in dogs; FeLV, FIP, and Toxoplasma in cats).

5. A CBC and biochemical profile may be helpful in evaluating the underlying health status of the female.

6. Thyroid hormone evaluation is indicated if other causes are not apparent.

7. Necropsy and stomach culture of the aborted fetus is recommended.

Treatment

1. Therapy should encompass supportive care for the female and specific treatment of any associated disease that is detected.

2. Administer oxytocin or ergonovine maleate to cause expulsion of uterine contents or involution of the uterus if necessary (see the previous section on Dystocia).

Prognosis

The prognosis is dependent on the associated etiology.

Disorders Associated with Abortion

Congenital defects (offspring)
Uterine defects (maternal)
Trauma
Abdominal surgery
Abnormal estrogen-to-progesterone ratios
Maternal starvation or malnutrition
Infectious causes (dog)
    Brucella canis
    Mycoplasma, Ureaplasma
    Other bacterial uterine infections
    Toxoplasmosis
    Herpesvirus
    Canine distemper virus
Infectious causes (cat)
    FeLV
    FIV
    FIP
    Toxoplasmosis
    Feline viral rhinotracheitis (FVR)
    Herpesvirus
    Feline panleukopenia virus
Any other severe maternal polysystemic
  disease

Persistent Estrus Following Ovariohysterectomy

Persistent estrus after ovariohysterectomy is an unusual disorder that may occur in the dog or cat.

Clinical Recognition

1. Signs of estrus recurring after ovariohysterectomy are historically obvious.

2. Estrogen and progesterone levels may be measured in the plasma (if available).

3. Occasionally, bitches with severe hepatic failure (e.g., vascular shunts) may exhibit constant estrus as a result of poor metabolism of estrogen. Bile acid assay may be indicated to rule out this possibility.

4. Ultrasonographic imaging or roentgenography may reveal ovarian masses.

Treatment

1. Perform surgical exploration for retained ovarian tissue. Explore the whole abdomen and any previous incision site. Perform a biopsy on any unusual tissue.

2. If this approach fails, try repositol progesterone (50-mg total dose SQ in the dog, administered every six months).

3. Do not use repositol progesterone in the intact female for estrus prevention, as pyometra may result.

Prognosis

The prognosis is excellent if tissue can be removed and the biopsy results show a nonneoplastic process.

Infertility in the Female

Problems with infertility require an investigation of both the male and the female, as well as of the breeding environment in question. More clinical research into fertility has been done in the dog than in the cat, and more is known about problems in the female than in the male. In this section, an approach to infertility in the female is discussed, with specific references to species when appropriate.

Evaluation of Female Infertility

1. Historical questions should include:
    A. Previous reproductive performance of this female and any related animals
    B. Medical and therapeutic histories, with emphasis on drugs used or surgeries performed, vaccinations, and so on
    C. Reproductive status of the male or males involved. (Have any of them successfully sired previous litters?)
    D. Environmental influences, both physical and disease-related (FIP, FIV, FeLV households for cat, Brucella exposure for dog)
    E. Socialization history, breeding behavior, and so on
2. A physical examination is always indicated, and should emphasize the following:
    A. Careful rectal and abdominal palpation
    B. Vaginal examination with a vaginoscope

3. Routine clinicopathologic tests should include:
    A. CBC
    B. Biochemical profile
    C. UA and fecal analysis
    D. Vaginal cytology
    E. Anterior vaginal bacterial and mycloplasma culture
    F. Serologic studies for infectious diseases (FeLV, FIP, FIV, toxoplasmosis for the cat; Brucella, toxoplasmosis for the dog)
    G. Mid-diestral progesterone levels (in the canine). This test is usually performed two to three weeks after estrus begins. Comparison with control samples is recommended.
    H. Thyroid hormone assay
4. Routine abdominal roentgenograms or ultrasonography may facilitate detection of uterine or ovarian pathologic processes.
5. Laparotomy with culture and biopsy of the uterus and ovaries is indicated if all else fails.

Specific Disorders Associated with Female Infertility

Atypical Estrus, "Silent" Estrus, or Breeding Management Failure

Variability in the length of appearance of proestrus or estrus may confuse owners, resulting in unsuccessful reproductive attempts.

Clinical Recognition

1. Atypical estrus may present as a short or long proestrus or estrus. "Silent" estrus refers to bitches who cycle but show no outward signs. Breeding management failure may be attributable to owners who follow ill-advised breeding schedules.
2. Physical examinations, clinicopathologic work-up, and roentgenographic/ultrasonographic studies are normal.

Treatment

1. Perform vaginal cytologic studies to determine optimal breeding time. Average lengths of proestrus and estrus are nine days for mature bitches, but ranges of 0 to 17 and

3 to 21 days may be normal, respectively, for proestrus and estrus.

2. Breed bitches every third or fourth day during the time when at least 90% of cornified epithelial cells are present on the vaginal swab. Allow at least one day between breedings. Allow the feline pairs to copulate several times during such breeding.

3. Teaser males may help determine when a bitch will be receptive.

4. Endoscopy of the vagina may help to determine the stage of the cycle.

5. Use artificial insemination if vaginal cytologic examination is indicative of optimal breeding time but natural reproductive performance is lacking.

Chronic Endometritis

1. Chronic endometritis is especially important in dogs, and represents an important treatable cause of infertility in the female.

2. Other than failure to conceive, no other signs are commonly noted.

Clinical Recognition

1. A history reveals that the female cycles normally, but fails to conceive. Normal reproduction may have occurred earlier in life. Stillbirths or abortions may also have occurred.

2. The physical examination is generally unremarkable.

3. The results of routine clinicopathologic evaluations are normal. (Occasionally, a heavy growth of some bacteria may be isolated from a cervical swab.)

4. Special transport and culture methods are necessary to demonstrate Mycoplasma and Ureaplasma infections in anterior vagina samples.

5. Abdominal roentgenography reveals normal anatomy. Ultrasonographic examinations are also normal.

6. This is most often a diagnosis of exclusion; thus, response to therapy may be required to identify the problem.

Treatment

1. Use vaginal cytologic results or teaser males, or both, to determine optimal breeding time (see above).

2. Allow breeding to occur. (Breed dogs as described under the section on Atypical Estrus.)

3. Several hours after each breeding, infuse the anterior vagina with broad-spectrum antibiotics in saline solution. (Use several times the normal daily adult systemic dose.)

4. Broad-spectrum oral antibiotics for one week before breeding and one week before and after parturition are also recommended in these cases.

5. Tetracycline or chloramphenicol should be used *prior* to breeding if Mycoplasma or Ureaplasma infections are demonstrated, along with a vaginal douche of 1% povidone iodine solution. *Do not* use these drugs during pregnancy.

Prognosis

1. Fair for viable offspring

2. Continue this procedure at each subsequent breeding if successful.

3. Consider therapy for ovulation failure (in the canine) if no response occurs.

Vaginitis

1. Vaginitis cannot be distinguished from chronic endometritis in most cases.

2. Clinical recognition and modes of treatment are identical to that for chronic endometritis.

3. Prognosis is good for viable offspring.

Brucellosis

1. Brucellosis is a problem in the dog. It has not been reported in the cat.

2. Transmission is by contact with infective fluids (vaginal, preputial, etc.).

3. Mild clinical infections have been documented in humans, but have been shown to respond quickly to therapy.

Clinical Recognition

1. The female dog may have a history of abortion, weak or dying puppies, or chronic vaginal discharge.

2. Physical examination may be unremarkable. Vaginal discharge or generalized lymphadenopathy may be present.

3. Abdominal roentgenograms are usually unremarkable.

4. CBCs may reveal a neutrophilic leukocytosis (either mature or with a mild left shift). Elevations of total protein levels secondary to increased globulins may occur.

5. Serologic tests for brucellosis yield positive results (high or rising titers). *Note:* The rapid-slide agglutination test is almost 100% effective in selecting infected animals (false-positive results may occur, but false-negative results have not been demonstrated). Further serologic studies or cultures are indicated when the animal tests positive.

Treatment

1. Inform the owner that infected dogs should no longer be used for breeding because presently, total elimination of the organism is almost impossible.

2. Treat pets or working dogs with oral tetracycline, 15 mg/lb t.i.d., in two separate three-week courses (with a one-month interval between courses). Streptomycin, 5 mg/lb t.i.d. IM, is added during the second course (during which renal function should be monitored).

Prognosis

1. Uniformly poor for return of fertility, but good for life

2. Advise owners of the public health significance of this disease.

Miscellaneous Infectious Diseases Associated with Infertility

1. FeLV
2. FIP
3. FIV
4. Toxoplasmosis (cat and dog)
5. Hemobartonellosis (cat)
6. Brucellosis (dog; see earlier section)

Clinical Recognition

1. Most often, only subtle historical clues or physical signs are present.

2. The diagnosis rests upon serologic studies (or culture in brucellosis)

3. In most cases, hemobartonellosis may be demonstrated by observation of a blood

smear. However, this disease entity is usually secondary to some underlying problem.

Treatment

1. Treatment exists for the viral diseases.

2. Treat hemobartonellosis with long-term tetracycline or chloramphenicol therapy.

3. Brucellosis (see earlier section)

Prognosis

1. Routinely poor for fertility (in these chronic infectious diseases)

2. To improve the prognosis for future reproduction in the environment, remove chronic carrier animals.

Underlying Noninfectious Systemic Diseases

1. The potential for underlying noninfectious systemic diseases justifies routine biochemical screening in cases of infertility.

2. Renal failure, hepatic failure, hyperadrenocorticalism, pancreatic insufficiency, and many other syndromes may be associated with poor fertility because of altered nutritional, normal, or homeostatic mechanisms.

Clinical Recognition

1. Clinical signs are usually nonspecific.

2. The problem becomes apparent after routine biochemical profile screening and follow-up clinicopathologic studies.

Treatment

If possible, treat the underlying condition.

Prognosis

1. Dependent upon the specific condition

2. Poor prognosis for fertility if the underlying condition is chronic (e.g., uremia)

Hypothyroidism

Infertility associated with hypothyroidism is likely in the dog (although theriogenologists cite the lack of scientific studies). The relationship in the cat is uncertain.

Clinical Recognition

1. The female may exhibit prolonged anestrus, abnormal cycles, minimal signs of estrus, or simply infertility.

2. Other signs of hypothyroidism (skin changes, obesity, heat-seeking behavior, "tragic" facial expression) may be present.

3. Physical examination reveals nothing specific unless overt signs of hypothyroidism are present (e.g., endocrine alopecia).

4. Roentgenographic examination of the abdomen is normal, as are ultrasonographic findings.

5. A thyroid stimulation test reveals both abnormally low resting triiodothyronine (T_3) and thyroxine (T_4) values and a poor response to intramuscular thyroid-stimulating hormone (TSH). Perform a stimulation test to confirm the diagnosis in borderline cases; obtain resting serum samples for T_3, T_4; inject 1 U/5 lb of TSH IM (up to a total of 10 U), and repeat the serum samples eight hours after injection. The poststimulation T_4 value should be two to four times the value of the resting sample. Radioimmunoassay is recommended; normal values vary with the laboratory.

Treatment

1. Oral levothyroxine (Synthroid) at 0.01 mg/lb, administered in divided doses b.i.d. ad infinitum

2. Test T_4 values periodically four to eight hours after dosage administration to determine the optimal dosage. However, clinical response is the most important guideline to follow.

3. Consider administering oral T_3, 5 to 10 μg/lb divided t.i.d., if measured T_3 levels alone are low, or if T_4 supplementation is not effective.

Failure to Cycle or Abnormal Estrus Cycles

1. Failure to cycle is primarily a problem in dogs.

2. Specific diagnosis is usually impossible.

Clinical Recognition

1. Anestrus, prolonged estrus, or extremely brief or prolonged diestrus may be recognized from the history. (Remember, basenji dogs normally cycle only once yearly.)

2. Physical examination and ancillary diagnostic tests are noncontributory. (Specific attention should be directed to thyroid hormone levels with these signs.)

3. Attempt to rule out previous ovariohysterectomy in the case of anestrus.

4. Serial vaginal cytologic studies do not reveal cornified epithelium consistent with estrus.

Treatment

1. For anestrus, administer 5 to 25 mg of follicle-stimulating hormone (FSH) IM once weekly until estrus occurs. Monitor vaginal cytologic findings. When estrus occurs, administer 5 to 10 mg of luteinizing hormone (LH) IM 24 hours prior to breeding. Breed twice.

2. For prolonged estrus, administer 5 to 10 mg of LH IM when vaginal cytologic findings reveal primarily cornified epithelium.

3. For short or long diestrus, initiate a 4- to 8-month regimen of mibolerone; then discontinue treatment and breed on the first ensuing estrus cycle.

Prognosis

1. Guarded in cases of anestrus

2. Fair in cases of abnormal estrus or abnormal diestrus

Failure to Ovulate and/or Hypoluteoidism

These are tenuous diagnoses, and are difficult to distinguish from subclinical endometritis.

Clinical Recognition

1. The history indicates normal estrus cycles and receptivity.

2. All physical findings and ancillary diagnostic test results may be normal.

3. Progesterone levels measured three weeks after the first day of estrus (in the female) may be decreased. (Use control values; a value of less than 5 ng/mL suggests this problem.)

Treatment

1. Administer 5 to 10 U of LH IM on day 1 of estrus. (Use a teaser male and check vaginal cytologic findings.) Breed twice two and four days later.

2. Administer repositol progesterone 2 mg/kg, every 3–5 days for 7 weeks.

3. Treat for endometritis if not successful.

Prognosis

1. The prognosis is guarded in terms of fertility.

2. The exogenous progesterone increases the chance of pyometra.

Lack of Libido

Clinical Recognition

1. A history of an unwillingness to accept the male may be elicited.

2. Physical examination and ancillary diagnostic test results are normal.

3. Vaginal cytologic findings and endoscopy can be used to determine whether estrus is present or impending.

Treatment

1. Administer 1 mg of oral DES daily at the onset of proestrus (as determined by vaginal cytologic findings if gross bleeding is not evident).

2. Bone marrow suppression may result from overzealous use of DES.

3. Artificial insemination performed every four days during the period when at least 90% of the vaginal epithelium is cornified is an option.

Prognosis

The prognosis is fair.

Miscellaneous Genetic or Congenital Anomalies

Consider any anatomic or chromosomal defect.

Clinical Recognition

1. Physical examination may reveal anatomic problems or evidence of pseudohermaphroditism.

2. Chromosomal determinations are not routinely available.

3. Hysterosalpingography is rarely used to evaluate reproductive anatomy.

4. Consider performing a laparotomy to check anatomy.

Treatment

Any obvious anatomic defect (e.g., persistent vaginal bands) may be surgically correctable.

Prognosis

The prognosis is usually poor in terms of fertility.

Psychogenic Infertility or Inexperience

Psychogenic infertility may be a problem in dogs or cats of either sex.

Clinical Recognition

1. The classical pampered toy breeds with no breeding experience are easy to recognize by their history. Cycles may be normal.

2. Physical examination and results of ancillary studies are normal.

Treatment

Breed the affected animal with an experienced male, or use artificial insemination at the appropriate time.

Prognosis

Prognosis is good in terms of fertility, but guarded for natural breeding ability.

Infertility in the Male

Inflammatory and endocrine problems may affect male fertility as well as that of the female. Very little is known about infertility in male cats. Evaluate male infertility as follows:

1. The animal's history of past performance and any previous or present systemic signs are important.

2. Physical examination centers on genital and prostatic (canine) anatomy. Scrotal width should be measured by caliper for future reference. Persistent frenulum or another anatomic anomaly may prevent the male from performing owing to pain.

3. Routine clinicopathologic studies should include a CBC, fecal and analysis, UA, biochemical profile, Brucella serologic testing, and T_3, T_4 serum measurements.

4. Collect semen for evaluation using a teaser female. The middle fraction of the ejaculum contains most of the sperm.

A. Perform a culture and sensitivity.

B. Immediately evaluate sperm motility and numbers (70% motility is normal).

C. Perform cytologic studies using eosin-nigrosin stain to detect sperm abnormalities.

5. Perform testicular biopsy if diagnosis or therapy is not successful by other methods. Special methods of specimen fixation are necessary.

6. Little information is presently available regarding the significance of hormonal levels in the male dog or cat.

Inflammatory Disease of the Genitourinary Tract

1. The scrotum, testicles, epididymus, prepuce, or prostate (canine) may be involved.

2. An acute problem may have occurred previously.

Clinical Recognition

1. Historical evidence of previous or present pain, swelling, or abnormal discharges from the genitalia may be elicited. Signs of prostatic disease (see earlier section in this chapter) may be present.

2. Physical examination may reveal specific evidence of inflammation.

3. Abnormal inflammatory cytologic results may be derived from examination of the ejaculum, or defective sperm or aspermia may be evident.

4. A neutrophilic leukocytosis with a left shift may occur.

5. Brucella serologic tests are positive if this organism is involved.

6. A culture and sensitivity often demonstrates significant growth if other bacteria are involved. Special transport and culture media are necessary to demonstrate Mycoplasma or Ureaplasma infections.

7. Testicular biopsy may reveal evidence of chronic or acute inflammation or neoplasia.

A. Immune mediate orchitis is characterized by lymphoplasmacytic cell types.

B. Special stains may reveal fungal or atypical mycobacterium organisms.

Treatment

1. High doses of appropriate antibiotics for long periods (at least six to eight weeks) are indicated for bacterial infections.

2. Tetracycline or chloramphenicol are indicated for Mycoplasma or Ureaplasma infections. Local preputial infusion with 1% povidone iodine solution is indicated in these cases.

3. Do not use animals testing positive for Brucella for further reproduction because of the threat of spreading infection. (Treatment is discussed in the earlier section on Female Infertility.) Consider castration.

4. Immunosuppressive dosages of prednisolone may control immune mediated orchitis. However, long-term glucocorticoids may cause infertility themselves.

5. Appropriate anti-infective drugs or castration may be indicated in fungal or mycobacterial inflammations.

Prognosis

The prognosis is guarded to poor for fertility.

Hormonal Disorders Causing Infertility

Except for hypothyroidism, most diagnoses of hormonal disorders are made on the basis of clinical impressions.

Clinical Recognition

1. Abnormal libido or failure to "settle" females may be reported.

2. Physical examination occasionally reveals soft or small testes.

3. Aspermia, oligospermia, or other sperm abnormalities are found in selected cases.

4. Ancillary diagnostic tests are not contributory except in the case of hypothyroidism, in which case T_3 and T_4 levels are decreased.

5. Testicular biopsy results may show tubular arrest or leydig cells decreased.

6. Plasma FSH, LH, and testosterone levels may be altered from normals.

Treatment

1. Thyroid replacement (levothyroxine), 0.01 mg/lb, administered orally b.i.d. is specific therapy for hypothyroidism.
2. Other therapeutic regimens are empirical.
  A. 25 mg of FSH IM once weekly for six weeks (dog or cat)
  B. 0.25 mg/lb of prednisolone daily for weeks (dog or cat)
  C. Pregnant mare serum gonadotropin (PMSG), 200 to 500 IU q3d SQ
  D. Reevaluate sperm or libido in one month.

Prognosis

The prognosis is poor in terms of fertility unless hypothyroidism is the underlying problem.

Failure of Spermatozoa Delivery Causing Infertility

Clinical Recognition

1. These males will have normal libido and normal mating behavior.
2. Testicular biopsies will reveal viable spermatozoa.
3. Ejaculate fractions will reveal azoospermia.
4. In males with a spermatocoele or bilateral spermatic duct obstruction, a sperm granuloma nodule may eventually be palpable.
5. In males with retrograde ejaculation, spermatozoa will be found in the urinary bladder by cystocentesis after ejaculation.

Treatment

1. Surgical bypass around an obstruction is theoretically possible but rarely performed.
2. Phenylpropanolamine or ephedrine may increase the tone of the internal urethral sphincter and allow for antegrade propulsion of spermatozoa in males with retrograde ejaculation.

Miscellaneous Disorders of Male Infertility

1. Overbreeding of the male (more than once every other day) has been associated with infertility.
2. Psychologic reasons have been proposed for lack of libido in some animals
3. Genetic abnormalities (e.g., XXY chromosomes) have been reported in the dog.
4. Neurologic abnormalities resulting in failure to ejaculate have been associated with infertility.
5. Seasonal decreases in sperm counts in the long-haired breeds have been reported (lower counts in the summer).
6. Anabolic steroids or chemotherapeutic agents are associated with decreased sperm production.

Suggested Readings

Barsanti SA (ed): Urinary disorders. In Kirk RW (ed): Current Veterinary Therapy IX, pp 1101–1209. Philadelphia, WB Saunders, 1986

Chew DJ, Dibartola SP, Fenner WR: Pharmacologic manipulation of urination. In Kirk RW (ed): Current Veterinary Therapy IX, pp 1207–1212. Philadelphia, WB Saunders, 1986

Chinn DR, Conley AJ, Evans LE: Bromocryptine as an abortifacient in the bitch (abstract). ACVIM Forum Proceedings, San Diego, 3: 137, 1985

Christie DW, Bell ET, Horth CE, Palmer RF: Peripheral plasma progesterone levels during the canine oestrous cycle. Acta Endocrinol 68: 543–550, 1971

Concannon P, Hansel W, McEntee K: Changes in LH, progesterone and sexual behavior associated with preovulatory luteinization in the bitch. Biol Reprod 17: 604–613, 1977

Feeney DA, Johnston GR, Klausner SS, et al: Canine prostatic disease—Comparison of radiographic appearance with morphologic and microbiologic findings: 30 cases (1981–1985). J Am Vet Med Assoc 190(8): 1018–1026, 1987

Feeney DA, Johnston GR, Klausner SS, et al: Canine prostatic disease—Comparison of ultrasonographic appearance with morphologic and microbiologic findings: 30 cases (1981–1985). J Am Vet Med Assoc 190(8): 1027–1034, 1987

Feldman EC, Nelson RW: Canine and Feline Endocrinology and Reproduction. Philadelphia, WB Saunders, 1987

Freshman JL, Amann RP, Soderberg SF, Olson PN: Clinical evaluation of infertility in dogs. Compend Contin Educ Pract Vet 10(4): 443–460, 1988

Gaudet DA, Kitchell BE: Canine dystocia. Compend Contin Educ Pract Vet 7(5): 406–416, 1985

Hardy RM, Osborne CA: Canine pyometra: Pathophysiology, diagnosis and treatment of uterine and extrauterine lesions. J Am Anim Hosp Assoc 10: 245–267, 1974

Jochle W, Anderson AC: The estrous cycle in the dog: A review. Theriogenology 7(3): 113–140, 1977

Johnston SD: Diagnostic and therapeutic approach to infertility in the bitch. J Am Vet Med Assoc 176(12): 1335–1338, 1980

Lein DH (ed): Reproductive disorders. In Kirk RW (ed): Current Veterinary Therapy IX, pp 1213–1258. Philadelphia, WB Saunders, 1986

Krawiec DR, Rubin SI: Urinary incontinence in geriatric dogs. Compend Contin Educ Pract Vet 7(7): 557–563, 1985

Lappin MR, Barsanti SA: Urinary incontinence secondary to idiopathic detrusor instability: Cystometrographic diagnosis and pharmacologic management in two dogs and a cat. J Am Vet Med Assoc 191(11): 1439–1442, 1987

Morrow DA (ed): Current Therapy in Theriogenology. Philadelphia, WB Saunders, 1980

Olsen P: Evaluating reproduction failure in the bitch. ACVIM Forum Proceedings, San Diego, 5: 103–110, 1987

Osborn CA, Low DG, Finco D: Canine and Feline Urology. Philadelphia, WB Saunders, 1972

Paisley LB, Fahning ML: Effects of exogenous follicle-stimulating hormone and luteinizing hormone in bitches. J Am Vet Med Assoc 168: 181–185, 1977

Phemister RD, Holst PA, Spano JS, Hopwood ML: Time of ovulation in the beagle bitch. Biol Reprod 8: 74–82, 1973

Schally AV, Kastin AS, Arimura A: Hypothalamic follicle-stimulating hormone (FSH) and luteinizing hormone (LH): Regulating hormone. Fertil Steril 22(11): 703–721, 1971

Scorgie NJ: The treatment of sterility in the bitch by the use of gonadotropic hormones. Vet Rec 51(9): 265–268, 1939

Shille VM, Stabenfeldt GH: Luteal function in the domestic cat during pseudopregnancy and after treatment with prostaglandin F_2. Biol Reprod 21: 1217–1223, 1979

Sokolowski JH: Evaluation of estrous activity in bitches treated with mibolerone and exposed to adult male dogs. J Am Vet Med Assoc 173(8): 983–984, 1978

Sokolowski JH: Prostaglandin F_2 alpha-THAM for medical treatment of endometritis, metritis, and pyometritis in the bitch. J Am Anim Hosp Assoc 16: 119–122, 1980

Stover DG, Sokolowski JH: Estrous behavior of the domestic cat. Feline Pract 8(4): 54–58, 1978

Verhage HG, Beamer NB, Brenner RM: Plasma levels of estradiol and progesterone in the cat during polyestrus, pregnancy and pseudopregnancy. Biol Reprod 14: 579–585, 1976

Wildt DE, Panko WB, Chakraborty PK, Seager SW: Relationship of serum estrone estradiol 17 and progesterone to LH, sexual behavior and time of evolution in the bitch. Biol Reprod 20: 648–658, 1979

Young B, Lai EV, Belbeck LW, Diamond P, Singh P: Testosterone production by ovarian follicles of the domestic cat. Horm Res 7: 91–98, 1976

CHAPTER FOURTEEN

Hyperadrenocorticism and Hypoadrenocorticism

Bernard Hansen

Hyperadrenocorticism

Spontaneous hyperadrenocorticism (Cushing's syndrome) is characterized by excessive secretion of corticosteroids—principally, cortisol (hydrocortisone)—by the adrenal cortex. This disorder results from either excessive pituitary secretion of adrenocorticotropic hormone (ACTH), termed pituitary-dependent hyperadrenocorticism (PDH), or from an autonomously secreting adrenal cortical tumor (adrenal-dependent hyperadrenocorticism [ADH]). Iatrogenic hyperadrenocorticism is a syndrome with similar clinical features caused by excessive or prolonged administration of glucocorticoids for therapeutic purposes.

Pituitary-dependent Hyperadrenocorticism

Pituitary-dependent hyperadrenocorticism is the most common cause of spontaneous canine and feline hyperadrenocorticism, accounting for 85% to 90% of all cases. Hypersecretion of ACTH by the pituitary results in excessive stimulation of the adrenal cortices,

bilateral hyperplasia, and overproduction of corticosteroids.

1. Causes

   A. In most species, corticotropic cells are located exclusively in the pars distalis of the pituitary gland.

   B. In the dog, however, the pars intermedia also contains corticotropic cells (β cells) (Fig 14-1). Some dogs with PDH have lesions involving this region of the pituitary.

   1) Pituitary hyperplasia

      a) Corticotropic hyperplasia of the pars distalis (and/or the pars intermedia in dogs)

   2) Pituitary neoplasia

      a) Adenomas of pars distalis

      b) Adenomas of pars intermedia in dogs

   3) The underlying reasons for development of hyperplasia and neoplasia are unknown. Excessive stimulation by the hypothalamus, either by hypersecretion of corticotropin releasing hormone or by direct stimulation from hypothalamic efferents to pars intermedia cells, may play a role. With excessive hypothalamic stimulation, the pituitary corticotropic cells hypersecrete ACTH and are abnormally resistant to feedback inhibition by circulating cortisol. The unrestrained secretion of ACTH stimulates excessive adrenal secretion of corticosteroids.

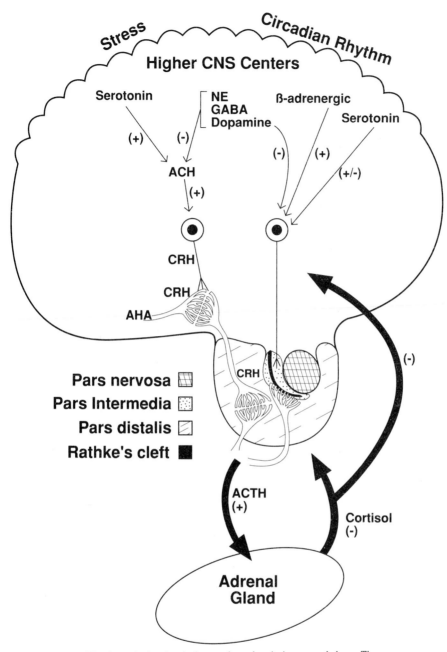

Figure 14-1. *The hypothalamic-pituitary-adrenal axis in normal dogs. The hypothalamus is subject to stimulation and suppression by higher CNS centers via excitatory (serotonin, β-adrenergic, acetylcholine [ACH] and others) or inhibitory (dopaminergic, norepinephrine [NE], gamma-aminobutyric acid [GABA]) neurons. Secretion of these substances is influenced by circadian rhythm, as well as environmental and internal stressors. When stimulated, neurons in the paraventricular nucleus and elsewhere synthesize and release corticotropin releasing hormone (CRH) to the portal circulation of the anterior hypophyseal artery (AHA). With stimulation of CRH, corticotropes in the pars distalis produce and secrete ACTH. Cells of the pars intermedia are directly controlled by neurons originating in the supraoptic nucleus, and are not influenced by CRH. With stimulation by ACTH, the adrenal cortex produces cortisol and other adrenocorticoids. Cortisol exerts a negative feedback effect on both pituitary corticotropes and hypothalamic neurons.*

Adrenocortical Neoplasia

Functional adrenal tumors are responsible for 10% to 15% of the cases of spontaneous hyperadrenocorticism in dogs and cats. These neoplasms are almost always unilateral and secrete cortisol autonomously, with no responsiveness to the normal control mechanisms. They occur in the right and left adrenal glands with equal frequency. Hypersecretion of cortisol suppresses pituitary secretion of ACTH which, in turn, results in contralateral adrenocortical atrophy. Rarely, a functional pituitary adenoma or pituitary hyperplasia is present at the same time and causes bilateral hyperplasia. It is possible that, in some cases, an adrenocortical tumor develops as a consequence of prolonged stimulation by ACTH in animals with PDH.

1. Types
    A. Adrenocortical adenomas and carcinomas occur with approximately equal frequency in the dog.
        1) Adrenocortical adenomas are generally benign, although they may be locally invasive.
        2) Adrenocortical carcinomas are generally malignant, and both local and distant metastases are common findings at the time of diagnosis. The liver is the organ most frequently affected by metastatic disease.

Pathogenesis

With either form of spontaneous hyperadrenocorticism, the pathophysiology of the disease results from prolonged elevation of plasma cortisol levels. Additionally, signs of local disease secondary to the expansive or metastatic properties of pituitary and adrenal tumors, respectively, may be present.

1. Effects of excessive circulating cortisol on other organ systems
    A. Endocrine functions
        1) Thyroid function
            a) Thyrotropin secretion in response to thyrotropin releasing factor is suppressed.
            b) There may be inhibition of peripheral tissue conversion of thyroxine (T_4) to triiodothyronine (T_3).
            c) There is reduced production of T_4-binding globulin. As a result, total plasma T_4 concentrations are low. However, free T_4, the physiologically active fraction, is present in normal concentrations, and the animal is likely to be euthyroid.
        2) Reproduction
            a) Animals with hyperadrenocorticism frequently exhibit reduced libido, testicular atrophy, or anestrus.
            b) Luteinizing hormone (LH) and follicle-stimulating hormone (FSH) secretion in response to gonadotropin releasing hormone (GRH) is suppressed.
            c) Reduced plasma concentrations of testosterone are partly attributable to suppressed LH release.
            d) There may also be direct suppression of gonadal function by glucocorticoids.
        3) Pancreatic endocrine function
            a) High circulating corticosteroid concentrations are associated with insulin resistance, glucose intolerance, and overt diabetes mellitus.
            b) This may be a result of both an insulin receptor defect (reducing insulin binding) and impaired coupling of cellular responses to the insulin receptor complex.
            c) Hyperinsulinemia is commonly present in dogs with hyperadrenocorticism. This is a normal pancreatic β cell response to counter tissue resistance to insulin and maintain plasma glucose concentrations in the normal range. However, if there is insufficient β cell reserves, overt hyperglycemia and ketosis may develop. With time, β cell exhaustion may develop, resulting in permanent diabetes mellitus.
        4) Calcemic hormones
            a) Cortisol excess impairs the activation of vitamin D to 1,25-dihydroxycholecalciferol.
            b) Reduced activity of 1,25-dihydroxycholecalciferol results in impaired intestinal calcium absorption, compensatory increases in serum parathyroid hormone (PTH) concentration, and increased bone reabsorption.

c) Cortisol also directly inhibits bone formation through a direct effect on osteoblasts.

d) Urinary excretion of calcium is enhanced.

5) Antidiuretic hormone

a) Cortisol interferes with the action of antidiuretic hormone at the distal collecting tubules of the kidneys. This results in an increase in free water clearance and compensatory polydipsia.

B. Intermediary metabolism

1) Increased protein catabolism

2) Hyperglycemia secondary to increased gluconeogenesis plus insulin antagonism

3) Increased caloric intake produces obesity.

4) Insulin resistance restricts plasma clearance of lipid, resulting in increased plasma triglyceride concentrations.

C. Inflammation and immunity

1) Acute inflammation

a) Metabolites of arachidonic acid are important chemical mediators of inflammation. The anti-inflammatory effects of glucocorticoids are mediated in large part by inhibition of arachidonic acid release from cell membranes. Corticosteroids induce the production of lipocortin, a protein that inhibits phospholipase A_2, the predominant enzyme responsible for arachidonate release from cell membrane phospholipids. As a result, production of prostaglandins, leukotrienes, and thromboxane is reduced.

i. Reduced capillary dilation

ii. Reduced transudation of serum and edema formation

iii. Reduced granulocytic migration, margination, and adherence

iv. Reduced fibrin deposition

v. Delayed and reduced fibroplasia and healing

vi. Impaired production of complement

2) Mononuclear cells

a) T and B lymphocytes, monocytes, and macrophages all possess cell membrane receptors for cortisol.

b) Hence, corticosteroids can modify cellular functions.

i. Impaired macrophage production of interleukin I.

ii. Cytotoxic for some subsets of T and B cells

iii. Suppression of immunoglobulin production

Signalment

Dogs

1. Breed

A. Although any breed of dog may develop spontaneous hyperadrenocorticism, several breeds appear to have a higher risk than others. In general, small breeds, especially terriers, are at increased risk, and large breeds and mixed breeds are at a much lower risk for development of this disorder. High-risk breeds include:

1) Silky terrier

2) Bull terrier

3) Boston terrier

4) Yorkshire terrier

5) Dachshund

6) Standard poodle

7) Toy and miniature poodle

B. Certain breeds may be prone to neoplasia associated with spontaneous hyperadrenocorticism.

1) Macroscopic pituitary tumor: boxers

2) Adrenal tumor: dachshunds

3) In general, large breeds may be more prone to adrenal tumors than small breeds.

2. Sex

A. Apparently, the sex of the animal or its neutering status has no bearing on the risk of developing spontaneous hyperadrenocorticism.

B. There may be a predisposition for adrenal neoplasia in females (75%) compared to males.

3. Age

A. Spontaneous hyperadrenocorticism generally affects middle-aged and older dogs.

The risk rises steadily until seven to nine years and then levels off.

B. Pituitary-dependent hyperadrenocorticism has been reported in dogs under one year of age.

Cats

1. Spontaneous hyperadrenocorticism appears to be a rare disease in cats; hence, absolute characterization is difficult.

2. There is no obvious breed predisposition.

3. There appears to be a much higher incidence in females (90%) than in males.

4. This condition appears to be more common in middle-aged and older cats than in younger ones.

5. The distribution of PDH and ADH in affected cats appears to be similar to that in dogs. Cats with PDH may have a higher incidence of macroscopic pituitary adenomas.

Table 14-1. **Approximate frequency of the clinical signs of Cushing's syndrome**

Sign	Percentage of Dogs Affected
Polyuria/polydipsia	85
Abdominal enlargement	75
Hepatomegaly	70
Alopecia	65
Lethargy	60
Polyphagia	60
Muscle weakness/atrophy	50
Obesity	50
Anestrus	50
Testicular atrophy	35
Comedones	30
Hyperpigmentation	25
Calcinosis cutis	15
Facial nerve palsy	<10

Historical and Clinical Findings

Dogs

Although dermatologic changes, polyuria/polydipsia, and abdominal enlargement are considered features of the "classic" Cushing's appearance, clinical signs in affected animals are variable (Table 14-1). Often, an individual animal will present with only one or two clinical signs predominating.

1. Polyuria/polydipsia

A. Often the initial sign noted by the owner; may precede other signs by weeks to months.

B. Probably secondary to cortisol antagonism of antidiuretic hormone, resulting in polyuria and secondary polydipsia

2. Abdominal enlargement

A. Attributable to a combination of abdominal muscle and skin atrophy, accumulation of intra-abdominal fat, and hepatomegaly

3. Hepatomegaly

A. Diffuse hepatomegaly is characterized on histologic examination by centrilobular vacuolization and perivacuolar glycogen accumulation within hepatocytes.

4. Dermatologic abnormalities

  A. Alopecia

    1) Bilaterally symmetrical, primarily truncal

    2) May develop relatively late in the course of disease

    3) About half of affected dogs have areas of complete alopecia; others exhibit thinning of hair. A "moth-eaten" appearance may be noted in short hair breeds.

    4) Hairs are easily epilated.

  B. Thin skin

    1) Secondary to dermal atrophy

    2) Skin appears inelastic owing to degeneration of collagen. The dog may appear dehydrated based on reduced skin pliability.

    3) Most easily recognized at alopecic regions where the skin tends to be thin normally (i.e., the ventral abdomen)

  C. Comedones

    1) Hair follicles become filled with keratin, usually becoming dark brown or black.

2) Seen most commonly on ventral abdominal, inguinal, dorsal midline, and cervical areas

  D. Hyperpigmentation

    1) Often focal, but can be diffuse

    2) The cause is unknown. ACTH may have some melanocyte-stimulating hormone (MSH) activity, or the pituitary may secrete excess MSH along with ACTH in dogs with PDH.

  E. Calcinosis cutis

    1) Secondary to dystrophic calcification of degenerating dermal collagen

    2) Seen most commonly in the ventral abdominal, inguinal, dorsal midline, and cervical areas

  F. Bruising, poor wound healing

    1) Associated with protein catabolic state and depressed fibroplasia. This contributes to poor wound healing and dehiscence postsurgically.

5. Polyphagia

  A. Possibly attributable to a direct appetite-stimulating effect of glucocorticoids

6. Neuromuscular abnormalities

  A. Muscle weakness/atrophy

    1) Generalized muscle atrophy develops as a result of protein catabolism.

    2) Owners often note reduced exercise tolerance, an inability to jump or play vigorously, or both.

  B. Myotonia

    1) An uncommon complication of hyperadrenocorticism associated with persistence of muscular contraction after cessation of voluntary effort

    2) Unilateral pelvic limb stiffness is often the initial clinical sign. The opposite limb and thoracic limbs become involved later and to a lesser extent. The pelvic limbs may be rigidly extended.

    3) Persistent "dimpling" of the muscle may be seen following percussion of the muscle belly as a result of prolonged contraction.

    4) Muscle catabolism, peripheral nerve lesions, and reduced myocyte potassium concentrations have all been implicated in this condition.

  C. Facial nerve paralysis

    1) An occasional finding, it may be bilateral or unilateral. It often improves following successful therapy for hyperadrenocorticism.

  D. Hypothalamic syndrome

    1) Neurologic abnormalities secondary to compression of the hypothalamic region by an expanding pituitary tumor

    2) The dog may develop vision disturbances with loss of pupillary light reflexes, abnormal thermoregulation, other hypothalamic-pituitary endocrine abnormalities, somnolence, circling, ataxia, and Horner's syndrome.

7. Obesity

  A. Results from cortisol-induced polyphagia. There is a tendency to accumulate fat in the abdomen and dorsal trunk. Abdominal distention may exaggerate the appearance of weight gain.

8. Reproductive abnormalities

  A. Anestrus in females

  B. Testicular atrophy in males

9. Cardiovascular disorders

  A. Hypertension (>180 mm Hg systolic or 95 mm Hg diastolic) is present in approximately 50% of affected dogs. This may be attributable to the mineralocorticoid activity of high concentrations of circulating corticosteroids, enhanced activity of the renin-angiotensin system, and increased vascular reactivity.

  B. Pulmonary thromboembolism occurs in some dogs and may be fatal. The incidence of subclinical pulmonary thromboembolism is unknown.

Cats

Spontaneous hyperadrenocorticism is an uncommon disease of cats. Hence, clinical information is scanty.

  1. The most common clinical signs include:

    A. Polyuria/polydipsia

      1) Often do not occur until secondary diabetes mellitus and glucosuria develop

    B. Polyphagia

    C. Pendulous abdomen

  2. Other, less common signs include:

    A. Thin skin

    B. Ventral alopecia

C. Hyperpigmentation
D. Recurrent infections
E. Muscle wasting
F. Obesity
G. Weight loss
H. Hepatomegaly

Routine Laboratory Evaluation

Hematologic and biochemical abnormalities are similar in both PDH and ADH.

Dogs

1. Hemogram
   A. Leukocytes
   1) Abnormalities include leukocytosis, mature neutrophilia, lymphocytosis, and eosinopenia. Of these, absolute eosinopenia is the most common finding.
   B. RBCs
   1) Mild elevations of hemoglobin, packed cell volume (PCV), and RBC counts are seen in some dogs.
2. Biochemical abnormalities
   A. Electrolyte measurements are routinely normal; however, some dogs may develop mild hypokalemia secondary to enhanced renal excretion. Mild hypophosphatemia develops in some dogs as a result of increased urinary excretion of phosphate.
   B. Alkaline phosphatase (ALP)
   1) Significantly elevated in 80% to 90% of dogs with spontaneous hyperadrenocorticism
   2) May see a 3- to 30-fold elevation
   3) This increase is largely attributable to the induction of a new ALP isozyme by the liver. The presence of this isozyme should alert the clinician to the possibility of previous exposure to glucocorticoids or of spontaneous hyperadrenocorticism. ALP serum electrophoresis is thus a useful screening test for spontaneous hyperadrenocorticism.
   C. Alanine aminotransferase (ALT)
   1) Mild to moderate increases in ALT may be seen in approximately 50% of dogs with spontaneous hyperadrenocorticism.
   2) The increase may result from a combination of altered cell metabolism, resulting in leakage, and an increase in enzyme production.
   D. Hypercholesterolemia
   1) Mild to marked elevations are seen in about 50% of the cases.
   2) This is related, in part, to abnormal lipid metabolism secondary to insulin resistance.
   E. Hyperglycemia
   1) Seen in about one third of cases
   2) Varies from mild increases in glucose level to severe hyperglycemia associated with diabetes mellitus
   3) Abnormal glucose tolerance test results may be seen in a much higher proportion of patients, indicating some degree of insulin resistance.
   F. Bromsulphalein (BSP) dye clearance
   1) Increased in about 50% of affected dogs
   2) Functional defect associated with steroid hepatopathy
   G. Low resting values of serum T_3 and T_4
   1) Result of depressed plasma concentrations of thyroid-binding globulin
   2) Free T_3 and T_4 concentrations remain normal; therefore the dog is not hypothyroid.
   3) Results of thyroid-stimulating hormone (TSH) stimulation testing are usually normal, although poststimulation T_4 concentrations are not as high as those recorded in normal dogs.
3. Urinalysis
   A. Dogs with polyuria/polydipsia may have a very low specific gravity (<1.010), but the range may be from approximately 1.002 to 1.045.
   B. There is usually at least a partial response to water deprivation testing.
   C. Urinary tract infection is a common finding, and females are more likely to be affected than males. Pyuria is often absent owing to the anti-inflammatory effect of cortisol.
4. Radiographic findings
   A. Hepatomegaly is seen in dogs with steroid hepatopathy.
   B. Osteopenia of vertebrae and flat bones is seen in a small number of cases.

C. Mineralization of one or more soft tissues, including the skin (calcinosis cutis), vasculature, and tracheal and bronchial rings, may be seen in most chronically affected dogs.

D. Adrenal calcification and adrenomegaly are evident on radiographic examination in about 50% of dogs with functional adrenocortical tumors. These findings are not evident in dogs with PDH, and so they are useful in differentiating dogs with adrenal tumors from those without. Adenomas and carcinomas appear equally likely to calcify.

5. Ultrasonography

A. Two-dimensional ultrasonography is a noninvasive means of imaging the adrenal glands. Normal adrenal glands are difficult to detect.

B. Dogs with ADH secondary to unilateral adrenal tumors may be readily identified. Dogs with PDH and bilateral adrenal hyperplasia may be differentiated from normal dogs if the hyperplasia is severe enough. Thus, ultrasonography may be useful both in diagnosing hyperadrenocorticism and in differentiating PDH from ADH in some cases.

6. Computed tomography (CT)

A. When combined with the results of specific endocrine testing, abdominal CT allows accurate determination of the site of adrenal gland disease.

B. The main indication of this procedure may be to determine the existence and location of pituitary or adrenal tumor, and to determine whether metastatic disease exists. Additionally, it is useful in distinguishing unilateral (ADH) from bilateral (PDH) adrenal changes in cases with equivocal endocrine function test results.

Cats

Routine laboratory abnormalities in cats with spontaneous hyperadrenocorticism are variable.

1. Hemogram

A. Leukocytes

1) As with dogs, there may be leukocytosis with absolute lymphopenia, eosinopenia, or both, but these findings are inconsistent.

B. RBC parameters are generally normal.

2. Biochemical abnormalities

A. Marked hyperglycemia (diabetes mellitus) is the most consistent finding.

B. Hypercholesterolemia is common, and is probably related to the altered lipid metabolism associated with diabetes mellitus.

C. Increased alkaline phosphatase is seen in only one third of affected cats.

1) This may be attributable to diabetes mellitus, as insulin therapy alone will often return values to normal.

3. Urinalysis

A. Glucosuria in hyperglycemic cats; reduced urine specific gravity secondary to osmotic diuresis.

B. Urinary tract infection may be present.

Associated Conditions

1. Diabetes mellitus

2. Acute pancreatitis

A. Chronic changes in serum lipids and direct effects of cortisol on the pancreas may predispose some dogs to recurrent pancreatitis.

3. Miscellaneous

A. Pathologic fractures in dogs with severe osteopenia

B. Gastrointestinal bleeding, ulceration, and possibly perforation secondary to high circulating levels of cortisol

C. Improvement of allergic dermatitis

D. Decreased pain from arthritis

Differential Diagnosis

1. For polyuria/polydipsia

A. Chronic renal disease

B. Chronic hepatic disease

C. Diabetes mellitus

D. Diabetes insipidus

E. Psychogenic polydipsia

F. Hypoadrenocorticism

G. Electrolyte disturbances

H. Hyperthyroidism

2. For dermatologic changes (Bilaterally symmetrical alopecia suggests an endocrine or metabolic abnormality.)

A. Hypothyroidism

B. Testosterone-responsive alopecia (castrated males)

C. Male feminizing syndromes (Sertoli cell tumor)

D. Castration-responsive alopecia

E. Estrogen-responsive alopecia (spayed females)

F. Hyperestrogenism, hyperprogesteronism

G. Growth-hormone–responsive alopecia

H. Acromegaly

I. Telogen effluvium

J. Feline endocrine alopecia

K. Alopecia areata

L. Color mutant alopecia

M. Congenital and idiopathic alopecia

Diagnosis

There is no single test that will reliably diagnose spontaneous hyperadrenocorticism in every patient. A suspicion of hyperadrenocorticism arises from supportive historical and physical findings, as well as ancillary test results. The next step toward diagnosis is the use of screening endocrine tests to confirm whether the animal does have spontaneous hyperadrenocorticism. Finally, PDH must be differentiated from the adrenal-dependent form.

Dogs

1. Assays for plasma cortisol

A. Plasma cortisol is assayed by three methods. With each method, normal values for the laboratory must be validated and established for that species. There is potential for cross-reactivity with any exogenous synthetic glucocorticoid except dexamethasone. With any method, it is advisable to wait at least one to two days after the last dose of any of these (longer if repository forms were given) before performing this test. Dexamethasone does not cross-react in any of these assays, and may be administered immediately prior to, or during, the ACTH stimulation test.

1) Radioimmunoassay (RIA)

a) Normal resting cortisol levels are approximately 1 to 8 μg/dL.

2) Fluorometric method

a) Normal resting cortisol levels are slightly higher (approximately 5 to 10 μg/dL) owing to concurrent measurement of corticosterone and nonspecific substances.

3) Competitive protein binding

a) Lower resting cortisol concentrations (approximately 1 to 2 μg/dL) are recorded with this method than with the other two methods.

B. Sample handling

1) Either plasma or serum may be used; however, use the one recommended by your laboratory.

2) Samples may be left uncentrifuged at 4°C for up to 40 hours without cortisol degradation.

3) Centrifuged and separated samples may be kept at room temperature for up to a week with no significant degradation of cortisol. Therefore, samples may be sent to the laboratory by routine mail.

2. Tests to diagnose spontaneous hyperadrenocorticism

A. Resting cortisol concentration

1) Not recommended because of considerable hour-to-hour variations in plasma cortisol concentrations in dogs with spontaneous hyperadrenocorticism. Because of this, a sizable proportion of random samples will lie within the normal range.

B. ACTH stimulation test

1) 80% to 90% of dogs with PDH and about 50% of those with ADH respond with excessive secretion of cortisol.

2) The advantages of this test include ease of use and high sensitivity.

3) The disadvantages include the possibility of false-positive results in clinically stressed dogs, false-negative results in about 15% of dogs with spontaneous hyperadrenocorticism, and the inability to distinguish between PDH and ADH.

4) Procedure

a) Follow the laboratory's advice for testing and sample handling.

b) Draw plasma samples at the beginning of the test (baseline sample) for cortisol determination.

c) Administer 0.25 mg of synthetic ACTH (cosyntropin, Cortrosyn) intravenously (IV) or intramuscularly (IM), or 2.2 U/kg (40 U maximum) of ACTH gel IM.

d) Obtain a second blood sample one hour (if IV cosyntropin was used) or two hours (if ACTH gel was used) after administration.

5) Interpretation

a) Normal dogs have a resting (0 hour) plasma cortisol concentration of 0 to 10 μg/dL (depending on which assay is used), and stimulate to a range of 6 to 16 μg/dL (a twofold to threefold increase over the resting value).

b) Although short-term stresses (e.g., overnight hospitalizations) do not appear to alter the response to ACTH significantly, some dogs with chronic nonadrenal illnesses (diabetes mellitus, renal failure, infectious disease, etc.) respond with cortisol values well above the normal response range. Therefore, the presence of coexisting disease must be taken into consideration when interpreting the results of this test. It is recommended that good control of diabetes mellitus be achieved with insulin therapy before attempting diagnosis of hyperadrenocorticism.

c) Poststimulation values greater than the normal response range are compatible with hyperadrenocorticism. This test does not distinguish between PDH and ADH; however, dogs with ADH tend to have the lowest prestimulation and poststimulation results.

C. Low-dose dexamethasone suppression test

1) Normal dogs respond to exogenous glucocorticoid administration with reduced production of ACTH and cortisol.

2) Dogs with hyperadrenocorticism lose the normal response of feedback inhibition by glucocorticoids; hence, they do not suppress production of cortisol following the administration of low doses of dexamethasone.

3) Approximately 90% of dogs with hyperadrenocorticism fail to suppress cortisol production.

4) The advantages and disadvantages of this test are similar to those of the ACTH stimulation test. However, of the two tests,

the low-dose suppression test may be slightly more sensitive. Chronically stressed dogs with nonadrenal illness may fail to suppress normally.

5) Procedure

a) Collect a baseline morning plasma sample.

b) Administer dexamethasone, 0.015 mg/kg IM or 0.010 mg/kg IV.

c) Additional plasma samples are drawn six and eight hours after injection.

6) Interpretation

a) Normal dogs suppress plasma cortisol concentrations to below 1.0 μg/dL for the entire duration of the test.

b) About 90% of dogs with hyperadrenocorticism respond with a diagnostic lack of suppression.

c) Of dogs with PDH, about 50% respond by suppressing to 50% of baseline or less two to six hours postinjection, but presuppression values are regained by six to eight hours postinjection. No cortisol suppression at all occurs in another 25%. In another 15%, cortisol concentration gradually declines to 50% of baseline by eight hours, but remains higher than 1.0 μg/dL.

d) A very small number of dogs with early PDH will suppress normally. These dogs may exhibit failure to suppress if tested again two to four months later.

e) Of dogs with ADH, 80% show no suppression at all. Another 15% show suppression to less than 50% of baseline (but still exceeding 1 μg/dL). About 5% partially suppress at two to four hours, but escape to presuppression values by eight hours.

3. Tests to distinguish PDH from ADH

A. High-dose dexamethasone suppression test

1) This test is based on the theory that dogs with PDH maintain sensitivity to plasma cortisol for feedback inhibition of ACTH release, although the hypothalamic-pituitary axis responds only to much higher concentrations of cortisol than normal. Therefore, they do not suppress ACTH and cortisol production with the low dose of dexamethasone used to diagnose spontaneous hyperadrenocorticism; however, they do respond with suppression to higher doses. In contrast, dogs with ADH show little to no response to even massive doses of dexamethasone because of the autonomous nature of cortisol secretion by the tumor.

2) The procedure is similar to that used for the low-dose suppression test.

a) Collect a baseline plasma sample.

b) Inject either 0.1 mg/kg or 1.0 mg/kg dexamethasone sodium phosphate IV. There is some evidence that the higher of the two doses will yield more reliable cortisol suppression in dogs with PDH.

c) Collect plasma samples six and eight hours postinjection.

3) Interpretation

a) PDH—Greater than 50% suppression is seen in 75% of affected dogs, and less than 50% suppression is seen in 25%.

b) ADH—No suppression is noted in 80%. Suppression to less than 50% of the baseline value is seen in the remainder, but values remain greater than 1.5 μg/dL.

B. Plasma ACTH determination

1) Determination of plasma ACTH concentration is a useful means of distinguishing between PDH and ADH in equivocal cases. Dogs with PDH tend to have a very high plasma concentration of ACTH; however, the concentration varies greatly during a 24-hour period owing to an episodic secretion pattern. As a result, some single determinations in dogs with PDH overlap with the normal range. Therefore, this is not a useful screening test for spontaneous hyperadrenocorticism. Plasma concentrations of ACTH tend to be very low in dogs with ADH. This represents an appropriate response by the hypothalamic-pituitary axis to chronic hypersecretion of cortisol by an adrenal tumor.

2) The disadvantages of this test include difficult sample handling, scarcity of veterinary endocrinology laboratories performing the test, and expense. Commercial laboratories that perform human ACTH determinations should not be used.

3) Procedure

a) Consult the endocrinology laboratory for specific instructions before performing this test.

b) Samples must be collected in cold, heparinized plastic syringes, spun immediately in a refrigerated centrifuge in plastic tubes, separated into plastic tubes, and stored by freezing until assayed.

4) The normal range for plasma ACTH concentrations is approximately 10 to 90 pg/mL.

5) The range in dogs with PDH is 40 to 600 pg/mL.

6) Dogs with ADH have ranges that are usually less than 20 pg/mL.

C. Combined dexamethasone suppression ACTH stimulation test

1) Designed to simultaneously diagnose hyperadrenocorticism and differentiate PDH from ADH

2) Procedure

a) Obtain a baseline cortisol sample.

b) Administer 0.1 mg/kg of dexamethasone IV.

c) Obtain a postdexamethasone sample two to four hours later.

d) ACTH is administered either as ACTH gel (IM) or cosyntropin (IV), as in a standard ACTH stimulation test.

e) A post-ACTH sample is taken one to two hours later.

3) The advantages of this test include ease of use, as only three blood samples are needed over a 3- to 6-hour period.

4) The disadvantages include a lower sensitivity for diagnosis of hyperadrenocorticism than either the ACTH stimulation test or low-dose dexamethasone suppression test. Additionally, the combined test (for which samples are obtained two to four hours postdexamethasone) is less discriminatory between PDH and ADH than the high-dose dexamethasone suppression test (which requires sampling of blood six to eight hours postdexamethasone administration). Dexamethasone may enhance or inhibit the adrenal response to exogenous ACTH, depending on the time interval between administration of the two agents.

D. Corticotropin releasing hormone (CRH) stimulation test

1) CRH is the hypothalamic polypeptide that modulates pituitary release of ACTH.

2) Procedure

a) 1.0 μg/kg of ovine CRH is administered IV.

b) Plasma samples are obtained for cortisol assay at 5, 15, 30, 60, 90, and 120 minutes postinjection.

3) Normal dogs respond with prompt increases in plasma cortisol concentration, peaking at 30 minutes.

4) Dogs with PDH respond with a doubling of plasma cortisol at 15 minutes postinjection.

5) Dogs with ADH show no increase in cortisol.

6) The advantages of the test include apparently good discrimination between PDH and ADH, and a relatively short test duration.

7) Among the disadvantages are the difficulty of obtaining CRH and its expense.

Cats

1. Cortisol assay

A. Plasma cortisol may be assayed by radioimmunoassay validated for this species. Be certain the laboratory employed has a validated assay.

B. Other methods of assay are not often employed clinically.

C. Normal resting cortisol concentrations in healthy cats ranges from less than 1 μg/dL to 8 μg/dL, and varies among laboratories. Refer to your laboratory's normal reference range.

D. There is no obvious circadian rhythm or detectable effect of different photoperiods on resting plasma cortisol concentrations.

2. Test to diagnose hyperadrenocorticism

A. ACTH stimulation test using ACTH gel

1) Collect baseline sample for cortisol assay.

2) Administer 2.2 U/kg of ACTH gel IM.

3) Collect blood samples at 90 to 120 minutes after administration.

4) Interpretation

a) There is considerable variation in response among cats

b) Normal cats respond with a peak increase in plasma cortisol to 4 to 18 μg/dL at 90 to 120 minutes.

c) Cats with diabetes, hyperthyroidism, or stressful illnesses do not appear to hyperstimulate consistently; however, results from some cats with these disorders may lie within the hyperadrenocorticism range.

d) Cats with spontaneous hyperadrenocorticism respond with increases well above the normal range.

B. ACTH stimulation test using synthetic ACTH

1) Collect a baseline sample for cortisol assay.

2) Administer 0.125 mg (1/2 vial) of cosyntropin (Cortrosyn) IV.

3) Peak cortisol responses occur earlier with this preparation as compared to ACTH gel; therefore, collect blood samples at 60 to 90 minutes after administration.

4) Interpretation

a) Similar to ACTH gel stimulation. Poststimulation cortisol concentrations are similar for the two tests in normal and stressed cats and, presumably, in cats with hyperadrenocorticism as well.

C. Dexamethasone suppression test

1) Not well standardized for cats

2) The low dose used for dogs (0.01 to 0.015 mg/kg) results in inconsistent suppression of plasma cortisol concentrations and may not be as useful in the cat.

3) The dose of 0.1 mg/kg of dexamethasone sodium phosphate provides more consistent suppression of plasma cortisol to low or undetectable concentrations. Significant suppression (<2 μg/dL) occurs by two hours, and maximal suppression is noted two to eight hours postinjection. Nonadrenal illness, such as diabetes, may cause a significant variation in response.

4) Procedure

a) Collect a baseline sample.

b) Administer 0.1 mg/kg of dexamethasone sodium phosphate IV.

c) Collect additional samples two to eight hours postinjection.

5) Interpretation

a) Significant suppression within two hours occurs in more than 90% of normal cats.

b) Most cats with spontaneous

hyperadrenocorticism fail to suppress to less than 50% of the baseline value.

  3. Test to differentiate ADH from PDH

  A. High-dose dexamethasone suppression

  1) The theory and principles for this test are the same for cats as in dogs.

  2) Procedure

  a) Same as low-dose test, except a dosage of 1.0 mg/kg of dexamethasone sodium phosphate is used.

  3) Interpretation

  a) All normal cats respond with cortisol suppression.

  b) Too few cats with hyperadrenocorticism have been evaluated to make firm statements concerning their response. Most cats with PDH suppress, whereas most cats with ADH fail to suppress.

  B. Endogenous ACTH assay

  1) The principles and procedure are the same for cats as for dogs.

  2) The normal range in cats is approximately 20 to 60 pg/mL.

  3) Cats with hyperthyroidism may have significantly elevated endogenous ACTH concentrations (approximately 200 ± 100 pg/mL).

  4) Cats with PDH have high concentrations, whereas cats with ADH have very low concentrations.

Treatment

Treatment of spontaneous hyperadrenocorticism is warranted because of the high frequency of complications of the disease and the likelihood of disease progression and death. Treatment modalities for PDH and ADH are quite different, emphasizing the need for accurate diagnosis.

Pituitary-dependent Hyperadrenocorticism in Dogs

  1. Surgery

  A. PDH may be managed either by bilateral adrenalectomy or hypophysectomy. Either method requires a skilled surgeon and intensive presurgical and postsurgical monitoring and care.

  B. Among the advantages of surgical therapy is the potential for permanent control of hyperadrenocorticism.

  C. The disadvantages include the high degree of skill required, the invasiveness of the procedure, a high likelihood of perioperative complications, and the necessity of lifelong hormone administration following either type of surgery.

  2. Drug therapy directed at the hypothalamic-pituitary axis

  A. Cyproheptadine (Periactin)

  1) A serotonin antagonist

  2) The rationale for its use is based on the fact that serotonin is a stimulus for hypothalamic release of CRF which, in turn, stimulates production and release of ACTH by the pars distalis.

  3) The dosage is 0.3 to 1.0 mg/kg/d, divided into three doses.

  4) Some success in the control of signs has been achieved in a small number of dogs.

  B. Bromocriptine (Parlodel)

  1) A dopamine agonist

  2) The rationale for its use is that hypothalamic dopamine appears to inhibit CRF release and ACTH formation in the pars distalis; it also inhibits ACTH release by the pars intermedia.

  3) The dosage is 24 to 50 μg/kg orally every 12 hours.

  4) Major drawbacks include apparently low efficacy and the development of severe side effects, including anorexia, vomiting, depression, and behavioral changes.

  3. Drug therapy directed at the adrenal glands

  A. Mitotane (o,p′-DDD, Lysodren)

  1) An isomer of the insecticide DDD

  2) Oral administration results in rather selective necrosis of the adrenocortical zona fasciculata and zona reticularis. Corticosteroid production in these regions rapidly declines. The zona glomerulosa, the site of aldosterone synthesis, is relatively resistant to the toxic effect of mitotane.

  3) Induction therapy: Initial dosage

is 30 to 50 mg/kg daily, divided into two doses, for 10 days.

a) In diabetic animals with insulin resistance, a lower dose of 20 to 25 mg/kg/d should help prevent a rapid reduction in plasma cortisol levels and corresponding difficulty in regulating insulin therapy.

4) The most common side effects of induction therapy include anorexia, lethargy, vomiting, and diarrhea. A small daily dose of oral prednisolone or prednisone (0.2 mg/kg) or cortisone (1.0 mg/kg) helps alleviate most of the problems associated with a rapid reduction in plasma cortisol levels. For diabetics, it may be beneficial to use twice the dose of oral glucocorticoids.

5) If significant adverse signs occur, induction therapy should be interrupted, and twice the daily dose of glucocorticoids should be administered, after which the dog should be reevaluated. Adverse effects from a rapid decline in plasma cortisol levels should be ameliorated within a few hours of administration of an oral dose of glucocorticoids.

6) Induction therapy is continued for 10 days. This phase of therapy can often be done at home, with outpatient reevaluations performed as needed. Daily water intake may be observed as a means of monitoring response to therapy.

a) Daily water intake is reduced significantly as circulating cortisol concentration is reduced. Prior to therapy, establish the animal's baseline 24-hour water consumption. Measure water consumption daily and discontinue induction therapy once there is a significant reduction in water intake.

7) After 10 days, or after noting a significant decline in daily water consumption, repeat the ACTH stimulation test. Discontinue oral glucocorticoids for at least 24 hours prior to testing.

a) Withhold further mitotane until cortisol results are available.

b) Both prestimulation and post-stimulation cortisol concentrations should be within the normal resting range—that is, the adrenal glands should be rendered unresponsive to ACTH.

8) If the results of the ACTH stimulation test suggest adequate control, proceed to maintenance therapy. If the adrenal glands are still capable of responding to ACTH, induction therapy should be resumed and the ACTH stimulation test should be repeated every 5 to 10 days until control is achieved. Although most dogs are under control by 10 to 15 days, a small number may require over a month of induction therapy.

9) Maintenance therapy begins immediately following successful induction. During this time, mitotane is administered at the rate of 50 mg/kg every seven days, divided into two to three doses over a single day. If mild side effects are encountered on treatment days, a small dose of oral glucocorticoid may be administered on that day.

10) Side effects of chronic maintenance therapy

a) Mild signs of cortisol deficiency occur in some dogs, and may include lethargy, partial anorexia, weakness, vomiting, and diarrhea. Maintenance therapy of the drug should be discontinued and glucocorticoid supplementation should begin. If the dog does not improve within a few hours of glucocorticoid supplementation, it should be evaluated for the possibility of acquired disease. Most dogs can resume maintenance therapy within two to six weeks.

b) A small number of dogs develop severe adrenocortical necrosis that includes the zona glomerulosa, causing aldosterone deficiency and classic signs of Addison's disease. In these dogs, maintenance therapy is discontinued and therapy for hypoadrenocorticism is begun (see the following section on hypoadrenocorticism). These dogs usually have permanent adrenal damage and do not require mitotane therapy again. Many will require lifelong therapy for hypoadrenocorticism.

c) Pituitary microadenomas or macroadenomas develop in some dogs receiving chronic mitotane therapy, and may result in neurologic signs resembling Nelson's syndrome in humans. One theory is that chronic hypersecretion of ACTH is enhanced by the loss of inhibition from hypercortisolism, and this stimulates (and possibly even initiates) growth of these tumors. Clinical signs may include stupor, head pressing, inability to maintain body temperature, behavioral changes, pacing, weakness, seizures, and primary adipsia.

11) Dogs receiving chronic maintenance therapy generally respond with resolution of clinical signs of Cushing's syndrome within four to six months. Dogs with diabetes mellitus will usually require continued insulin therapy for life; however, the insulin dose required for control is usually lower, and hyperglycemia is more easily managed. Rarely, a diabetic will have enough β cell reserve to allow discontinuation of insulin therapy following successful control of hyperadrenocorticism.

12) About 50% of the dogs that successfully undergo induction and initial maintenance therapy suffer a relapse of signs within the first 12 months of therapy. ACTH stimulation testing should be repeated every three to six months to monitor control of the disease. If the dog develops an adrenocortical response to ACTH, induction therapy should be resumed for 5 to 10 days, followed by a higher weekly maintenance dose (75 mg/kg weekly). Some dogs may require a dosage as high as 100 to 300 mg/kg weekly to achieve successful long-term control.

B. Ketoconazole

1) Interferes with adrenocortical corticosteroid production. Because of this property, the drug has been used in a small number of dogs with hyperadrenocorticism and has shown promising results.

2) The dosage is 15 mg/kg twice daily.

3) Most dogs treated thus far have responded with remission of clinical signs within 2 to 11 months. Side effects include vomiting, but appear to be minimal. There does not appear to be a compensatory increase in pituitary ACTH production in treated dogs whose clinical signs are controlled.

4) The disadvantages of this mode of therapy include its high expense for large dogs. Only a small number of dogs have been treated thus far, making long-term comparisons with mitotane difficult at this time.

Pituitary-dependent Hyperadrenocorticism in Cats

1. Medical management

A. Mitotane therapy is infrequently used in cats because of their sensitivity to chlorinated hydrocarbons. However, a daily dosage of 25 mg/kg for 25 days, with repeated ACTH stimulation testing during the induction period, has been used in some cats.

B. Ketoconazole appears to be ineffective in cats, and may be hepatotoxic.

C. Metapyrone inhibits conversion of 11-desoxycortisol to cortisol, and has been tried in some cats at a dose of 200 to 250 mg/d. This treatment has been associated with minimal side effects, but only slight clinical improvement in the small number of cats so treated thus far.

2. Surgical management

A. Bilateral adrenalectomy via midline celiotomy is currently the most successful therapy for PDH in the cat. As in the dog, this treatment requires a skilled surgeon and intensive perioperative care.

Adrenal-dependent Hyperadrenocorticism in Dogs

1. Surgical treatment

A. The treatment of choice when possible

B. Midline celiotomy is often the approach of choice, as this allows inspection of both adrenal glands and exploration for evidence of metastases.

C. Because the contralateral adrenal gland is atrophied, plasma cortisol concentrations will be dramatically reduced following removal of a functional adrenal tumor. Therefore, high doses of glucocorticoids (dexamethasone sodium phosphate, 0.1 to 0.2 mg/kg or prednisolone sodium succinate, 1.0 to 2.0 mg/kg) are administered IV immediately prior to surgery. High doses (three to five times the maintenance dose) of glucocorticoids are continued, and are gradually tapered over a period of 7 to 10 days. Maintenance doses of glucocorticoids are continued for one to three months postoperatively and are gradually discontinued as the remaining adrenal gland returns to normal function, as determined by ACTH stimulation testing.

2. Medical management

A. Indicated when the owner refuses surgery or when metastases from an adrenocortical carcinoma are identified.

1) Mitotane therapy has limited success in affected dogs. It is administered at a daily dose of 50 to 150 mg/kg. ACTH stimulation testing is performed at two-week intervals, and the dosage of mitotane is reduced once suppression of poststimulation cortisol concentrations is achieved. If successful control is achieved, daily maintenance therapy with oral glucocorticoids may be necessary.

2) Ketoconazole therapy, similar to that used for PDH, has controlled clinical signs in a small number of dogs with ADH. A dose of 15 mg/kg has resulted in control of signs by two to six months. It does not appear to affect tumor growth.

Adrenal-dependent Hyperadrenocorticism in Cats

Surgical treatment is the therapy of choice for cats. Surgical and perioperative care considerations are the same for cats as for dogs.

Prognosis

Without therapy, hyperadrenocorticism is generally a progressive disorder that results in death. Death is usually caused by complications associated with chronically elevated plasma cortisol concentrations, including diabetes, infection, hypertension, and thromboembolism. Death may occasionally result from progressive expansion of a pituitary adenoma, or from metastatic disease associated with adrenal carcinoma.

With therapy the prognosis is often more favorable. However, many affected dogs are older and may have concurrent illness. In some, particularly those with mild signs of hyperadrenocorticism, it may be advisable to forgo treatment in the face of severe concurrent illness, advanced age, or likely poor owner compliance.

Dogs and cats that undergo surgical treat-

ment for adrenal adenomas may achieve a permanent cure. The prognosis for adrenal carcinoma is often very poor, as many of these dogs have metastases present at the time of diagnosis and die within a few weeks to months. The prognosis for dogs with PDH that are managed with mitotane is considerably improved over that for untreated dogs, with an average survival of approximately 22 months. Some chronically treated dogs survive for six to seven years.

···

Hypoadrenocorticism

Adrenocortical insufficiency is characterized by inadequate secretion of corticosteroids by the adrenal cortex, either as a result of insufficient secretion of ACTH (secondary adrenal insufficiency), or because of partial or complete destruction of the adrenal glands (primary adrenal insufficiency).

Primary Adrenocortical Insufficiency (Addison's Disease)

Primary hypoadrenocorticism develops as a result of the loss of most functional adrenal cortical tissue, either because of destruction or replacement with abnormal tissue. Subtotal loss of the adrenal cortices causes partial adrenal insufficiency characterized by inadequate adrenal reserve that may manifest itself only during times of stress. Complete loss of the adrenal cortices causes a metabolic crisis, regardless of other stressors.

1. Most common causes

A. Idiopathic atrophy of the adrenal cortex is the most common form of the disorder. Destruction by an autoimmune process is suspected.

B. Bilateral destruction secondary to toxicity to o,p'-DDD (Lysodren) during therapy for hyperadrenocorticism.

2. Rare causes

A. Inflammatory disease with infiltration and replacement by granulomatous tissue
   1) Histoplasmosis
   2) Blastomycosis
   3) Tuberculosis
B. Metastatic neoplasia
C. Infarction secondary to disseminated intravascular coagulation
D. Hemorrhagic necrosis secondary to sepsis
E. Bilateral adrenalectomy

Secondary Adrenocortical Insufficiency

Secondary hypoadrenocorticism develops when reduced secretion of ACTH by the pituitary results in atrophy of the zona fasciculata and reticularis, resulting in impaired ability to secrete glucocorticoids.

   1. Causes
   A. Treatment with pharmacologic doses of glucocorticoids is the most common cause, occurring most often during chronic administration of potent glucocorticoids (e.g., dexamethasone) or repeated use of long-acting forms of glucocorticoids.
   B. Destructive lesions of the pituitary gland or hypothalamus
      1) Neoplasia
      2) Inflammation
      3) Trauma

Pathogenesis

   1. Aldosterone acts primarily on the renal cortical collecting tubules to increase reabsorption of sodium and chloride and to increase secretion of hydrogen ion and potassium.
   A. Aldosterone deficiency results in:
      1) Excessive renal loss of sodium and chloride with subsequent hyponatremia
      2) Decreased extracellular fluid volume and hypovolemia secondary to decreased total body sodium content
         a) Reduced cardiac output reduces the renal glomerular filtration rate (GFR) and may result in prerenal azotemia.

         b) Reduced cardiac output promotes muscular weakness. Signs of circulatory shock appear when severe.
      3) Hyperkalemia secondary to reduced GFR and impaired distal tubular capacity to excrete potassium
      4) Normal anion gap metabolic acidosis secondary to impaired distal tubular renal excretion of H^+ ion
   2. Cortisol influences the function of many different tissues in the body. In the kidney, it plays primarily a permissive role—that is, a basal amount is required to maintain renal blood flow and GFR—but variations in cortisol secretion are not necessary for normal renal function.
   A. Glucocorticoid deficiency results in:
      1) Neurologic abnormalities
         a) Lethargy, depression
      2) Gastrointestinal signs
         a) Anorexia
         b) Vomiting, diarrhea, or both
            i. May aggravate water and electrolyte imbalances
         c) Colic
      3) Impaired gluconeogenesis resulting in fasting hypoglycemia
      4) Altered hemodynamics
         a) Reduced cardiac output
         b) Hypotension
            i. Hypotension stimulates ADH secretion; subsequent water retention aggravates hyponatremia.
         c) Reduced renal blood flow and GFR
      5) Muscular weakness
         a) Secondary to reduced cardiac output and hypoglycemia
      6) Hematologic abnormalities
         a) Lymphocytosis
         b) Eosinophilia

Signalment and History

Dogs

   1. Primary hypoadrenocorticism is an uncommon disorder in the dog. There is no apparent breed predisposition. Approximately 70% of affected dogs are female. The age at onset ranges from 10 weeks to 14 years; most dogs with idiopathic primary hypoadrenocorticism are middle-aged (four to eight years).

2. Abnormalities result from a deficiency of glucocorticoids, aldosterone, or both. In primary hypoaldosteronism, the history may be one of acute collapse, although more commonly, there is a history of intermittent (waxing and waning) signs. Signs may become apparent only after a precipitating stressor, and improvement may be seen after veterinary care with parenteral fluids or glucocorticoids. Historical signs may be quite vague, resembling those of gastrointestinal or renal diseases. In dogs with secondary adrenal insufficiency, there may be a history of prior glucocorticoid use or signs referable to a mass lesion in the pituitary region. Historical problems, listed in decreasing order of frequency, include:

  A. Lethargy/depression
  B. Gastrointestinal signs
   1) Decreased appetite
   2) Vomiting
   3) Diarrhea
  C. Muscular weakness
  D. Weight loss
  E. Trembling/shaking
  F. Polyuria/polydipsia

Cats

1. Primary hypoadrenocorticism is rare in cats.

2. All reported cats were neutered domestic shorthair (DSH). Their age at onset ranged from one to nine years, with an average age of five years.

3. Historical abnormalities include lethargy, anorexia, weight loss, weakness, vomiting, polyuria, and polydipsia.

Physical Examination

Dogs

Depression and weakness are, by far, the most common abnormalities noted on physical examination. Other abnormal physical findings, in order of decreasing frequency, include:

1. Dehydration
2. Bradycardia
3. Weak pulse
4. Hypothermia
5. Trembling/shaking
6. Sensitivity to abdominal palpation

Cats

The abnormal physical findings in cats, listed in decreasing order of frequency, include:

1. Depression
2. Weakness
3. Dehydration
4. Slow capillary refill time
5. Weak pulse

Routine Laboratory Evaluation

Dogs

1. Hemogram changes may be seen in both the primary and secondary form of the disease.

  A. Mild normochromic, normocytic, nonregenerative anemia is present in one third of cases. This may be masked initially by dehydration.

  B. Normal or elevated absolute lymphocyte and eosinophil counts are often noted. The presence of a normal lymphocyte or eosinophil count in a stressed or ill animal is inappropriate and suggests loss of the restraining effect of cortisol.

2. Serum biochemical abnormalities are generally seen only in primary hypoadrenocorticism.

  A. Electrolytes
   1) Hyponatremia
    a) Serum [Na$^+$] less than 140 mEq/L, attributable to enhanced renal and gastrointestinal losses
   2) Hyperkalemia
    a) Serum [K$^+$] greater than 6.0 mEq/L, attributable to diminished urine excretion and acidosis
   3) The ratio of sodium to potassium is less than or equal to 27:1.
    a) The normal ratio is 27–32:1.

b) A ratio of less than 24 : 1 is suggestive of primary hypoadrenocorticism and is more sensitive than the concentration of either electrolyte alone. However, a ratio of less than 24 : 1, by itself, is not diagnostic for hypoadrenocorticism. The diagnosis must be confirmed with more specific tests.

B. Azotemia

1) The increase in BUN may be greater than the increase in serum creatinine concentration, reflecting the fact that the azotemia is prerenal in nature.

C. Hypercalcemia

1) Seen in up to 25% of dogs with primary hypoadrenocorticism. The etiology is unclear.

2) In general, the severity of hypercalcemia parallels the severity of other electrolyte imbalances.

D. Hypoglycemia

1) Seen in only 5% to 10% of dogs with primary hypoadrenocorticism

2) Mild hyperglycemia is seen more often than hypoglycemia

E. Metabolic acidosis

1) Observed in 40% to 50% of dogs with primary hypoadrenocorticism

2) Acidosis is generally associated with a normal anion gap, and is caused by a failure of distal tubule secretion of H^+ (i.e., loss of $NaHCO_3^-$).

3) In dogs showing signs of circulatory shock, lactic acidosis may develop, causing an increase in the anion gap.

3. Urinalysis

A. The urinalysis may help distinguish prerenal azotemia from primary renal azotemia if the urine specific gravity is between 1.025 and 1.050. However, the urine specific gravity is frequently lower in dogs with primary hypoadrenocorticism. The reason for impaired maximal urine concentrating ability in these dogs is unclear.

4. Radiographic findings

A. Microcardia and decreased size of the intrathoracic veins are suggestive of hypovolemia.

5. Electrocardiogram

A. An ECG is a useful and rapid means of monitoring the physiologic effects of hyperkalemia and hyponatremia. Although there may be considerable variability between dogs, the ECG allows a reasonable estimation of the degree of hyperkalemia, and may be used to guide treatment prior to receiving laboratory confirmation of electrolyte abnormalities.

1) Serum $[K^+]$: 5.5 to 6.5 mEq/L

a) Increased amplitude of T waves, which may become thin and peaked

2) Serum $[K^+]$: 6.5 to 7.0 mEq/L

a) Prolongation of QRS and P–R intervals; decreased amplitude of R wave; S–T segment depression

3) Serum $[K^+]$: 7.0 to 8.5 mEq/L

a) Decreased amplitude of P wave with increased duration; longer QRS and P–R intervals; prolongation of Q–T interval

4) Serum $[K^+]$: 8.5 to 10.0 mEq/L

a) Disappearance of P waves; sinoventricular rhythm. Heart rate may be slow (<80 beats/min), particularly when interpreted relative to the degree of hypovolemia.

5) Serum $[K^+]$: >10.0 mEq/L

a) Increasing width of QRS until a smooth biphasic curve is seen; terminal ventricular flutter, fibrillation, or asystole

B. Hyponatremia alone can cause similar changes in the ECG; however, in dogs with Addison's disease, this is usually accompanied by hyperkalemia.

C. These ECG changes are not always reliable; some dogs with marked hyperkalemia may have minimal changes on their ECG. Since the ECG shows the physiologic effects of hyperkalemia on the heart, it may serve as an indicator of how severely the hyperkalemia is affecting that patient.

Cats

1. Cats with primary hypoadrenocorticism have similar laboratory abnormalities as dogs.

A. Hematology

1) Mild normocytic, normochromic, nonregenerative anemia

2) Relative or absolute lymphocytosis and/or eosinophilia

B. Serum biochemistry

1) Hyponatremia

2) Hypochloremia

3) Hyperkalemia

4) Azotemia

5) Hyperphosphatemia

C. Urinalysis
    1) Urine specific gravity lower than expected
D. Radiographs
    1) Microcardia
E. ECG
    1) May show changes similar to those associated with hyperkalemia in the dog

Differential Diagnosis

Dogs

1. Primary renal disease
2. Postrenal azotemia, uroabdomen
3. Primary gastrointestinal disease can produce hyponatremia, hyperkalemia, a low Na : K ratio, and similar clinical signs, including vomiting, diarrhea, weakness, lethargy, depression, dehydration, weak pulses, and abdominal sensitivity to palpation.
    A. Trichuriasis
    B. Salmonellosis
    C. Duodenal ulceration
4. Neuromuscular disease causing weakness
5. Other metabolic diseases—diabetes mellitus
6. Overuse of diuretics
7. Pseudohyperkalemia (in Akitas)

Cats

1. Cardiomyopathy
2. Urethral obstruction, uroabdomen
3. Primary renal disease
4. Others similar to dogs?

Diagnosis

Definitive diagnosis depends on documentation of reduced plasma cortisol concentrations or hyporesponsiveness to administered ACTH.

Dogs

1. Cortisol concentration is usually measured, instead of aldosterone, because of its greater availability and lesser expense.

2. The ACTH stimulation test generally yields more information than a single resting plasma cortisol concentration measurement.
    A. The procedure for the ACTH stimulation test is similar to that used to identify hyperadrenocorticism.
        1) Draw a plasma sample at the beginning of the test (baseline sample) for cortisol determination.
        2) Administer 0.25 mg of synthetic ACTH (cosyntropin, Cortrosyn) IV or IM or 2.2 U/kg (maximum of 40 U) of ACTH gel IM.
        3) Withdraw a second blood sample at one hour (if IV cosyntropin was used) or two hours (if ACTH gel was administered).
        4) Follow the recommendations of your laboratory if they differ from those listed here.
    B. It is advisable to avoid administering any exogenous glucocorticoid preparation within two days of performing this test (longer if repository forms are used). Dexamethasone does not cross-react in any assay, however, and may be given immediately prior to, or during, the ACTH stimulation test.
    C. Normal dogs have a resting (0 hour) plasma cortisol concentration of 0 to 10 μg/dL (depending on which assay is used), and stimulate to a range of 6 to 16 μg/dL (a twofold to threefold increase over the resting value).
    D. Dogs stressed with nonadrenal illness may have mild to moderate elevations of resting plasma cortisol concentrations and may exhibit an exaggerated response to stimulation (8 to 40 μg/dL).
    E. Dogs with primary hypoadrenocorticism have low resting plasma cortisol concentrations and show no response to ACTH.
    F. Dogs with secondary hypoadrenocorticism resulting from hypopituitarism may have low to normal resting values and demonstrate a slight to normal response to administered ACTH, depending on the degree of adrenocortical atrophy present.
3. Plasma ACTH concentration
    A. Endogenous ACTH concentrations are helpful in distinguishing hypothalamic-pituitary disorder from primary adrenocortical deficiency once a diagnosis of hypoadrenocorticism is established. This is particularly

true in cases in which serum electrolyte values are normal.

B. This test is not widely available and is expensive. Consult a veterinary endocrinology laboratory that performs this assay for specific instructions before performing this test.

C. Samples must be collected in cold, heparinized, plastic syringes; spun immediately in a refrigerated centrifuge in plastic tubes; separated into plastic tubes; and stored by freezing until assayed.

D. Plasma concentration varies greatly during a 24-hour period owing to an episodic secretion pattern, as well as dynamic responses to stress. The normal canine range is 10 to 90 pg/mL.

E. Plasma concentrations of ACTH are low in animals with secondary hypoadrenocorticism (0 to 20 pg/mL) and high in those with primary hypoadrenocorticism (500 to 3700 pg/mL).

4. Modified Thorn test

A. The modified Thorn test is a crude but rapid screening test for hypoadrenocorticism.

B. Based on changes in lymphocyte and eosinophil counts in response to elevations in plasma cortisol levels

C. Perform a baseline CBC.

D. Administer 0.25 mg of cosyntropin IV. Perform a CBC four hours after administration.

E. In normal dogs, the neutrophil/lymphocyte (N:L) ratio increases, whereas absolute eosinophil counts decrease.

F. Dogs with hypoadrenocorticism do not show increased N:L ratios and show only mild reductions in the number of eosinophils.

G. Dogs that fail both to increase N:L ratios by at least 30% and to decrease the number of eosinophils by at least 50% should be assumed to have hypoadrenocorticism until results of plasma cortisol assays become available.

Cats

1. The small number of reported cases in cats makes absolute guidelines difficult to establish.

2. ACTH stimulation test

A. Refer to the previous section on Hyperadrenocorticism.

B. The average poststimulation plasma cortisol concentration in cats with hypoadrenocorticism is 0.5 ± 0.2 μg/dL.

3. Plasma ACTH determination

A. The theory and principles underlying this test in cats are identical to those in dogs.

B. Plasma ACTH concentrations in cats with spontaneous hypoadrenocorticism are usually high (1460 to 8000 pg/mL; normal: 5 to 125 pg/mL), consistent with primary hypoadrenocorticism.

Treatment of the Acute Crisis

Dogs

1. Hypovolemia

A. IV infusion of 0.9% NaCl

1) Infuse NaCl through a large-gauge IV catheter or, if venous access is difficult, through a large bone marrow aspiration needle placed in the proximal diaphyseal marrow of the femur.

2) Treat with large volumes for shock, if present (40 to 90 mL/kg/h) until adequate intravascular volume is achieved.

3) Consider monitoring central venous pressure and urine production.

2. Electrolyte balance

A. Lowering serum K^+ concentration

1) Saline infusion and mineralocorticoid therapy are often all the therapy that is required to correct hyperkalemia.

2) $NaHCO_3$ therapy may be initiated to drive K^+ intracellularly.

a) Empirical dose: 1 to 2 mEq/kg IV over a period of 15 minutes

b) Alternatively, the same dose as that used for treating acidosis may be administered

3) Dextrose and insulin infusion

a) Glucose added to IV saline infusion: 0.5 to 1.0 g/kg over a period of 30 to 60 minutes

b) Alternatively, IV regular crystalline insulin (0.5 IU/kg) may be administered with 2 g of glucose per unit of insulin over 30 to 60 minutes.

    c) Monitor blood glucose concentration. Administer glucocorticoid therapy before giving insulin to assist gluconeogenesis.

    4) Calcium gluconate

    a) Calcium directly antagonizes the effects of hyperkalemia at the cell membrane. It will not reduce the plasma concentration of potassium. It is given IV only in animals with hyperkalemic crisis in which cardiotoxicity is severe. Dilute 10% solution in 5% dextrose solution and administer 0.5 mL/kg IV (of the 10% solution) slowly (over 10 to 20 minutes) while monitoring an ECG. This treatment may be contraindicated in the presence of known existing hypercalcemia.

    B. Raising serum sodium concentration

    1) Use only IV solutions that contain physiologic concentrations of sodium and no (or small amounts of) potassium, such as 0.9% sodium chloride or lactated Ringer's solution.

    C. Hypercalcemia

    1) Animals with hypercalcemia generally respond rapidly to saline infusion and glucocorticoid replacement therapy. Glucocorticoids promote urinary calcium excretion, impair intestinal calcium absorption, and impair release of calcium from bone.

    3. Acidosis

    A. Treatment is only necessary if acidosis is moderate to severe.

    B. Ideally, the decision to treat should rest on clinical evaluation along with laboratory evaluation of acid–base balance. Serum total carbon dioxide (TCO_2) concentration is the most widely available measurement of bicarbonate.

    1) Dogs with venous TCO_2 concentrations of less than 10 mEq/L should probably be treated. Estimate the required dose of $NaHCO_3$ according to the following formula:

$$\text{mEq of } NaHCO_3 \text{ needed} = (\text{body weight in kg}) \times 0.4 \times (22 - \text{patient's } TCO_2)$$

Administer 25% to 50% of this estimate over the first six hours and reevaluate. If treating for hyperkalemia, this amount may be given over a period of 15 minutes to one hour.

    4. Hormone deficiency

    A. Glucocorticoids

    1) Initial doses should be high enough to at least approximate normal cortisol production during times of severe stress. It is probably better to overdose initially with glucocorticoids than to undertreat.

    a) Dexamethasone sodium phosphate: 0.5 to 1.0 mg/kg IV. A solution of 4 mg/mL of dexamethasone sodium phosphate contains 3.3 mg of dexamethasone base per milliliter. It will not interfere with plasma cortisol determinations.

    b) Prednisolone sodium succinate: 2 to 10 mg/kg IV

    c) Hydrocortisone sodium succinate: 1 to 10 mg/kg IV

    2) These doses may be repeateed in two to six hours if needed.

    3) As the dog improves, reduce the dosage to maintenance levels of prednisolone (0.2 mg/kg/d) or hydrocortisone (1 mg/kg/d) over a period of three to five days. Continue parenteral administration until the dog tolerates oral medications.

    B. Mineralocorticoids

    1) Desoxycorticosterone acetate (DOCA) in oil: 0.2 to 0.4 mg/kg IM every 24 hours. Do not exceed a 5-mg total daily dose. This drug is currently available.

    2) As soon as the patient tolerates oral medications, fludrocortisone (Florinef) may be administered at the same dosage used for maintenance therapy.

    5. Continue therapy until laboratory abnormalities normalize and the dog begins to eat and drink without vomiting. At this point, change the regimen to maintenance therapy.

Cats

    1. Treat similarly to dogs.

    A. The dosage of DOCA for cats is 0.5 to 1.0 mg once daily.

    2. The initial response to therapy is apparently much slower in cats than it is in dogs. Cats often require three to five days of treatment before they show signs of improvement.

Maintenance Therapy for Chronic Adrenocortical Insufficiency

1. Mineralocorticoid replacement therapy
   A. Fludrocortisone (Florinef)
   1) 0.1-mg tablets dosed at 0.1 mg/5 kg orally, divided twice daily for dogs, and 0.1 mg once daily for cats
   2) Monitor serum electrolyte levels frequently to gauge initial response.
   3) This drug has some glucocorticoid activity, so there is usually no need to supplement with glucocorticoids.
   B. DOCA pellets
   1) A surgically implanted, slow-release pellet form of DOCA
   2) Initial dosage is one pellet for every 0.5 mg of daily DOCA that was required for initial maintenance. If DOCA injection is used, it may be difficult to establish a safe and effective dose for a patient.
   3) Each pellet lasts approximately six to eight months.
   4) The advantages of this drug form include improved owner compliance and the ability to deliver the drug during periods of anorexia or vomiting when the animal may not tolerate oral medications.
   5) The disadvantages of DOCA pellets include wide variations in patient response, the necessity of surgical implantation, the risk of infection at the implantation site, and the long time required for correction of dosage owing to the slow release of the drug.
   C. Desoxycorticosterone pivalate (DOCP) injection
   1) A suspension delivered by deep IM injection
   2) Dosage: 25 mg for every 1 mg of DOCA needed initially to maintain normal serum electrolyte concentrations
   3) The dosage range is generally 12.5 to 100 mg once a month for dogs, and 10 to 12.5 mg once a month for cats.
   4) The drug's advantages are the same as those for DOCA pellets.

5) The disadvantages include the long periods required for correction of the dosage owing to the slow release of the drug, and the necessity of monthly office visits. DOCP injection is available only directly from the manufacturer (Ciba-Geigy Animal Health).
2. Glucocorticoid supplementation
   A. Most animals that are treated with fludrocortisone do not require additional glucocorticoid supplementation.
   B. Some animals receiving DOCA appear to benefit from physiologic doses of glucocorticoid.
   C. Administer prednisolone or prednisone (0.2 mg/kg) or cortisone (1.0 mg/kg) every morning.
   D. Dogs with secondary hypoadrenocorticism generally require only glucocorticoid supplementation, without supplemental mineralocorticoid. If secondary hypoadrenocorticism is attributable to chronic administration of glucocorticoids, the animal may be able to be weaned off of the drug over a period of one to six months.
   E. Owners may need to increase the dose of glucocorticoids during times of illness or stress.
3. Salt supplementation
   A. Dietary supplementation with 0.5 to 5 g of NaCl per day will often reduce the requirement for mineralocorticoid supplementation, particularly when large doses of fludrocortisone are required for control.

Follow-up

1. The first follow-up visit should be one week after discharge.
   A. Perform a physical examination, as well as electrolyte and creatinine determinations.
   B. Adjust the dose of fludrocortisone upward, if necessary, based on serum electrolyte concentrations.
2. The second follow-up visit should be scheduled one month after discharge.

A. Increase the dose of fludrocortisone if necessary; consider decreasing it if electrolyte levels are normal or if there is a tendency for hypokalemia or hypernatremia.

3. Reevaluate the animal's status every four to six months thereafter.

Prognosis

The prognosis for dogs and cats with idiopathic primary hypoadrenocorticism is excellent with administration of proper corticosteroid therapy. Patients with adrenal or pituitary destruction secondary to tumor, infection, or vascular disease are often very ill at the time of diagnosis and have a poor prognosis. Patients with secondary hypoadrenocorticism caused by chronic glucocorticoid administration have an excellent prognosis for recovery of adrenal function once the medication is carefully withdrawn.

Suggested Readings

Hyperadrenocorticism

Feldman EC, Nelson RW: Hyperadrenocorticism. In Feldman EC, Nelson RW (eds): Canine and Feline Endocrinology and Reproduction. Philadelphia, WB Saunders, 1987

Peterson ME: Canine hyperadrenocorticism. In Kirk RW (ed): Current Veterinary Therapy IX. Philadelphia, WB Saunders, 1986

Hypoadrenocorticism

Feldman EC, Nelson RW: Hypoadrenocorticism. In Feldman EC, Nelson RW (eds): Canine and Feline Endocrinology and Reproduction. Philadelphia, WB Saunders, 1987

Schrader LA: Hypoadrenocorticism. In Kirk RW (ed): Current Veterinary Therapy IX. Philadelphia, WB Saunders, 1986

CHAPTER FIFTEEN

Dermatologic Disorders

Patricia D. White and Kenneth W. Kwochka

Dermatologic Disorders

The skin is the largest organ of the body. In addition to being affected by specific cutaneous disorders, the skin can serve as a "mirror" reflecting the functional integrity of internal organ systems. Dermatologic disorders often constitute up to 50% of patient presentations and owner complaints.

Advances in diagnostics and therapeutics have resulted in a change in focus from treating cutaneous diseases symptomatically to discovering the etiopathogenesis of disease syndromes. When a specific diagnosis has been made, appropriate treatment protocols can be employed. A systematic approach that can be routinely employed provides the best opportunity for a successful diagnosis and prevents misdiagnosis of the common skin problem that may present with unusual clinical symptoms.

There are five broad categories of cutaneous diseases that have both prominent clinical features and represent owners' primary complaints:

Hair loss (alopecia or hypotrichosis)
Pruritus (excessive licking, biting, chewing, or scratching)
Blistering and ulceration
Scaling and crusting
Skin masses

Of course, there are overlaps between these presentations. How can you, as the clinician, untangle and organize clinical information regarding an animal that has a long, complex course and questionable therapeutic response? The following discussion provides an outline of routine diagnostic techniques. Then, each of the broad categories just described is addressed, with special attention to specific diagnostics and therapeutics.

This chapter is not intended to provide comprehensive information about specific dermatologic diseases, but rather is designed to provide a quick, logical, and systematic approach to diagnosing and treating dermatologic disorders. Although therapeutic trials are often as diagnostic as specific laboratory tests, they should only be employed after logical and systematic evaluation of the presented information.

Clinical Approach

History

A complete history will yield approximately 70% of the information needed to make a diagnosis.

1. Age of animal at onset of problem
   A. Very young (younger than 18 months)—Likely diagnoses include demodicosis, dermatophytosis, food allergy, canine scabies, notoedric mange, food allergy, and flea bite dermatitis.

B. Young adult (one to six years)—Likely conditions include allergies (atopy, food allergy, flea allergic dermatitis).

C. Mature adult (older than six years)—Likely diagnoses include endocrine dermatosis, autoimmune diseases, and neoplasia.

2. Seasonality

A. In what season does the problem present and is there a pattern?

B. Nonseasonal?—Possible entities include parasitism, food allergy, infections, psychogenic, autoimmune, or endocrine disorders.

C. Did it start as a seasonal problem and stay seasonal, or progress to a year-round problem (e.g., flea allergy, atopy)?

3. Diet

A. Brand and type of dog food (canned versus semi-moist versus dry); types of table scraps and treats

B. Changes in dog food (Has the diet been fed long enough for sensitization to occur?)

4. Distribution pattern (where on the body did the problem start and how did it spread?)

A. Focal (localized demodicosis; dermatophytosis; chin acne), multifocal (pyoderma; dermatophytosis; pemphigus foliaceus) or diffuse (generalized demodicosis or pyoderma)

B. Regional (atopy; black hair follicle dysplasia)

C. Symmetric (endocrine) or asymmetric

5. Determine whether the problem was initially one of only pruritus without a dermatitis (allergies), or whether lesions were seen first, with pruritus developing as the dermatitis progressed (pyoderma, autoimmune disorders).

6. Inquire about items in the environment (bedding, plastic bowl) which may indicate contact dermatitis. Indoor (carpeting, cleaning products) versus outdoor (parasites, vegetation, fertilizers) environments may offer diagnostic clues.

7. Question owners about previous therapy and response. Home remedies and prescriptions are of equal importance.

8. Question the owner carefully about previous response to corticosteroids and antibiotics. Have antibiotics ever been given *without* steroids, and if so, what was the response (allergy versus pyoderma as cause of pruritus)?

9. Are other animals or family members affected? (If so, consider infectious and parasitic causes such as dermatophytes or scabies.)

10. Are there concurrent signs of systemic disease (vomiting, diarrhea, polyuria (PU), polydipsia (PD), polyphagia)? Consider metabolic (hepatic, pancreatic), endocrine (thyroid, adrenal), or neoplastic causes.

11. Question the owner carefully about previous medical or surgical problems including congenital abnormalities.

A. Cryptorchid—Consider Sertoli cell tumor with feminization and hyperpigmentation.

B. Females—Consider estrogen excess or deficiency.

12. Reproductive-history (decreased libido, aspermia, failure to cycle or conceive)—Consider endocrine abnormalities.

Physical Examination

1. Perform a *complete* general physical examination before evaluating the integument. Major clues to the diagnosis may lie in the results of this examination.

2. Evaluate the integument with regard to the:

A. Presence or absence of symmetry of lesions (e.g., a bilateral presentation involving the trunk may indicate an endocrine disorder)

B. Distribution pattern (e.g., a caudal dorsum pattern may suggest flea allergy dermatitis)

C. Configuration of lesions (linear, annular, serpiginous, etc.)

3. Upon closer inspection, determine whether the predominant skin lesions are papules, pustules, or nodules reflecting a primary disease process, or crusts, scales, or excoriations that may have occurred as a result of maturation of primary lesions or self-inflicted trauma.

4. Remember that the skin is often just an innocent bystander, and that the major problem may be attributable to problems deeper than the skin.

Diagnostic Tests

1. Skin scraping

A. An easy, quick, inexpensive procedure used to diagnose cutaneous parasitic infestations (demodicosis, cheyletiellosis, and sarcoptiform mite infestations), as well as dermatophyte infections

B. It should be performed on *every* case.

C. Equipment needed: No. 10 scalpel blade, heavy mineral oil, microscope glass slides and coverslips, and a microscope.

D. Scrape a *minimum* of three sites.

E. Choose the periphery of a typical, unexcoriated lesion for scraping, as most parasites, such as *Sarcoptes* and *Cheyletiella*, move away from sites of inflammation and excoriation. Careful trimming of the hair around the chosen site with scissors may facilitate scraping.

F. Place a drop of mineral oil on the skin and glass slide. Squeeze the chosen site before scraping.

G. Hold the blade perpendicular to the skin. For deep scrapings (*Demodex*), excoriate deeply enough to cause *mild* capillary bleeding. Superficial scrapings (*Sarcoptes, Cheyletiella*, etc.) require that only the superficial layers of the epidermis be removed.

H. Transfer the material (epidermal debris and mineral oil) to the glass slide using your blade as a spatula. Add a coverslip and examine under low (×10) microscopic power.

I. Rule of thumb—Scrape a wide area (superficial), and multiple sites if you suspect scabies; scrape to the level of the follicle (deep) if demodicosis is suspected.

2. Wood's light

A. A UV light source used on a suspicious lesion in a darkened room to screen for some dermatophytes

B. Positive fluorescence is characterized by a bright apple-green color associated with hair shafts

C. Only *Microsporum canis, M. audouini,* and *M. distortum* fluoresce. *M. canis* is the only significant veterinary pathogen that fluoresces.

D. *M. canis* fluoresces only 50% of the time. Positive fluorescence provides a quick

diagnosis, whereas negative fluorescence is inconclusive.

E. False-positive results are common (i.e., dirt and dust may impart a bluish-white fluorescence; scale, crust, or medication may yield a pale yellow fluorescence).

F. Suspicious areas should be sampled for potassium hydroxide (KOH) preparation and fungal culture.

3. KOH Preparation

A. Samples are obtained via skin scrapings without mineral oil or by *gently* plucking a few hairs with hemostats. Ideally, areas exhibiting positive or suspicious fluorescence are sampled.

B. A small amount of the hair and epidermal debris is placed on a glass slide with two to three drops of 10% KOH. Allow the sample to clear for 20 to 30 minutes at room temperature, or heat with the light from the microscope for 10 minutes.

C. An alternative clearing agent is chlorphenolac (equal parts of liquefied chloral hydrate, phenol, and lactic acid). It is used in the same manner as KOH, but requires only 5 to 10 minutes to clear.

D. Scan slide under low power (×10) for abnormal hair, then examine under high dry (×40) for ectothrix spores along hair shafts and hyphae in epidermal debris.

E. Requires practice for consistent results

F. Negative findings do not rule out dermatophytosis.

4. Fungal culture is the best method for diagnosing a dermatophyte infection.

A. Confirmation of fungal infection is mandatory before instituting a long course of systemic antifungal therapy. This diagnosis should be ruled out prior to instituting corticosteroid therapy for pruritic dermatoses.

B. Select the area to be sampled and clip the hair short ($\frac{1}{8}$ to $\frac{1}{4}$ inch). Gently swab the area with 70% alcohol and allow it to air-dry. Sterile hemostats are then used to gently tease hair from the follicle.

C. Plucked hair, scale, and epidermal debris, obtained from the periphery of the lesion or from an area exhibiting positive fluorescence, provide the best samples.

D. Sabouraud's dextrose agar or derma-

tophyte test media (DTM) are used most frequently for dermatophyte culture. Make sure
the sample hairs are embedded in the surface
of the culture media.

    E. A modified Mackenzie brush tech-
nique is a rapid and reliable means of collecting samples from catteries and asymptomatic cats in an infected household.

        1) A sterile or new toothbrush is
used to brush the animal on several areas of
the body.

        2) The DTM is then inoculated by
gently pressing the bristles of the brush into
the culture media.

    F. DTM contains gentamicin, chlortetra-
cycline, and cycloheximide to inhibit non-
pathogenic fungi and bacteria, as well as
phenol red, which serves as a color indicator
of positive (alkaline pH) dermatophyte
growth.

    G. Early in their growth, the metabolic
products of dermatophyte colonies are alkaline from protein metabolism changing the
media's color to red. As the protein in the
media becomes exhausted, the dermatophytes utilize carbohydrates to maintain
growth, resulting in an acid environment and
a return to yellow media color. Other fungi
utilize carbohydrates first, then proteins; old
DTMs (older than 2 weeks) may be red in
color when contaminated by saprophytic
fungi. Occasionally, rapidly growing sapro-
phytes will change the media color earlier.

    H. The DTM is held at room temperature
and read daily for 7 to 10 days. The media
color will change to red with colony growth.
Dermatophytes colonies of veterinary importance are generally white to beige in color.

    I. A definitive diagnosis is made by
microscopic examination of hyphae and conidia. Use clean forceps and a piece of cellophane tape to remove hyphae and conidia
from the top of the colony and transfer them
to a glass slide. A drop of lactophenol cotton
blue stain facilitates microscopic identification.

  5. Bacterial culture

    A. Superficial pyoderma

        1) Sample an unexcoriated lesion,
choosing an intact pustule if possible.

        2) Do not use strong antiseptic prod-

ucts or alcohol on the site prior to sampling,
as these may sterilize the pustule.

        3) Use a sterile 25-gauge needle to
prick the top of the pustule.

        4) Touch the culture swab to the
fluid contents, being careful not to touch the
surrounding skin.

        5) If only a crust is present, it may be
gently peeled back and the fluid under the
crust swabbed for culture.

    B. Deep pyoderma

        1) May be cultured from an intact
pustule or furuncle by sampling expressed
purulent material collected after *gently*
cleansing the surface with 70% alcohol

        2) If a lesion is nonexudative, then a
culture is best obtained by biopsying a piece
of skin.

        3) Skin surface should be gently
cleaned with an antiseptic soap, such as
povidone iodine or chlorhexidine.

        4) A skin biopsy is then obtained
using sterile technique. A 4-mm to 6-mm
biopsy punch instrument provides an adequate sample for culture.

        5) The biopsy sample should be
minced with a sterile scalpel blade prior to
placing it in the culture media.

  6. Cytology

    A. Cytologic examination of primary
lesions can often yield a rapid presumptive
diagnosis in many conditions (neoplasms,
pemphigus complex, infections).

    B. Sample intact vesicles and pustules if
possible. All nodular lesions and deep, draining lesions should also be sampled.

    C. Samples may be obtained by impres-
sion smear or fine-needle aspiration (FNA)
technique.

    D. Secondary lesions may be sampled by
removing the overlying crust and making an
impression smear of the material underneath.

    E. Cutaneous masses may be evaluated
by FNA or by making an impression smear of
the cells from the cut surface of a biopsy
sample. The tissue should be blotted with a
dry gauze sponge to remove excessive RBCs
before making the smear.

    F. Stain slides with a suitable Wright's,
Giemsa, or Gram stain. Diff-Quik is a good
all-around stain. Examine for microorganisms,

inflammatory cells, and neoplastic cells under high dry (×40) and with oil emersion.

G. Suspected neoplasms and autoimmune dermatoses *must* be confirmed by biopsy.

7. Skin biopsy

A. It is best to biopsy all obviously neoplastic lesions, lesions that are unusual, or lesions that have not responded to logical therapy.

B. Two basic techniques are commonly employed.

1) Localized skin masses are removed by excisional biopsy; this is both diagnostic and therapeutic.

2) Four- to 8-mm surgical punches (disposable biopsy instrument) are used when sampling multiple lesions.

C. Do *not* cleanse or surgically prepare the skin before biopsy, as this will alter surface architecture.

D. Locally anesthetize the proposed biopsy site with approximately 0.5-1.0 mL of 2% lidocaine subcutaneously (SQ).

E. Obtain specimens from several lesions in different stages of development if possible, and include "normal skin" on at least one specimen. Include only the most representative primary lesion if obtaining only one biopsy sample.

F. Carefully label each specimen with the site of biopsy and a brief description of the lesion. Be sure to indicate which sample contains normal skin.

G. The key to diagnosis often is hidden in the crust or superficial layers of the epidermis; therefore, extreme care should be exercised in handling the lesion during biopsy. Include the crust in the biopsy sample, even if it falls off during the procedure, and inform the pathologist that it has been included in the sample.

H. Wounds created by 4- to 8-mm punches may be sutured using nonabsorbable suture material.

I. Gentle aseptic preparation is indicated only in severely contaminated lesions and on specimens that will be submitted for deep bacterial or fungal culturing procedures.

J. Place biopsy samples for histologic examination in 10% formalin. Samples for direct immunofluorescent assay (IFA) should be fixed in Michel's media.

K. Select a good veterinary dermohistopathologist to examine the biopsy samples. Discuss with the consulting pathologist the appropriate handling of the samples for immunofluorescence or electron microscopy.

8. Allergy testing

A. Often indicated in pruritic skin conditions

B. Intradermal skin testing is the most common and reliable method used to diagnose allergic inhalant dermatitis (atopy).

C. In vitro testing (enzyme-linked immunosorbent assay [ELISA] or radioallergosorbent test [RAST]) is also being used in the diagnosis of atopy.

D. A food elimination diet, which may be used to diagnose food allergy, involves feeding a protein source that the animal has never eaten.

E. Patch tests may be used to identify contact allergens.

F. These tests will be discussed in greater detail under the section on Allergies.

9. Routine clinical pathologic tests

A. Dramatically visible skin problems may represent manifestations of underlying metabolic disease or endocrinopathies.

B. Routine clinicopathologic tests are important to identify specific clinical syndromes, as well as to provide support for diagnoses based on clinical findings.

1) A CBC, biochemical profile, and urinalysis are required in all animals with long-standing dermatopathies, in animals with apparent systemic illness, or in those in whom the diagnosis is elusive.

2) Examination of blood and feces for parasites may demonstrate an underlying problem.

3) Radiographic evaluation of the body cavities may be helpful in demonstrating neoplasia and organomegaly.

4) Endocrine abnormalities may be diagnosed definitively with provocative testing (i.e., with the thyroid-stimulating hormone [TSH] test, the adrenocorticotropic hormone [ACTH] stimulation test or dexamethasone suppression test).

a) The TSH test is the most reliable, widely available method for identifying the functionally thyroid-deficient animal. Baseline total triiodothyronine (T_3) and thyroxine (T_4) values are appropriate screening tests, but marginal values must be interpreted with caution. The diagnosis of hypothyroidism in borderline cases should not be made without the support of a TSH response test. Intravenous (IV) bovine TSH (0.1 IU/kg), coupled with a pre-TSH and a 6-hour post-TSH serum sample for T_3 and T_4 values is one of the most popular and reliable protocols for performing this provocative test.

   b) An ACTH response test. (ACTH, gel 1.0 IU/lb, not to exceed 40 IU/dog, administered intramuscularly [IM]) with a pre-ACTH and a 2-hour post ACTH plasma cortisol sample) is an excellent screening test for differentiating iatrogenic Cushing's disease from pituitary-dependent or primary hyperadrenocorticism. Iatrogenic Cushing's disease is a common problem seen in dogs with chronic allergic skin diseases that have been receiving long-term corticosteroid therapy.

   c) Low-dose (0.015 mg/kg IV) and high-dose (0.1 mg/kg IV) dexamethasone suppression tests help confirm a diagnosis of and differentiate between primary and pituitary-dependent hyperadrenocorticism. These tests are discussed in detail in the section on endocrine causes of alopecia that follows.

Alopecia

Alopecia is a term used to describe hair loss of any magnitude. There are many causes of alopecia. For simplicity, they may be divided into two groups: those caused by internal factors (i.e., genetic or metabolic factors) and those caused by external factors (i.e., nutritional, environmental, infectious/inflammatory, pruritic, toxin- or drug-induced, stress-induced, or psychogenic causes). It is important that the clinician differentiate between self-induced alopecias and those that reflect a primary pathologic process affecting the hair-follicle. Remember that a bilaterally symmetrical alopecia may be the primary manifestation of pruritus, especially in cats.

The clinical history (age of onset, presence or absence of pruritus, seasonality, therapeutic response) and the physical examination (alopecia with or without concurrent dermatitis, pattern of hair loss) will provide the best clues for formulating a logical list of differential diagnoses and a solid diagnostic plan (Fig. 15-1).

Congenital/Hereditary Causes

Feline Alopecia Universalis (Sphinx Cat)

   1. Emerging as a "new breed," sphinx cats are born to normal litters.
   2. There are no primary or guard hairs; secondary hairs are short and epilate easily. Nails are frequently abnormal.
   3. Sebaceous and apocrine glands open directly onto the skin's surface and function normally.
   4. Affected cats are greasy as a result of the glandular activity and these cats' reluctance to groom themselves with their rough tongues.
   5. On histologic examination, the condition is characterized by a thickened (8 to 10 cells) epidermis, glands opening on the surface, and a normal dermis.
   6. Treatment consists of frequent bathing with a mild sulfur/salicylic acid shampoo and careful trimming of the deformed nails.

Canine Hairless Breeds

   1. These dogs are alopecic as a result of a genetic mutation, and are seen rarely in the general population.
   2. The Chinese crested dog is totally alopecic except for the top of its head and its feet.
   3. The Mexican hairless breed has variable degrees of alopecia with a great deal of individual variation.
   4. Other alopecic breeds include the Xoloitzcuintl, African sand dog, and Peruvian hairless dog.
   5. Problems that occur secondary to the alopecia include dry, scaly skin, or very greasy skin. Amelioration of these conditions can be attempted with weekly sulfur/salicylic acid shampoos.

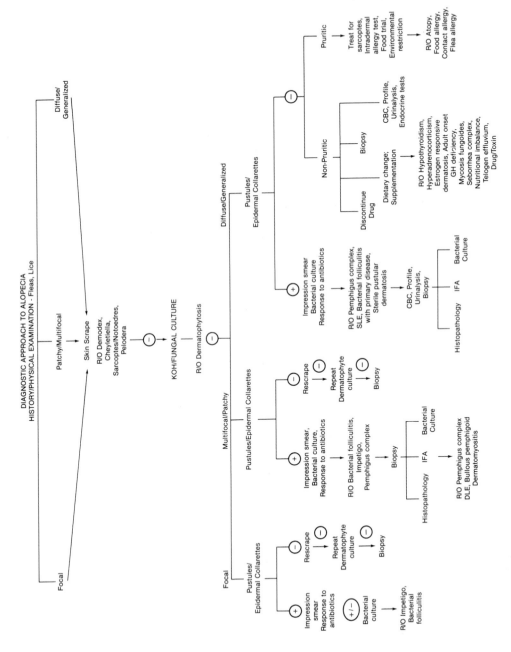

Figure 15-1. *Diagnostic approach to alopecia. R/O, rule out; DZ, disease; DLE, discoid lupus erythematosus; PE, pemphigus erythematosus; BP, bullous pemphigoid; LSA, lymphosarcoma; IFA, direct immunoflourescent assay; SLE, systemic lupus erythematosus; GH, growth hormone.*

Color-Mutant Alopecia

Clinical Signs

1. Hereditary follicular dystrophy in color mutants of specific breeds. Blue, fawn, and red Doberman pinschers, blue Great Danes, fawn Irish setters, blue dachshunds, blue chow chows, and blue whippets have been described. A milder form is suspected in some black and tan Doberman pinschers.

2. Dogs are born with normal hair coats. The syndrome usually manifests itself in young adults and tends to spare the normal-colored tan points.

3. The first clinical signs are a dull, dry hair coat with a moth-eaten appearance and scaly skin. Papules caused by cystic follicles with secondary pyodermas develop next.

4. Without therapy, many dogs will progress to an almost complete truncal alopecia with comedones and persistent pyoderma. Although the alopecia is usually irreversible, secondary problems can be controlled with therapy.

Diagnosis

1. Scaly, papular dermatitis with a moth-eaten hair coat in a color-diluted dog

2. Differential diagnoses should include primary hypothyroidism, demodicosis, dermatophytosis, bacterial folliculitis, and all the diseases of the seborrhea complex.

3. The results of appropriate diagnostic tests (skin scraping, fungal culture, measurement of T_4 levels, TSH response test) are normal or negative.

4. A trial of thyroid hormone supplementation for two to three months is ineffective unless the dog is concurrently hypothyroid.

5. Histologic findings are diagnostic, and include hyperkeratosis and keratin-filled hair follicles devoid of hair, large aggregates of melanin in the cortex and medulla of remaining hairs, and a diffuse perifolliculitis to furunculosis with a perivascular dermatitis.

Treatment

1. Directed at improving the condition of the skin and hair coat. Owner should be advised that there is no cure, and that man-agement of the condition will be a lifelong battle.

2. Benzoyl peroxide shampoos (Pyoben [Allerderm/Virbac]; OxyDex [DVM]) are recommended once to twice weekly to flush the follicles and keep secondary pyodermas in check.

3. Antiseborrheic shampoos (SebaLyte [DVM]; Sebolux [Allerderm/Virbac]) may be used once a week to remove crust and scale.

4. An after-bath humectant spray (Humilac [Allerderm/Virbac]), veterinary bath oil (Hy-Lyt EFA [DVM]; Sesame Oil Rinse [Veterinary Prescription]), or human bath oil used as a rinse (Alpha Keri [Westwood]; 1 capful/gallon of water) will help rehydrate the skin.

5. Oral daily essential fatty acid supplements (Derm Caps [DVM] or EFAVET [VetKem]) may be helpful. Administer for at least two months before evaluating response.

Black Hair Follicular Dysplasia

Clinical Signs

1. Broken hairs, hypotrichosis, and alopecia involving the black-haired areas of the skin

2. The condition has been observed in mixed breed dogs, bearded collies, a dachshund, a basset hound, a beagle, and a schipperke. No breed predisposition has been identified.

Diagnosis

1. Based on clinical presentation

2. Histologic findings

    A. Biopsy of areas of white-haired skin yields normal results.

    B. Black-haired skin demonstrates distortion and dilatation of hair follicles, hairs broken at the infundibulum, and follicular keratosis with blockage from keratin debris. Melanin-laden macrophages surround the base of affected hair follicles.

Treatment

1. There is no effective therapy for this disease.

2. A benzoyl peroxide shampoo may be somewhat palliative in keeping hair follicles open.

Acquired Alopecias

Pattern Baldness

1. Occurs primarily in the dachshund; other breeds affected include the Manchester terrier and miniature pinscher.
2. Affects adult male and female dogs
3. Characterized in the male by a bilaterally symmetrical pinnal alopecia that progresses caudally. Thinning of the hair coat on the ventral abdomen progresses to complete alopecia of the ventrum, especially in females.
4. Differential diagnoses include hypothyroidism, hyperadrenocorticism, estrogen-responsive dermatosis, black hair follicular dysplasia, congenital alopecia, ear margin dermatosis, pinnal alopecia, and color-mutant alopecia. The primary differential diagnosis in spayed females is estrogen-responsive alopecia.
5. The diagnosis is one of exclusion. Biopsy provides the best supportive information.
6. Determining the animal's response to a course of estrogen therapy (0.1 to 1.0 mg of oral diethylstilbestrol [DES] q24h; treatment should continue for three weeks with a rest period for one week; this regimen is maintained for three to four months), is an appropriate approach to this syndrome. If a good response is seen after three to four months of DES administration, then reduce the dose interval to once a week. Benign neglect is an acceptable alternative approach if the metabolic causes for this condition have been eliminated.

Pinnal Alopecia

1. A spontaneous process of ear margin alopecia of unknown etiology seen in both dogs and cats
2. Dachshunds, Boston terriers, and Chihuahuas older than 1 year of age are often affected, usually permanently.
3. A tentative diagnosis may be made on the basis of the history and physical examination. Rule out ear margin dermatosis, vasculitis, pattern baldness, and estrogen-respon-

sive dermatosis. Biopsy confirms the diagnosis.
4. Siamese cats and miniature poodles can develop a spontaneous, periodic alopecia of the ears. The alopecia may last for several months, but the hair will grow back in almost every case.
5. No treatment is necessary.

Periauricular Alopecia of Cats

1. Symmetrical alopecia between the ear and eye in the temporal region of the head
2. A normal coat pattern is observed in cats. Hair coat color (black) or hair length (short) may make this condition more noticeable in some cats.
3. Rule out dermatophytosis, demodicosis, and bacterial folliculitis.
4. No treatment is necessary.

Infectious/Parasitic Causes

The three major differential diagnoses for this category of alopecia are bacterial folliculitis, dermatophytosis, and demodicosis. Bacterial folliculitis and dermatophytosis are discussed in detail in the pruritic and scaling dermatoses sections, respectively.

Demodectic Mange (Red Mange, Demodicosis)

The demodectic mange mite normally lives in the hair follicles and sebaceous glands of all domestic animals and humans without signs of clinical disease. The mite is species-specific, with *Demodex canis* being the species of origin in dogs. *D. cati* (follicular dwelling) and a short, stubby-bodied, unnamed second species (surface dwelling) occur in the cat. The pathogenesis of clinical demodicosis is unknown, but is thought to be associated with a disordered immune system.

Clinical Signs

1. Canine
   A. Localized
      1) Usually affects young dogs (<1 year of age)

2) Circumscribed areas of alopecia, erythema, pustular eruptions, and scale appear, involving the head and extremities.

3) The condition is generally non-pruritic and spontaneously resolves in 90% of the cases.

  B. Generalized

    1) Affects young dogs (<1-1/2 years of age)

    2) Lesions begin locally, but progress to involve the entire body. The most common lesions include macules, edema, erythema, with crusting, scaling and pustules. Secondary pyodermas are common, and are caused by Staphylococcus species, Proteus species, and Pseudomonas species. Signs of systemic illness (fever, lymphadenopathy, etc.) are common.

    3) Breeds that are overrepresented include the Dalmatian, English bulldog, Chinese Shar Pei, Old English sheepdog, Great Dane, Doberman pinscher, and boxer.

    4) Since a hereditary predisposition has been identified, animals with generalized demodicosis should not be bred. Any adult dog with generalized demodicosis should be neutered once the disease is controlled.

    5) Adult onset (>5 years of age) demodicosis demands investigation for underlying disease (e.g., neoplasia, diabetes mellitus, hepatic disease, hyperadrenocorticism, etc.), stress-related incidences (estrus, whelping, etc.), or drug use (corticosteroids).

    6) Generalized demodicosis can become a chronic problem that becomes resistant to many types of therapy. The prognosis for cure is guarded, and owners should be warned that maintenance therapy (monthly amitraz dips) may be needed to keep the disease controlled.

    7) Dogs younger than 18 months of age may undergo a spontaneous cure.

    8) Differential diagnoses include bacterial folliculitis, dermatophytosis, chin and muzzle acne, pemphigus complex, and dermatomyositis.

  2. Feline

    A. Demodicosis, focal or generalized, is rare in the cat. Clinical presentation includes focal areas of alopecia, erythema, and papulocrustous eruptions, with or without pruritus.

The generalized form caused by either mite can affect the trunk, and may be characterized by scaling and hyperpigmentation.

    B. *D. cati* affects the eyelids, periocular area, ear canals, head, and neck. The occurrence of the generalized form warrants an investigation for an underlying disease (feline leukemia virus [FeLV], diabetes mellitus, systemic lupus erythematosus [SLE], neoplasia, etc.).

    C. The surface living mite is generally more pruritic than the follicular one, and may affect the head, neck, and ventral abdomen. Clinical disease caused by this form has not been associated with systemic disease.

    D. Differential diagnoses for feline demodicosis include dermatophytosis, cheyletiellosis, notoedric mange, otodectic mange, food allergy, and pemphigus complex.

Diagnosis

  1. Skin scraping

    A. *D. cati* and *D. canis*—The cigar-shaped mites or football-shaped eggs may be detected on deep skin scrapings, ear swabs, fecal examination, or biopsy.

    B. Surface living mite in cats—Short, stubby, cigar-shaped mites with a blunted abdomen or football-shaped eggs may be detected on superficial scrapings.

  2. Biopsy

    A. Chronic demodicosis complicated with deep folliculitis or furunculosis, especially of the feet, may occasionally yield negative findings on skin scrapings.

    B. Histopathologic examination may reveal mites deep within the hair follicle.

Treatment

  1. Localized demodicosis can best be treated by cleansing with 2.5% to 3% benzoyl peroxide shampoo, followed by daily topical rotenone cream (Goodwinol ointment [Goodwinol Products Corp.] or Canex lotion [Pitman–Moore]). Rescrape the skin in two weeks and examine for decreasing numbers of mites. These cases often spontaneously cure, with or without treatment, within six to eight weeks.

  2. Generalized demodicosis is a serious,

potentially life-threatening disease if not treated appropriately.

A. Evaluate the animal for underlying disease (perform a heartworm test, fecal examination, CBC, urinanalysis, and chemistry profile), especially older patients.

B. Treat the pyoderma. Initiate a regimen of broad-spectrum bactericidal antibiotic and continue treatment for four to six weeks. In systemically ill patients, in those with long-standing conditions, or those with deep pyodermas, a bacterial culture with sensitivity is prudent.

C. A total body clip, removing all of the hair, is mandatory to ensure maximal efficacy of dip therapy.

D. Bathe the animal for a minimum of 10 to 15 minutes with an antibacterial, keratolytic, or follicular flushing shampoo, such as benzoyl peroxide, prior to dipping.

E. For animals with severe suppurative pyoderma, daily chlorhexidine (Nolvasan) whirlpool baths or bathtub soaks for 20 to 30 minutes, continued for a period of one week, may be indicated prior to initiating dips.

F. Amitraz (Mitaban [Upjohn] diluted 1 bottle/2 gallons water) is the most effective approved acaricide for dogs. Wearing gloves, sponge the amitraz (0.025%) onto affected areas once a week after the bath. Allow the animal to air-dry.

G. Continue weekly dips for *at least* six weeks *and* until two consecutive weekly skin scrapings are negative for mites or eggs. Follow-up care includes monthly skin scrapings for at least six months after clinical cure.

H. Warn owners about the side effects associated with amitraz, such as anorexia, vomiting, diarrhea, and severe sedation.

I. People who are taking monoamine oxidase-inhibiting medications, such as some antihypertensive drugs, should not handle amitraz. The safest and most efficacious approach is to have the animal dipped at the veterinary clinic.

4. Pododermatitis is perhaps the most difficult to treat. It may be treated with weekly, 15-minute foot soaks during the amitrax dip. If this approach is unsuccessful, mix 0.5 mL of amitraz with 30 mL of mineral oil or propylene glycol and have the owner paint this on the feet weekly after the dip.

5. Vitamin E therapy (400 IU q6–12h) has had mixed results, but is worth a try in refractory cases.

6. Ivermectin does not appear to work, but the newer Avermectin compounds (i.e., Milbamycin) are being evaluated.

7. In the cat, therapy for localized demodicosis involves topical rotenone cream (Goodwinol ointment) or the use of lime sulfur (2%) dips q5d for three to five treatments or until two consecutively negative skin scrapings are obtained.

8. Amitraz dips (0.0125%), administered on a weekly basis for three treatments, have proven effective for generalized feline demodicosis. However, this product is not approved for use in the cat. A 2% lime sulfur dip, as described earlier, is safe and effective.

9. There is *no* indication for corticosteroid therapy of any kind with any form of demodicosis.

Endocrine Causes

Hypothyroidism

1. Hypothyroidism is the most common cause of endocrine dermatosis in dogs; it is an exceedingly rare, naturally occurring, congenital disorder in cats. Naturally occurring, adult-onset hypothyroidism has not been documented in the cat.

2. The Irish wolfhound, Chow chow, Great Dane, Doberman pinscher, Old English sheepdog, Irish setter, English bulldog, boxer, dachshund, Newfoundland, Alaskan malamute, and golden retriever breeds are over-represented, although this disease may occur in any breed.

3. Affects mature dogs of either sex.

Etiology

1. Decreased functional thyroid tissue. Lymphocytic thyroiditis is the most common form in dogs.

2. Lack of thyroid stimulation from decreased TSH (secondary) or thyroid releasing hormone (TRH) (tertiary)

3. Precursor (iodine) deficiency

4. Peripheral abnormalities (problems with

conversion of T_4 to T_3, receptor site, or auto-antibody production)

5. Decreased binding proteins

6. Drug interference or systemic illnesses—"euthyroid sick syndrome"

Clinical Signs

1. Hypothyroidism may mimic a variety of diseases, not be associated with any, and may show one or more of the following clinical symptoms:

A. Systemic signs—Lethargy, mental dullness and neurologic abnormalities, bradycardia, ocular abnormalities, weight gain leading to obesity, recurrent infections, cold intolerance, reproductive problems

B. Cutaneous signs—dry, dull hair coat that epilates easily; poor hair growth; loss of primary hairs with retention of a thick undercoat; symmetrical alopecia; excessive dry or greasy scale; tissue myxedema; hyperpigmentation; and frequent or persistent superficial pyoderma

C. Pruritus, when present, is generally associated with pyoderma or xerosis. Dogs with unexplained pyoderma, seborrhea, or both should be evaluated for hypothyroidism.

D. The differential diagnoses are varied and are dependent on clinical presentation.

Diagnosis

1. Based on history and physical findings

2. CBC and serum biochemical studies may reveal a mild anemia, as well as elevated cholesterol, alanine aminotransferase (ALT), and creatinine phosphokinase (CPK) levels.

3. Histologic findings may reveal hyperkeratosis, follicular keratosis, follicular atrophy, absence of anagen follicles, sebaceous gland atrophy, and dermal myxedema.

4. Radioimmunoassay (RIA)

A. The most reliable method of determining total T_3 and T_4 concentrations

B. A value well within the normal range for the laboratory performing the test should be considered normal.

C. Low baseline total T_4 values (< 1.0 μg/dl) are generally diagnostic in the *uncomplicated* hypothyroid patient.

D. A borderline total T_4 value (1.0 to 2.0 μg/dl) warrants a TSH response test.

E. Because of hourly fluctuations, T_3 values are unreliable and should never be used alone to diagnose hypothyroidism.

F. Free T_4 concentrations tend to reflect the amount of hormone available to cells and may be a more reliable screening test than total T_4.

5. The following pitfalls must be taken into consideration before ordering a T_4 test:

A. The RIA techniques utilized must be specific to canine and feline sera. Test results from analyses utilizing human tests kits are often inaccurate and should not be used.

B. Certain drugs can interfere with thyroid function/metabolism (i.e., phenylbutazone, phenobarbital, corticosteroids).

C. Make sure that concurrent illness (infections, hepatic disease, renal disease, severe nutritional deficiency, autoimmune disease, diabetes, Cushing's disease, neoplasia, etc.) is not a factor in lowering basal T4 values. Sick dogs with low T4 values may be "euthyroid sick" and will stimulate normally with TSH.

D. Do not overinterpret low normal basal values as daily fluctuations commonly occur.

E. Follow the normal range established for the laboratory performing the test.

6. When in doubt, perform a TSH response test.

7. Provocative tests

A. TSH response test

1) Blood samples are taken immediately before and six hours after TSH administration (0.1 IU/kg IV bovine TSH for the dog not to exceed 5 IU/dog; 1.0 IU IV for the cat), and the serum is immediately separated.

2) An acceptable response is a doubling of the T_4 value over baseline and *into the normal range*. T_3 values are extremely variable and are, therefore, unreliable.

3) Dogs with euthyroid sick syndrome and those receiving nonthyroidal medications will have a normal response. Dogs with very low T_4 concentrations secondary to corticosteroid therapy may not achieve expected poststimulation concentrations, but the magnitude of the response will be normal.

4) Dogs that have previously been receiving thyroid replacement medication should be taken off of the drug for at least six weeks prior to performing a TSH response test.

   B. TRH response test

      1) Used to distinguish between euthyroid and primary hypothyroidism

      2) Serum T_4 concentrations are determined immediately before and six hours after IV administration of 200 to 500 μg of TRH. Unaffected dogs at least double the baseline. Cholinergic side effects have been seen with higher doses of this drug.

   C. Antithyroglobulin antibodies may be elevated in approximately 50% of hypothyroid dogs.

   D. Thyroid gland biopsy

  8. A *significant* improvement in clinical signs should be seen following an 8-12 week supplemental trial.

Treatment

  1. Sodium levothyroxine (T_4)—0.1 mg/10 lb of body weight (0.022 mg/kg) up to a total dose of 0.8 mg for any size dog. Administer the drug every 12 hours initially; then reduce the dosing interval to every 24 hours once post-pill serum samples and physical examination indicate the disease is controlled (generally within four to six weeks).

  2. A post-pill T_4 determination 30 days after starting therapy is often desirable to monitor the therapeutic concentration of the levothyroxine. A serum sample should be obtained four hours after administration of the medication. Post-pill values should be in the high normal range.

  3. Reevaluate post-pill T_4 serum concentrations one month after reducing the dose to once a day. Adjust the dose based on clinical response as well as test results.

  4. Provide the supplement for a minimum of three months before determining efficacy.

  5. Warn owners that the cutaneous abnormalities (hairloss, scales, etc.) may get worse before they improve with therapy.

  6. If managing another disease (seizures, diabetes, cardiac disease, etc.), a lower dose of levothyroxine should be administered initially. Appropriate adjustments in drug therapy, as outlined earlier, are indicated once the hypothyroidism is controlled. Medications given for concurrent disease may also have to be adjusted.

Hyperadrenocorticism (Cushing's Disease)

  1. Common disease of dogs associated with excessive endogenous or exogenous glucocorticoids. It is rare in cats.

  2. May be characterized by polyuria, polydipsia, neurologic signs, excessive panting, abnormal estrus cycles, weight gain associated with an increase in appetite, thin hair coat, bilaterally symmetrical alopecia, thin skin, hepatomegaly, and muscle wasting.

  3. May occur naturally (pituitary-dependent, adrenal tumor) or it may be iatrogenic. More than 50% of the cases with chronic dermatologic disease are iatrogenic in origin.

  4. Some animals may present with only cutaneous signs.

Clinical Features Involving the Integument

  1. Bilaterally symmetrical alopecia with ease of epilation of hair

  2. Hyperpigmentation

  3. Poor wound healing; animal is easily bruised

  4. Thin, wrinkled skin

  5. Calcinosis cutis in dogs

  6. Pyoderma

  7. Pruritus is generally absent except with calcinosis cutis, in which case pruritus is moderate to severe.

  8. Demodicosis may be an additional secondary problem.

  9. Differential diagnoses include renal disease, hepatic disease, diabetes mellitus, hypothyroidism, sex hormone imbalance, and growth hormone deficiency.

Diagnosis

  1. Suggested by history and clinical signs

  2. Stress leukogram; elevated cholesterol, ALT, and alkaline phosphatase levels; low urine specific gravity and occasionally bacteriuria are identified in dogs

  3. Cats are frequently diabetic with persistant hyperglycemia, glucosuria, and are unresponsive to insulin.

  4. If glucocorticoids have been used in the past, the first adrenal function test to perform is the ACTH stimulation test. In dogs administer ACTH gel (1.0 IU/lb) up to a total dose of 40 IU IM. Obtain a preinjection and 2-hour postinjection plasma sample to measure cortisol concentrations. In cats administer 0.125 mg synthetic ACTH (Cortrosyn-Organon, Inc) or 2 IU ACTH gel IM. Obtain a 30 minute and 1 hour post stimulation plasma sample.

5. Iatrogenic Cushing's disease is confirmed by low prestimulation cortisol concentrations with little or no response. Hyperadrenocorticism is suspected with an exaggerated cortisol response.

6. A low-dose dexamethasone (0.01 mg/kg IV) suppression test in dogs and cats will usually confirm the diagnosis. A normal animals plasma cortisol level should suppress to less than 1.0 μg/dL at six and eight hours postadministration. However, a low percentage of normal animals will not suppress adequately.

7. Differentiation between pituitary-dependent and primary adrenal Cushing's disease (adrenal tumor) can be accomplished with the high-dose dexamethasone (0.1 mg/kg IV in dogs and 1.0 mg/Kg in cats with a six- and eight-hour postadministration sample) suppression test. Animals with pituitary dependent hyperadrenocorticism should suppress with this test while animals with functional adrenal tumors will not suppress.

8. Abdominal ultrasound may reveal bilateral adrenomegaly with pituitary dependent Cushing's, unilateral adrenomegaly with contralateral adrenal atrophy with an adrenal tumor.

9. Plasma ACTH concentrations are elevated with pituitary tumors.

10. Skin biopsy reveals changes that are consistent with an endocrinopathy, including dermal, epidermal, and follicular atrophy; follicular dilatation with hyperkeratosis; and follicular telogenization. Dystrophic mineralization (calcinosis cutis) is highly suggestive of hyperadrenocorticism in dogs.

Treatment

1. o,p'-DDD (mitotane; Lysodren) at an initial dosage of 25 to 50 mg/kg, PO delivered in divided doses q12h for 7 to 10 days, causes selective necrosis and atrophy of the zona fasciculata and zona reticularis of the adrenal gland. Monitor response by performing an ACTH response test biweekly. Once normal cortisol concentrations are reached, a weekly maintenance dose of 50 mg/kg should be effective.

2. Side effects related to op' DDD are associated with cortisol deficiency and include vomiting, diarrhea, anorexia, and lethargy. It is prudent to administer prednisolone (0.2 mg/kg q24h PO) concurrent with the op'DDD to reduce the incidence of these side effects.

3. Although cats appear to tolerate mitotane, clinical response to this drug is poor.

4. Ketaconazole has demonstrated adrenocortical steroidogenesis suppression activity in humans and dogs. This drug may be used in cases where mitotane has been ineffective. A dosage of 15 mg/kg/d is suggested. It has not shown the same efficacy in cats.

5. Nothing specific can be done for calcinosis cutis but to allow it to regress on its own (usually within three to six months) once the cause has been controlled. In an effort to relieve the associated pruritus, cool water soaks with colloidal oatmeal (Aveeno [Rydelle Laboratories]), or use of a sulfur-based shampoo, may be helpful. These measures may be employed twice a week, or as often as the owner finds necessary to provide relief.

6. Iatrogenic Cushing's disease requires a gradual reduction in glucocorticoid therapy. Patients are, in fact, adrenocorticoid-deficient, and this condition may persist for 3 to 12 months after the excessive doses have been discontinued.

Pituitary Dwarfism (Growth Hormone Deficiency)

1. An autosomal recessive hereditary hypopituitarism seen in German shepherds. There is no sex predilection.

2. Characterized by proportionate dwarfism, hyperpigmentation, and bilaterally symmetrical alopecia. Affected animals may also be hypothyroid, addisonian, and have reproductive abnormalities.

3. Symptoms manifest at approximately three months of age. The affected animal fails to grow, retains its puppy coat, and develops progressive alopecia, hyperpigmentation, and thinning of the skin.

4. Diagnosis is confirmed by performing a growth hormone stimulation test. Administer clonidine (30 μg/kg IV) or xylazine (100 to 300 μg/kg IV) and obtain a 0-, 15-, 30-, 45-, 60-, and 90-minute plasma sample for growth hormone evaluation. A failure to stimulate is seen in pituitary-deficient animals. It may be difficult to find this test commercially available.

5. Therapy utilizing porcine growth hormone (2 IU SQ every 48 hours for four to six weeks) or bovine growth hormone (10 IU SQ every 48 hours for four weeks) will result in an improvement in skin and hair coat within six to eight weeks; regulations on these hormones make them difficult to obtain. Human or synthetic growth hormones may also be tried; availability or expense may preclude their use. Concurrent endocrine abnormalities should also be treated.

Adult-onset Growth-Hormone–Responsive Dermatosis

1. Bilaterally symmetrical alopecia that develops in young adult male chow chows, Pomeranians, miniature poodles, and keeshounds. The alopecia usually involves the trunk, neck, caudal medial thighs, tail, and ears.

2. Differential diagnosis include hypothyroidism, sex hormone abnormalities, and Cushing's disease.

3. The diagnosis is based on signalment, history, normal laboratory tests, and response to growth hormone therapy.

4. Because growth hormone is difficult to obtain and the availability of the growth hormone assay is poor, response to castration is an appropriate diagnostic and therapeutic approach. Castration of male dogs will often result in a partial to complete regrowth of hair. The mechanism for this phenomenon is unknown.

5. Diagnosis is confirmed by performing a growth hormone stimulation test. Administer clonidine (30 μg/kg IV) or xylazine (100 to 300 μg/kg IV) and obtain 0-, 15-, 30-, 45-, 60-,

and 90-minute plasma samples for growth hormone evaluation. Because abnormal growth hormone assays have been described in Pomeranians with normal coats, abnormal growth hormone assays are suggestive of, but not diagnostic for, growth hormone deficiency.

6. Despite procurement difficulties, treatment with procine or bovine growth hormone (2.5 IU SQ q48h < 14 kg; 5 IU SQ q48h > 14 kg) is both diagnostic and therapeutic.

7. The side effects of growth hormone therapy include diabetes mellitus (reversible with discontinuance of therapy), acromegaly, and anaphylaxis.

Hyperestrogenism

1. A rare disorder characterized by bilaterally symmetrical alopecia, hyperpigmentation, gynecomastia, and reproductive abnormalities. The disorder generally affects middle-aged female dogs and older male dogs.

2. Rule out sertoli cell tumor in a retained testicle in males.

3. Rule out estrogen/testosterone imbalance in male dogs with normal physical examinations.

4. Rule out cystic ovaries or ovarian tumor in females.

5. Neutering is both diagnostic and therapeutic.

Estrogen-responsive Dermatosis

1. An adult-onset alopecia affecting female dogs that have undergone premature ovariohysterectomy

2. Characterized by bilaterally symmetrical alopecia involving the perineum, ventral abdomen, flanks, thorax, pinnae, and neck.

3. Rule out hypothyroidism, Cushing's disease, and pattern baldness.

4. Estrogen therapy (0.1 to 1.0 mg of DES q24h for three weeks, followed by discontinuation of the drug for one week, followed by a repeat of the cycle) for a period of three months is both diagnostic and therapeutic.

5. Because the problem is primarily one of esthetics, benign neglect is also an appropriate approach.

Miscellaneous Causes

Feline Psychogenic Alopecia

1. An alopecia that occurs with or without chronic inflammation of the skin, and that is caused by excessive grooming. Siamese, Burmese, and Abyssinian cats are predisposed to this condition.

2. Affected areas include the medial thigh, ventral abdomen, lateral thorax, center of the back, the extremities, and the tail. Hair does not epilate easily, and microscopic examination of the hairs reveals broken shafts.

3. This is a rare condition in cats. The diagnosis is made only after eliminating other causes of alopecia and pruritic dermatoses.

4. Rule out atopy, flea or food allergy, dermatophytosis, and demodicosis.

5. Therapy includes administration of behavior-modifying drugs (Valium, 1 to 2 mg orally every 12 to 24 hours; phenobarbital, 8 to 12 mg orally q12h), use of Elizabethan collars or body stockingettes, and benign neglect.

Telogen Effluvium

1. Stress-induced abrupt cessation of hair growth (secondary to surgery, parturition, illness, or drug therapy) with synchronization of hairs in catagen and telogen

2. Hairs are shed en masse, after which there is a two- to three-month period of no hair growth.

3. Spontaneously resolves without therapy

Pruritus

Pruritus is the most common dermatologic complaint in small animal practice. Behavioral manifestations of pruritus include licking, chewing, biting, scratching, personality changes, and owner harassment (i.e., the owner unable to sleep at night owing to the pet's constant licking). Obvious clinical signs of pruritus include erythema, excoriated skin with broken hair in areas that are easily accessible, hair loss, and saliva staining of the hair coat. Chronic pruritus may be characterized by lichenification and hyperpigmentation with alopecia. In cats, miliary dermatitis, bilaterally symmetrical alopecia, eosinophilic plaque, eosinophilic granuloma, or mild erythema without alopecia are common presentations.

The causes of pruritus are numerous, and include a long list of parasitic, infectious, and allergic/immunologic causes. A complete history, with emphasis on whether the pruritus or dermatitis came first, as well as the animal's response to previous corticosteroid therapy, is invaluable in reducing the differential list. Table 15-1 provides a brief outline of steroid- versus nonsteroid-responsive dermatoses.

Determining the severity of pruritus based on historical information can be difficult, as it is based on the owner's subjective evaluation of degree and frequency. For example the cat who is genuinely pruritic but is a "closet licker" may be overlooked while the poodle

Table 15-1. **Steroid- and nonsteroid-responsive dermatoses**

Corticosteroid-responsive	Nonresponsive to Corticosteroids
Acute moist dermatitis	Acral lick dermatitis
Flea allergy dermatitis	Sarcoptiform mite infestation
Allergic inhalant dermatitis	Food allergy
Pyoderma (+/−)	Neurodermatitis
Miliary dermatitis (+/−)	Metabolic/hormonal
Seborrhea complex (+/−)	

who licks for attention (psychogenic) is presented for this problem. Observing the animal in the examination room may help with this determination.

Infectious Causes

Pyoderma

Defined as "bacterial infection in the skin," pyoderma is a very common but often overlooked cause of pruritus. An impression smear made from the contents of an intact pustule, stained with Diff-Quik and examined under a microscope for cell type and presence of microorganisms, is a quick and reliable way of evaluating a pyoderma. Although most pyodermas do not require culture and sensitivity testing at first presentation, this procedure is mandatory for the chronic, nonresponsive, or recurrent case. Knowledge of normal and abnormal cutaneous bacteriology in both the dog and cat will help with interpreting culture results.

General Considerations

1. Primary cutaneous pathogenic bacteria in the dog include *Staphylococcus intermedius* and *S. aureus.* Organisms, such as Pseudomonas species or Proteus species, usually reflect an opportunistic infection, and may signal the presence of an underlying, immunosuppressive disease process. Each case should be scraped carefully for demodicosis.
2. Primary cutaneous bacterial pathogens in the cat include *S. aureus*, *S. intermedius,* and Pasteurella spp., with *Escherichia coli* and β-hemolytic streptococci occurring secondarily. Pyoderma is rare in cats.
3. Pyoderma is a common secondary problem in dogs associated with some underlying disease in which the integrity of the epidermis is disrupted.
4. Pyodermas can contribute significantly to the intensity of the pruritus; therefore, an appropriate course of an antibiotic and use of antibacterial shampoo therapy can be both diagnostic and therapeutic. No corticosteroids should be used during antibiotic therapy.
5. Once the pyoderma is under control, the

patient can be reevaluated for other causes of residual pruritus.

Surface Pyoderma

1. Presents as very superficial erosions of the skin precipitated by an irritant.
2. The associated pruritus is usually intense.

Pyotraumatic Dermatitis

Clinical Signs

1. Also called hot spot, acute moist dermatitis, or summer eczema, pyotraumatic dermatitis affects any age, breed, or sex, although it is most prevalent in long-haired, thick-coated breeds during hot weather
2. Rapid onset and progression of alopecia, erythema, and superficial exudation with self excoriation. Lesions may occur anywhere on the body.
3. Consider possible underlying causes (poor grooming, inadequate nutrition, or filthy environment; allergic disease [flea, atopy, food]; parasite infestation [fleas, scabies, ear mites], or infection [bacterial or fungal]).

Skin Fold Dermatitis (Intertrigo)

1. Also called frictional dermatitis
2. Associated with an array of presentations, but all are precipitated by anatomical predispositions.
3. Pruritus is generally mild to intense.

Clinical Signs

1. Lip fold pyoderma
  A. Prevalent in cocker and springer spaniels, setters, Newfoundlands, and St. Bernards.
  B. Primary complaint is usually halitosis.
2. Facial fold pyoderma
  A. Affects primarily brachycephalic breeds.
  B. Primary complaint is excessive tearing and corneal ulcers secondary to self-trauma.
3. Vulvar fold pyoderma
  A. Most common in obese, spayed bitches
  B. Primary complaints include scooting,

excessive licking, concurrent urinary tract infection (UTI), and odor

    C. Perform a cystocentesis, followed by a urine culture and sensitivity to rule out UTI.

  4. Tail fold (screw tail) pyoderma

    A. Prevalent in bulldogs and Boston terriers

  5. Body fold pyoderma

    A. Affects Shar Peis and obese dogs

    B. Primary complaints include body odor and moist dermatitis.

Diagnosis

1. A complete history, physical examination, skin scrape, flea comb, and dermatophyte culture will confirm or eliminate precipitating causes.

2. Consider allergy testing if it is a chronic, recurring problem and parasitic, management-related, and infectious causes have been eliminated.

Treatment

1. Clip hair locally.

2. Clean the affected area with an antiseptic soap or a benzoyl peroxide shampoo.

3. Dry the affected area with aluminum acetate (Domeboro or Burow's solution) soaks.

4. Apply a topical antibiotic cream that does not contain corticosteroids (steroids may interfere with epithelial and collagen synthesis and, therefore, healing).

5. Break the itch-scratch-itch cycle.

    A. Elizabethan-collar

    B. A short course of oral prednisolone (0.55 mg/kg/d for three to five days).

6. A three-week course of systemic antibiotics is recommended for chronic or refractory cases that are unresponsive to the treatment just described. If there is still no response, a biopsy should be performed.

7. Institute a weight loss program in obese animals.

8. Identify the underlying cause.

9. Surgical ablation of the anatomic defect is the most effective treatment, but results are variable and the problem may recur.

Superficial Pyoderma

1. A bacterial infection of the epidermis characterized clinically by papules, pustules, and crusting dermatitis

2. A diagnosis may be quickly established by making an impression smear of the fluid contents of a pustule, staining the slide with Diff-Quik stain, and examining the smear for the presence of a mixture of polymorphonuclear leukocytes (PMNs) and intracellular bacteria, lymphocytes, and macrophages.

3. A 3-week course of an appropriate systemic antibiotic and weekly shampoo therapy containing either benzoyl peroxide or chlorhexidine generally results in clinical resolution of the pyoderma.

Impetigo (Puppy Pyoderma)

1. Characterized by nonfollicular pustular eruptions in the groin, axilla, and ventral abdomen

2. The disease affects prepubescent dogs, and the associated pruritus is generally mild.

3. Evaluate the animal for nutritional status, endoparasites and ectoparasites, environment (sanitation).

4. Generally responsive to weekly benzoyl peroxide or chlorhexidine containing shampoos or topical benzoyl peroxide gel.

5. Systemic antibiotics (for 10 to 14 days) may be indicated in refractory cases.

6. Feline impetigo is seen in young kittens. Lesions generally occur around the neck and are believed to be secondary to "mouthing" by the queen. The treatment is the same as for canine impetigo.

7. Rule out demodicosis, dermatophytosis, and flea allergy.

Superficial Bacterial Folliculitis

1. The most underdiagnosed condition in veterinary dermatology

2. The clinical presentation includes a papular to pustular eruption through which a hair shaft emerges.

3. Lesions progress to circumscribed areas of alopecia collared by a peeling back of stratum corneum and a central area of hyperpigmentation (epidermal collarette). This presentation is frequently erroneously diagnosed as ringworm.

4. The primary differential diagnoses include demodicosis and dermatophytosis. Therefore, skin scraping and fungal culture should always be performed.

5. Therapy consists of a three- to four-week course (or one week beyond clinical cure) of appropriate systemic antibiotics and weekly shampoos with a follicular flushing agent, such as benzoyl peroxide.

6. If there is a recurrence, look for a precipitating cause (allergies, metabolic disorders, endocrine conditions).

Folliculitis of Short-coated Dogs

1. This condition presents with discrete patches of alopecia and small bumps affecting primarily the dorsal trunk. It is frequently confused with hives.

2. Seen in the boxer, English bulldog, Doberman pinscher, weimaraner, dachshund, Great Dane, and Dalmatian. Both sexes are represented.

3. Pruritus is mild to intense.

4. Therapy involves a three to six-week course of systemic antibiotics and weekly benzoyl peroxide shampoos. Control of this problem may require a lifelong regimen of frequent benzoyl peroxide shampoos. No corticosteroids should be used.

5. Rule out fungal causes or demodicosis. Consider hypothyroidism, allergic disease, or seborrheic syndrome as underlying precipitators of the bacterial folliculitis.

Deep Pyoderma/Furunculosis

Clinical Signs

1. A bacterial infection that extends beyond the hair follicle to involve the dermis.

2. Seen in adult dogs with no age or sex predilection. The German shepherd may be overrepresented.

3. The clinical picture includes multiple pustules, suppurative nodules, and fistulous tracts. A primary cause is frequently demodicosis.

4. An underlying disease process must be considered in every case. Primary differential diagnoses include hyperadrenocorticism (primary or iatrogenic); hypothyroidism; immune abnormalities (demodicosis, neoplasia, autoimmune disorders, immune deficiency syndrome; atopy); and infection (atypical mycobacteria, or fungal).

5. The degree of pruritus may range from absent to intense.

A. Muzzle pyoderma—Folliculitis and furunculosis involving the chin and muzzle of short-coated breeds; often resolves with puberty.

B. Pressure point pyoderma—Folliculitis and furunculosis of the lateral stifle, hocks, lateral digits, and elbows. Caused by constant trauma and associated with the development of ingrown hairs. Large breed dogs are predisposed to this condition.

C. Interdigital pyoderma—Characterized by suppurative nodules (furuncles) that progress to tracts draining serosanguinous to purulent material (cellulitis). *Always* scrape the skin deeply and sample multiple sites for demodicosis.

Diagnosis

1. Deep skin scraping to detect demodicosis

2. CBC, urinanalysis, biochemical profile, measurement of T_4 levels with TSH response

3. Impression smear of exudate stained with Diff-Quik and a Gram stain

4. Cutaneous biopsy of a surgically prepared lesion for deep culture and sensitivity (fungal and bacterial)

5. Cutaneous biopsy of an unprepared lesion for histopathologic examination. Save a sample obtained from a site adjacent to a primary lesion in Michel's media for IFA if autoimmune disease is suspected.

Treatment

1. Directed at controlling the bacterial component while identifying the underlying cause.

2. Six-week course of systemic antibiotics (bactericidal) selected according to the results of the Gram stain and culture and sensitivity.

3. Chlorhexidine or povidone iodine whirlpool baths or soaks daily for three to seven days.

4. Weekly to twice weekly chlorhexidene or benzoyl peroxide shampoos.

5. In addition to appropriate systemic antibiotics, pododermatitis may be managed with chlorhexidine (Nolvasan) or povidone iodine (Betadine) foot soaks every 12 to 24 hours.

6. Treatment for pressure point pyoderma includes benzoyl peroxide medicated baths and a three- to six-week course of systemic antibiotics.

7. Therapy for muzzle pyoderma involves daily cleansing with 2.5% benzoyl peroxide (Pyoben; Oxydex) shampoo and daily application of a 2.5% benzoyl peroxide gel.

Antibiotic Selection

1. In the dog, most superficial pyodermas are caused by *S. intermedius* and respond well to a three-week course of systemic antibiotics. This isolate typically will *not* respond to ampicillin, penicillin G, or tetracycline.

2. Deep pyodermas may have a gram-negative component; antibiotic selection should be based on culture and sensitivity results when possible.

3. Specific antibiotics

A. Erythromycin (11 to 18 mg/kg q8h; administer half of the dose with food for the first two to three days to avoid vomiting, then administer the full dose with food for three weeks) and lincomycin (22 mg/kg q12h) are bacteriostatic, narrow spectrum antibiotics that are generally chosen for their specificity for skin pathogens. Resistance develops quickly with these antibiotics, and resistance to one usually means resistance to the other.

B. Oxacillin (22 mg/kg q8h) and cloxacillin (22 mg/kg q8h) which have a narrow, gram-positive spectrum, are expensive but effective. Administer on an empty stomach.

C. Trimethoprim-sulfadiazine (22 mg/kg q12h) has a gram-negative and gram-positive spectrum. Some dogs, especially Doberman pinschers, may exhibit polysystemic hypersensitivity reaction (myalgia, joint pain, stiff gait, neurologic abnormalities). Keratoconjunctivitis sicca is a common side effect of sulfa drugs. Discontinuation of the drug usually will reverse these signs.

D. Amoxicillin-clavulenic acid (22 mg/kg q12h) is used against β-lactamase–producing Staphylococcus spp.

E. Cephalosporins (cefadroxil, cepha-lexin, 33 mg/kg q12h or 22 mg/kg q8h) are considered the "big guns" of cutaneous antibiotics and should be reserved for cultured resistant cases.

F. Quinolone antibiotics (enrofloxacin [Baytril] 2.2 mg/kg q12h; norfloxacin [Noroxin] 5 to 10 mg/kg q12h). These are *absolutely* reserved for the bacterial infections that have been cultured and are resistant to other appropriate antibiotics. This group of antibiotics is most helpful with gram-negative organisms.

3. *Never* use concomitant corticosteroid and antibiotic therapy. A false sense of improvement is derived as inflammation is decreased by the cortisone. At the same time, the immune system is suppressed, preventing resolution of the bacterial infection.

4. Base further diagnostic steps and therapeutics on a follow-up examination, monitoring the animal's degree of improvement. Resolution of the pyoderma and pruritus simultaneously suggests that the pyoderma caused the pruritus. If pruritus still exists, then pursue other causes (e.g., allergies).

Parasitic Causes

Fleas and Flea Bite Dermatitis

1. The most common cause of pruritic dermatitis in dogs and cats

2. Characterized by infestation with a large number of fleas, resulting in papular to crusting dermatitis from the flea bite and self-excoriation

3. The usual distribution of lesions is on the head, neck, and dorsum in the cat (miliary dermatitis), and the lumbosacral and caudomedial thigh region in the dog. Concurrent findings include hot spots, lumbosacral alopecia, and superficial pyoderma.

Flea Allergy Dermatitis

1. Flea allergy dermatitis (FAD) affects dogs and cats that are hypersensitive to one or more of a number of antigenic products in flea saliva.

2. Characterized by both an immediate (type 1) and a delayed (type 4) hypersensitivity reaction upon intradermal challenge in dogs, and an immediate (type 1) hypersensitivity reaction in cats.

3. Manifestation of the disease has no correlation to the population of fleas found on the animal; one flea that bites the allergic animal can cause an allergic reaction and intense pruritus.

4. Remember that the flea spends most of its life cycle off the host, so complete environmental control is paramount to successful treatment.

Clinical Signs

1. The age of onset is older than six months (except in Chinese Shar Pei dogs, which may show signs earlier).

2. The problem occurs seasonally summer to fall, except in areas where the climate is warm and humid year-round.

3. Remember that because the hypersensitive animal is allergic to flea saliva, the animal must first be bitten for the allergy to manifest itself. Not all animals with fleas are allergic to the saliva.

4. Clinical signs include an intensely pruritic, erythematous, papular, and crusting dermatitis involving the caudal-medial thighs, lumbosacral area, ventral abdomen, perineum, and neck. Alopecia may or may not occur.

   A. In the dog, the pattern of distribution typically involves the caudal dorsum and posterior-medial thigh area.

   B. A caudal and cervical distribution of miliary dermatitis is the most typical presentation of FAD in the cat. Bizarre or agitated behavior is a common owner complaint in addition to the cutaneous signs.

5. Cats may also present with any one or a combination of eosinophilic ulcer, eosinophilic plaque, and lip granuloma.

6. Confirmation may be based on results of an intradermal skin test for fleas and resolution of the lesion with flea control.

7. Secondary superficial pyodermas, pyotraumatic dermatitis, miliary dermatitis, and seborrhea are common concurrent problems.

Diagnosis

1. Diagnosis may be based on any one of the following:

   A. Physical findings (fleas, eggs, or debris).

   1) Use a flea comb and thoroughly comb through the hair coat.

   2) Use a water-moistened gauze sponge to wipe debris from the examining table. Flea excreta (digested blood) will dissolve and stain the sponge a rusty brown color.

   B. Presence of tapeworm segments in the stool

   C. Intradermal skin test results using an aqueous preparation of flea antigen (Greer Laboratories 1 : 1000 W/V solution flea antigen), histamine as a positive control, and saline as a negative control. Immediate reactions are seen within 10 to 15 minutes. Delayed reactions (24 to 48 hours) are common.

2. Response to flea control

3. Rule out atopy, food allergy, intestinal parasite hypersensitivity, ectoparasites (scabies, notoedric mange, demodicosis, etc.), bacterial dermatitis, and dermatophytosis. Many animals may have multiple, concurrent problems.

Treatment

1. Flea control therapy must be directed toward client education.

   A. Make sure the owner understands the importance of persistent flea control practices, even if fleas are no longer being seen.

   B. Remember that the flea-allergic pet will be allergic for life.

2. The three-pronged approach to treatment that provides the best success involves treating the indoor environment, the outdoor environment, and the affected animal along with all in-contact pets.

   A. Vacuum and mop the pet's environment thoroughly, discarding the vacuum bag after use, and wash all bedding. Exterminate the house utilizing an adulticide (chlorpyrifos or a synthetic pyrethrin) with methoprene (growth inhibitor) every two weeks for one month, then monthly or every two months throughout the flea season. A professional exterminator is often employed in heavily infested areas and large homes. Premise sprays and foggers are best in small apartments or in situations in which the affected animals are confined to a limited area.

B. Weekly dipping of *all* animals with approved organophosphates, pyrethrins, or pyrethroids is recommended. Use caution when combining products, as their effects may be undesirably additive, leading to toxicity.

C. Daily or alternate day pyrethrin sprays between dips provide added protection and are safe. Animals with concurrent skin lesions may be irritated by alcohol-based flea products; water-based sprays may reduce the discomfort.

D. Flea shampoos are rarely helpful in the flea-allergic pet, as there is no residual activity; a cleansing shampoo will be as effective in removing fleas and debris. Flea collars are essentially useless.

E. The outdoor environment frequented by pets should be sprayed every two to three weeks with a garden insecticide (diazanon; carbaryl; malathion). Diazanon granules may require less frequent application.

F. Microencapsulation of products such as chlorpyrifos, permits its use outdoors.

3. Initial therapy should be directed at controlling secondary superficial pyodermas with the use of weekly antibacterial shampoos (Nolvosan or Pyoben) and a three-week course of systemic antibiotics.

4. Symptomatic therapy for pruritus utilizing antihistamines or anti-inflammatory doses of corticosteroids may provide some relief for the flea-allergic dog or cat.

A. Diphenhydramine HCl (Benadryl) or hydroxyzine HCl (Atarax), 2.2 mg/kg every 8 to 12 hours (The response is usually fair to poor.)

B. Oral corticosteroids (prednisolone or prednisone, 0.55 mg/kg q12h for five days, q24h for five days, then q48h for 10 days) may be used as adjunctive therapy to help control pruritus. It should only be employed after the secondary pyoderma has been controlled.

5. Currently, there is no reliable method available for hyposensitizing the flea-allergic pet.

6. Oral organophosphates (Cythioate) have been used with some success in the nonal-lergic dog. Fenthion (ProSpot) has some repellant activity, and may be helpful. Both have questionable efficacy in the allergic animal.

Sarcoptic Mange (Sarcoptes scabiei, *Canine Scabies*)

Clinical Signs

1. This highly contagious, intensely pruritic dermatitis is characterized by papular eruptions, thick scale, crusts, and alopecia involving the elbows, ear margins, hocks, legs, chest, and ventral abdomen. It may become generalized.

2. Lymphadenopathy is common.

3. The condition may present with only mild erythema with intense pruritus.

4. The response to anti-inflammatory doses of corticosteroids is usually poor.

5. Human infections usually spontaneously resolve once the affected animal is treated.

Diagnosis

1. Based on history and clinical presentation. History often reveals that other in-contact dogs and humans also have a pruritic dermatitis.

2. Multiple skin scrapings yield negative results in more than 50% of the cases.

3. Fecal examination may reveal mites, eggs, or both.

4. Ear swabs may yield mites, eggs, or both.

5. There may be a positive or negative pinna-femoral reflex (rubbing of the margin of an ear against itself results in the dog scratching at the ear).

6. Response to therapy is often the most reliable diagnostic aid. If you suspect scabies, treat it!

7. Rule out fly bite, atopy, food allergy, otodectic dermatitis, dermatophytosis, autoimmune disease.

8. Because unusual presentations are possible, scabies should be considered a primary differential with every pruritic dog.

Treatment

1. Clip hair if necessary.

2. Precede parasiticidal therapy with shampooing with a good cleansing, keratolytic, antiseborrheic shampoo (e.g., SebaLyt [DVM]; Sebulux-[Allergroom]) to remove loose crusts.

3. Whole body parasiticidal sponge-on dips

A. Phosmet (Paramite) weekly for 6 weeks (resistance may occur)

B. Amitraz (Mitoban) every two weeks for three treatments (effective therapy but not approved for this use in dogs)

C. Lime sulfur (1 : 30) q5d for six to eight treatments or until two weeks after clinical cure. This product is especially appropriate for sick, debilitated, or very young (younger than six weeks of age) affected animals.

4. Ivermectin (cattle formulation), 200 μg/kg orally or SQ every two weeks for two to three treatments (effective therapy but not approved for this use in dogs). Do not use in Collies, Shelties, or collie crossbreeds.

5. Prednisolone, 0.55 mg/kg/d for three to five days to break the itch-scratch-itch cycle.

6. Wash bedding and treat all in-contact animals to prevent reinfestation.

Notoedric Mange (Notoedres cati, Feline Scabies)

Clinical Signs

1. History and clinical signs are similar to scabies in the dog. The infestation involves the face, head, ear margins, feet, and perineum. Rare occurence.

2. Lesions are characterized by thick scale and crusts with severe pruritus.

3. Rule out food allergy, pemphigus foliaceus/erythematosus, Otodectes infestation, dermatophytosis, demodicosis.

Diagnosis

1. Mites and eggs in skin scrapings are found commonly.

2. Fecal examination may reveal eggs and/or mites or mite parts.

3. Eliminate other differential diagnoses and evaluate the animal's response to therapy.

Treatment

1. Parasiticidal dips—Lime sulfur (1 : 30) (Lym-Dyp), weekly for three to six treatments; ivermectin (cattle formulation), 200 μg/kg SQ

every two weeks for two treatments (not approved for use in cats)

2. This parasite is highly contagious to other cats therefore, clean and treat the environment (flea foggers or premise sprays are effective) and treat in-contact animals.

Otodectic Mange (Otodectes cynotis)

Clinical Signs

1. Affects dogs and cats of all ages and breeds

2. Pruritus and otitis externa are characterized by head shaking, ear scratching, head tilt, periauricular excoriation, and a dark brown to black, thick, ceruminous exudate.

3. Infestation may involve the head, face, neck, feet, perineum, and tail head. Ear involvement is usually bilateral, but may be unilateral.

4. In cats, infestation may be accompanied by a miliary dermatitis.

Diagnosis

1. Ear swab and microscopic examination of exudate for mites and eggs

2. Otoscopic examination for mites and eggs

3. Fecal examination

4. Skin scraping

Treatment

1. Ear cleaning (may require sedation or general anesthesia)

A. Soften debris with a ceruminolytic agent and remove with a cotton tipped swab.

B. Cleansing can be achieved by *gentle* flushing with dilute povidone-iodine or chlorhexidine solution, using a rubber-tipped pediatric bulb syringe.

2. Otic preparations

A. A mitocidal product such as Mitox Liquid (Norden) is excellent for the uncomplicated infection.

B. A combination product with anti-inflammatory, antiparasitic, and antibacterial activity is the best choice for secondarily infected ears; (Tresederm [MSD Agvet]).

C. Treat both ears twice a day for one week, once a day for one week, then two to three times a week for two weeks. Re-evaluate two weeks after discontinuing the medication.

3. Ivermectin (cattle formulation), at a dosage of 200 μg/kg SQ, repeated in two weeks, is an especially effective drug for both dogs and cats. Its use is most appreciated in barn cats, multi cat households, or difficult-to-handle pets. It is not approved for this use.

4. Topical antiparasiticides (i.e., a good flea shampoo) should be used to prevent reinfestation of the ears by mites that have inhabited the haircoat.

5. All in-contact animals should be examined and treated.

6. Rule out bacterial otitis, Malassezia (Pityrosporon) otitis, atopy, food allergy, foreign body, and fly bite.

Cheyletiellosis ("Walking Dandruff")

1. Found in dogs, cats, rabbits, and humans, this highly contagious parasitic infestation is transmitted among young animals by direct contact or from a contaminated environment.

2. Clinical signs are variable, but classically include diffuse dry scale over the dorsum. The condition may or may not be accompanied by pruritis.

3. The diagnosis is established on the basis of skin scrapings, use of a flea comb or cellophane tape to remove scale for microscopic examination, or visualization of the moving mites.

4. Rule out scabies, Notoedres infestation, atopy, FAD, and seborrheic dermatitis.

5. This mite succumbs to most parasiticides; therefore, therapy involves the use of any approved parasiticidal dip or shampoo for *all* in-contact animals. Ivermectin (200 μg/kg SQ), repeated once in two-weeks, is also effective. Ivermectin is not approved for this use.

6. Environmental cleaning, followed by use of an environmental insecticide for fleas (foggers/premise sprays), is required in every case.

7. This mite can cause a severe pruritic dermatitis in humans, so affected owners should seek the care of a physician.

Allergic and Immunologic Causes

Allergic Inhalant Dermatitis (Atopy)

1. A common disease in dogs that is estimated to involve up to 15% of the canine population

2. Age of onset is between one and two years. Both sexes are represented. The Chinese Shar Pei may develop signs of atopy as early as two to three months of age.

3. Occurs in both purebred and mixed breed dogs. Breeds that are overrepresented include terriers, golden retrievers, Irish setters, Dalmatians, Lhasa apsos, English bulldogs, and Shar Peis.

4. The history includes a seasonal occurrence that may progress to a nonseasonal problem.

5. Feline atopy occurs, but is specifically diagnosed less frequently than in the dog.

Clinical Signs

1. Pruritus is the hallmark of atopic disease.

2. The classic historical complaints in dogs include face rubbing, foot licking or chewing, and scratching the axillae and ears. The history is generally supported by signs of erythema, inflammation, and self-excoriation detected on physical examination.

3. Hyperpigmentation, lichenification, and superficial pyoderma are common secondary problems.

4. In cats, atopy may present as symmetrical alopecia without dermatitis, miliary dermatitis, pruritus of the head and neck, or a generalized scaling dermatosis. Atopy may also present as eosinophilic granuloma, eosinophilic ulcer, or as eosinophilic plaque.

Diagnosis

1. Historical clues (breed, season, steroid-responsiveness)

2. Negative results on skin scrapings

3. Elimination or identification of other causes of pruritus, such as fleas or food allergy.

4. Intradermal skin test results

A. Can be performed in both dogs and cats

B. Determines the presence of antigen-specific immunoglobulin E (IgE) in the skin

C. Indications

1) When other differential diagnoses have been eliminated

2) When the problem has progressed from a seasonal to a nonseasonal pattern

3) When the owner or clinician believe that symptomatic therapy is not the best approach for controlling the disease

D. Preparations for skin test

1) Discontinue all corticosteroids (prednisolone for a minimum of three weeks; methyl prednisolone acetate and megestrol acetate for at least three months), antihistamines (for two weeks), and aspirin (for at least one week) prior to skin testing.

2) Perform an intradermal histamine (1 : 100,000)/saline (diluent) control test when the animal has been receiving anti-inflammatory drugs. Wait until a good histamine response (4+) occurs prior to performing the full intradermal test.

3) Control secondary bacterial infections with antibiotics *prior to the skin test.*

4) Allergens used should include pollens chosen according to regional vegetation and perennial substances, such as house dust, epidermals, and molds. All should be in an aqueous, nonglycerinated, base to reduce the risk of irritant reactions.

E. Proper interpretation of skin test reactions depends on the skill of the tester/examiner.

5. Two in vitro tests are commercially available for dogs.

A. RAST (A & M Biosciences, Inc., Mesa, Arizona; Spectrum Laboratories, Texas).

B. ELISA (Bioproducts for Medicine, Inc., Tempe, Arizona)

C. Both utilize anti-canine IgE to detect circulating IgE group specific antibodies.

D. These tests have a high incidence of false-positive results, but are a welcome alternative when intradermal skin testing is unavailable or difficult to perform.

E. In-vitro allergy testing has not been developed for cats because feline IgE has not been immunochemically identified.

6. Provocative testing is the ultimate in allergy testing for both dogs and cats, but difficult to achieve in most cases. It is an excellent method for identifying allergies to products such as cigarette smoke or cat dander. The test requires eliminating the animal's exposure to the suspected allergen for two to three weeks, observing improvement, then reexposing the animal and observing a recurrence or exacerbation of the pruritus.

Treatment

1. Antihistamines have variable effects in controlling pruritus, but should be tried before instituting long-term corticosteroid therapy.

A. Hydroxyzine HCl (Atarax or generic), 2.2 mg/kg q8h for dogs only

B. Diphenhydramine (Benadryl or generic), 2.2 mg/kg q8h for dogs only

C. Chlorpheniramine (Chlor-Trimeton or generic), 2 to 4 mg (total dose) every 12 hours. Best for toy breeds and cats.

D. Doxepin HCl, 0.5 to 1.0 mg/kg gl2h for dogs only

E. Individual responses to specific antihistamines vary. It may be helpful to prescribe a two-week course for each of three different antihistamines, then choose the one with the best response for maintenance.

2. Corticosteroids—the treatment of choice for some animals

A. When hyposensitization is not an attractive option to the owner and when antihistamine/fatty acid combinations have been unsuccessful

B. Animals with a short (8 to 12 weeks) allergy season.

1) Prednisone or prednisolone, 0.55 mg/kg q12h for three to five days, q24h for three days, then administered on alternate days. Reduce to the lowest dose possible to control clinical signs.

2) Long-acting corticosteroids (methylprednisolone acetate) have no place in managing atopy in the dog unless the season is very short (4 to 6 weeks) and one or two treatments control the symptoms completely.

3) Methylprednisolone acetate (Depo-Medrol, 20 mg SQ or IM) is effective in controlling pruritus in cats, but the duration of effect may appear to shorten with extended use. Megestrol acetate's (Ovaban) detrimental effects (diabetes mellitus, pyometra/metritis, adrenal suppression, mammary hyperplasia/ neoplasia, etc.) preclude its routine use for symptomatic therapy in the cat.

3. Buffered aspirin (5 mg/kg q12h), administered with food may be helpful in some dogs. Discontinue if gastrointestinal (GI) upset occurs. Do not use in cats.

4. Essential fatty acid supplements (Derm Caps [DVM]; Efavet [Vetkem]

    A. Administer alone at twice the manufacturer's recommended dose, for a minimum of six weeks before assessing response.

    B. May result in an enhanced anti-inflammatory response when used in combination with corticosteroids or antihistamines.

5. Hyposensitization is the method of choice in the young patient or the animal with nonseasonal pruritus. Although improvement is rarely seen before three months after initiation of therapy, it is effective in about 65% of the cases within the first year. This form of therapy is required for life, but allows a decrease in or elimination of adjunctive therapy. Vaccines should be tailored to the needs of the animal and based on the results of either an intradermal skin test, RAST, or ELISA.

6. Antibiotic therapy is indicated to control secondary pyodermas in all cases.

7. Once to twice a week therapeutic bathing utilizing a benzoyl peroxide, sulfur/salicylic acid, or chlorhexidine shampoo helps combat the pruritus and will help keep secondary seborrheas and pyodermas under control.

Food Allergy

History and Clinical Signs

1. Usually affects young animals (dogs and cats of all breeds) approximately one year of age, but may occur at any age

2. Should be ruled out before pursuing intradermal skin testing in young animals

3. Not generally associated with a recent change in diet, but may be associated with a diet that the animal has consumed for some time

4. Characterized by intense pruritus that involves the face, head, caudal dorsum, and perineum. The pruritus is generally non-steroid-responsive.

5. In dogs, there may be general erythema and pruritus without severe dermatitis, a flea allergy-like lumbosacral distribution of alopecia and dermatitis, an atopy-like distribution pattern, or a seborrheic dermatitis.

6. In cats, the problem may present as miliary dermatitis, any of the eosinophilic granuloma complex presentations (plaque, ulcer, or granuloma), an intensely pruritic head and neck seborrheic condition, or self-induced symmetrical alopecia without dermatitis.

Diagnosis

1. A food elimination diet is the best means of establishing the diagnosis of food allergy. A home-cooked diet insures complete control of content.

2. Feed a protein source that the animal has never been exposed to, such as lamb, deer, rabbit, fish, or tofu for a period of *at least* three weeks. During this time, no other snacks, rawhide chew bones or meat flavored/chewable medications should be given.

    A. Home-cooked diet

        1) Mix one cup of the cooked protein source with three cups of cooked, regular long-grain brown rice.

        2) Approximately one cup of the mixture for every 10 pounds of body weight per day, divided into two feedings, will meet the daily caloric requirements.

    B. Hill's d/d Prescription Diet (canned lamb protein; dried egg protein); Annergen (Wysong–lamb and chicken); Nature's Recipe non-meat kibble

3. After the three-week trial, the animal is challenged with the normal diet and observed (a minimum of 48 hours) for returning pruritus.

4. Should the pruritus recur, then the hypoallergenic diet should be reinstituted until the pruritus again resolves. Specific proteins (i.e., beef, egg, chicken, etc.) are fed individually for a period of three days in an attempt to identify the offending allergen. Return to the hypoallergenic diet between challenges.

5. Cats are difficult to test, but will often eat preservative-free lamb baby food or the canned Hill's Prescription canine diet d/d. Taurine, a dietary requirement for cats on a home-cooked diet, has been added to the Hill's d/d diet. The dietary trial period is the same as in dogs.

Treatment

1. Avoidance of the offending dietary allergen

2. Feeding the home-cooked diet with vitamin and mineral supplements or a commercial hypoallergenic diet

3. Be careful. Preservative-free and "designer" dog foods containing lamb will often have other protein products (egg, whey, chicken, etc). Although they *may* be adequate for maintenance, the ingredients list of these diets should be carefully screened and compared with the results of the dietary challenge before feeding.

4. Corticosteroids are of little help.

Contact Hypersensitivity

1. Occurs rarely in the dog or cat owing to the protection afforded by the long fur

2. May either be an allergic or an irritant reaction

Clinical Signs

1. Hairless or sparsely haired body parts, such as the ventrum, axillae, ventral aspect of the feet, and scrotum, are most commonly affected by both irritant and allergic reactions.

2. Irritant contact dermatitis is characterized by acute, painful dermatitis that may progress to ulceration. More than one pet or human is commonly affected.

3. Allergic contact dermatitis begins as a pruritic, papular to macular, eruptive dermatitis that progresses to crust and scale with self-trauma. It is characterized by a chronic and progressive course over months to years in a single animal.

Diagnosis

1. History of exposure

2. Exposure to the suspected allergen through patch testing is a reliable method of diagnosis.

3. The suspected antigens must be held in close contact with a shaved area of skin for 48 hours and observed for urtication or erythema at the site of contact.

4. Another approach is to remove the suspected allergen from the environment. Once the dermatitis has resolved, the animal should be challenged by re-exposure to confirm the diagnosis.

5. Rule out contact irritant dermatitis, scabies, demodicosis, hookworm dermatitis, pelodera, pyoderma.

Treatment

1. Avoidance of allergen

2. Some relief may be achieved with the use of topical corticosteroids or systemic corticosteroids administered at an anti-inflammatory (0.5 mg/kg q12h) dose.

3. Treat secondary pyodermas with a three-week course of systemic antibiotics and weekly antibacterial shampoos.

Drug Eruption (Drug Allergy)

1. Rare; variably pruritic; poorly steroid-responsive

2. Cutaneous eruptions +/− mucocutaneous involvement

3. May be dose-dependent and predictable based on the drug's pharmacologic behavior, or may be an idiosyncratic or hypersensitivity reaction

4. Clinical manifestations vary widely, and may include erythema, depigmentation, erosions, mucocutaneous ulcerations, petechia to ecchymoses, urticaria, angioedema, and papulocrustous dermatitis.

5. May mimic any dermatologic problem

6. Because a drug-induced dermatopathy may occur days to months after drug use, and may persist for months after discontinuation of the offending drug, a carefully screened medical history provides the best evidence that a drug may be the precipitator of the dermatitis.

7. Provocative challenge with the suspected offender confirms the diagnosis, but is generally too dangerous to attempt.

8. Therapy is directed at:

A. Discontinuing the offending medication

B. Providing symptomatic therapy (antibiotics, gentle shampoo therapy, etc.) as needed. Corticosteroids may not be helpful but should be considered if life-threatening signs develop.

C. Avoiding related drugs

Miscellaneous Pruritic Dermatosis

Feline Miliary Dermatitis

1. Also known as papulocrustous dermatitis, or "scabby cat" disease
2. May affect cats of any age, breed, or sex. Represents approximately 38% of feline dermatologic presentations
3. Intensely pruritic, papulocrustous dermatitis
4. The distribution pattern may be localized (neck or lumbosacral region) or diffuse.
5. This pattern of dermatitis in cats reflects a cutaneous response to an immunologic, infectious, or irritant agent. It is *not* an entity in and of itself. A search for an underlying disease process is warranted.
6. Differential diagnoses include flea allergy (> 54%), food allergy (10.6%), atopy (12%), bacterial folliculitis, drug eruption, intestinal parasite hypersensitivity, ectoparasites (Notoedres, Otodectes, etc.), dermatophytes, or a dietary imbalance (essential fatty acid, biotin).
7. The diagnostic plan should include flea combing, skin scraping, use of Wood's light, fecal examination, fungal culture, food trial, and intradermal skin testing.

Pruritic/Psychogenic Dermatosis

Acral Lick Dermatitis (Lick Granuloma)

1. Adult male dogs are overrepresented.
2. Doberman pinschers, Great Danes, golden retrievers, German shepherds, and Labrador retrievers are overrepresented.
3. Seen in high-strung or bored adult animals. Often a sudden environmental change (death in the family, new baby, etc.) will precipitate the behavior.
4. Characterized by a single, focal, alopecic, nodular plaque that is usually located on the anterior surface of the carpus or metacarpus.
5. Caused by the constant licking of the site, leading to erosion and finally, thickening of the skin. Pruritus is usually severe.
6. Rule out neoplasia, allergic disease (atopy, FAD, food), deep bacterial infection, dermatophytosis, subcutaneous mycosis, osteomyelitis, foreign body reaction, meta-

bolic/endocrine disease, and psychogenic causes.
7. The diagnostic plan should include a CBC, chemistry profile, skin scraping, dermatophyte culture, biopsy, and radiographs. This tends to be a diagnosis of exclusion.
8. Treatment
   A. Identify and treat the underlying problem.
   B. Change the environment or modify the animal's behavior.
      1) Phenobarbital, 2.2 to 6.6 mg/kg q12h
      2) Tranquilizers may be helpful when a stressful situation is anticipated.
      3) Megestrol acetate (Ovaban) 1 mg/kg PO q24h. Do not use in intact females.
      4) Naltrexone (Trexan [DuPont Pharmaceuticals] an endorphin blocker), 2.2 mg/kg orally q24h
   C. Topical corticosteroid and antibiotic preparations have had variable, but generally poor, results.
   D. Systemic antibiotics are required if a deep infection is present and should be used for a minimum of six to eight weeks.
   E. Surgical removal, cryosurgery, and radiation therapy have all yielded variable results.

Blistering/Ulcerative Dermatoses

Diseases in this category include syndromes whose primary lesions range from papular and pustular to those with an erosive to ulcerative appearance. Again, a thorough history, including previous drug therapy and response, a complete physical examination, as well as the performance of carefully selected diagnostic tests provide the best route to identifying the cause and formulating a sound therapeutic plan (Fig. 15-2).

Eosinophilic Granuloma Complex

Eosinophilic granuloma complex is probably a misnomer for a group of diseases that frequently are not characterized by eosinophils and histologically may not be granulomas.

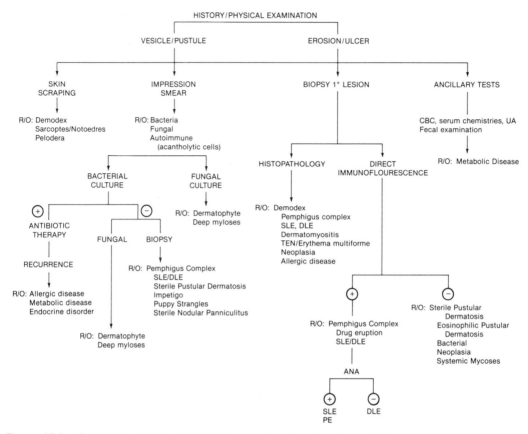

Figure 15-2. *Diagnostic algorithm for blistering or ulcerative dermatoses.* SLE, *systemic lupus erythematosus;* DLE, *discoid lupus erythematosus;* TEN, *toxic epidermal necrolysis;* DTM, *dermatophyte test media;* UA, *urinalysis;* STAPH, *staphylococcus;* T_4; *thyroxine;* TSH, *thyroid-stimulating hormone.*

Although a group of specific pathogen-free cats with a high incidence of eosinophilic granuloma were studied and revealed evidence to support a heritable mode of transmission for these presentations, the etiology of this syndrome remains elusive. As with miliary dermatitis, presentations that fall within the eosinophilic granuloma complex of diseases usually reflect a cutaneous response to some underlying primary problem. It is important to investigate the possibilities and attempt to treat the primary problem, rather than sentence the cat to a lifetime of systemic corticosteroids without alternatives.

Feline Indolent Ulcer (Lip Ulcer, Rodent Ulcer)

Clinical Signs

1. Raised, red, glistening, alopecic lesions on the upper lip or in the oral cavity of cats
2. There is no age or breed predilection, but female cats may be overrepresented.
3. Strong evidence exists that suggests that many of these ulcers are a manifestation of a hypersensitivity response (atopy, food allergy, flea allergy).
4. Some of these lesions may be precancerous (e.g., squamous cell carcinoma).

5. Differential diagnoses should include infectious (bacterial, fungal, FeLV- or FIV-associated viral diseases), neoplasia (mast cell, squamous cell carcinoma, melanoma, and cutaneous lymphoma), metabolic disorders (diabetes mellitus, renal disease), and psychogenic or traumatic causes.

Diagnosis

1. Biopsy usually reveals a hyperplastic or ulcerated epidermis, mononuclear perivascular dermatitis, and dermal fibrosis. Tissue eosinophilia generally does not occur.

2. A history of a chronic or seasonally recurring problem that is responsive to glucocorticoids should prompt diagnostic testing for allergic disease.

3. Response to flea control, hypoallergenic diet, intradermal allergy test

Treatment

1. First, try to identify and treat the underlying cause (e.g., flea control, hypoallergenic diet).

2. Prednisone or prednisolone (1.1 to 2.2 mg/kg q24h or divided q12h) or methylprednisolone (Depo-Medrol) (20 mg/cat every two weeks for three treatments) is often effective in controlling lesions.

3. Progestational compounds (e.g., megestrol acetate) are *not* recommended because of the severity of their potential side effects.

4. Immunomodulation (oral levamisole, mixed bacterial vaccine) has been tried on a limited basis. These drugs have not been approved for use in the cat.

5. Other methods of therapy include irradiation, cryosurgery, chrysotherapy (goldsalts), excision, and laser treatments. The response has been variable.

Feline Eosinophilic Plaque

Clinical Signs

1. Common; often associated with allergic disease

2. There is no age or breed predisposition; females may be overrepresented.

3. The most common sites of occurrence

are the medial thigh, ventral abdomen, and oral cavity. Lesions also occasionally affect the ear tips and foot pads.

4. Oral and cutaneous lesions are circumscribed, moist, red, raised, alopecic, and often, ulcerated.

5. With cutaneous lesions, pruritus is generally intense.

6. The differential diagnoses are the same as for the lip ulcers discussed earlier.

Diagnosis

1. Histologic evaluation reveals a hyperplastic superficial, and deep perivascular eosinophilic dermatitis with or without eosinophilic microabscessation

2. CBC frequently reveals a circulating blood eosinophilia.

3. Cat skin normally responds to an allergen with a large number of tissue mast cells. Have biopsy samples examined by a reliable veterinary histopathologist to avoid the false diagnosis of cutaneous mastocytosis or neoplasia.

Treatment

1. Same as for indolent ulcer

Feline Eosinophilic Granuloma (Linear Granuloma)

Clinical Signs

1. Common cutaneous and oral mucosal lesion seen in cats. Many affected cats are younger than one year of age. There is no breed or sex predilection.

2. On the caudal thigh, the lesions are raised, firm, nodular plaques that often take on a linear configuration and are usually nonpruritic and nonulcerated.

3. In the oral cavity and on the face, these lesions take on a papular configuration.

4. Chin granulomas present as a "fat chin and lip" syndrome as a result of the asymptomatic swelling that occurs.

Diagnosis

1. Clinical presentation

2. Biopsy. Histologic examination reveals

that these are true collagenolytic granulomas. Biopsy reveals nodular to diffuse granulomatous dermatitis with collagen degeneration. Eosinophils and multinucleated giant cells may also be seen.

3. The differential diagnoses for the oral and face lesions are the same as for the eosinophilic plaque and lip ulcer.

Treatment

1. As for the eosinophilic plaque and lip ulcers.

2. Benign neglect for the caudal thigh linear granuloma is an appropriate approach. May spontaneously regress.

Feline Plasma Cell Pododermatitis

Clinical Signs

1. No age, breed, or sex predilection

2. Mild to severe swelling of multiple footpads on multiple feet

3. The pads may or may not be painful.

4. The plantar surfaces of the pads may demonstrate a scaly dermatitis to severe hyperkeratosis (hard pads). Progression may lead to ulceration.

5. Cats may present with associated lameness or lymphadenopathy.

6. Some cats will have concurrent plasma cell stomatitis.

7. Historically, the problem may wax and wane, or may have a seasonal pattern.

Diagnosis

1. Clinical presentation

2. Fine-needle aspirate and cytologic examination reveals a large number of plasma cells and low numbers of lymphocytes and neutrophils.

3. Biopsy reveals a superficial to deep perivascular to nodular plasma cell dermatitis.

4. Fungal and bacterial cultures of tissue yield negative results.

5. As with the two preceding dermatopathies, plasma cell pododermatitis may be a manifestation of an underlying immunologic abnormality. Rule out fungal, bacterial, neoplastic (mast cell, squamous cell), allergic (food, atopy, flea, mosquito), and autoimmune disease (pemphigus foliaceus, SLE).

6. Strongly consider a contact irritant or allergen (carpet cleaner/deodorizer, perfumed cat litter, grass fertilizer, etc.).

7. May be idiopathic

Treatment

1. Identify and eliminate or treat the underlying cause.

2. Immunosuppressive doses (prednisolone, 2 to 4 mg/kg/d) of systemic glucocorticoids may be required for animals with idiopathic presentations. This is gradually tapered to an alternate-day dose.

3. Chrysotherapy (aurothioglucose; sodium thiosulfate)—1 mg IM at week one, 2 mg IM at week two, then 1 mg/kg IM weekly for six to eight weeks or until clinical signs abate. The maintenance dose is 1 mg/kg IM every other week. Rare side effects in cats include anemia, neutropenia, glomerulonephritis, and toxicepidermal necrolysis (TEN) therefore, a biweekly CBC and urinalysis are suggested during induction.

Canine Eosinophilic Granuloma

Clinical Signs

1. Affects male dogs older than three years of age. Siberian Huskies are overrepresented.

2. Palatine ulcers and plaques, as well as lingual vegetative masses, are the primary clinical presentations.

3. Nonpruritic papular eruptions and plaques on the ventral abdomen and flanks occur less commonly.

4. The etiology is unknown. Rule out bacterial or fungal disease, as well as neoplasms (mast cell tumor, squamous cell carcinoma, melanoma, or cutaneous lymphoma).

Diagnosis

1. Biopsy reveals a granulomatous dermatitis with foci of collagen degeneration and diffuse, eosinophilic, cellular infiltration.

Treatment

1. Canine eosinophilic granuloma is extremely responsive to glucocorticoids (0.5 to 2.2 mg/kg/d).

2. The lesions regress spontaneously in some animals.

Pemphigus Complex

The pemphigus complex is a group of rare blistering autoimmune skin diseases that may also affect the mucous membranes and mucocutaneous junctions in dogs and cats. The deposition of autoantibody in the desmosomes between keratinocytes results in proteolysis of the intercellular cement. Subsequent separation of keratinocytes leads to vesicle and bullae formation and the development of acantholytic cells. Because of the thinness of canine and feline epidermis, the primary vesicles/bullae are transient, resulting in predominantly pustules, crusts, and ulcers on clinical presentation.

Pemphigus Vulgaris

Clinical Signs

1. Occurs in both dogs and cats without age, breed, or sex predisposition
2. Ulcers may affect the oral cavity and any mucocutaneous junction (eyes, lips, nares, vulva, prepuce, anus). Ulcerative or erosive lesions may occur alone or in conjunction with cutaneous lesions. Cutaneous lesions occur primarily in the groin and axilla, but may be diffuse.

Diagnosis

1. Diagnostic plan
   A. CBC, chemistry profile, urinalysis
   B. Impression smear of the contents of an intact pustule to determine the presence or absence of neutrophils (PMNs), eosinophils, and acantholytic cells
   C. Biopsy
      1) Histopathologic examination of a biopsy specimen from an intact vesicle or pustule reveals *suprabasilar cleft formation* with acantholytic cells. Basal cells remain attached to the basement membrane zone (BMZ), giving the appearance of "a row of tombstones."
      2) Direct IFA of a sample obtained from biopsy of the skin adjacent to a primary lesion (vesicle or pustule). The pattern of immunofluorescence is intercellular.
2. The differential diagnoses include bullous pemphigoid, SLE, TEN, drug eruption, necrolytic migratory erythema (diabetes dermatopathy) and causes of ulcerative stomatitis (FeLV, FIV, candidiasis, uremia, spirochetes).

Treatment

1. Glucocorticoids (prednisone; prednisolone)
   A. Immunosuppressive doses (2.2 to 4.4 mg/kg q12h in the dog; 4.4 to 6.6 mg/kg q12h in the cat) for the first two weeks, then half that dosage every 10 to 14 days until a very low (0.55 mg/kg/d) alternate-day dose is achieved. Corticosteroids alone rarely control the disease.
   B. Associated side effects include iatrogenic hyperglucocorticoidism, acute pancreatitis, hepatopathy, polyuria, polydipsia, polyphagia, weight loss or gain, muscle weakness, diarrhea, and an increased susceptibility to infections.
   C. Serum biochemical studies may demonstrate a fivefold to tenfold elevation in ALT and alkaline phosphatase. These values are a result of the chemotherapy, are not usually associated with patient morbidity, and tend to return toward normal after six to eight weeks of therapy. Monitor bi-weekly.
   D. Reducing the dose too rapidly or discontinuing therapy prematurely may result in a relapse.
2. Azathioprine (Imuran)—2.2 mg/kg orally every other day.
   A. Used in conjunction with prednisone in dogs; Allows reduction in or discontinuation of prednisone.
   B. Obtain a CBC weekly during induction (first six weeks) to screen for leukopenia and thrombocytopenia. This drug reaction may be fatal and warrants immediate discontinuation and initiation of broad spectrum antibiotics.
   C. Metabolized by the liver; causes elevation in ALT and alkaline phosphatase. These parameters should be monitored, but therapy should not be discontinued unless an elevation in enzymes correlates with clinical illness.
   D. Cats are very susceptable to the toxic side effects, therefore it should *not* be used in this species.
3. Chrysotherapy (aurothioglucose

[Solganal]; gold sodium thiomalate [Myochrisine])

A. Gold salts are used in conjunction with corticosteroids. Two test doses are given a week apart prior to initiating therapeutic doses. (Dogs weighing less than 10 kg and cats: 1 mg IM first week; 2 mg IM second week. Dogs weighing more than 10 kg: 5 mg IM first week; 10 mg IM second week)

B. The therapeutic dose is 1 mg/kg/week until the disease is controlled. The dose is reduced to biweekly administration for three treatments, then monthly dosing for maintenance. Six to 12 weeks will elapse before resolution of signs is seen.

C. This is the adjunctive therapy of choice for cats, as toxicity is rarely seen. Blood dyscrasias (anemia, thrombocytopenia, leukopenia) may occur.

D. TEN reactions have been reported in dogs. To avoid an increased risk of toxicity, do not use shortly after or along with cytotoxic drugs (azathioprine, cyclophosphamide, etc.).

Pemphigus Vegetans

1. Benign variant of pemphigus vulgaris that is rarely reported
2. Characterized by verrucous or vegetative hyperkeratosis of the skin
3. Histologic characteristics include epidermal hyperplasia and eosinophilic microabscessation.
4. Rule out bacterial, fungal, and neoplastic (e.g., cutaneous lymphosarcoma) causes.
5. The treatment is the same as for pemphigus vulgaris.

Pemphigus Foliaceus

1. The most common form of the pemphigus complex
2. Affects dogs and cats with no age or sex predilection
3. Akitas, chow chows, and collies are predisposed to this disease.

Clinical Signs

1. Presents as vesiculobullous eruptions that may be diffuse in distribution
2. The primary lesions are fragile; conse-

quently, the most common presentation is an exfoliative dermatitis.
3. Erosions at the mucocutaneous junctions occur infrequently. Oral lesions are rare. Hyperkeratotic footpads occur frequently in dogs and cats and may be the only presenting problem.
4. Head and neck pruritus with erosive dermatitis is a common presentation in cats.
5. Secondary pyodermas are common.

Diagnosis

1. Differential diagnoses include bacterial folliculitis, dermatophytosis, zinc-responsive dermatosis, necrolytic migratory erythema (older dogs), and dermatomyositis (young dogs).
2. Diagnostic plan
    A. An impression smear reveals PMNs, possible eosinophils, and acantholytic cells.
    B. Biopsy
        1) Histopathologic examination reveals *intragranular to subcorneal vesicles* with acantholytic cells and eosinophilic microabscessation in the outer root sheath of hair follicles.
        2) IFA—intercellular fluorescence

Treatment

1. Treatment is the same as for pemphigus vulgaris.

Pemphigus Erythematosus

Clinical Signs

1. Benign variant of pemphigus foliaceus, may be a crossover disease with SLE.
2. Reported in dogs and cats. German shepherds, collies, and Akitas may be predisposed to development of the disease.
3. This vesiculopustular disease tends to be confined to the face and ears.
4. Depigmentation and ulceration of the nasal planum and nares is common. Oral ulceration is rare.
5. Sunlight and stress may precipitate or exacerbate the condition.

Diagnosis

1. Diagnostic testing is the same as for pemphigus foliaceus.

A. IFA—positive intercellular fluorescence and at the BMZ.
B. Frequently ANA-positive.

Treatment

1. The treatment approach is the same as for pemphigus foliaceus. Lesions confined to the nose and face can often be managed with topical corticosteroids and waterproof sunscreen (SPF-15 or greater), applied frequently when sun exposure is anticipated.
2. The differential diagnoses are the same as for pemphigus foliaceus.

Bullous Pemphigoid

Clinical Signs

1. No age or sex predilection
2. Collies and Doberman pinschers may be predisposed.
3. Bullous eruptions and ulcers commonly occur at mucocutaneous junctions, in the oral cavity, and skin (especially the axilla and groin). Paronychia and footpad ulceration may also be seen.
4. Secondary problems include anorexia, fever, and infections.

Diagnosis

1. Diagnostic plan
   A. Impression smear—inflammatory cells without acantholytic cells.
   B. Biopsy should be performed on primary eruptions, if possible, or on perilesional skin.
      1) Histopathologic examination reveals intact vesicles without acantholysis, as well as a lichenoid band of inflammation at the dermoepidermal junction.
      2) IFA reveals linear fluorescence at the BMZ.
2. Differential diagnoses include pemphigus vulgaris, SLE, TEN, drug eruption, lymphoreticular neoplasia, and causes of ulcerative stomatitis.

Treatment

1. The treatment approach is the same as for pemphigus vulgaris. Combination immunotherapy (i.e., prednisone and azathioprine) provides the most satisfactory results. This condition may require a lifetime of therapy. Sunlight may exacerbate the problem.

Systemic Lupus Erythematosus

Clinical Signs

1. Multisystemic autoimmune disorder affecting dogs and cats
2. No age or sex predilection. Collies, shelties, and German shepherds are predisposed.
3. The etiology is multifactorial (viral, genetic, immune-related, idiopathic) and the disease can be triggered by a variety of factors (drugs, vaccinations, sunlight).
4. Clinical presentation
   A. Cutaneous lesions may include vesiculobullous to erosive dermatitis, mucocutaneous and oral ulceration, paronychia, pododermatitis and footpad ulceration. Lesions may be pruritic or painful.
   B. Animals frequently are systemically ill (fever, anorexia, depression).
   C. One or more other systems are usually involved, as may be reflected by anemia and thrombocytopenia (hematopoietic), proteinuria (renal), polyarthritis, polymyositis, diffuse lymphadenopathy, and splenomegaly.

Diagnosis

1. The diagnostic plan is the same as for other autoimmune diseases. Because the disease presentation is so variable, diagnostic test results also vary depending on which organ systems are involved. An ANA and lupus erythematosus cell preparation test (LE prep—steroid-labile) may be positive and will confirm the diagnosis. Laboratories vary in their level of sensitivity in performing these tests.
2. The differential diagnoses depend on the specific presenting signs, and may include dermatophytosis, demodicosis, bullous pemphigoid, pemphigus complex, lymphoreticular neoplasia, allergic disease (food, atopy), and bacterial folliculitis.
3. The dermatohistopathologic changes most frequently seen include a lichenoid or interface dermatitis (a mononuclear dermal inflammatory cell infiltrate that hugs the dermoepidermal junction) that involves the outer root sheath of hair follicles; hydropic

degeneration of basal cells; and thickening of the BMZ.

4. IFA reveals a positive "lupus band" at the BMZ.

Treatment

1. The treatment approach is chosen to fit the presenting set of problems, but includes immunomodulating drugs (see the section on pemphigus vulgaris). Chrysotherapy is typically not helpful with this variant. The prognosis is variable and is dependent on the severity of the disease and the organ systems involved.

Discoid Lupus Erythematosus (DLE)

1. Benign variant of SLE in which systemic involvement is absent

2. No age predilection

3. German shepherds, shelties, Siberian huskies, and Akitas are overrepresented.

4. Clinical features include nasal planum erythema, depigmentation, erosion, ulceration, and crusting. Occasionally, periocular areas, ear margins, lip margins, and the oral cavity may also be involved. Sunlight exacerbates the condition.

5. Histologic findings are characterized by an interface dermatitis and ballooning degeneration of basal epidermal cells.

6. IFA results are positive at the BMZ.

7. Treatment

    A. Daily application of waterproof sunscreens and sun avoidance

    B. Topical glucocorticoids

    C. Vitamin E, 400 to 800 IU orally q12h

    D. Immunosuppressive doses of glucocorticoids q24h–48h

Scaling Dermatoses

Dermatoses manifested clinically by excess scale formation and histologically by abnormalities of the epidermis can be characterized as keratinization disorders (Table 15-2). These disorders may be associated with the skin, keratinizing portions of the hair follicle, and the hair itself. Clinical signs associated with keratinization disorders include dry, waxy, or greasy scaling, and comedones or follicular casts. Secondary problems occur frequently and include inflammation, alopecia, crusts, pruritus, and pyoderma. Unfortunately, the term seborrhea is used as a descriptive term for any dermatosis manifested clinically by dry or greasy scaling. The term "seborrhea" should be reserved for primary idiopathic keratinization defects and idiopathic abnormalities in the production of epidermal or sebaceous lipids (Table 15-3).

Table 15-2. **Breed-related keratinization disorders**

Disorder	*Breed*
Primary idiopathic seborrhea	Cocker spaniel, springer spaniel, Labrador retriever, Irish setter, basset hound, Doberman pinscher, West Highland white terrier
Follicular dystrophy	Doberman pinscher
Vitamin A-responsive dermatosis	Cocker spaniel, others
Zinc-responsive dermatosis	Alaskan Malamute, Siberian huskie
Sebaceous adenitis	Vizsla, akita, Samoyed, standard poodle
Comedo syndrome	Miniature schnauzer
Ear margin dermatosis	Dachshund
Acne	Short-coated breeds in dogs; cats
Epidermal dysplasia	West Highland white terrier
Ichthyosis	Terrier breeds

Table 15-3. **Primary idiopathic seborrhea—breed presentations**

Breed	Type	Distribution	Conditions to Be Ruled Out
Cocker spaniel	Greasy	Lips, ears, periocular areas, ventral cervical and ventral trunk regions, tail, interdigital skin	Dermatophyte Demodicosis Folliculitis Hypothyroidism Vitamin A-responsive dermatosis
Irish setter	Dry	Diffuse scale with sparse, dry hair coat	As above, plus allergic dermatosis
Basset hound	Greasy	Legs, feet, skin folds, ventral cervical region	As above, plus allergic dermatosis
Doberman pinscher	Dry/waxy	Trunk	As above, plus color-mutant alopecia
Labrador retriever	Dry with intense pruritus	Face, ears, ventral trunk, lateral thigh, distal extremities	As above, plus scabies, allergic dermatosis
West Highland white terrier	Greasy with hyperpigmentation and lichenification	Periocular areas, ventral trunk, distal extremities	As above, plus allergic dermatosis and epidermal dysplasia

Clinical Approach

Signalment

1. Age

A. Young animals—hereditary disorders (idiopathic seborrhea, epidermal dysplasia, ichthyosis). Rule out infectious or parasitic causes.

B. Middle aged animals—Rule out primary causes of secondary scaling (endocrinopathies, allergies, autoimmune diseases).

C. Older animals (>9 years)—Rule out cutaneous neoplasms and endocrinopathies.

2. Sex—sex-hormone–related keratinization disorders

3. Breed—primary keratinization disorders (primary idiopathic seborrhea, follicular dystrophy, epidermal dysplasia, ichthyosis, vitamin A- and zinc-responsive dermatoses, sebaceous adenitis, comedo syndrome, ear margin dermatoses, acne).

History

1. Provides the most important information for diagnosis

2. Determine the following:

A. Exposure to other animals—parasitic conditions or dermatophytosis

B. Diet—deficiencies

C. Seasonal pruritus—flea allergy or inhalant allergy

D. Systemic signs (polyuria/polydypsia [PU/PD], lethargy, abnormal estrus cycles, etc.) suggest endocrinopathies.

E. Response to previous therapy

Physical Examination

1. Focal, multifocal, or diffuse; dry, waxy, or greasy scaling dermatoses

2. Inflammation may be moderate to severe.

3. Erythematous plaques covered by thick, yellow scales and crusts

4. Secondary pyoderma, comedones, follicular casts, alopecia, and ceruminous otitis externa are concurrent findings.

Diagnostic Techniques

1. Skin scrapings (mineral oil and KOH) should be performed in every case to rule out parasitic and infectious causes (Fig. 15-3).

2. Dermatophyte culture

Diagnostic Algorithm - Scales and Crusts

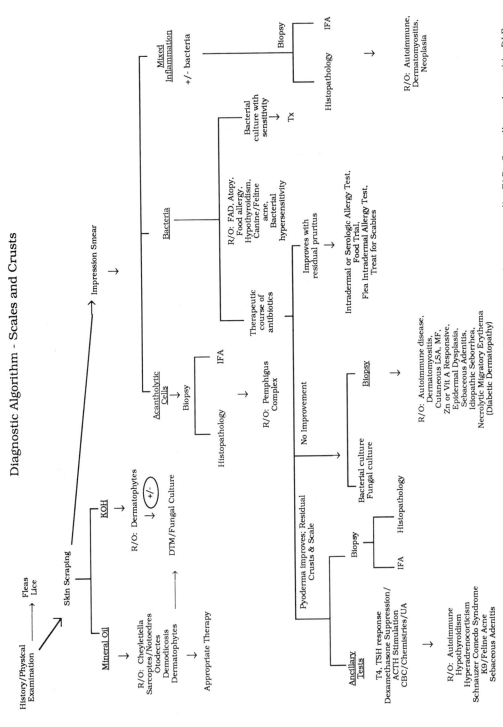

Figure 15-3. *Diagnostic algorithm for scales and crusts. R/O, rule out; DTM, dermatophyte test media; FAD, flea allergy dermatitis; DLE, discoid lupus erythematosus; SLE, systemic lupus erythematosus; Cut. LSA, Cutaneous lymphosarcoma; MF, Mycosis fungoides; IFA, direct immunofluorescent assay; T₄, L-thyroxine; TSH, thyroid-stimulating hormone; ACTH, adrenocorticotropic hormone; UA, urinalysis; Zn, zinc; Vit A, vitamin A; TEN, toxic epidermal necrolysis.*

3. Intradermal, RAST, or ELISA allergy tests
4. Elimination diet
5. Hormone assays, serum biochemistries, fecal parasite and fat examination
6. Bacterial culture
7. Vitamin or mineral supplementation
8. Skin biopsy—probably the most important diagnostic tool for primary disorders

Treatment

1. Directed at identifying the primary cause, normalizing the excessive scaling, and controlling the secondary problems.
2. Primary keratinization disorders are controlled, not cured.
   A. Greasy scale
     1) High-concentration tar-sulfur-salicylic acid shampoos (Lytar [DVM]; Allerseb-T [Allerderm/Virbac]), alternated with benzoyl peroxide shampoos (Pyoben [Allerderm/Virbac]; OxyDex [DVM]). When these do not work, selenium sulfide shampoos (Selsun Blue [Abbott]; Selenium Sulfide Shampoo [Vet-Kem]) may be helpful.
     2) Low-dose, alternate-day prednisone or prednisolone may be administered for severe, erythematous, pruritic, seborrheic dermatitis.
     3) Antibiotics are prescribed for secondary pyoderma.
     4) A balanced diet is important; essential fatty acid supplements may help.
     5) The synthetic retinoids isotretinoin (13-*cis*-retinoic acid, Accutane [Roche]) and etretinate (Tegison [Roche]), 1 mg/kg every 12 to 24 hours, have been utilized with variable results. These drugs are very expensive, but when they work, they are very effective.
   B. Dry scale
     1) Sulfur-salicylic acid shampoos (SebaLyt [DVM]; Sebbafon [Winthrop]; Sebolux [Allerderm/Virbac]), moisturizing hypoallergenic shampoos (Allergroom [Allerderm/Virbac]; HyLyt [DVM]) and frequent emollient bath oil rinses (Alpha Keri [Westwood]; Hylyt-EFA [DVM]; Humilac [Allerderm/Virbac])
   C. Benzoyl peroxide shampoos, although drying, are helpful for severe folliculitis and comedones.
   D. Treat primary problems.

Vitamin A-Responsive Dermatosis

1. Rare, nutritionally responsive dermatosis
2. Clinical signs include generalized scaling, dry hair coat with easy epilation, ceruminous otitis externa, prominent comedones, and hyperkeratotic plaques.
3. Diagnosis is based on biopsy findings of marked follicular keratosis without comparable epidermal (nonfollicular) hyperkeratosis.
4. The diagnosis is confirmed by response to therapy.
   A. Vitamin A alcohol (Aquasol-A [Armour]), 10,000 IU orally q24h
   B. Improvement is seen within four to six weeks.
   C. Therapy is continued for life.

Zinc-Responsive Dermatosis

1. Rare, nutritionally responsive dermatosis
2. Two clinical syndromes
   A. Zinc-responsive dermatosis of Siberian huskies and Alaskan malamutes; also seen in Doberman pinschers and Great Danes
     1) Lesions develop before puberty.
     2) Alopecia, erythema, crusting, and scaling involving the face, head, scrotum, and legs, with hyperkeratotic footpads
     3) May be precipitated by stress, estrus, GI disorders affecting absorption, high-calcium diets, and diets high in phytates
     4) Malamutes have a genetic defect affecting zinc absorption from the intestine.
   B. Zinc-responsive dermatosis of rapidly growing puppies
     1) Seen with zinc-deficient diets and/or oversupplementation with vitamins and minerals, especially calcium
     2) Great Danes, Doberman pinschers, beagles, German sheperds, German short-haired pointers, Labrador retrievers, and Rhodesian ridgebacks are commonly affected.
     3) In addition to the crusting and scaling, these dogs exhibit secondary infections, lymphadenopathy, depression, and anorexia.
   C. Generic dog food dermatosis may also represent a zinc deficiency.

3. Diagnosis

    A. Based on dietary history, physical examination, and biopsy

    B. Skin biopsy reveals a marked, diffuse, and follicular parakeratotic hyperkeratosis.

4. Treatment

    A. Zinc sulfate or zinc gluconate, 10 mg/kg administered orally every 12 to 24 hours with food

    B. Zinc methionine, 1.7 mg/kg q24h orally

    C. Correct dietary imbalances; provide good quality dog food.

    D. Lifetime therapy is required in huskies and malamutes.

Epidermal Dysplasia of West Highland White Terriers

1. Also called Armadillo disease and idiopathic seborrhea of West Highland white terriers

Clinical Signs

1. Heritable keratinization disorder characterized by erythema and pruritus of the ventrum and extremities in young Westies of either sex

2. Rapidly progresses to a generalized disorder with severe pruritus and erythema, alopecia, hyperpigmentation, lichenification, lymphadenopathy, greasiness, and malodor

Diagnosis

1. Biopsy reveals hyperplastic perivascular dermatitis, excessive keratinocyte mitosis, crowding of basilar keratinocytes, epidermal buds, and parakeratosis.

2. Often accompanied by a Malassezia dermatitis, which may be confirmed by microscopic examination of a skin swab or histopathologically.

3. Differential diagnoses should include atopy, FAD, scabies, and ichthyosis.

Treatment

1. Poorly responsive to medical therapy

2. Management includes antibiotics for secondary pyodermas, systemic glucocorticoids, and topical antiseborrheic therapy with high-concentration tar and benzoyl peroxide shampoos once to twice a week.

3. Ketoconazole (10 mg/kg, qizh) may be used for the yeast infection.

Sebaceous Adenitis

Clinical Signs

1. Affects young to middle-aged dogs

2. Any breed may be affected, but vizslas, akitas, Samoyeds, and standard poodles appear to be overrepresented.

3. Lesions in short-coated breeds are characterized by circular, expanding areas of trunkal scaling and alopecia which may coalesce, dry hair coat and hypotrichosis, and recurrent secondary bacterial folliculitis.

4. Long-coated breeds develop a severe, dry to greasy crusting and scaling dermatosis with progressive thinning of the haircoat. Recurrent pyodermas are common.

Diagnosis

1. Biopsy reveals granulomatous destruction of the sebaceous glands (early), multinodular or diffuse granulomatous inflammation (later), or complete absence of the sebaceous glands (latest).

2. Differential diagnoses include demodicosis, dermatophytosis, bacterial folliculitis, hypothyroidism, and idiopathic seborrhea.

Treatment

1. Prednisone or prednisolone, 2.2 to 4.4 mg/kg orally q24h, then q48h as needed.

2. Isotretinoin (13-*cis*-retinoic acid, Accutane [Roche]), 1 mg/kg orally every 12 to 24 hours. This drug is expensive.

3. Cyclosporin A (Sandimmune [Sandoz]), 10 mg/kg orally q12h. This drug is also expensive.

4. Symptomatic therapy with antiseborrheic agents and emollient bath oil rinses

5. Topical 75% propylene glycol with 25% Humilac Spray [Allerderm/Virbac]

6. The prognosis is poor unless the condition is diagnosed and treated early.

Schnauzer Comedo Syndrome

Clinical Signs

1. Inherited defect of miniature schnauzers characterized by multiple comedones along the dorsum

2. Pustule formation with secondary bacterial folliculitis

3. Pain and/or pruritus may accompany the infection.

Diagnosis

1. Gross observation of follicular comedones

2. Biopsy reveals dilated hair follicles filled with keratinous debris, dilated or cystic sebaceous or apocrine glands, folliculitis, perifolliculitis, and furunculosis.

3. Differential diagnoses include demodicosis, dermatophytosis, and bacterial folliculitis.

Treatment

1. Benzoyl peroxide shampoos or gels, as needed, to flush follicles and control secondary bacterial folliculitis

2. If there is no response to topical therapy, isotretinoin (13-*cis*-retinoic acid, Accutane [Roche]), 1 to 2 mg/kg orally q24h has proven to be effective, but is expensive.

Idiopathic Nasodigital Hyperkeratosis

1. Nasal hyperkeratosis, digital hyperkeratosis, or a combination of the two may be seen at any age and in any breed.

2. Dry, focal to diffuse pattern of hyperkeratosis accompanied by fissures, erosions, or ulcers

3. Differential diagnoses include distemper, ichthyosis, pemphigus foliaceous or erythematosus, DLE, SLE, zinc-responsive dermatosis, and necrolytic migratory erythema (diabetic dermatosis; hepatocutaneous syndrome).

4. Treatment

    A. Surgical removal of excessive hyperkeratotic scale

    B. Hydration of the hyperkeratotic tissue by water soakings or dressings, followed by application of petrolatum jelly to help seal in the moisture.

    C. KeraSolv Gel [DVM]

    D. Retin-A [Ortho]

    E. Corticosteroid-antibiotic ointments, creams, or gels

Canine Ear Margin Dermatosis

1. Affects only the pinna of the ear; occurs primarily in dachshunds.

2. Greasy plugs of keratinaceous debris adhere tightly to the skin surface and hair shafts of the pinnal margins.

3. May progress to severe inflammation, ulceration, and thrombosis of the capillaries supplying the ear margins

4. Biopsy reveals hyperkeratosis and parakeratosis.

5. Treatment includes frequent keratolytic shampoos and topical glucocorticoid creams.

6. Advanced cases may require cosmetic surgical correction of permanently damaged ear margins.

Canine/Feline Acne

1. Common follicular keratinization disorder resulting in secondary bacterial folliculitis, furunculosis, comedo formation, and pustules involving the chin, lips, and muzzle.

2. Common in short-coated breeds, such as English bulldogs, boxers, Great Danes, and Doberman pinschers; also seen in cats

3. Differential diagnoses include demodicosis, dermatophytosis, and bacterial folliculitis.

4. Treatment includes benzoyl peroxide shampoos or gel, a systemic antibiotic if needed, and warm soaks and hot packs. A short course of glucocorticoids may help to reduce inflammation.

Dermatophytosis

Clinical Signs

1. Affects dogs and cats of all ages, but especially puppies and kittens

2. Persian and Himalayan cats are overrepresented.

3. The common species affecting dogs and cats are *Microsporum canis, M. gypsum,* and *Trichophyton mentagrophytes.* In cats, 98% of the infections are caused by *M. canis.* Transmission is by direct contact with spores.

4. The classic presentation is a focal, circular area of alopecia with mild scale. The lesions typically appear to spread centripetally as healing occurs centrally. Often, several animals or people in the environment are affected.

5. Little or no inflammation or pruritus is seen with *M. canis,* whereas *T. mentagrophytes* and *M. gypsum* usually produce moderate pruritus and inflammation.

6. Differential diagnoses include bacterial folliculitis, demodicosis, seborrheic dermatitis, sebaceous adenitis, black hair follicle dysplasia, and color mutant alopecia.

Diagnosis

1. Wood's light examination—Only *M. canis* fluoresces, and then only 50% of the time.

2. Skin scraping and KOH preparation for microscopic examination—Findings are variable and dependant on the examiner's experience.

3. Carefully chosen hair and debris should be cultured using Sabouraud's dextrose agar or DTM.

A. Make sure hair and debris are embedded in the surface of the test media.

B. Be sure to keep DTM at room temperature, read plates daily for 10 days, and examine suspected colony growth microscopically, utilizing lactophenol cotton blue mounting media.

C. The MacKenzie brush technique (p 15-5) is an excellent means of collecting samples from a multiple-cat household, or when an asymptomatic carrier is suspected.

D. Biopsy and histopathologic examination—Examine samples for ectothrix spores and hyphae in hair follicles.

Treatment

1. Solitary lesions

A. Often self-limiting and may resolve without therapy within four to six weeks.

B. Miconazole (Conofite [Pitman Moore]) or clotrimazole (Lotrimin [Shering]), applied twice daily to focal lesions, may facilitate their resolution. Clip hair from around the lesion(s) first.

2. Generalized dermatophytosis—topical therapy

A. Whole body clips may be required to remove infected hair.

B. Lime sulfur (Lym-Dyp [DVM]; 2% to 4% solution q5d), povidone iodine solution (Betadine; 1:4 in water, daily), or chlorhexadine (Nolvasan shampoo [Fort Dodge]; q5d) are appropriate topical treatments. They should be used in conjunction with systemic therapy.

3. Systemic therapy

A. Griseofulvin (microsize formulation—Fulvicin U/F [Shering]), 60 to 120 mg/kg/d (cats) 25–60 mg/kg/d (dogs) in divided doses given twice a day with a fatty meal.

1) May cause a potentially fatal idiosyncratic bone marrow suppression syndrome in cats. Does not appear to be dose- or time-dependent. This reaction not been reported in the dog.

2) Monitor CBCs weekly for anemia, leukopenia, and/or thrombocytopenia.

3) Treatment involves early identification of toxicity, discontinuation of the griseofulvin, and supportive care (antibiotics and fluid therapy).

4) May also cause GI upset, hepatotoxicity, and drug eruptions; may be teratogenic

B. Ketoconazole

1) A fungistatic imidazole antibiotic that may be as effective as griseofulvin without the bone-marrow suppression. Side effects include anorexia, GI upset, and hepatotoxicity, especially in cats.

2) Dosage: 10 mg/kg q12h

3) Usually reserved for those cases in which the dermatophyte is resistant to, or the patient cannot tolerate, griseofulvin.

C. Prognosis is excellent if systemic therapy is instituted at the correct dose, frequency, and duration.

D. Continue therapy for a minimum of six weeks. Reculture at the end of the therapeutic course. If the culture results are positive, continue systemic therapy two weeks beyond clinical cure and reculture.

4. Environmental considerations

A. Infected hair and epidermal debris in the environment are the primary sources for reinfection.

B. Wash all bedding and the sleeping area with bleach, if possible.

C. Vacuum and steam-clean carpet, furniture, and drapery to remove infected hairs. Change air filters.

D. If the problem is a recurring one, check for asymptomatic carrier animals.

Cutaneous Masses

Cutaneous masses and nodular dermatoses are common dermatologic complaints. The causes are multiple and run the gamut from bacterial furunculosis and sterile granulomas (Table 15-4) to neoplasia. Although skin tumors are the most common presentation (25% to 30%) of all neoplastic processes seen in veterinary medicine, it is often difficult to differentiate inflammatory disease from a neoplastic process, as inflammation can be severe with neoplasia. With severe inflammation, careful examination must be made to determine whether a uniform type of pleomorphic cell population (spindle versus round

Table 15-4. **Differential diagnoses: nonneoplastic nodular or draining wounds in dogs and cats**

Infectious

Bacterial folliculitis/furunculosis
Abscess
Kerion, pseudomycetoma
Atypical mycobacteriosis
Pythiosis (oömycosis), phaeohyphomycosis, zygomycosis
Nocardiosis
Sporotrichosis
Systemic mycosis (cryptococcosis, blastomycosis, histoplasmosis, coccidiodomycosis
Feline leprosy

Parasitic

Demodicosis
Cuterebriasis

Noninfectious

Hematoma
Foreign body
Bullous diseases
Calcinosis cutis
Cutaneous histiocytosis
Idiopathic sterile nodular panniculitis

cell) is present, signaling the presence of a neoplastic process.

A discussion of all the etiologic origins of nodular dermatoses is beyond the scope of this chapter. Detailed information on diagnostic and therapeutic approaches for specific diseases can best be obtained from a comprehensive small animal dermatology or oncology text. However, a good general approach to these lesions will allow an accurate diagnosis to be made, prognosis to be determined, and appropriate therapy to be instituted early in the course of the disease. Effective diagnostic techniques include exfoliative cytologic examination (tissue impression smear, FNA, or smear of exudate) or tissue biopsy. The best and most definitive means of diagnosis is the biopsy.

Diagnostic Approach

Cytologic Examination

1. FNA is a fast, safe, and efficient method of establishing a presumptive diagnosis for cutaneous masses. It requires no anesthesia and minimal equipment. Equipment includes a 22-gauge, one-inch needle; a 10-cc syringe; microscope slides; and a modified Wright's stain, such as Diff-Quik.

2. Slides prepared in this manner should be examined for cell type(s), as well as for the presence of organisms (parasites, bacteria, fungi).

3. Impression smears of an ulcerated surface may be helpful, but most frequently demonstrate a mixed inflammatory or suppurative picture as a result of secondary bacterial infection.

4. Impression smears from the cut surface of a surgical specimen (after blotting to remove blood and fluid) may provide a quick tentative diagnosis while awaiting the histopathologic report.

5. Skin neoplasms are often secondarily inflamed; therefore, the slide should be examined carefully for a uniform population of noninflammatory cells.

6. Once the lesion has been identified as neoplastic, it must then be determined whether it is benign or malignant.

A. Benign tumors are usually slow growing, lack ulceration/inflammation, well circumscribed, and noninfiltrative

B. Malignant tumors are generally fast growing, inflamed and/or ulcerated to necrotic, and infiltrative, with adherence to surrounding tissue

Histologic Examination

1. Biopsy is mandatory for definitive identification of the cause of a skin mass.

2. Samples may be obtained by punch biopsy (4- to 8-mm), excisional, or incisional techniques. All procedures may be performed under local anesthesia if the mass is small.

3. If several types of lesions are present, samples representing the range of lesions should be obtained. At least one sample should include normal skin and must be identified as such for the histopathologist.

4. Surgical excision can be both diagnostic and therapeutic. Wide and deep margins (greater than 1 cm if possible) should be taken.

5. Samples obtained for histologic examination are preserved in 10% formalin. Histologic interpretations should be made by a veterinary pathologist.

Ancillary Diagnostic Tests

1. Bacterial culture and sensitivity of exudate or tissue (obtained aseptically)

2. Fungal culture of exudate or tissue (obtained aseptically)

3. CBC, serum biochemistries, urinalysis

4. ANA, LE cell prep, tissue immunofluorescence

5. Chest and abdominal radiographs

6. FNA of enlarged lymph nodes

Inflammatory Nodular Dermatoses

Cutaneous Histiocytosis

Clinical Signs

1. Benign histiocytic proliferation disorder in dogs. No age, breed, or sex predilection has been reported.

2. Multiple erythematous, raised, firm, nodular masses that are 1 to 5 cm in diameter; may appear anywhere on the body

3. Affected animals are not sick, and no evidence of systemic involvement can be found.

Diagnosis

1. Diagnosis is based on histologic findings, which include dermal to subcutaneous infiltration with normal-appearing histiocytes.

2. Differential diagnoses include malignant histiocytosis, cutaneous lymphoma, fibrous histiocytosis (affecting collies and shelties), mycosis fungoides, and mast cell tumor.

Treatment

1. Treatment with immunosuppressive doses of glucocorticoids has had variable results. Lesions may wax, wane, or spontaneously regress.

Calcinosis Cutis

Clinical Signs

1. Uncommon cutaneous disorder caused by the deposition of mineral salts (primarily calcium) in the skin and subcutis

2. The primary cause is excessive glucocorticoids, either endogenous or iatrogenic.

3. Other proposed causes include chronic inflammatory/infectious disease, neoplasia, metabolic disorders (diabetes mellitus, chronic renal disease), or idiopathic causes (large breeds and young dogs).

4. Cutaneous lesions range from yellowish papules to nodules that are very firm, often ulcerated, frequently infected, and almost always pruritic. Lesions may occur anywhere on the body, but are most frequently seen in the axillae, groin, and dorsum.

Diagnosis

1. Confirmation of the diagnosis is made by histologic examination.

Treatment

1. Therapy is directed at treating the secondary infection with antibiotics. Corticosteroids have no place in the treatment of this syndrome.

2. Correcting the underlying cause will allow the mineral deposits to resolve eventually. This process may take as long as 6 to 12 months.

Panniculitis

Clinical Signs

1. Inflammation of the subcutaneous fat
2. Occurs in both dogs and cats. No age, breed, or sex predilection has been reported.
3. Characterized by solitary to multiple, fluctuant to firm, cutaneous nodules of various sizes. Some nodules will break open to the surface, draining a fatty, purulent material.
4. Lesions tend to occur on the lateral thorax, ventral abdomen, and chest. Healing may result in scarring.

Diagnosis

1. Animals are rarely systemically ill except with idiopathic sterile nodular panniculitis. Patients with this disease may be anorectic, febrile, and lethargic.
2. Diagnosis can only be made through histopathologic examination.
3. FNA of an intact nodule will demonstrate many foamy macrophages and neutrophils. Sudan stain reveals ingested fat in macrophages and neutrophils. Microorganisms are absent. These bench-top tests should prompt the following studies:
  A. Excisional biopsy is mandatory to establish the histologic diagnosis of panniculitis.
  B. Request special stains for higher bacteria and fungal organisms, and polarizing light studies for a suspected foreign body. These tests typically yield negative results.
  C. Bacterial and fungal cultures of tissue and exudate yield negative results.
  D. The results of tissue immunofluorescence (IFA) may be positive or negative.
  E. Other diagnostic tests (CBC, serum biochemistries, urinalysis, blood culture if fever is a factor, ANA, and LE cell prep) are chosen on the basis of the suspected underlying etiology.
4. Differential diagnoses include abscess, neoplasia, deep bacterial dermatoses, deep fungal dermatoses, autoimmune conditions (lupus, drug eruption, vasculitis), foreign body, vitamin E deficiency (pansteatitis), metabolic disorders (pancreatitis), and idiopathic disease (sterile nodular granulomatous dermatitis, puppy strangles).

Treatment

1. Control the primary cause of the condition.
2. Solitary lesions can be excised surgically.
3. Multiple lesions are best treated with immunosuppressive doses of prednisone or prednisolone. The initial dosage is 2 to 4 mg/kg orally q24h; this is gradually tapered over a 6- to 8-week period. Remission usually occurs.
4. Vitamin E, 400 IU q12h, administered orally two hours before or after a meal, may be helpful.

Suggested Readings

Advances in Clinical Dermatology. The Veterinary Clinics of North America: Small Animal Practice. 20:6, 1990

Feldman EC, Nelson RW: Canine and Feline Endocrinology and Reproduction. Philadelphia, WB Saunders, 1987

Goorman NT, Halliwell REW: Veterinary Clinical Immunology. Philadelphia, WB Saunders, 1989

Muller GH, Kirk RW, Scott DW: Small Animal Dermatology. 4th ed. Philadelphia, WB Saunders, 1989

Parasitic Infections. The Veterinary Clinics of North America: Small Animal Practice. 17:6, 1987

Pruritis. The Veterinary Clinics of North America: Small Animal Practice. 18:5, 1988

CHAPTER SIXTEEN

Orthopedic and Neurologic Emergencies

James M. Fingeroth

Orthopedic Emergencies

True orthopedic emergencies are uncommon, but many animals with orthopedic injuries frequently have suffered violent trauma, necessitating a comprehensive, systematic, and logical approach to the entire emergency scenario. Most orthopedic injuries themselves are not life-threatening, and so good first aid may be all that is indicated while the patient is initially evaluated for more severe problems. This is especially important to bear in mind when a traumatized patient is rushed in for treatment; an open bleeding fracture may be the most obvious injury present, and is almost certainly the one the owner is anxious to have treated, but clinicians must discipline themselves to evaluate the rest of the patient first. Remember that a tremendous amount of energy is usually required to luxate a joint or create a comminuted fracture; this energy is transmitted to the bone through the soft tissues, and it is absorbed by all structures in the body, including the thoracic and abdominal cavities. Because general anesthesia is frequently indicated for the repair of an orthopedic injury, it is incumbent on the veterinarian to ensure that no complicating injuries (such as pneumothorax, traumatic myocarditis, ruptured viscus, etc.) are present, and to plan for dealing with such complications if they become apparent.

Although fracture hematomas can be extensive (especially with comminuted femoral fractures), these rarely are the sole source of hypovolemic shock in animals. If shock is present, other causes should be looked for, and treatment initiated.

Relative orthopedic emergencies include articular fractures, open fractures, and septic arthritis. The concept of relativity is important to bear in mind; early treatment is warranted, but only after more life-threatening problems have been addressed.

Articular Fractures

Anatomic reduction and fixation of articular fractures is necessary to prevent long-term sequellae, such as arthritis and decreased limb function.

1. Because of muscle contraction, early callus formation, and ongoing damage to articular cartilage, delay of more than two to three days after injury is often accompanied by greater difficulty in achieving successful reduction and fixation. However, although it is desirable to repair the fracture quickly, it is best to delay treatment until the patient is otherwise stable.

2. Many articular fractures can be successfully repaired even a week or more after injury, albeit warranting a more guarded prognosis.

Open Fractures

An open fracture often represents an urgent orthopedic emergency. Open fractures are also termed compound fractures, denoting that both bone and soft tissue structures, including skin, have been traumatized. A variety of classification schemes have been developed to guide the clinician in management. It is important to remember that a continuum of injuries exist, and that individual fractures may possess features from several of the more rigidly defined classes.

1. First aid instructions given to clients over the telephone should urge them to cover the wound with a clean dry dressing, and to transport the patient to the hospital promptly. If a bone fragment is seen protruding, it should be kept moist and covered, but need not be pushed back under the skin until seen by the veterinarian. Loose bone fragments should be preserved.

2. Veterinarians seeing open fractures should also apply basic first aid, even if they intend early referral to another facility. The area around the wound should be clipped thoroughly (sterile aqueous gel can be placed in the wound bed to prevent hair from penetrating the wound), and a light surgical scrub should be performed. The wound should then be covered by a sterile bandage and, if practical, an external support (e.g., splint) should be applied during transportation. Modified Shroeder-Thomas splints should not be used for fractures above the elbow or stifle.

3. Veterinarians receiving patients as referrals should remove any bandages and inspect the wound as soon as possible. It is not unheard of for a nondebrided, highly contaminated wound to be covered by a textbook-quality bandage. Also, a small open fracture can easily be missed if covered by fur, and the referring veterinarian may have overlooked it.

Grade I Open Fractures

1. A grade I open fracture is the mildest of this type of fracture.

2. It is usually produced by the penetration of the fractured end of the bone from the inside out, through the skin surface. Often, there is a recoil action and the bone end spontaneously returns to the inside, leaving behind a puncture wound on the skin surface.

3. There is minimal soft tissue injury with grade I open fractures.

4. Treatment consists of early clipping, shaving, and cleansing of the wound, taking advantage of the so-called "golden period" before bacterial infection becomes established. If appropriately managed in the first few hours after injury, grade I open fractures can be handled as if they were closed fractures, including use of external coaptation (e.g., casts), if indicated. Depending on the delay between injury and treatment, and the extent of bone/soft tissue injury, systemic antibiotics may be prescribed.

Grade II Open Fractures

1. A grade II open fracture usually is caused by penetration to the bone from the outside in. The degree of contamination is greater than a grade I fracture because dirt and debris are tatooed into the wound at the time of injury.

2. Soft tissue injury is moderate, but can include crushing, laceration, devascularization, and compromise of neurovascular bundles.

3. Such wounds should be debrided and irrigated promptly. A shocky patient often has a dulled sensorium, and may tolerate initial debridement without the need for sedation. All gross debris and obviously devitalized tissues should be excised. Injured nerves or major vessels should be preserved and tagged for later repair.

4. Microbiologic cultures from the depths of the wound should be obtained in order to determine appropriate antibiotic therapy.

5. Frequently changed moist dressings are applied until definitive bone and soft tissue repair can be accomplished safely.

Grade III Open Fractures

1. The worst open fractures are classified as grade III. Such injuries involve extensive in-

jury to or loss of soft tissues, and possible loss of bone fragments as well.

2. Close-range shotgun blasts, high-velocity rifle projectiles, and dragging motor vehicle encounters frequently induce grade III open fractures.

3. The initial goals of treatment are debridement of dead tissues and contamination, preservation of blood supply, identification of vital structures (tendons, ligaments, nerves, vessels, large bone fragments), and stabilization. These injuries may also involve one or more joints (e.g., tarsometatarsal shear wounds), and attention must be focused on preservation of joint integrity.

A. Animals with grade III open fractures should be moved into the operating room as soon as practical after life-threatening injuries have been stabilized.

B. Grade III injuries are not adequately treated by quick flushing in the emergency room. Optimal results are achieved only if meticulous surgical management is employed.

C. Frequently, more time will be spent debriding a grade III wound than in applying any fixation devices for stabilization. The latter can be delayed while soft tissues are managed over a period of several days. The reward for such aggressive, time-consuming care will be healthy granulation beds and restored viability.

4. Systemic antibiotics are indicated for grade III open fractures, based on the results of deep cultures obtained at the time of initial debridement.

5. When lavaging large open wounds, antiseptics or antibiotics may be added to the lavage fluid; however, the key to lavage is mechanical dilution of dirt and microorganisms. Copious amounts (liters) should be expended in flushing out all nooks and crevices. Moderate pressure (7 to 8 psi) can be achieved by using a 35-ml syringe and an 18- or 19-gauge needle.

6. Primary closure of grade III open fractures is usually not possible because of extensive skin and muscle loss, and probably should not be performed anyway. Frequent, repeated debridement, lavage, and bandage changes encourage second intention healing. Skin grafting may be needed in some cases to cover large denuded granulation beds at the end of the wound contraction period.

Septic Arthritis

1. Septic arthritis demands early treatment because of rapid enzymatic damage incurred by cartilage in the presence of degenerating leukocytes and bacteria.

2. The initial goals of therapy should include decompression drainage in order to allow escape of these cartilage-destroying elements.

3. Joint fluid should be collected aseptically for cytologic and microbiologic analyses.

4. Through-and-through joint lavage or open drainage and flushing should be instituted, depending on the severity and duration of the condition.

5. As with open fractures, the volume of lavage is probably more important than the composition of the lavage fluid (i.e., whether or not it contains antibiotics or antiseptics). Sterile, isotonic intravenous fluids are generally adequate as lavage fluids.

Neurologic Emergencies

Head Trauma

Despite the prevalence of trauma in animals, including a high incidence of motor vehicle accidents, veterinarians are not frequently confronted with the spectrum and severity of the head injuries seen in humans. Part of the explanation is anatomic, owing to the relatively thicker calvaria and overlying muscles in dogs and cats. Subdural hematomas, a common sequella to head trauma in people, are infrequently recognized in veterinary medicine.

Clinical Signs

1. The hallmark of brain injury seen in animals is alteration in the state of consciousness.

2. Some animals may be hyperexcited and thrashing, whereas most have depressed sensoria ranging from mild stupor to coma.

3. Infratentorial signs, such as nystagmus and balance loss, are common and do not necessarily reflect a poor prognosis.

4. Many of the signs spontaneously clear within the first 48 hours after injury.

5. Evidence of brain stem injury (pupillary changes, abnormal breathing patterns, non-arousable state, or absent cerebrocortical electrical activity) carries a guarded to grave prognosis.

6. The mechanisms of brain dysfunction include concussion, edema, and hemorrhage.

Treatment and Evaluation

1. If hemorrhage is suspected, drugs such as urea or mannitol should be used sparingly or not at all, as they may potentiate intracranial bleeding.

2. The drugs of choice for head trauma are corticosteroids. Large intravenous (IV) bolus doses should be administered several times in the first 24 to 48 hours after injury. The efficacy of steroids wanes beyond this time, and the dosages should be quickly tapered, especially if signs of improvement are noted.

3. If the animal is thrashing or rolling, it should be gently padded and restrained to prevent self-inflicted injuries.

4. An indwelling IV catheter should be aseptically maintained to provide an easy route for administration of medications.

5. Crystalloid fluids should be administered to maintain hydration, as the animal may be unable to imbibe on its own.

6. Urine output should be monitored.

7. The head should be palpated or radiographed to document any evidence of skull fracture.

A. Nondisplaced fractures may be treated conservatively.

B. Obviously depressed fragments of bone cause brain compression and should be stabilized or removed surgically.

8. Animals with acute head injury rarely have seizures. Seizures, especially epileptiform (recurrent) seizures, may represent a

sequella to chronic brain injury and resultant scarring. Seizures, if they occur, would not be expected for weeks to months after a brain injury.

Spinal Emergencies

The common thread underlying all situations that induce emergency conditions of the spinal cord is rapidly progressive loss of function. Thus, the etiology, whether it be an acute spinal fracture/luxation or the latter stages of a previously slow compressive mass lesion, is less important than the recognition of diminishing function and initiation of appropriate diagnostic and therapeutic measures.

1. The spinal cord has an exquisitely balanced, self-regulating, homeostatic mechanism for maintaining its structural and functional health. This mechanism can be disrupted by a lesion that directly compresses neural parenchyma, or that interrupts the vascular integrity of the cord.

2. The goal of the clinician is to deduce from the signalment, history, neurologic and ancillary examinations the location of the lesion, the nature of the lesion, and its likely future course.

General Approach

Diagnosis and Clinical Status

1. The nature of the lesion (e.g., luxation, disk extrusion, infarct, tumor) is suggested by the history and radiographic findings.

2. When managing a patient with spinal dysfunction, the clinician must monitor the progression of the neurologic deficits. If deficits are worsening, especially in the face of vigorous medical treatment, then more aggressive measures, such as surgery, may be warranted. It is inexcusable to delay treatment or referral of a patient with spinal cord injury until after it has lost sensory function.

Treatment

1. A major part of patient management in spinal cord injury cases is nursing care.

A. Nursing care should be initiated preoperatively, and continued in the postoperative period.

B. It is important to review the various forms of urinary and fecal incontinence, and to remember that patients with upper motor neuron bladder dysfunction will reflexively void urine, but incompletely. If not regularly expressed or catheterized, the bladders of these animals may become chronically overstretched (leading to possibly permanent incontinence even if the neurologic disease is eliminated), and the animal will be at great risk for the development of fulminant bacterial cystitis.

C. Urine and fecal scalding, as well as decubital ulcers, are the other major consequences of paralysis, and should be addressed in the care plan.

2. Medical management of spinal cord injury is based mainly on the use of corticosteroids.

A. Osmotic diuretics, such as mannitol, are effective for brain edema, but are notoriously unreliable for reducing spinal cord edema.

B. Other drugs, such as dimethyl sulfoxide (DMSO), naloxone, and thyrotropin-releasing hormone, can be effective for acute spinal cord injury, but usually only when massive doses are administered either before (moot) or within one hour after the onset of spinal cord injury.

C. The potential side effects of high-dose corticosteroid therapy should be kept in mind when treating spinal cord injury.

1) If high (total doses of greater than 2 to 3 mg of dexamethasone in small patients, or 5 to 10 mg in larger patients) doses of steroids are used, they should only be given for one or two treatments in the first 24 hours after injury.

2) After one or two high-dose treatments, or beyond 24 hours after injury, the efficacy of steroids diminishes, but the risk of fatal complications (e.g., colonic ulceration) increases. Steroid dosages should be drastically reduced after this point.

3) If definitive therapy (i.e., decompressive mass removal) is achieved, steroids should not be continued beyond 24 hours

(maximum) postoperatively, if at all, unless there is a specific indication for ongoing use.

Prognosis

1. The three major functional elements of spinal cord function are nociception (pain perception), voluntary motor activity, and proprioception (position sense).

2. Because of relative fiber size and myelination, animals with spinal cord injury from any cause typically lose proprioception first, followed by voluntary motor activity, and finally, nociception. Because the small pain fibers that ascend in the spinal cord are relatively invulnerable, loss of nociception (so-called "loss of deep pain") generally warrants a grave prognosis for recovery. If this condition persists beyond 24 to 48 hours, it is highly improbable that neurologic recovery will occur, despite medical or surgical intervention.

Quick Assessment of Spinal Cord Status

When presented with a patient in which spinal cord injury is suspected, a clinician may want to gain an early, rough insight into the degree of neurologic deficit. It is usually cumbersome to perform a complete, detailed neurologic examination, or to classify the patient according to some textbook scheme. These things may be done subsequently, but because it may not be immediately apparent how emergent a spinal cord problem is, the clinician should strive to obtain meaningful data in a short period of time.

Signalment

Because certain etiologies are most commonly associated with certain ages or breeds of animals, the clinician should be thinking about these associations when examining the patient.

History

If possible, the clinician should ascertain the onset of the problem (peracute, acute, etc.) and the course of the disorder (progressive, nonprogressive, waxing/waning). Does the owner think the condition is painful to the animal? Also the clinician should attempt to determine whether the deficits were lateralizing, especially if, at the time of the initial examination, the animal has symmetrical dysfunction.

Neurologic Examination (Abbreviated)

1. Observe the animal. This is best accomplished by placing the unrestrained patient on the floor while obtaining the history. Is the animal ambulatory or not? Which limbs are affected? Are the deficits lateralizing? Does the animal appear to be in discomfort? If the patient is nonambulatory, observe whether there are any purposeful (voluntary) movements of the affected limb(s).

2. If the patient is ambulatory, check for proprioceptive deficits. If the animal is nonambulatory, it is moot to check for loss of proprioception, so move on.

3. If the patient is nonambulatory, check for voluntary motor activity. Support the animal and move it forward or backward. Tickle the digits and look for deliberate movement of the limb.

4. If the patient is nonambulatory and has no voluntary motor activity, it becomes critical to test for nociception.

A. The presence of the former two signs indicates that there is a severe spinal cord injury, but it may be reversible (especially if it is attributable to extramedullary compression).

B. Complete sensorimotor plegia (loss of pain perception and motor ability), however, often indicates an irreversible spinal cord injury.

    1) Pain perception is checked by pinching a toe with fingers or hemostats, or by applying a sharp pin to the limb.

    2) Pain perception is subjectively measured by observing a conscious response by the patient (struggling to get away, whining, turning to look at or bite the examiner, etc.).

    3) *Simple withdrawal of a limb can be purely reflexive and, by itself, does not indicate intact deep pain perception.*

    4) Always check multiple toes.

    5) Check sensation from the tail and perineum as well.

    6) Again, movement of these structures may be reflexic (and with upper motor neuron [UMN] injuries, these reflexes may be exaggerated), so rely only on conscious responses.

    7) Because of the severity of injury usually needed to produce sensorimotor plegia, it is extremely rare to find animals with sensorimotor tetraplegia, as such patients usually die before they can receive medical attention.

5. If the patient has diminished (hypalgesic) or absent (analgesic) pain responses from the tail or digits, try to establish the boundary between normal and abnormal responsiveness. This is termed the sensory level and, if found, is highly localizing.

A. Using a pin or hemostat, stimulate the skin from distal to proximal and cranial.

B. Animals with a measurable sensory level will be nonchalant about stimulation caudal/distal to the line of transition, but will turn around vigorously when stimulated proximal/cranial to the line.

C. Repeat the test. If the results are reproducible, confidence in this subjective test grows, and the line may be traced up to the spine in order to determine the segmental level of the spinal cord lesion.

D. Keep in mind that the spinal cord segments do not always reside in the vertebral canal of the same number, and the nerve roots usually angle caudally as they emerge from the foramina. Thus, a sensory level found at the location of the L-2 vertebra may indicate a spinal cord lesion at the level of the T-13–L-1 segments.

E. Note that the sensory level is different from the panniculus reflex.

    1) The sensory level measures the conscious recognition of a noxious stimulus.

    2) The panniculus reflex is a complex-reflex arc involving the spinal cord, cervical intumescence, lateral thoracic nerve, and cutaneous trunci muscle.

F. Although the panniculus can be helpful in suggesting a level of normal versus abnormal function, it is not totally reliable. For example, some animals have poorly developed cutaneous trunci muscles in the caudal lumbar region. The absence of a panniculus reflex in such a patient may be normal, and may not represent a severe spinal cord injury or a transition level at that location.

6. Reflex examination should be performed to augment other findings with respect to the level of the spinal cord lesion.

A. Diminished or absent segmental reflexes indicate injury to the grey matter (cell bodies) that subserves the nerves involved in the reflex arc. These are lower motor neuron (LMN) injuries.

B. Normal or increased segmental reflexes usually are seen with supersegmental (UMN) injuries.

C. In the rear limbs, the patellar, cranial tibial, and withdrawal reflexes are the ones to assess quickly.

1) The patellar reflex tests the femoral nerve and its spinal cord segments (predominantly L-4 and L-5). An exaggerated patellar reflex is consistent with either an injury above L-3 or L-4, or an injury involving lower lumbar segments (L-6, L-7), which largely subserve sciatic nerve function. Damage to these segments would cause decreased function in the muscles that antagonize and oppose the quadriceps, causing an exaggerated response to patellar tendon tapping.

2) The cranial tibial and lateral withdrawal reflexes test the sciatic nerve and its segments. Remember not to confuse intact withdrawal with intact pain perception. Pinching the medial digit stimulates the saphenous nerve endings, which are terminal branches of the femoral nerve.

D. After the normal segmental reflexes are tested, the rear limbs should be checked for the presence of abnormal reflexes. These include the crossed-extensor reflex and the Babinski-like reflex.

1) The crossed-extensor reflex is a pathological display of the righting reflex that is normally present only in the standing, weight-bearing animal. When present, these reflexes indicate the presence of a UMN injury with respect to the tested extremity. They are not localizing and have absolutely no prognostic significance. The absence of a crossed-extensor reflex contributes nothing in any way, and cannot be used to localize a lesion (UMN versus LMN).

2) The Babinski-like reflex (fanning of the digits in response to tactile stimulation of the plantar surface of the metatarsus) is interpreted in exactly the same way as the crossed-extensor reflex.

E. In tetraparetic patients, the forelimbs are tested as well, although it is generally harder to elicit normal segmental (triceps, biceps, etc.) reflexes. It may be best to rely on muscle tonicity and degree of spasticity (or flaccidity) as clues to the level of the lesion. Crossed-extensor reflexes may be found with UMN lesions to the forelimbs, but Babinski's test only applies to the rear limbs.

7. A rectal examination should be performed to assess the function of the external anal sphincter and anal tone.

A. Animals with spinal cord lesions above the sacral segments will have intact or exaggerated anal tone and perineal and sphincter reflexes.

B. The presence of a dilated or hypotonic anus indicates injury to the sacral segments or pudendal nerves.

8. The spine should be palpated for a region of hyperpathia.

A. Spinal pain is the hallmark of extradural disease, but some intramedullary diseases, such as granulomatous meningoencephalomyelitis (GME), can cause intense hyperpathia.

B. Although in some patients it is possible to localize the painful area to a particular vertebra, usually a zone (e.g., thoracolumbar, midlumbar, low cervical, etc.) will be identified as being hyperpathic. This zone should agree with the other findings of the neurologic examination (UMN versus LMN reflexes, sensory level).

C. The presence of a hyperpathic level and sensory level at the T-L junction in a patient with LMN deficits in the rear limbs, tail, and anus is indicative of diffuse spinal cord injury, and usually signifies the presence of descending myelomalacia.

9. At the conclusion of the examination, the patient should be described (e.g., "left-lateralizing, nonambulatory, UMN paraparetic with moderate voluntary motor ability" or "non-lateralizing, nonambulatory, UMN sensorimotor paraplegic"). Keep in mind that this is a static assessment of the patient; it may have been quite different (better or worse) several hours earlier, and may also be quite different several hours hence. It is, therefore, imperative for the clinician to consider the known progression of the deficit, and to examine the patient serially if it is decided to pursue a conservative course of therapy. Any historical or current suggestion that the deficits are rapidly worsening should prompt a change to a more aggressive form of treatment, especially if nociception is being encroached upon.

10. There are no absolute rules when considering the issue of lost deep pain perception. The 24- to 48-hour period is a general guideline; recovery beyond this time is usually not seen. However, some dogs with loss of nociception only minutes before definitive therapy may have permanent paralysis. Similarly, anecdotes abound about dogs with "no deep pain for a week" who eventually recover with (or without) treatment.

A. The seeming contradiction is partly explained by remembering that assessments as to whether the animal can feel a hemostat pinching its toe are subjective. A stoic animal that is experiencing intense spinal pain may not care very much about a hemostat on its toe if it is hypalgesic; it may not, therefore, react consciously to our noxious stimulus; and may, therefore, be diagnosed as being analgesic. With time, therapy, or both, this patient may recover, and the logical (but erroneous) conclusion would be that it regained deep pain perception. This animal was in a "grey zone" that made it impossible to differentiate severe hypalgesia from analgesia clinically.

B. The prognostic significance of this distinction, however, is overwhelming, as true loss of deep pain represents an irreversible degree of spinal cord injury.

C. Currently, objective measurement of spinal cord integrity using evoked response testing is being investigated and may be available at appropriately equipped institutions in the near future. For the present, or in hospitals without electrodiagnostic capabilities, reliance on the clinical examination is still

paramount, and the caveat offered here should be constantly borne in mind.

Differential Diagnoses in and General Approach to Treatment of Neurologic Emergencies

1. Head trauma
  A. Concussion/edema—treat with corticosteroids, mannitol, and supportive care.
  B. Intracranial hemorrhage; hematoma—Minimize use of mannitol; consider surgical evacuation of hematoma.
  C. Depressed skull fracture—surgical decompression
  D. Brain stem injury; brain herniation—emergency decompression; hyperventilation

2. Acute tetraparesis*/tetraplegia
  A. Lesion above the foramen magnum (supratentorial or infratentorial)—Assess cerebrum, cerebellum, and cranial nerve functions.
  B. Atlantoaxial luxation—Usually affects small breeds of dogs; forelimbs may be weaker than rear limbs.
  C. Cervical intervertebral disk extrusion—usually severe hyperpathia
  D. Fibrocartilagenous embolic (ischemic) myelopathy—peracute onset; may be painful for first few seconds or minutes, but thereafter, there may be no hyperpathia; nonprogressive
  E. Granulomatous meningoencephalomyelitis (GME, reticulosis)—profound hyperpathia; progressive deficits; intramedullary lesion detected on myelogram; CSF analysis may be abnormal. Treat with steroids.
  F. Spinal fracture/luxation—may be obvious or subtle; look for displaced ("locked") articular facets. Treatment involves reduction and stabilization. The urgency with which fixation is achieved and the type of fixation used are dependent on the animal's neurologic status and progression of deficits.

3. Acute paraparesis/paraplegia
  A. Intervertebral disk extrusion—most common in thoracolumbar region, but can

---

* Any lesion that causes acute tetraparesis may compromise muscles of respiration, including the diaphragm. Affected animals will have weakened voices, as they are less able to move air through the glottis.

occur anywhere in lumbar spine. Rarely, extrusions may occur cranial to T10–T11. Treatment is based on the severity of neurologic deficits, anticipated progression, and a consideration of the animal's past history. Be very suspicious of animals that present with a past history of "multiple disk problems;" it may be that a single disk has been herniating and subsiding intermittently. This disk, even if only producing back pain at the present, is a "time bomb;" it may subsequently extrude and paralyze the patient. More aggressive therapy (myelography, diskectomy, decompression) may be indicated for such a patient. The frequency of occurrence of second or third disk extrusions is not really known. Published figures range from less than 3% to as high as 40%. The actual figure is likely to lie between these extremes (10% to 15%). *Note:* Mineralized disks seen on plain roentgenograms, unless obviously displaced into the spinal canal, may be red herrings. Patients with mineralized disks (chondrodystrophoid dogs; aged dogs and cats) may require myelography or computed tomography to localize the actual site of spinal cord or nerve root compression.

B. Spinal fracture/luxation—occurs most commonly at thoracolumbar, lumbosacral, and sacrococcygeal junctions. The latter often results in signs of fecal and urinary incontinence (LMN) and tail paralysis. Rear limb dysfunction is possible if traction injury to the spinal cord was sustained. Treatment involves reduction and stabilization. Decompressive laminectomy is rarely warranted (unless there is conclusive evidence of spinal cord compression by mass), and may be contraindicated because of further destabilization. Urgency of treatment and prognosis are dictated by the neurologic status.

C. Pathologic fracture—occasionally seen with primary or metastatic extradural tumors that invade the vertebral body and pedicles. The history usually lacks sufficient evidence of trauma to explain radiographic injury. Treatment is based on the severity of neurologic deficits and consideration of the underlying etiology.

D. Spinal cord infarction (fibrocartilagenous embolic myelopathy)—peracute onset of signs, often while the animal is playing, jumping, running, or climbing. The affected animal may vocalize loudly for the initial few seconds or minutes; thereafter, the condition is not painful. Neurologic deficits are frequently very lateralizing. Myelography may reveal spinal cord swelling or normal findings. Treatment involves medical therapy (corticosteroids) and observation. Lesions producing UMN dysfunction will often spontaneously regress, allowing restoration of partial or total function. LMN injuries carry a graver prognosis.

E. Spinal cord tumor—Although a progressive history is usually extracted from owners with dogs having spinal cord tumors, some may be presented for acute, rapidly progressive paraparesis. Extradural tumors may predispose to pathologic fracture (see **C,** above). Intradural/extramedullary or intramedullary tumors may grow slowly, allowing the spinal cord to adapt to progressive compression without obvious clinical deficit; however, beyond a certain threshold, the compression may lead to an acute decompensation of spinal cord function. Diagnosis is based on myelography, computed tomography, and magnetic resonance imaging. CSF analysis may yield normal results, and is not a sensitive indicator. Treatment involves surgical excision of the tumor, if possible, and appropriate adjunctive therapy (e.g., chemotherapy, irradiation).

Suggested Readings

Arnoczky SP: Musculoskeletal system. In Slatter DH (ed): Textbook of Small Animal Surgery. Philadelphia, WB Saunders, 1983

Delahunta A: Veterinary Neuroanatomy and Clinical Neurology, ed. 2. Philadelphia, WB Saunders, 1983

Oliver JE, Horlein BF, Mayhew IG (eds): Veterinary Neurology. Philadelphia, WB Saunders, 1987

CHAPTER SEVENTEEN

Neurologic Disorders

William R. Fenner

This chapter consists of three major sections. The first is a review of the neurologic examination, presenting a method of performing the examination and discussing what portions of the nervous system are tested by each portion of the exam. The second section is a discussion of signs and symptoms with which animals present when they have a neurologic disease. These signs and symptoms are divided into historical and physical findings; each of these categories subdivides further into abnormalities seen on general observation, gait, examination of the head and spinal reflexes, and sensory examination. We discuss these abnormalities in terms of their site(s) of origin in the nervous system. The final section lists the nervous system by regions and lists differential diagnoses affecting each portion.

If you feel uncomfortable performing a neurologic examination, review the first section of this chapter before beginning to evaluate a patient with a neurologic disorder. The signs and symptoms section will then help you arrive at a neuroanatomic diagnosis. After you have reached the best possible diagnosis, turn to the third section for a discussion of the diseases of concern.

General Approach to Patients with Neurologic Disease

Diagnosis of neurologic disease should not be any more difficult than diagnosis of diseases involving other organ systems. When you evaluate the patient, you attempt, by your clinical method, to create a set of deductions that explains the specifics you obtained in the history and on physical examination. Your diagnosis rests on selecting the single explanation that is most compatible with all of the clinically observed facts. First, you secure the clinical data by history and physical examination. Next, you interpret the data to determine the best anatomic location to explain your clinical and historical signs. Finally, you run laboratory tests and interpret their results in light of your clinical data. The coupling of the historical and physical diagnosis with the results of appropriate diagnostic tests allows you to arrive at an etiologic diagnosis.

History

In the patient with disease of the nervous system, the history is of paramount importance. The history, if used properly, provides both etiologic and anatomic information. The format of the neurologic history does not differ greatly from the general medical history. Attempt to characterize the patient's symptoms according to the following scheme:

1. Date of onset and temporal course of disease
2. Initial site and spread of signs
3. Character of disease
   A. Intensity
   B. Severity
   C. Aggravating factors
4. Effects of previous treatment

Ask general screening questions about all areas of nervous function. If you receive a positive answer, further characterize the nature of the complaint by detailed specific questioning. Too much questioning about normal areas tires the owner and burdens you with meaningless information.

Owners usually volunteer a history centering on obvious difficulties, such as blindness, epileptic fits, head tilts, or paralysis. However, they often neglect to mention other, more subtle abnormalities; you have to bring these out by careful questioning. Owners also may misinterpret certain signs or symptoms. They may report to you that an animal is bumping into walls because it is blind, when in actuality the animal has loss of balance and is bumping into walls because of ataxia. Thus, you must be able to separate clinical fact from clinical fiction.

As you obtain the history, keep in mind that certain types of lesions have characteristic features. For example, vascular disease has a sudden, cataclysmic onset with maximal severity of signs at the onset of the disease; neoplastic diseases have a slow progression of focal neurologic deficits; degenerative diseases have slow, progressive, diffuse deficits; inflammatory diseases generally have an acute onset of multifocal signs; and metabolic diseases tend to have waxing and waning multifocal signs. So, the age of the patient and the duration and mode of progression of the signs (all part of the natural history of the patient's disease) limit the possible diagnoses even before the examination takes place. Figure 17-1 is a sample of a neurologic history form that lists specific types of questions you should ask.

· ·
The Neurologic Examination

The neurologic examination consists of observing an animal, watching its gait, carefully palpating it for abnormal muscle tone or atrophy, performing tests of reflexes and reactions in that animal, and, finally, interpreting the information you have gained to answer a series of questions about that patient. The questions, simply put, are as follows: does the patient have disease of the nervous system or not? If so, does it involve one or more parts of the nervous system, and if only one part, which part? These questions are presented in algorithmic form in Figure 17-2.

Before you perform the examination, remember these general comments. The localization of a lesion is important because, in neurology, the clinical signs reflect the anatomy, not the pathologic nature, of the lesion. Cerebral disease has little variation whether the disease process is caused by a tumor, inflammation, degeneration, or vascular disease. When performing the neurologic examination, remember that you wish to explain all of the clinical signs by a lesion in one location. If you cannot do this, then the patient must be defined as having a multifocal or diffuse disease process. As you perform the neurologic examination, always try to be logical, methodical, and consistent. Develop your own order and always follow it. If you are going to perform a test that is painful to the animal, perform it last, because pain alters a patient's response to you and so alters the remainder of the neurologic examination. Proceed from the general to the more specific. When you perform a test, remember that a normal response requires the presence of both sensory input and motor output. An animal may have an abnormal reflex because of either an inability to perceive the stimulus or an inability to respond to the stimulus.

The neurologic examination may be divided into six parts: general observations, gait, cranial nerve examination, attitudinal and postural examination, spinal reflexes, and sensory evaluation.

General Observations

Evaluate the animal's behavior, level of consciousness, and alertness. Divide consciousness into the brain stem and the cerebral portion. The brain stem portion (arousal) is centered in the reticular activating system

```
                                              Date_____
                                              Clinician_____
                                              Vaccination status_____
```

1. Primary complaint_____
2. Date of onset_____
3. Onset of signs Sudden_____ Gradual_____
4. Onset of signs associated with Exercise_____ Trauma_____ Toxins_____
                                   Medical Therapy_____ Other Illness_____
5. Signs are Improving_____ Static_____ Deteriorating Steadily_____
                                                             Intermittently_____
6. The signs Do_____ Do Not_____ include weakness.
    If so, which limb was weak first?_____
    Has this changed?_____
    Which limb(s) are weak now?_____
7. The signs Do_____ Do Not_____ include an unsteady or an ataxic gait?
8. The signs Do_____ Do Not_____ include an unsteady or uncoordinated head?
9. Does your pet walk in circles?_____ If so, in what direction?_____
10. Have you noticed any change in your pet's ability to see?_____ If so, in one or both
    eyes?_____
11. Has your pet started to be incontinent in the house?____Has there been any other change in his
    toilet habits?_____
12. Describe any Personality Changes_____
                  Behavior Changes_____
                  Changes in Sleep Habits_____
                  Changes in Alertness_____
13. Have you noticed that your pet is in pain?_____
    If so, is it constant?_____
    Is it associated with movement?_____
    Was it present at the beginning of the illness?_____
14. Does your pet lick, chew, or bother his feet in any unusual way since the start of
    his illness?_____
15. Has your pet had any epileptic fits, fainting spells, seizures, or episodes of unconsciousness?____
    When did they start?_____
    How often do they occur?_____
    Are they being treated?_____ With what?_____
    What do they look like?_____
    How long does each one last?_____
    How long are the after-effects?_____
    Do they occur at any special time of day?_____
    Do you know when they are going to happen?_____
16. Please list every medication that your pet is currently taking, why he is taking it, and if it has
    helped the problem._____
17. Were you referred to this hospital, and if so by whom?_____

Figure 17-1. *Neurologic history*

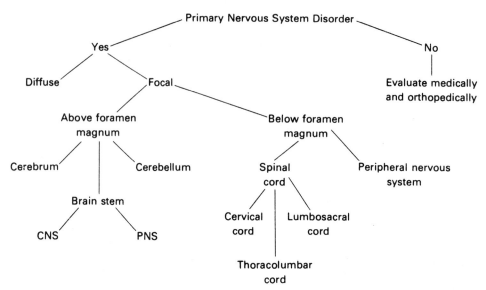

Figure 17-2. *A simple algorithm for determining the site of origin of a neurologic disorder*

(RAS) located in the midbrain and rostral pons. The RAS controls sleep–wake cycles, and dysfunction of this center causes decreased ability to be aroused. With advancing disease, the animal appears to go into a progressively more advanced sleeplike state (coma). Like brain stem lesions, those involving the entire cerebrum cause decreased arousal because there is no normal cortex for the RAS to regulate. Therefore, consider animals with stupor or coma as having disease of the brain stem or the entire cerebrum until proven otherwise.

The second portion of consciousness is cerebral in origin; it may be called content or higher integrative function. It is the sum of mental function, and disorders here cause confusion, delirium, or dementia. Perception of these subjective states is often dependent upon the owner's history. Dementia is a sign of cerebral disease.

Observe the animal for head tilts, circling, or other postural abnormalities that would indicate a disturbance in vestibular or cerebellar function.

Observation of Gait

Normal gait requires use of almost the entire nervous system. A disturbance of gait may be either sensory or motor. Sensory disturbances causing abnormalities in gait reflect a loss of proprioception. Therefore, a sensory gait disturbance is seen clinically as ataxia. Sensory gait disturbances are most frequently seen with lesions of the peripheral nervous system (PNS)—including cranial nerve 8—and spinal cord. They are seen rarely in cerebral disease.

Motor disturbances of gait may be of two types. They may be cerebellar in origin (involuntary motor), affecting coordination of muscle activity and manifesting as ataxia. In addition, they may be voluntary motor, causing paresis (partial loss of voluntary activity) or paralysis (complete loss of voluntary activity). Voluntary motor abnormalities in gait manifest as weakness or an inability to use the affected limbs.

Cerebral disease is not usually associated with an abnormal gait. If you do see an abnormal gait secondary to cerebral disease, the signs will be contralateral to the diseased hemisphere.

Brain stem diseases may cause hemiparesis or tetraparesis, as well as ataxia. The signs are usually ipsilateral to the diseased portion of the brain stem.

Cerebellar dysfunction may cause hemiataxia or ataxia of all four limbs. In addition, there is dysmetria of limb movement. Cerebellar signs are ipsilateral to the diseased hemisphere of the cerebellum. There should be no demonstrable weakness in cerebellar disease.

Spinal cord signs may be unilateral or bilateral and may include both ataxia and weakness. Either tetraparesis or hemiparesis is seen with cervical cord diseases, and caudal paresis or monoparesis is seen with lumbar spinal cord diseases.

Cranial Nerve Examination

In the cranial nerve examination, test the function of each cranial nerve. Cranial nerve I (olfactory nerve) originates in the cerebrum; testing it tests cerebral function. Cranial nerve II (the optic nerve) originates in the diencephalon and is concerned with both vision and pupillary light accommodation. Test this cranial nerve in two ways. Perform the visual evaluation to test cerebral function and the light reflex evaluation to test brain stem function. Cranial nerve III (the oculomotor nerve) originates in the mesencephalon. This nerve is concerned with pupillary constriction (light accommodation), which is a parasympathetic function, and with eye movement. Evaluation of this nerve tests brain stem function. Cranial nerve IV (the trochlear nerve) is concerned with eye movement and originates in the mesencephalon. Evaluation of this nerve also tests brain stem function. Cranial nerve V (the trigeminal nerve) originates in the metencephalon or pons. This nerve has two functions, sensory to the face and motor to the muscles of mastication. Evaluation of this nerve tests the brain stem and the cerebral connections for sensation. Cranial nerve VI (the abducens

nerve) originates at the metencephalic–myelencephalic (pontomedullary) junction. It is concerned with eye movement and retraction of the eye. Evaluation of this nerve tests brain stem function. Cranial nerve VII (the facial nerve) is concerned with the movement of the muscles of facial expression. This nerve also originates at the pontomedullary junction; evaluation of this nerve tests brain stem function. Cranial nerve VIII (the vestibulocochlear nerve) originates in the myelencephalon or medulla and is concerned with hearing, balance, and involuntary eye movements. Evaluation of this nerve tests brain stem function. Cranial nerve IX (the glossopharyngeal nerve) originates in the medulla and is concerned with innervation of the muscles of swallowing. Testing of this nerve evaluates brain stem function. Cranial nerve X (the vagus nerve) originates in the medulla and is concerned with swallowing. Evaluation of this nerve tests brain stem function. Cranial nerve XI (the spinal accessory nerve) originates in the cranial cervical spine and the medulla and is concerned with elevation of the head. Evaluation of this nerve tests brain stem and cervical spinal cord function. Cranial nerve XII (the hypoglossal nerve) originates in the medulla and is concerned with innervation of the muscles of the tongue. Evaluation of this nerve tests brain stem function. Refer to Table 17-1 for a review of cranial nerves.

When testing the cranial nerves, you stimulate a sensory nerve to cause a response in a motor nerve. To determine whether the sensory or the motor nerve is dysfunctioning, test each sensory nerve with two different motor responses, and test each motor nerve with two different forms of sensory innervation. In addition, you must determine whether this dysfunction is peripheral, nuclear, or supranuclear. By peripheral we mean along the course of the peripheral nerve, after it has left the brain stem and before it reaches the organ of innervation. A lesion may be peripheral and still be in the skull. Nuclear means involving the brain stem grey matter or nucleus of origin of the nerve. Supranuclear means a cerebral dysfunction causing an

Table 17-1. **The cranial nerves**

Cranial Nerve	Site of Origin	Function	Functional Area Tested
I (Olfactory)	Rhinencephalon	Smell	Cerebrum
II (Ophthalmic)	Diencephalon	Vision Light perception	Cerebrum Diencephalon
III (Oculomotor)	Mesencephalon	Eye movement Pupil constriction Eyelid elevation	Brain stem
IV (Trochlear)	Mesencephalon	Eye movement	Brain stem
V (Trigeminal)	Metencephalon	Facial sensation	Brain stem
VI (Abducens)	Myelencephalon	Eye movement Globe retraction	Brain stem
VII (Facial)	Myelencephalon	Facial expression Tear production Taste	Brain stem
VIII (Vestibulo-cochlear)	Myelencephalon	Equilibrium Hearing Ocular position	Brain stem
IX (Glossopharyngeal)	Myelencephalon	Swallowing Taste	Brain stem
X (Vagus)	Myelencephalon	Swallowing Heart rate/rhythm Gastrointestinal motility	Brain stem
XI (Spinal accessory)	Cervical cord	Shoulder elevators	Cervical cord
XII (Hypoglossal)	Myelencephalon	Tongue movement	Brain stem
Ocular sympathetic nerve	Thoracic cord	Pupil dilation Eyelid elevator Retraction of nictitans	Cervical cord

Table 17-2. **Tests of cranial nerves**

Maneuver	Sensory Nerve	Motor Nerve	Normal Response	Portion of CNS Tested
Menace	II	VII	Blink	Cerebrum
Pupillary light reflex	II	III	Pupil constriction	Midbrain
Doll's eye	VIII	III, IV, or VI	Nystagmus	Brain stem
Lid blink	V	VII	Lid closure	Pons or medulla
Retractor oculi	V	VI	Eye retraction	Pons or medulla
Gag reflex	IX or X	IX or X	Swallow	Medulla
Eye position at rest	VIII	III, IV, or VI	Normal conjugate position	Vestibular brain stem
Temporal muscle palpation	—	V	Full, symmetrical muscles	Pons or brain stem
Positional nystagmus	VIII	III, IV, and VI	No eye movements	Cerebellum or vestibular nerve
Tongue examination	V	XII	Normal movement, no atrophy	Caudal medulla

upper motor neuron (UMN) dysfunction of the nerve being tested. *Note,* in small animal veterinary medicine to date, only cranial nerves (CNs) V and VII have been shown reliably to manifest supranuclear dysfunction.

1. Animals have 12 pairs of cranial nerves.

A. CN I and the visual portion of CN II test cerebral function.

B. CN II (reflex portion) and all remaining cranial nerves test brain stem nuclei and their connections.

2. Abnormalities in function may indicate a lesion of the:

A. Peripheral nerve, ipsilateral (except CN IV)

B. Nucleus in the brain stem, ipsilateral (except CN IV)

C. Loss of cerebral influence, contralateral (CNs V and VII)

1) Review Tables 17-2, 17-3, and 17-4 for tests of cranial nerves.

2) For a more complete discussion of the evaluation of cranial nerves, consult any standard text of neurology.

Attitudinal and Postural Reactions

Attitudinal and postural reactions test the integrity of the proprioceptive pathways, their cerebral and cerebellar components, and the motor pathways responsible for correcting postural deficits. The technique involved in all of these tests is to place a limb in an abnormal posture and see if the animal corrects its position.

Lesions in the cerebrum, brain stem, spinal cord, and peripheral nerves all cause a diminished ability to correct for a postural abnormality. With cerebral disease, the signs are opposite to the involved hemisphere; with involvement in the other areas, the signs are ipsilateral. A lesion involving the cerebellum generally does not cause loss of proprioception. Instead, the correcting movement is ataxic. With disease of the vestibular system, the correcting response is often preserved, but the animal falls or rolls to the diseased side when it moves to correct the postural

deficit. Refer to Table 17-3 for a review of the postural reactions.

Spinal Reflexes

Proceed to the spinal segmental examination and test the reflex arc. The most specific abnormality—loss of reflexes—is seen with lower motor neuron (LMN) disease and localizes the lesion. This is called an LMN reflex change. A lesion in any part of the reflex arc delays or abolishes the reflex.

Exaggerated reflexes only localize a lesion to the central nervous system (CNS) above the reflex arc; these are called upper motor neuron (UMN) reflexes or UMN reflex changes. They indicate the presence of CNS disease but are not as localizing as LMN reflex changes. Any lesion between the brain and the reflex arc may cause the reflex to be hyperactive. Refer to Table 17-5 for a review of the spinal reflexes.

Sensory Evaluation

Animals may have two types of sensory disturbance. The first—decreased awareness of pain—is of prognostic value in spinal cord disease. The second—an increased awareness of pain—is usually a sign of nerve root disease or meningeal irritation and is of localizing value. Test the digits for awareness of pain perception to test spinal integrity. Then test the dermatomes along the back to localize any painful areas (see Table 17-3).

Interpretation of Findings

Once you know how to perform a neurologic examination, consider again how you interpret your findings so as to localize disease, as well as what you have gained by performing the examination.

Begin by making a list of abnormal findings in different regions of the nervous system (Table 17-6).

Table 17-3. **Overview of the neurologic examination**

	General Parameters		
Test Performed	Neuroanatomic Site(s) Evaluated	Functional System	Reliability
General observations			
Mental status			
Level of consciousness	Brain stem/cerebrum	Consciousness	*****
Content consciousness	Cerebrum	Consciousness	*****
Head posture	Brain stem/cerebellum/CN VIII	Special proprioception	***
Head coordination	Cerebellum	General proprioception	****
Circling	Cerebrum	Unknown	***
	Cerebellum/brain stem/CN VIII	Special proprioception	***
Gait	Cerebellum/brain stem/CN VIII/spinal cord/spinal nerves	Motor/proprioception	****
Ataxia			
Weakness	Cerebrum/brain stem/spinal cord/spinal nerves	Motor	***
Stance	Brain stem/CN VIII/cerebrum/ cerebellum/spinal cord/ spinal nerves	Motor/proprioception	***
Attitudinal reactions			
Delayed	Cerebrum/brain stem/spinal cord/spinal nerves	Motor/general proprioception	****
Ataxic	Cerebellum/brain stem/CN VIII/spinal cord/spinal nerves	Proprioception	****
Cranial nerve evalution (see detailed explanation that follows)	Cerebrum Brain stem/cranial nerves	UMN LMN	**** *****
Spinal reflex evaluation (see detailed explanation that follows)	Cerebrum/brain stem/spinal cord	UMN	****
	Spinal cord/spinal nerves	LMN	*****
Nociceptive evaluation			
Hyperesthesia	Nerve roots	Nociception	****
Analgesia	Cerebrum/spinal cord	Nociception	****
	Spinal nerves	Nociception	*****

Abbreviation Key: CN, cranial nerve; UMN, upper motor neuron; LMN, lower motor neuron
Reliability Key: *****, Highly localizing/abnormality indicates neurologic dysfunction;
       **** , Somewhat localizing/abnormality indicates neurologic dysfunction;
       ***   , Somewhat localizing/abnormality often indicates neurologic dysfunction;
       **   , Somewhat localizing/abnormality sometimes indicates neurologic dysfunction;
       *   , Rarely localizing/abnormality sometimes indicates neurologic dysfunction.

1. Ask yourself the following questions:

A. Does the patient have a neurologic disease? (This question cannot always be answered accurately.) If there are pluses after any of these signs, this question is answered in the affirmative.

B. Is the disease above or below the foramen magnum? If the animal has any abnormality of the cranial nerves, a history of seizures, abnormal head posture or coordination, or an abnormal level of consciousness, the answer to this question is yes. If there is

Table 17-4. **The cranial nerve evaluation**

Test Performed	CN Tested	Central Integration	Reliability
Menace response	II (Sensory) VII (Motor)	Cerebrum Brain stem (Cerebellum)	*****
Pupillary light reflex	II (Sensory) III (Motor)	Brain stem	*****
Pupillary size	II (Sensory) III (Motor) Symp (Motor)	Brain stem Brain stem/cervical cord	****
Pupillary symmetry	III (Motor) Symp (Motor)	Brain stem Brain stem/cervical cord	***
Oculovestibular reflex	VIII (Sensory) III (Motor) IV (Motor) VI (Motor)	Brain stem	*****
Pathologic nystagmus	VIII (Sensory)	Brain stem Cerebellum	*****
Palpebral reflex	V (Sensory) VII (Motor)	Brain stem Cerebrum	*****
Corneal reflex	V (Sensory) VII (Motor)	Brain stem Cerebrum	*****
Retractor oculi reflex	V (Sensory) VI (Motor)	Brain stem	*****
Jaw tone	V (Sensory) V (Motor)	Brain stem	***
Facial symmetry	V (Motor) VII (Motor)	Brain stem	***
Gag reflex	IX/X (Sensory) IX/X (Motor)	Brain stem	***
Tongue symmetry	V (Sensory) XII (Motor)	Brain stem	***

Reliability Key: *****, Highly localizing/abnormality indicates neurologic dysfunction;
**** , Somewhat localizing/abnormality indicates neurologic dysfunction;
*** , Somewhat localizing/abnormality often indicates neurologic dysfunction;
** , Somewhat localizing/abnormality sometimes indicates neurologic dysfunction;
* , Rarely localizing/abnormality sometimes indicates neurologic dysfunction.

only involvement of the limbs, then the lesion is below the foramen magnum.

C. Is the disease in the CNS or PNS? If the animal has cranial nerve deficits, use your evaluation of attitudinal and postural reactions, spinal reflexes and mentation to answer this question. If there are only isolated cranial nerve deficits with no other signs, then the lesion is probably in the PNS. If there are multiple cranial nerve deficits with the presence of UMN signs, the disease is probably in the CNS. If the disease is below the foramen magnum and any UMN reflex changes are present, then the lesion is in the CNS. If all spinal reflexes are LMN, then the lesion is in the PNS.

D. Now that you have localized the lesion as CNS or PNS and as above or below the foramen magnum, try to arrive at a specific localization based on your findings.

2. By localizing the disease, you know whether the animal has focal or diffuse dis-

Table 17-5. **The spinal reflex evaluation**

Reflex Tested	PNS Tested	CNS Tested	Response	Interpretation	Reliability
Triceps	Radial nerve	**C-7, C-8, T-1,** (T2)	Exaggerated	UMN lesion	****
			Normal	±No lesion	**
			Diminished	LMN lesion	*****
Biceps	Musculocutaneous nerve	C-6, **C-7,** C-8	Exaggerated	UMN lesion	****
			Normal	±No lesion	**
			Diminished	LMN lesion	*****
Thoracic flexor	Musculocutaneous axillary, median ulnar, and radial nerves	C-6, **C-7, C-8, T-1,** (T2)	Normal	±No lesion	**
			Diminished	LMN lesion	*****
Patellar	Femoral nerve	L-4, **L-5,** L-6	Exaggerated	UMN lesion	****
			Normal	±No lesion	**
			Diminished	LMN lesion	*****
Cranial tibial	Sciatic nerve	**L-6, L-7, S-1,** (S2)	Exaggerated	UMN lesion	****
			Normal	±No lesion	**
			Diminished	LMN lesion	*****
Pelvic flexor	Primarily sciatic nerve; some femoral nerve	**L-6, L-7, S-1,** (S2) L-4, **L-5,** L-6	Normal	±No lesion	**
			Diminished	LMN lesion	*****
Perineal	Pudendal nerve	**S-1, S-2, S-3**	Normal	±No lesion	**
			Diminished	LMN lesion	*****
Crossed extensor	—	**UMN** to limb	Present	UMN lesion	*****

Abbreviation Key: CN, cranial nerve; PNS, peripheral nervous system; CNS, central nervous system; UMN, upper motor neuron; LMN, lower motor neuron

Spinal Reflex Key: **Boldface entries:** essential to reflex; regular typeface entries: always supplies axons to nerve, but not essential to reflex; parenthetical entries (): supplies axons to nerve in some animals, but not essential to reflex.

Reliability Key: *****, Highly localizing/abnormality indicates neurologic dysfunction;
    ****, Somewhat localizing/abnormality indicates neurologic dysfunction;
    ***, Somewhat localizing/abnormality often indicates neurologic dysfunction;
    **, Somewhat localizing/abnormality sometimes indicates neurologic dysfunction;
    *, Rarely localizing/abnormality sometimes indicates neurologic dysfunction.

Table 17-6. **Example of abnormal neurologic findings**

Signs	Cerebrum	Brain Stem	Cerebellum	Cord
Seizures	++			
Ataxia	++	++	++	++
Paresis	+	++		++
Visual loss	++			
Dementia	++			

ease. Stop and think about which diseases of the nervous system cause diffuse or multifocal signs and which cause focal signs.

A. Multifocal diseases are often inflammatory, metabolic, or degenerative.

B. Focal diseases tend to involve masses, such as vascular lesions, granulomas, or tumors.

3. The localization of the disease helps you determine the type of diagnostic aid to use. Think of the nervous system in an overview, then list diagnostic aids for cerebral disease, spinal cord disease, and peripheral nerve disease. Some are of value in many cases, but some have limited application. It is as important to know what not to use as it is to know what to use.

4. Finally, the neural examination may automatically exclude certain diagnoses. For example, an animal with focal cerebral disease probably does not have a lumbar disk protrusion that is causing its sign. From this, it follows that there are two more questions to ask.

A. Based on the examination and history, what class of diseases must be considered?

B. What diagnostic aids serve best to differentiate those diseases?

5. The neurologic examination is now complete. Figure 17-3 is a sample of a neurology examination form that may help you in evaluating your patients.

··

Signs and Symptoms of Neurologic Disease

Historical Complaints

Seizures

Seizures are paroxysmal electrical discharges from the brain associated with periods of clinical abnormality. If the seizures are recurring, the animal is diagnosed as an epileptic.

1. Seizures indicate a cerebral abnormality that may arise from a structural lesion in the brain, a systemic metabolic illness, or a func-

tional abnormality in the brain. Other disorders that may cause similar signs and be confused with epilepsy include:

A. Fainting (syncope)

   1) Cardiovascular disease

   2) Respiratory disease

B. Narcolepsy, a sleep disorder

C. Vertigo, dizziness secondary to vestibular disease

D. Eclampsia (postparturient hypocalcemia)

2. Vertigo, narcolepsy, and epilepsy are covered more fully later in this section.

3. Eclampsia is discussed in the genitourinary section (see Chapter 13).

4. Syncope is covered in the cardiovascular section (see Chapter 9).

Dizziness, Vertigo, or Disorientation

Acute lesions of the vestibular system cause profound loss of orientation to gravity. This causes rolling, circling, dizziness, and severe disorientation. Animals with these signs may have a lesion of the inner ear, cranial nerve VIII, brain stem, or cerebellum. Lesions of the peripheral nerve or inner ear usually cause the most profound loss of balance.

1. If the lesion is in the inner ear, there may be an associated paralysis of facial muscles, Horner's syndrome, or both.

2. If the lesion is in the eigth cranial nerve, there are usually no other signs.

3. If the lesion is in the brain stem, there are usually multiple cranial nerve deficits, proprioception deficits, and spinal reflex changes.

4. If the lesion is in the cerebellum, there is usually associated tremor, postural ataxia, and dysmetria.

Loss of Balance

Balance in an animal is controlled primarily by the vestibular system. This includes the inner ear, the peripheral eighth cranial nerve (which connects the inner ear to the brain stem), the brain stem vestibular nuclei, and the cerebellar nuclei that coordinate vestibular motor responses. The function of the ves-

Date _____

Examiner _____

GENERAL OBSERVATIONS:

Personality/Mentation/Consciousness (cerebrum/brain stem)_____

Head posture (vestibulo-cerebellar)_____

Head coordination (cerebellar)_____

Limb posture (conscious proprioception)_____

Limb coordination (unconscious proprioception/cerebellar)_____

GAIT: Requires that vision/balance/proprioception/motor function all be intact and integrated.

Description of gait: _____

CRANIAL NERVE EXAM:

	L. eye	R. eye	
Menace (2,7)	____	____	Facial symmetry;
Pupil size (2,3,Sym.)	____	____	Temporal/Masseter (5)_____
			Expressive muscles (7)_____
Pupil symmetry (3,Sym.)	____	____	Palpebral reflex (5,7)_____
PLR (2,3)	____	____	Retractor oculi (5,6)_____
Doll's eye (8,3,4,6)	____	____	Gag reflex (9,10)_____
Ocular position (8,3,4,6)	____	____	Tongue (12)_____
Pathologic nystagmus (8)	____	____	

EVALUATION OF THE LIMBS:

	LEFT	RIGHT
Hemistanding (strength)	_____	_____
Proprioception		
Front	_____	_____
Rear	_____	_____
Segmental reflexes		
Front: Biceps	_____	_____
Triceps	_____	_____
Crossed Extensor	_____	_____
Rear: Patella	_____	_____
Anterior tibial	_____	_____
Anal	_____	_____
Crossed extensor	_____	_____

SENSORY EXAMINATION:

Sensory deficits (loss of pain perception)_____

Hyperpathia/Sensory level_____

Neck pain_____

ANATOMIC DIAGNOSIS:_____

RECOMMENDATIONS:_____

ETIOLOGIC CONSIDERATIONS:_____

Key: Numerals in parentheses correspond to CNN tested; *SYM,* sympathetic nerve; PLR, pupillary light reflex.

Figure 17-3. *Sample neurologic examination form.*

tibular system is to maintain posture and to correct for changes in body position. Any disease process that damages the inner ear, the peripheral eighth cranial nerve, the brain stem vestibular nuclei, or the cerebellum is capable of causing a disorder of balance.

1. Clinical presentation—Animals with balance disorders tend to have certain similar signs, regardless of where in the vestibular system the pathologic process occurs. These unifying clinical signs include the following:

A. Circling—Animals with vestibular dysfunction walk in tight circles, usually toward the affected side.

B. Head tilt—Vestibular dysfunction causes the head to be tilted, generally with the affected side held lower than the normal side.

C. Rolling or falling—Vestibular dysfunction makes animals fall toward the affected side. Often these animals cannot stop themselves after falling and they continue to roll.

D. Dizziness (vertigo)—Animals with loss of balance may appear disoriented, confused, excited, or restless as a result of vestibular dysfunction.

E. Abnormal nystagmus—Affected animals exhibit an involuntary rhythmic oscillating eye movement. This results from imbalance in the resting muscle tone in the extraocular muscles. The resting tone is determined by the vestibular apparatus. Thus, in most clinical cases, nystagmus is a sign of vestibular dysfunction. Nystagmus is classified both according to the direction of eye movement and according to when nystagmus is present.

1) Direction of nystagmus

a) *Horizontal nystagmus*. The eyes move in a plane parallel to the animal's head (side to side), with the eyes going faster in one direction than the other. This type of nystagmus is most commonly seen in peripheral vestibular disease or inner ear disease. The fast component of the nystagmus is away from the diseased side.

b) *Vertical nystagmus*. The eyes move in a plane perpendicular to the head (up and down). Vertical nystagmus is most

commonly seen with disease involving the central vestibular system (the brain stem and the cerebellum).

c) *Rotary nystagmus*. The eyes move in a clockwise or counterclockwise direction in the orbit. Thus, they may appear to have both a horizontal and a vertical component. Rotary nystagmus may be seen with disease in any portion of vestibular system.

d) *Direction-changing nystagmus.* If the direction of the nystagmus changes with changes in head position, it usually indicates a CNS disease.

2) Nystagmus may also be classified by the time of its appearance in an animal.

a) *Constant nystagmus*. Constant nystagmus is present at all times and in all body positions. An animal that has constant nystagmus shows evidence of involuntary eye movements any time you look at the animal. Constant nystagmus is most frequently seen with peripheral vestibular disease.

b) *Positional nystagmus*. Positional nystagmus is present only when the animal is in certain body positions. It is also called induced nystagmus because it is initiated when the examiner lays the animal on its back or its side. Positional nystagmus is most commonly seen in central vestibular disorders, but may be seen in the recovery phase of peripheral diseases.

2. There are additional signs with vestibular disease that narrow the pathologic process to specific neuroanatomic sites.

A. Facial paralysis—The seventh cranial nerve leaves the brain stem at the same level as the eighth nerve and travels adjacent to it to the level of the inner ear. For this reason, CN VII paralysis may be seen with diseases of the inner ear, the peripheral eighth nerve, or the brain stem eighth nerve. The facial paralysis is on the same side as the pathologic process.

B. Horner's syndrome—The sympathetic innervation to the eye passes through the middle ear. Diseases of the middle ear are capable of causing an associated Horner's syndrome, which is characterized by an abnormally small pupil in the affected eye, enophthalmos, and protrusion of the third eyelid. The pupillary light reflex (PLR) should be present in both eyes. The affected eye is on the same side as the pathologic process.

C. Other cranial nerve paralysis—With lesions involving the brain stem, such as tumor or granulomatous diseases, there may be involvement of many cranial nerves. Cranial nerves V, VI, IX, X, and XII are the ones most commonly affected. They are usually affected on the same side as the pathologic process.

D. Proprioceptive deficits—A lesion in the brain stem can cause damage to both the conscious and unconscious proprioceptive pathways. This results in ataxia or loss of coordination of gait. In addition, the animal stands with the limbs in an abnormal position (i.e., knuckled over).

E. Tremor—A lesion in the cerebellum may cause tremor. The tremor that results from failure to coordinate fine motor movement, such as eating, is called *intention tremor*. The tremor that is seen while attempting to maintain an erect body posture is called *postural tremor*.

F. Weakness—With lesions of the brain stem there may be damage to the motor pathways. This injury causes loss of voluntary function of the affected limbs. As the lesion removes UMN control from the affected limb, increased tone and exaggerated reflexes (signs of UMN disease) occur.

3. Loss of balance is generally a sign of vestibular injury. The first step in diagnosis is to decide whether the lesion is in the inner ear, peripheral nerve, brain stem, or cerebellum. Because the vestibular signs are the same regardless of location of the disease, it is the associated signs that are used to localize the lesion.

Head Tilt

1. Head tilt is most commonly seen with vestibular dysfunction. It may be either central (brain stem or cerebellar) or peripheral (inner ear or CN VIII). See the preceding section on loss of balance for features that separate them.

2. Nonneurologic causes of head tilt include otitis externa, ear lacerations, and other facial injuries.

Circling

1. Animals may circle as a result of disease of any portion of the CNS above the foramen magnum (cerebrum, brain stem, cerebellum), as well as with peripheral vestibular disorders. In general, cerebral disorders are associated with circling in large circles and aimless wandering, whereas with vestibular, brain stem, and cerebellar disease, circling tends to be in tight circles. Regardless of the site of origin of the circling, animals generally circle toward the diseased side of the nervous system.

2. Cerebral disease that causes circling may also cause seizures, visual deficits, proprioceptive deficits, or hemiparesis.

3. Brain stem disorders may be associated with tetraparesis or hemiparesis, head tilts, multiple cranial nerve deficits, proprioceptive changes, or abnormal levels of consciousness.

4. Cerebellar disorders may be associated with head tilts, tremor, or dysmetria.

5. Peripheral vestibular disease may be associated with facial paralysis, head tilts, or Horner's syndrome.

Abnormal Consciousness and Dementia

1. Definitions
   A. *Stupor* is a state of extreme depression or drowsiness from which an animal can be aroused only with a strong noxious or painful stimulus. When the stimulus is removed, the animal returns to a nonresponsive state.
   B. *Coma* is a condition of persistent unresponsiveness from which the animal cannot be aroused.
2. Normal consciousness includes both appropriate content of consciousness and level of arousal.
   A. Disorders in content of consciousness involve an animal's mentation, ability to remember commands, personality, and so forth.
      1) Controlled by the cerebrum
      2) Abnormalities in mentation or content of consciousness:
         a) Result in dementia
         b) Imply a cerebral disorder

c) May result from any of the disease processes that affect the cerebrum

3) Examples of disorders causing dementia include:

a) Functional cerebral disorders (i.e., idiopathic epilepsy)

i. The dementia is a manifestation of postictal behavior.

ii. It is seen only in association with, or immediately following, a seizure.

b) Metabolic disorders affecting the cerebrum

i. Dementia may be the only clinical abnormality seen.

ii. Dementia in metabolic disease generally waxes and wanes.

iii. In liver disease, the dementia is often related to meals.

c) Structural cerebral disease

i. Dementia is generally a constant finding.

ii. There are usually other neurologic deficits in addition to the dementia.

4) The clinical manifestations of dementia may include:

a) Unusual or aggressive behavior

b) Bumping into objects

c) Loss of continence

d) Failure to recognize people

e) Abnormal performance of any learned or voluntary activity

B. Disorders affecting arousal produce a progressive sleeplike state.

1) In their mildest forms, they produce depression or lethargy. An animal in this condition can be aroused easily.

2) Stupor is seen with more serious injuries.

3) Coma is seen with very serious injuries.

C. Alterations in the level of arousal may arise from lesions in two parts of the nervous system.

1) Sleep–wake cycles are controlled by the ascending RAS.

a) This is located in the rostral brain stem.

b) Focal injury to the rostral brain stem may damage the RAS and result in a disease process characterized by coma.

2) The RAS is responsible for arousing or activating the cerebrum. Any diffuse process that affects the cerebrum:

a) Makes it unable to respond to activation by the RAS

b) May result in stupor or coma

c) Acute cerebral processes cause more mental changes than do chronic cerebral processes.

Diseases that may cause alterations in consciousness can be subdivided into three basic groups, including structural mass lesions, structural generalized lesions, and metabolic diseases. Each of these tends to have certain features that allow the clinician to arrive at a tentative diagnosis based on the clinical examination (Table 17-7).

Behavioral or Personality Changes

Behavioral changes and alterations in personality that result from neurologic disease are usually a sign of a cerebral lesion. A large number of behavioral and personality abnormalities are a result of environment, training, endocrine abnormalities, and so on. A careful neurologic examination should allow differentiation between neurologic disorders and purely behavioral abnormalities.

Ataxia

A normal gait is characterized as swift, accurate, graceful, and smooth. With an ataxic gait, the animal may have a broad base. The animal may cross its legs over the midline and scrape the dorsal aspect of its toes when walking. The limb movements may be dysmetric, with hypermetric gait (overstepping) or hypometric gait (understepping). All of these actions combine to create a staggering, swaying, clumsy gait that is described as *ataxic.* Ataxia may be sensory (from proprioceptive deficits) or motor (from cerebellar deficits).

Table 17-7. **Classification of coma**

Neurologic Findings	Etiologic Considerations
Focal or lateralizing neurologic signs*	
Asymmetrical motor signs	CNS hemorrhage secondary to systemic bleeding disorders
Abnormal pupils	
Abnormal eye movements	CNS infarction secondary to thrombosis or embolism (hypothyroidism, feline ischemic encephalopathy)
Orderly progression of signs	
Often abnormal CSF examination	Epidural and subdural hemorrhage secondary to brain trauma
	CNS neoplasia
	Focal encephalomyelitis
	Granulomatous disease (granulomatous meningoencephalitis, fungal infections, parasite migration)
	Rocky Mountain spotted fever
Meningeal irritation†	
Neck pain present	Encephalitis
Abnormal CSF examination	Toxoplasmosis
Abnormal reflexes	Cryptococcosis
	Feline infectious peritonitis
	Canine distemper
	Other infections
	Meningitis
	Subarachnoid hemorrhage
No focal or lateralizing neurologic signs‡	
Usually normal reflexes	Intoxication
Normal pupils	Metabolic disturbances (diabetic acidosis, uremia, addisonian crises, hepatic coma, hypoglycemia, hypoxia)
Normal CSF examination	
	Severe systemic infections
	Circulatory collapse (shock) from any cause
	Epilepsy (postictal behavior)
	Hyperthermia or hypothermia
	Concussion

* With or without changes in the CSF

† With blood or an excess of white cells in CSF; usually without focal or lateralizing signs

‡ No alteration of cellular count of CSF

From Thorn et al: Harrison's Principles of Internal Medicine, New York, McGraw-Hill, 1974. Used with the permission of McGraw-Hill Book Company.

1. Sensory ataxia

A. Special proprioception (the vestibular system)

1) Special proprioceptive deficits are characterized by ataxia with associated loss of balance.

2) Animals have vestibular dysfunction characterized by:

a) Head tilt

b) Circling

c) Disorientation

d) Pathologic nystagmus

e) Often normal postural reactions

B. General proprioception (the spinal proprioceptive pathways)

1) Ataxia from general proprioceptive disorders is associated with lesions involving pathways in the peripheral nerves, spinal cord, brain stem, or cerebrum. These disorders are usually accompanied by some degree of weakness from simultaneous involvement of motor pathways. In addition, animals with general proprioceptive disorders usually have abnormal postural reaction, as well as ataxia.

2) Cerebral lesions rarely cause ataxia; they may cause abnormal postural reactions.

3) Brain stem ataxia

a) Usually associated with cranial nerve deficits

b) Frequently associated with vestibular signs in addition to ataxia

c) May have alterations of consciousness

d) Signs are ipsilateral to disease process

4) Spinal cord ataxia

a) No evidence of cranial nerve abnormalities (except in Horner's syndrome)

b) Usually associated with weakness

c) Associated with abnormal postural reactions

d) Clinical signs are ipsilateral to the pathologic process.

e) Usually associated with abnormal spinal reflexes

5) Peripheral nerve ataxia

a) Ataxia is usually overshadowed by profound weakness.

b) Decreased spinal reflexes are usually seen.

c) Associated cranial nerve deficits with some disorders

2. Motor ataxia is the primary characteristic of cerebellar disease.

A. Clinically, this disorder is associated with marked abnormalities of gait.

1) Wide-based gait

2) Irregular, deviating gait

3) Ataxia accentuated by circling or turning

4) A gait characterized by veering when attempting to walk a straight line

B. Ataxia of head and trunk

C. Normal strength and normal reflexes

D. Normal postural reactions

E. Affected animals may have associated vestibular signs (i.e., head tilt, pathologic nystagmus, circling).

Weakness

1. An abnormal gait characterized by weakness is a gait that has decreased strength, power, or endurance of the muscles responsible for the gait. Neurologic causes of weakness may be associated with two sets of clinical signs. There may be a loss of voluntary activity, with preservation of reflex activity (UMN lesion), or there may be loss of both reflex and voluntary activity (LMN lesion).

A. UMN dysfunction

1) A UMN is defined here as each of the motor neurons that originates in the brain and synapses on an LMN to initiate voluntary or postural motor activity.

2) Signs of UMN dysfunction include:

a) Weakness

b) Loss of voluntary function (partial to total)

c) Preservation of reflex function with exaggeration of reflexes

d) Increased tone to the innervated muscles

e) Decreased ability to flex the limbs

f) Occurrence of abnormal reflexes (i.e., Babinski's or crossed extensor reflexes)

B. LMN weakness

1) An LMN is defined as a motor neuron that sends its axon to terminate directly upon a muscle fiber. The LMN is thus responsible for both voluntary and reflex activity.

2) Clinical signs of LMN dysfunction include:

a) Weakness

b) Loss of voluntary activity

c) Loss of reflex activity

d) Decreased tone in the muscle

e) Decreased ability to extend the limbs

f) Atrophy of muscles

2. Neuroanatomic lesions—Lesions at certain neuroanatomic sites may cause injury to motor pathways, resulting in weakness.

A. Cerebrum

1) Character of motor deficits

a) All limb deficits are UMN.

b) Weakness is usually mild.

c) Deficits are either contralateral *hemiparesis* (weakness in one front limb and one rear limb on the same side) or *tetraparesis* (weakness in all four limbs).

2) Other associated deficits

a) Seizures

b) Personality changes

c) Visual loss

d) Endocrine abnormalities

B. Brain stem

1) Motor deficits

a) All limb deficits are UMN.

b) Weakness may be severe.

c) Weakness may manifest as hemiparesis or tetraparesis.

2) Other deficits

a) Multiple cranial nerve signs

b) Alterations in consciousness

c) Alterations in heart rate and respiration

d) Head tilts and loss of balance

e) Ataxia

C. Spinal cord

1) Injuries of the cervical spine may cause tetraparesis or hemiparesis.

a) Caudal cervical—If the injury is in the caudal cervical spine, the animal will have LMN reflex changes in the front limb and may have signs of Horner's syndrome in the ipsilateral eye.

b) Cranial cervical—If the injury is in the cranial cervical spine, the animal will exhibit UMN signs in both the front and rear limb.

2) Animals with thoracolumbar disease present with *caudal paresis* (weakness of both rear legs) or *monoparesis* (weakness of one rear leg).

a) Disease of the thoracic or cranial lumbar spine is associated with UMN signs in the involved limbs.

b) Disease of the lumbosacral spine is characterized by signs of LMN disease in the affected limbs.

c) Other signs commonly seen with thoracic and lumbar spinal cord disease include urinary incontinence, fecal incontinence, and decreased tail function. If the lesion is in the thoracic or cranial lumbar spine, the incontinence is associated with a normal anal reflex. If the disease is in the caudal lumbar or sacral spine, the incontinence is associated with loss of anal tone and reflex.

3) If the weakness is of pure spinal cord origin, there should be no historical signs referable to the head.

4) Animals with spinal cord disease usually have a combination of weakness and ataxia, rather than pure weakness or pure ataxia.

D. Peripheral nerve

1) Weakness associated with peripheral nerve injuries may result from focal or diffuse neuropathies.

a) If the injury is focal, the signs are confined to one limb.

b) If the process is diffuse, all limbs are usually affected; frequently, the rear limbs are more severely affected than the front ones.

2) Weakness caused by a peripheral nerve abnormality is characterized by:

a) Loss of muscle tone

b) Decreased or absent reflexes

3) In most cases, there are no cranial nerve signs seen with disease processes that involve spinal nerves. Exceptions include:

a) Polyradiculoneuritis

b) Myasthenia gravis

c) Botulism

Abnormal Findings Derived from Either Historical or Clinical Observations

Pain

1. Pain as a sign of neurologic disease may be manifested as self-mutilation (e.g., tail biting), carrying of a limb, an arched back,

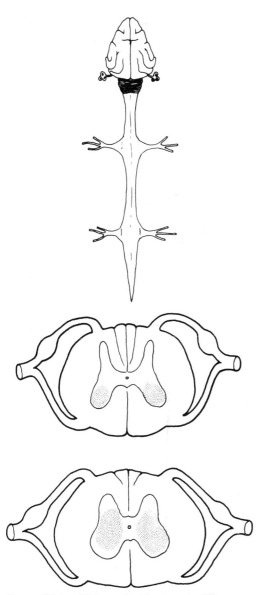

A. Cerebral disease

1) Lead poisoning, some forms of encephalitis, and, rarely, mass lesions involving the thalamus or hypothalamus may cause pain.

2) Affected animals tend to have unlocalized pain and cry out with any movement. They usually have other signs as well (i.e., seizures, visual changes, circling, personality changes).

Figure 17-4. *With meningitis, there is diffuse pain and fever. With myelitis, there is weakness, diffuse pain, and fever (i.e., feline infectious peritonitis and canine distemper).*

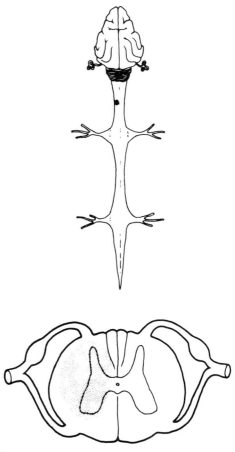

Figure 17-5. *Chronic pain associated with the nervous system usually indicates inflammation of the nerve roots or meninges. Focal cervical disorders include intervertebral (IV) disk disease, tumors, infections, and vertebral fractures; the other signs associated with these disorders are weakness and ataxia.*

nuchal rigidity, or crying, growling, or attempting to bite when moved.

2. Pain of nervous system origin may be seen with certain cerebral diseases and with lesions involving meninges or nerve roots (Figs. 17-4 to 17-6).

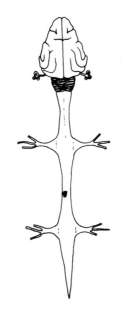

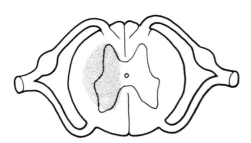

Figure 17-6. *With focal thoracic or lumbar disorders, the associated signs are weakness, pain, and ataxia. The disorders are caused by IV disk disease, tumors, infections, and vertebral fractures.*

B. Meningeal and nerve root (radicular) pain

1) Inflammatory diseases of the meninges (meningitis, meningoencephalitis) and compressive, traumatic, or inflammatory lesions of the nerve roots may cause severe back or neck pain.

2) These animals show an arched back or nuchal rigidity. They are reluctant to move and often cry out or snap at sudden movement.

3) They may mutilate the portion of the body that is innervated by the diseased nerve or nerve root.

4) They may appear lame and often attempt to carry the affected limb.

5) These signs may be caused by any disorder that affects the meninges and any extramedullary process affecting the spinal cord.

6) If there is involvement of the cord, additional signs (weakness or ataxia) are seen.

7) If the disease is purely meningeal or radicular, usually no other clinical signs are seen.

C. Nonneurologic causes of pain must always be ruled out in dogs showing pain without other neurologic signs. These include:

1) Musculoskeletal disorders
2) Pancreatitis
3) Steatitis (in cats)
4) Pyelonephritis
5) Colic

Urinary and Fecal Incontinence

1. Complex reflexes control both urination and defecation, requiring cerebral, brain stem, spinal cord, and PN integration and a healthy bladder and colonic musculature to occur properly.

2. *Incontinence* is a term that may be used to describe both the inability to store urine or feces and the inability to void urine or feces.

3. Signs of incontinence may include constant dribbling of urine or stool without apparent knowledge of the act, involuntary spontaneous urination or defecation at an abnormal time or place with apparent control between episodes, or repeated attempts to urinate with voiding of only small amounts and retention of a large residual volume.

A. Cerebral disease

1) Incontinence is usually manifested as loss of normal urinary/fecal control and normal residual volumes.

2) Associated with other clinical signs of cerebral disease

B. Brain stem and spinal cord disease (not including sacral segments)

1) Incontinence in such conditions involves spontaneous defecation or urination, initiated reflexively when the bladder or colon fills, with inability to relax the sphincter. Voiding is incomplete, difficult to initiate by manual expression, and associated with a large residual volume. Other signs of UMN spinal cord or brain stem disease are seen as well.

C. Sacral cord and peripheral nerve disease

1) There are no attempts at urination or defecation in affected animals. The bladder and colon are constantly overdistended, and there is loss of sphincter tone. This causes constant dribbling of urine. The bladder is easily expressed on manual palpation.

2) Other signs include paralysis of the tail and LMN changes in the rear limbs.

D. Nonneurologic causes of incontinence must be ruled out; these include chronic cystitis, prostatic disease, and overdistention of the bladder following obstruction.

Visual Deficits

Visual deficits (blindness) may be unilateral or bilateral. In addition, the loss of vision may be either ophthalmic or neurologic in origin. Often these causes may be differentiated by a careful neurologic and ophthalmic examination. In other cases, special diagnostic tests (electroretinography) may be required. Only neurologic causes of blindness are discussed here.

1. Unilateral blindness

A. Visual loss in one eye or in one visual field may result from a unilateral lesion involving the retina, optic nerve, optic tract, optic radiation, or cerebral cortex.

1) If the deficits originate in the optic nerve, there is a one-sided blindness and a loss of PLR in both eyes when the blind eye is illuminated. There is normal PLR when the normal (visual) eye is illuminated. There may be no other signs of neurologic disease. The pupils may be symmetrical, or the pupil in the blind eye may be minimally larger than the pupil in the sighted eye.

2) If the lesion occurs in the optic tracts, the optic radiations, or the cerebral cortex, there is a visual field deficit (apparent blindness on one side) with normal PLR.

There will also be other signs of cerebral disease in association with lesions in this area. The visual loss is on the opposite (contralateral) side from the disease. The pupils are equal in size.

2. Bilateral visual loss

A. If the lesion is in the retina, optic nerve, or optic tract, there is complete blindness with pupils that are maximally dilated and do not respond to light. There are no other signs of neurologic disease.

B. If the lesion is in both optic radiations or visual cortex, there is complete absence of vision, but the pupils are normal in size and still respond normally to light stimulation. The reason for this is that the visual and light reflex pathways separate at the lateral geniculate nucleus. A lesion rostral to this causes both abnormal vision and an abnormal PLR. A focal lesion caudal to this causes only a visual deficit or light reflex changes.

Abnormal Findings Derived from the Neurologic Examination

Cranial Nerve Signs

Pupil Abnormalities

1. Abnormal pupil size

A. Pupil size is regulated by the relative tone of two antagonist muscles.

1) The pupillary constrictor is innervated by CN III. Increased tone in the constrictor is the basis of the PLR.

2) The pupillary dilator is controlled by the sympathetic nerve. Tone in the dilator is increased by noxious stimuli (i.e., pain, fear, etc.).

B. Abnormally large pupils may be caused by:

1) Loss of function of the third cranial nerve

a) Usually with associated loss of eye movement

b) Loss of PLR

c) May result from a pathologic process or from drugs (e.g., atropine)

2) Loss of light (which would require a bilateral retinal or optic nerve lesion so the animal would be blind as well)

3) Excess sympathetic tone

a) Seen with frightened animals or those in pain; dilation can be overridden with a bright light source

b) Drugs, such as neosynephrine, instilled into the eye

C. Abnormally small pupils may be caused by:

1) Excessive light

2) Loss of sympathetic function

a) Other associated signs

i. Enophthalmos

ii. Prolapse of third eyelid

b) May arise from brain stem, spinal cord, or peripheral nerve injury, with signs referable to them as well

3) Excessive tone of third nerve

a) Bright light

b) Parasympathomimetic drugs (i.e., organophosphates)

2. Unequal pupil size

A. Practically speaking, unequal pupil size reflects an asymmetrical lesion of either the sympathetic or parasympathetic innervation to an eye. To separate these, perform a PLR test.

B. If the lesion is in the third nerve (parasympathetic), the large pupil is the abnormal pupil; it does not respond to light stimulation, regardless of which eye is illuminated. The smaller (normal) pupil responds appropriately when either eye is illuminated.

C. If the lesion is in the sympathetic nerve (Horner's syndrome), the smaller pupil is abnormal and both it and the larger (normal) pupil respond to light stimulation when either eye is illuminated. There are no visual deficits in either of the above cases.

1) A lesion of the third nerve may arise from:

a) Brain stem injuries

i. Other cranial nerve deficits

ii. Abnormal consciousness

iii. Weakness

iv. Ataxia

b) Peripheral nerve injuries—cavernous sinus

i. Combined paralysis of CNs III, IV, V, VI, and Horner's

syndrome of the affected eye

ii. No other signs are seen.

c) Isolated third nerve lesion

i. Has been reported (anecdotally) in cats testing positive for feline leukemia virus (FeLV) with no other signs

ii. Idiopathic internal ophthalmaplegia may be seen, more commonly in cats than in dogs. They have no other signs and may improve spontaneously.

iii. May result from inadvertent medication of the animal's eye with parasympatholytic drugs

2) Horner's syndrome—A sympathetic lesion to the eye may result from:

a) Brain stem injuries

i. Rarely occur

ii. Associated with other brain stem signs

b) Cranial spinal cord signs

i. Rarely occur

ii. Associated UMN weakness and ataxia in all four limbs

c) Caudal cervical cord, nerve root lesion

i. Associated with LMN injury to the front limb on the same side (brachial plexus avulsion).

ii. If the lesion is in the spinal cord, there is an associated UMN weakness and ataxia in the rear limbs.

d) Peripheral nerve

i. Middle ear—associated vestibular and facial paralysis on same side

ii. Isolated paralysis—no other associated signs

iii. Cavernous sinus ipsilateral CNs III, IV, V, VI

3. Abnormal PLR

A. An abnormal PLR may arise from a lesion in the retina or optic nerve, or from a lesion in the third cranial nerve.

B. If the lesion is in one optic nerve,

1) The pupils are equal in size at rest (or the diseased eye may have a slightly enlarged pupil).

2) When the diseased eye is illuminated, there is no response in either eye.

3) When the light source is directed into the normal eye, both pupils constrict.

4) When the light source is moved back to the diseased eye, both pupils dilate. This is called the *swinging flashlight test*.

5) A visual deficit exists in addition to the abnormal PLR.

C. If the lesion involves both optic nerves, the pupils are equal in size, the animal is totally blind, and there is no PLR.

D. If the lesion involves CN III on one side, the pupils are unequal in size at rest.

1) When the large (diseased) pupil is illuminated, only the small (normal) pupil responds.

2) When the light source is directed into the normal pupil, only that pupil responds.

3) In another sense, the large (diseased) pupil is refractory to light stimulation, regardless of which eye is illuminated. The small (normal) pupil responds normally, regardless of which eye is illuminated.

4) No visual deficits are seen.

E. If the third nerve is involved bilaterally, the pupils are both dilated and are equal in size. There is no PLR, regardless of which eye is illuminated, but no visual deficits are seen.

F. Third nerve lesions may arise from injuries to the:

1) Brain stem—other signs of CNS involvement

2) Peripheral nerve—cavernous sinus

a. Associated ipsilateral CN IV, V, VI, paralysis, and Horner's syndrome in affected eye

b. No other signs

3) Isolated CN III lesion

a) No other signs

b) May see as part of FeLV-related disease

c) May result from medication of eye

d) May be idiopathic

Abnormal Eye Movement

Abnormal eye movement may be manifested in one of two ways; there may be paralysis and inability to move the eye(s), or there may be spontaneous abnormal eye movement (*pathologic nystagmus*).

1. *Strabismus* is a deviation of one eye from its normal conjugate position.

A. Strabismus may result from paralysis of CN II, IV, VI, or VIII.

B. Ventrolateral deviation of the eye

1) May result from paralysis of CN III or VIII

2) If the lesion involves the third cranial nerve, the eye is fixed in its position, so no eye movement occurs with movement of the head. In addition, there is usually paralysis of the pupil.

3) Lesions of the third cranial nerve may result from:

    a) Brain stem lesions

        i. Altered consciousness

        ii. Weakness of limbs

        iii. Ataxia

        iv. Other CN deficits

    b) Peripheral lesions

        i. Cavernous sinus, with associated paralysis of CNs IV, V, and VI, and sympathetic innervation to that eye

4) If the lesion is in the eighth cranial nerve, the eye responds to head movement with a normal physiologic nystagmus (doll's eye response) in most cases.

5) Lesions of the eighth cranial nerve cause head tilts, pathologic nystagmus, circling, and strabismus.

6) These lesions may result from

    a) Brain stem abnormalities

        i. Altered consciousness

        ii. Weakness

        iii. Proprioceptive loss

        iv. Other cranial nerve deficits

    b) Peripheral lesions

        i. May have associated paralysis of CN VII and the sympathetic nerve to same side, or no other signs

C. Medial deviation of the eye

1) Results from paralysis of the sixth

cranial nerve. The eye maintains its fixed position during head movement.

    2) Lesions of the sixth cranial nerve may result from:

        a) Brain stem lesions

            i. Abnormal consciousness

            ii. Associated cranial nerve paralysis

            iii. Weakness

            iv. Ataxia

            v. Proprioceptive loss

        b) Peripheral lesions

            i. Isolated; extremely rare; associated with no other signs

            ii. Cavernous sinus with involvement of CNs III, IV, and V, and sympathetic innervation to the same eye.

D. Various forms of strabismus may be seen as a result of congenital anomalies of the extraocular muscles. Affected animals usually have normal eye movement and no other clinical signs.

2. Abnormal doll's eye (physiologic nystagmus)

A. Principles of the doll's eye—Eye movement during head turning is initiated in the semicircular canals. The semicircular canals convert acceleration into a neural signal proportional to the head velocity. This information is passed to the vestibular nuclei, which project into the pontine paramedian reticular formation (PPRF). The velocity information is converted to a positional signal and projected to the ocular motor neurons by way of the medial longitudinal fasciculus (MLF) to determine final eye position. The response of the eyes to vestibular stimulation is a slow tonic deviation of the eyes away from the vestibular apparatus being stimulated. If either the stimulus is removed or the eyes deviate to their maximal degree, there is a rapid return of the eyes to normal position. If the stimulus continues or is initiated again, the slow tonic deviation of the eyes is repeated. When rotating an animal, you are stimulating the vestibular apparatus on the side toward which you turn the animal. Spinning an animal from left to right stimulates the right

vestibular apparatus and causes a slow and tonic deviation of the eyes to the left. When the eyes reach their maximal degree of excursion to the left, there is a rapid correcting phase and the eyes jerk back to the right. Stimulating the right vestibular apparatus by head turning creates a physiologic nystagmus with a slow tonic deviation to the left and a rapid jerk back to the right (fast phase in the direction of movement).

    B. Abnormal doll's eye may be failure of one eye or both eyes to respond to head turning.

    1) Failure in one eye indicates a paralysis of one or more of the extraocular muscles. This may be caused by a lesion of CN III or VI.

    2) Cranial nerve III

        a) There is an associated paralysis of the pupil.

        b) There is an associated strabismus.

        c) Location of the lesion

            i. Brain stem

                A. Altered consciousness

                B. Abnormal proprioception

                C. Weakness

                D. Other cranial nerve signs

            ii. Peripheral

                A. Cavernous sinus—Associated paralysis of CNs IV, V, VI, and the sympathetic nerve to the same eye; dilated pupil

                B. Isolated peripheral lesion; dilated pupil

    3) Cranial nerve VI

        a) There is an associated medial strabismus.

        b) Location of the lesion

            i. Brain stem

                A. Associated, other cranial nerve signs

                B. Proprioceptive changes

            ii. Peripheral nerve

                A. Cavernous sinus—Associated paralysis of CNs III, IV, V, and the sympathetic nerve to the same eye; no other signs

B. Isolated, no other signs

4) Failure of eye movement in both eyes indicates a lesion of the vestibular system—either a bilateral peripheral injury or a lesion in the brain stem.

    a) Associated signs include:

      i. Head tilt

      ii. Pathologic nystagmus

      iii. Other cranial nerve paralysis

      iv. Weakness

      v. Proprioceptive deficits

3. Pathologic nystagmus is nystagmus that is present without head turning and is a sign of vestibular disease. Pathologic nystagmus is present in both peripheral vestibular disease and central vestibular disease. If you damage one vestibular apparatus, nystagmus occurs. The reason for the nystagmus is asymmetry in muscle tone of the extraocular muscles. If you remove the right vestibular apparatus, you stimulate only the left vestibular apparatus; this causes a slow, tonic deviation of the eyes to the right with a rapid jerking back (or correcting phase) to the left and then a slow tonic deviation to the right and a rapid, jerking-back phase to the left. So, with peripheral vestibular disease nystagmus occurs, the fast phase of which is away from the side of the lesion. The origin of the fast-correcting phase is believed to be cerebral. One of the characteristics of vestibular nystagmus is that it is not related to vision and is present even in blind animals, so vestibular nystagmus may be present either with the eyes open or with the eyes closed.

A. Pathologic nystagmus may be characterized in one of two ways: by its direction and by how it is induced. Each of these has some localizing significance.

    1) Nystagmus is classified by its direction relative to the plane of the animal's head.

      a) Horizontal—Nystagmus from side to side usually implies peripheral disease; the fast component is away from the side of the lesion.

      b) Rotatory—The eyes rotate clockwise or counterclockwise in the orbit, with no specific localizing significance.

      c) Vertical—Eyes move ventral to the plane of the head; this is usually seen with central disease.

      d) Direction changing—If the direction of the nystagmus changes with different head positions, it indicates central disease.

    2) Form of induction

      a) Constant nystagmus is present when the animal's head is in a normal position. It is usually seen in peripheral disorders.

      b) Position-induced nystagmus is present when the head is not parallel to the ground. It persists more than 60 seconds after head movement stops. Usually, positional nystagmus is seen in central disease.

B. Pathologic nystagmus indicates vestibular disease. Associated signs include head tilt, ataxia, circling, and vertigo.

    1) Peripheral—The pathologic nystagmus of peripheral vestibular disease is maximal at the onset of the disease and diminishes during the course of the disease. Therefore, it is rare for nystagmus of peripheral vestibular disease to be present in an animal for more than a few weeks.

      a) The nystagmus of peripheral vestibular disease tends to be spontaneous, so it is present at all times, regardless of head position.

      b) It tends to be unidirectional and to maintain that direction, regardless of the animal's head position.

      c) Finally, it is most frequently horizontal in direction.

      d) If it is caused by lesions of the inner ear, CN VII paresis and Horner's syndrome are observed; if the lesion is in the peripheral nerve, there are no other signs.

    2) Central—The pathologic nystagmus of central origin tends to be persistent. As long as the animal has the disease, nystagmus can be induced. The nystagmus with central vestibular disease often is progressive and becomes more severe with the passage of time. The direction of the nystagmus may change with changing head postures, and it frequently has a vertical component. Central vestibular disorders may arise from lesions of the:

      a) Brain stem

        i. Other cranial nerve deficits

    ii. Weakness
    iii. Proprioceptive deficits
  b) Cerebellum
    i. Hypermetria
    ii. Tremor
    iii. Absent menace reflex with normal vision

Facial Paralysis

Paralysis of the muscles of facial expression (eyelid, lips, and ear) results from injury to the seventh cranial nerve. The paralysis may be either unilateral or bilateral. The clinical signs include inability to blink the eye, drooping of the lip, weakness of the ear, excessive drooling from one side of the mouth, and, occasionally, contracture of the facial muscles on one side. These signs may occur with cerebral lesions (supranuclear), brain stem lesions (nuclear), or peripheral lesions.

1. Unilateral facial paralysis, in which the facial weakness only involves one side of the face. The lesion may involve the:
  A. Peripheral nerve
    1) This is the most common cause of unilateral facial paralysis. The lesion is usually complete (there is total paralysis), and facial reflexes are lost. If the lesion is in the inner or middle ear, there may be associated vestibular signs (head tilt, nystagmus, etc.) and a Horner's syndrome in the eye on the affected side.
    2) With most peripheral seventh nerve injuries, there are no other signs.
  B. Brain stem
    1) Associated with other cranial nerve signs, weakness, proprioceptive deficits, and so on.
    2) The lesion may be complete or incomplete.
  C. Cerebrum
    1) The seventh nerve signs are partial (incomplete). There is weakness but not paralysis of the involved muscles. Facial reflexes are spared.
    2) There are other signs of cerebral dysfunction (i.e., seizures, dementia, weakness, visual changes).
2. Bilateral facial nerve paralysis

  A. The signs involve all of the facial muscles.
  B. The lesion is usually peripheral.
    1) It is usually isolated with no other clinical signs.
    2) It may be associated with otitis media interna (vestibular signs, Horner's syndrome).
  C. If the lesion involves the brain stem, the animal has other cranial nerve signs (weakness, loss of proprioception).
  D. If the lesion involves the cerebrum, the animal has other signs (seizures, dementia, visual changes, etc.).

Facial Sensory Loss

Anesthesia or analgesia of the head indicates a lesion of the fifth cranial nerve. A lesion in the peripheral nerve, brain stem, or the cerebrum may cause this sign.

1. Peripheral nerve lesion
  A. The signs may be unilateral or bilateral.
  B. The loss of pain perception is complete.
  C. Reflex facial movement is lost.
  D. There are usually no other associated signs.
2. Brain stem lesion
  A. The sensory loss is only partial.
  B. Some facial reflexes may be decreased.
  C. Other signs of brain stem dysfunction are seen.
    1) Other cranial nerve signs
    2) Weakness
    3) Ataxia
3. Cerebral lesion
  A. There is no conscious perception of the painful stimulus, but facial reflexes are preserved.
  B. Other signs of cerebral disease are seen (seizures, visual changes, weakness, etc.).

Jaw Paralysis

Paralysis of the motor branch of CN V may occur. Paralysis of the jaw is associated with inability to close the mouth (dropped jaw) and inability to eat. The lesion may arise from:

1. Peripheral nerves
   A. No other neurologic signs are seen.
   B. Atrophy of temporal muscles may occur.
2. Brain stem, in which case other neurologic signs may include:
   A. Abnormal consciousness.
   B. Other cranial nerve paralysis
   C. Weakness
   D. Ataxia
   E. Proprioceptive loss

Abnormal Swallowing

1. The neurologic cause of dysphagia is paralysis of CNs IX and X. Clinically, the animals choke, gag, may have an abnormal-sounding voice, and may regurgitate.
   A. Peripheral nerve lesions
      1) Isolated; no other signs are seen.
      2) May be associated with myasthenia gravis and generalized weakness
   B. Brain stem lesions
      1) Associated with other cranial nerve signs
      2) Accompanied by weakness, ataxia, and proprioceptive deficits
2. Nonneurologic forms of swallowing difficulty must be ruled out (e.g., oral or esophageal foreign bodies).

Paralysis of the Tongue

Paralysis of the tongue may arise from injury to the 12th cranial nerve. The signs include atrophy, deviation of the tongue from the midline, inability to retract the tongue, and inability to eat or drink properly. Lesions causing tongue paralysis may arise in the:

1. Peripheral nerve
   A. There are usually no other signs.
   B. There is marked loss of function.
   C. There is atrophy of the tongue.
2. Brain stem
   A. The loss of tongue function is not as severe as it is with lesions in other locations.
   B. There are other cranial nerve signs.

   C. Other signs include weakness, ataxia, and proprioceptive deficits.
3. Cerebrum
   A. The primary tongue sign is inability to pull the tongue back into the mouth.
   B. Atrophy does not occur.
   C. Other signs usually include visual deficits, seizures, and weakness.

Limb Signs

Proprioceptive Loss

Loss of proprioception causes abnormal placement reactions in the limbs, abnormal limb posture at rest (limb crossed over, nails turned under) and abnormal wearing of the toes. Loss of proprioception is a nonspecific indication of neurologic disease. Lesions involving the cerebrum, brain stem, spinal cord, and peripheral nerve all may cause loss of proprioception. The pattern of proprioceptive loss may prove helpful in localizing a disease process.

1. Proprioceptive loss in all four limbs may be seen with:
   A. Bilateral cerebral disease—Other signs include seizures, abnormal consciousness, weakness, and visual changes.
   B. Brain stem disorders—Other signs include abnormal consciousness, multiple cranial nerve deficits, and weakness.
   C. Spinal cord disorders
      1) Must be in cervical spine
      2) May see associated weakness or Horner's syndrome
      3) Should not be any other cranial nerve signs.
   D. Peripheral nerve disorders
      1) Accompanied by generalized weakness with atrophy and diminished reflexes
      2) Occasionally, facial weakness and decreased swallowing are noted.
2. Proprioceptive loss in one front and one rear limb on the same side may be seen with:
   A. Focal cerebral disorders—Associated signs include weakness, circling, seizures, visual changes, and so on.
   B. Focal brain stem disorders—Associated signs include multiple cranial nerve

deficits and weakness on the same side as the proprioceptive deficit.

C. Focal spinal cord disorders

1) The lesion must be in the cervical spine.

2) There may be an associated weakness or Horner's syndrome on the same side as the proprioceptive deficit.

3) There should be no other cranial nerve signs.

3. Proprioceptive loss confined to the rear limbs

A. Proprioceptive loss in both rear limbs is almost always an indication of a spinal cord lesion in the thoracic or lumbar spinal cord.

B. Associated signs include weakness, urinary or fecal incontinence, or pain.

4. Proprioceptive loss confined to one limb

A. Forelimb—A proprioceptive loss confined to a single forelimb is usually a sign of a peripheral nerve injury. Associated signs include absent reflexes, sensory loss, atrophy, and loss of muscle tone.

B. Rear limb—Loss of proprioception confined to one rear limb may result from either a unilateral thoracolumbar spinal cord lesion or a peripheral nerve injury.

1) Spinal cord lesion—Associated signs include weakness, spasticity, pain, and UMN reflexes.

2) Peripheral nerve injury—Associated signs include weakness, atrophy, decreased reflexes, and loss of muscle tone.

Paresis or Paralysis

Paresis or paralysis indicates that there is decrease in voluntary motor activity of a limb with associated weakness. Lesions in the cerebrum, brain stem, spinal cord, or peripheral nerves are all capable of causing motor weakness. With cerebral and brain stem lesions, the paresis is always UMN in the affected limbs, and so is associated with increased tone (spasticity), loss of voluntary motor activity and weakness, normal or increased spinal reflexes, and release of abnormal reflexes (i.e., Babinski's and crossed extensor). With lesions of the peripheral nervous system, the signs are always LMN in the affected limbs and are characterized by loss

of both voluntary activity and reflex activity, weakness, and loss of muscle mass (atrophy). With spinal cord disease, the reflex changes seen are dependent upon the location of the lesion within the cord.

1. Tetraparesis (weakness of all four limbs) may result from:

A. Cerebral lesions (require a bilateral or diffuse process)

1) Limb signs are usually mild.

2) Reflexes are UMN.

3) Associated signs include seizures, visual signs, personality changes, and dementia.

B. Brain stem lesions

1) The limb signs may be severe.

2) Reflexes are UMN.

3) Associated signs include abnormal consciousness, multiple cranial nerve deficits, abnormal postural reactions, and ataxia.

C. Spinal cord lesions (The lesion must be in the cervical cord.)

1) Cranial cervical cord (C1–C5) lesions

a) Limb reflexes are all UMN.

b) Associated signs would be ataxia, abnormal postural reactions, or neck pain.

2) Caudal cervical cord (C6–T2) lesions

a) Front limb reflexes are LMN.

b) Rear limb reflexes are UMN.

c) Associated signs may include neck pain, ataxia, abnormal postural reactions, or Horner's syndrome.

D. Peripheral nerve lesions

1) With a diffuse peripheral nerve lesion, the signs are predominantly profound weakness with decreased or absent spinal reflexes and decreased muscle tone.

2) Associated signs in certain diffuse motor unit disorders may include involvement of the cranial nerves as well as of the spinal nerves.

2. Hemiparesis (weakness in a front limb and rear limb on the same side) may result from a focal lesion involving the:

A. Cerebrum

1) The signs are opposite the diseased cerebral hemisphere.

2) Associated signs may include seizures, dementia, and personality changes, as well as visual deficits, abnormal postural reactions, and sensory deficits on the same side as the motor signs.

3) Reflexes in the affected limbs are UMN.

B. Brain stem

1) The reflexes in the affected limbs are UMN.

2) Associated signs include abnormal consciousness, as well as cranial nerve deficits and decreased postural reactions on the same side as the affected limbs.

C. Spinal cord (For the signs listed above to arise from a focal spinal cord lesion, the lesion would have to be in the cervical cord.

1) Cranial cervical cord (C1–C5) lesions

a) There are no cranial nerve deficits.

b) There may be associated ataxia and abnormal postural reactions in the affected limbs.

c) There may be neck pain.

d) All limb reflexes are UMN.

2) Caudal cervical cord lesions

a) There may be anisocoria from a Horner's syndrome in the eye on the same side as the affected limbs.

b) The front limb exhibits LMN reflexes.

c) The rear limb exhibits UMN reflexes.

d) Associated postural deficits and ataxia are present in the affected limbs.

e) There may be neck pain.

3. Paraparesis (weakness limited to the rear limbs) may be a result of a thoracic or lumbar spinal cord injury.

A. There are no cranial nerve deficits.

B. Back pain may be present.

C. Associated signs include ataxia and abnormal postural reactions in the affected limbs.

D. If the lesion is cranial to L3, the rear limb reflexes are UMN.

E. If the lesion is caudal to L3, the rear limb reflexes are LMN.

F. In both cases, the front limb reflexes are normal.

4. Monoparesis (paralysis of one limb) is always a sign of LMN injury if confined to the front limb. If one rear limb is involved, the lesion may be either spinal cord or peripheral in origin.

A. Front limb

1) LMN reflexes

2) Associated signs

a) Abnormal postural reaction in that limb

b) Possible pain

c) Possible Horner's syndrome in the eye on the same side as paralysis

B. Rear limb

1) T2–L3 spinal cord lesions

a) Affected limb has UMN reflexes.

b) Associated signs include ataxia and abnormal postural reaction in the affected limb.

2) L4–S3 or peripheral nerve lesions

a) Reflexes are LMN.

b) Associated signs are abnormal postural reactions and atrophy in the affected limb.

Changes in Spinal Reflexes

Abnormal spinal reflexes are among the easiest part of the neurologic examination to overinterpret or misinterpret. Be aware that abnormal spinal reflexes are simply indicators of an injury to a motor pathway; they are not prognostic tools.

Dramatically asymmetrical reflexes (reflexes in one limb that differ markedly from those in the opposite limb) are generally more significant than a mild generalized increase or decrease in reflex activity. Front limb reflexes are generally less consistent and harder to demonstrate than rear limb reflexes, and so are less reliable.

Each person's description of a reflex is highly subjective. This can be further explained with two truisms: (1) one person's normal is another person's abnormal; (2) the best way to make a mistake is to accept the results of someone else's neurologic examination. With those warnings in mind, we continue our discussion.

1. Increased spinal reflexes

A. An increase in the force or degree of excursion of tendon reflexes (i.e., biceps, triceps, or patella) is usually a sign of UMN injury in the motor pathways to the tested limb. The primary exception to this results from injury to the sciatic nerve (as seen in cauda equina lesions). This type of injury removes the antagonist muscles that oppose the quadriceps muscle group. As a result, the patellar reflex is artificially exaggerated, giving a "false localizing sign" or the appearance of UMN disease (injury cranial to the reflex being tested), when the disease is actually caudal to the tested reflex.

B. An increase in flexor reflexes (spastic flexor) is highly subjective and its significance is questionable.

2. Decreased spinal reflexes, whether tendon, flexor, or perineal, are a sign of a lesion in the reflex arc.

A. These lesions may be in the sensory peripheral nerve, spinal cord grey matter, or motor peripheral nerve.

B. Decreased reflexes are of highly specific localizing value.

3. Development (release) of abnormal reflexes—With UMN injuries, two reflexes that are not normally seen become unmasked. These are Babinski's sign and the crossed extensor reflex. Both are indicators of UMN injury to motor pathways. They should not be interpreted as meaning more.

A. Babinski's sign is an elevation and spreading out of the toes of the rear limb when the plantar aspect of the metatarsus is stroked. When seen in humans, it is a sign of UMN disease. Its significance is more debatable in subprimates.

B. The crossed extensor reflex is elicited when a flexor reflex is initiated in one limb and the contralateral limb involuntarily extends. This may occur in the front or back limb. It is a sign of UMN release to the limb that extends.

Tail Paralysis

Paralysis of the tail may result from thoracic or lumbar spinal cord disease, as well as from disease of the peripheral nerves.

1. With spinal cord disease, the paralysis usually occurs late in the course of the disease. Associated signs include rear limb weakness, urinary or fecal incontinence, or pain.

2. With a peripheral nerve lesion, there is loss of muscle tone in the tail, as well as a loss of voluntary activity.

A. With diffuse peripheral nerve lesions, such as occur from botulism, tick paralysis, and coonhound paralysis, the associated clinical signs include generalized weakness with loss of all spinal reflexes.

B. In focal peripheral nerve injuries (lesions in the cauda equina), associated signs include pain, urinary or fecal incontinence, loss of proprioception in the rear limbs, and weakness in the rear limbs.

Sensory Loss

Animals may develop sensory deficits with cerebral, spinal cord, or peripheral nerve lesions.

1. Sensory loss confined to one side of the body implies a lesion in the cerebrum, with the affected portion of the brain being contralateral to the sensory deficit exhibited.

A. The sensory deficit is characterized by an inability to localize painful stimuli or an abnormal response to stimuli, rather than by a loss of the ability to feel.

B. Associated signs include seizures, weakness, visual deficits, and personality changes.

C. All reflexes are preserved.

2. Sensory loss confined to both rear limbs is an indication of thoracic or lumbar spinal cord disease. It is also an indicator of a severe or advanced pathologic process. Associated signs include back pain, paralysis of both rear limbs, and urinary or fecal incontinence.

3. Sensory loss confined to one limb is an indication of a peripheral nerve or grey matter lesion. Associated signs include paralysis of the limb with loss of tendon reflexes and atrophy of the limb.

Specific Neurologic Disorders Classified According to Location

Motor Unit Disorders

The motor unit consists of a motor neuron, its axon, and the muscle that it innervates; it is the basic functional unit of the nervous system. As motor units may arise from all motor neurons, signs of motor unit disease may be seen in muscles innervated both by cranial nerves and by spinal nerves.

To understand the clinical signs connected with motor unit or LMN diseases, it is important to remember two functions of the motor unit. First, the motor unit is the "final common pathway" for all neural activity. If the LMN is lost, the ability to carry out both voluntary activity and reflex activity is lost. Second, the LMN has a trophic function that maintains the integrity of muscle. Without this trophic influence, atrophy or loss of muscle mass would occur.

LMN diseases are characterized by paralysis, areflexia, and atrophy.

Focal Motor Unit Disorders

Cranial Nerve Lesions

When evaluating animals with lesions of the cranial nerves, you must first decide whether the lesion involves the CNS or the PNS (Fig. 17-7). This is best accomplished by a complete neurologic examination. With a PNS lesion, the signs are totally confined to the affected nerves. With CNS disease, there are other signs in addition to the cranial nerve deficits.

Lesions Involving Cranial Nerve V

1. Idiopathic trigeminal neuropathy (dropped jaw syndrome)

A. This is a syndrome of acute onset in which there is a temporary paralysis of the muscles of mastication. The disease is self-limiting, may be inflammatory in nature, and (in the author's experience) usually occurs in late fall.

B. Clinical presentation

1) There is no breed, age, or sex predilection.

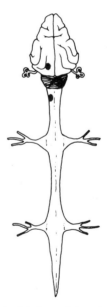

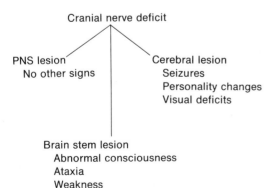

Figure 17-7. *Isolated cranial nerve paralysis may result from brain stem injury. If it does, weakness, ataxia, and altered consciousness will be seen. Any cause of brain stem injury may bring about paralysis. Paralysis of any individual nerve may also represent peripheral nerve injury associated with no other clinical signs. In this case, the causes may be idiopathic and are (usually) self-limiting (such as in seventh cranial nerve paralysis and fifth cranial nerve injury [manifested by a dropped jaw], tumors, or trauma).*

2) Dogs have an acute inability to close the mouth.

3) The owners complain of dysphagia.

4) There are usually no other complaints.

C. Diagnosis—The animal is normal except for paralysis of the jaw.

D. Diagnostic approach

1) Electromyography (EMG) may reveal evidence of denervation.

2) All other tests are normal.

E. Treatment

1) Teach the owners to feed the dog with its head elevated.

2) Steroids should not be given because they artificially increase the appetite in an animal that is having difficulty eating.

F. The prognosis is excellent; all affected animals reported have improved spontaneously within two months.

2. Other causes of CN V paralysis

A. The most common causes are tumors involving CN V and trauma.

B. These processes are usually unilateral.

C. Clinical presentation

1) The usual presenting complaint is acute onset of unilateral atrophy of the temporal muscles.

2) Animals that have neoplasia develop signs of other cranial nerve paralysis (usually CNs VII and VIII) over a period of weeks or months.

3) The mass eventually compresses the brain stem and causes CNS signs.

D. Diagnostic approach

1) Skull roentgenograms may show evidence of lysis from tumors.

2) An EMG may reveal evidence of denervation.

3) A CSF tap will yield abnormal results after the tumor grows into the cranial vault.

a) Elevated pressure

b) Elevated protein

c) Elevated cell count if there is tumor necrosis

E. Treatment—No therapy is currently available.

F. Prognosis

1) Animals with trauma usually neither progress nor improve.

2) Animals with neoplasia eventually exhibit brain stem compression and die.

Lesions Causing Facial Paralysis

1. Either unilateral or bilateral paralysis of the facial muscles (eye, lip, ear) may be seen.

2. Clinical presentation

A. An acute onset of excessive salivation, lip droop, inability to blink the eye, or other evidence of facial paralysis

B. Some animals have an antecedent history of respiratory illness.

C. There are no others signs.

3. Diagnostic considerations

A. Most cases are idiopathic. This condition has also been associated with endocrine dysfunction (hypothyroidism, Cushing's disease), trauma to the face, or tumors of the nerve.

B. Diagnostic approach

1) An EMG reveals denervation.

2) Skull roentgenograms may show lysis if a peripheral nerve tumor is present.

3) Testing of blood for thyroid function and adrenal function should be performed.

4. Treatment

A. If an etiology can be determined, treat the underlying cause appropriately (e.g., thyroid hormone replacement in animals with hypothyroidism).

B. If no etiology can be determined, no treatment is indicated.

5. Prognosis

A. In most idiopathic cases, a gradual return of function has occurred within one to two months. In some affected animals, muscle contracture will occur on the denervated side. If the eye blink does not return, a dry eye may result.

Lesions Involving Cranial Nerve II

1. Lesions of CN II may cause an acute onset of unilateral or complete blindness. This may result from primary ocular disorders or primary lesions of the optic nerve.

2. These lesions are covered in Chapter 18.

Sympathetic Nerve Lesions Involving the Eye

1. Because of its long course, the sympathetic nerve appears to be prone to injury. Most cases of sympathetic nerve dysfunction involving the eye (Horner's syndrome) result from lesions of the brachial plexus, middle ear, or cavernous sinus, and are associated with other clinical signs. However, idiopathic Horner's syndrome may also be seen.

2. Clinical presentation—Abnormally small pupils that are responsive to light, in association with prolapse of the third eyelid, enophthalmos, and a decrease in intraocular pressure

3. Diagnostic considerations

    A. This condition may be seen following soft tissue injuries of the head and neck, mild upper respiratory diseases, or with no associated history of illness.

    B. Diagnosis may be confirmed by pharmacologic testing of the eye with sympathomimetic drugs.

4. Treatment—No treatment is available.

5. Prognosis—If the signs are idiopathic or related to trauma, they usually resolve spontaneously.

Focal Cranial Nerve Disorders (Miscellaneous Comments)

1. All the cranial nerves are susceptible to trauma. The rules of degeneration and regeneration of peripheral nerves apply to cranial nerves as well.

2. All cranial nerves, like spinal nerves, may become involved in a neoplastic process, such as neurofibrosarcoma, meningioma, or lymphoma, and specific cranial nerve syndromes may result.

3. As cranial nerves exit the various foramina of the skull, they have an increased susceptibility to trauma, tumors, or infection.

Lesions Causing Multiple Cranial Nerve Signs

1. Cavernous sinus syndrome

    A. The cavernous sinus lies lateral to pituitary and provides venous drainage to the orbit.

    B. The cavernous sinus contains CNs III, IV, V, and VI, and is the site of sympathetic innervation to the eye.

    C. Signs

        1) Midrange pupil—no response to any stimulus

        2) Loss of all eye movements in that eye

    D. Etiology

        1) Cavernous sinus tumor—hemangiosarcoma; usually no other signs

        2) Pituitary tumor—Visual deficits are also seen.

        3) Fungal infections—diffuse CNS disease

    E. Diagnosis—infraorbital venography

    F. Treatment—Treat the underlying disease.

2. There are several disorders (discussed in the section on disorders of the spinal nerves) that may have cranial nerve signs associated with them. They include:

    A. Acute polyradiculoneuritis (coonhound paralysis)

    B. Chronic polyneuritis

    C. Tick paralysis

    D. Botulism

    E. Myasthenia gravis

    F. Polymyositis

    G. Other chronic polymyopathies

    H. The major cranial nerve complications seen with these are:

        1) Glossopharyngeal and vagal nerve paresis

            a) Dysphagia

            b) Aspiration pneumonia

        2) Facial paralysis

        3) Weakness of jaw tone

        4) Paralysis of pupils (in botulism)

Focal Spinal Nerve Injuries

Focal injuries of a spinal nerve usually result from trauma or compression. If a result of trauma, there is usually an antecedent history of trauma. If compressive lesions are the cause, the history is often more vague. The major causes of compressive or entrapment-type nerve injuries are bony lesions involving the spine, and nerve root tumors. These both tend to have slowly progressive histories and may be quite painful. In addition, the site of the injury along the nerve may help to determine the etiology. Table 17-8 should assist in this determination.

Peripheral Nerve Neoplasia

1. Clinical presentation

 A. Slow progressive disuse of the affected limb over a period of weeks to months

  1) An enlargement in the affected area of the nerve may be palpated.

  2) Area of tumor may be painful owing to irritation of sensory nerve fibers (neurofibrosarcoma).

 B. Signs of LMN (peripheral nerve) dysfunction

  1) Loss of function of the muscles denervated

  2) Severe atrophy of the muscles supplied by the diseased nerve

  3) Occasional fasciculations of the muscles supplied by the diseased nerve

  4) Signs vary with the specific nerve involved and the degree of involvement.

 C. Signs associated with specific nerve damage of the forelimb

  1) Suprascapular nerve—atrophy of supraspinous and infraspinous muscles

  2) Radial nerve

   a) Atrophy of triceps, extensor carpi radialis, and other extensors of the carpus and digits

   b) Inability to bear weight on limb

   c) Elbow is dropped.

  3) Musculocutaneous nerve

   a) Atrophy of biceps and brachials

   b) Decreased flexion of elbow

  4) Medial and ulnar nerves—atrophy of superficial and deep digital flexors

 D. Signs associated with specific nerve damage of the hindlimb

  1) Obturator nerve—atrophy of external obturator, pectineal, abductor, and gracilis

  2) Femoral nerve

   a) Inability to bear weight on limb or fix (extend) the stifle

   b) Atrophy of quadriceps

  3) Sciatic nerve

   a) Atrophy of gluteal, semimembranous, semitendinous, gastrocnemius, and anterior tibial

   b) Inability to flex stifle

   c) Proprioceptive deficit

   d) May be associated with a dropped hock

  4) Tibial nerve

   a) Atrophy of gastrocnemius

   b) The hock joint remains flexed when animal walks or stands (dropped hock).

2. Differential diagnosis

 A. Neurofibrosarcoma is the most common neoplasia in adult dogs.

Table 17-8. *Principles for localizing mononeuropathies*

	Spinal Cord	**Nerve Root**	**Nerve**
Distribution of weakness	Segmental muscles innervated by several nerves involved	Segmental	Restricted to muscles innervated by affected nerve
Severity of weakness in affected limb	Mild weakness	Mild weakness	Severe weakness
Limbs caudal to affected limbs involved	Yes	No, early on; yes, late	No
Muscle tone	Decreased	Decreased	Decreased
Reflexes	Decreased	Decreased	Decreased
Atrophy	Entire limb, mild	Entire limb, mild	Focal, severe
EMG changes	+	+	+
Nerve conduction velocity (NCV)	Normal early, decreased late	Normal early, decreased late	Decreased or absent

B. Lymphosarcoma (LSA) is most common in young cats (1 to 2 years of age), but may be seen in cats and dogs at any age.

C. The brachial plexus is a common site for both neurofibrosarcoma and LSA.

D. The cauda equina (L6–S3) is also a common site for LSA.

E. Both tumors may involve any peripheral nerve.

  3. Diagnostic approach

    A. Roentgenography

      1) May reveal no abnormalities, or may show a soft tissue swelling in the area of the tumor

      2) Thoracic roentgenograms may show nothing or may show large lymph nodes that are compatible with LSA.

    B. EMG

      1) Confirms which nerves are involved

      2) Nerve conduction studies determine whether the nerves are intact.

    C. Hematologic studies

      1) Blood test for FeLV

      2) Bone marrow biopsy if LSA is suspected

  4. Treatment

    A. Exploration, removal of tumor, and anastomosis of nerve, if possible

    B. In the case of brachial plexus involvement, the limb usually must be amputated.

    C. Postsurgical radiation therapy may decrease the likelihood of recurrence.

  5. Prognosis

    A. Neurofibrosarcoma

      1) If the lesion is isolated, the tumor may be removed and the animal may have no further problems.

      2) This tumor is known to occur in multiples, so the animal must be watched for development of any new signs.

    B. LSA

      1) Metastatic from some other site

      2) The prognosis for correcting the problem is grave, but you may be able to prolong the animal's life.

Cauda Equina Syndrome

  1. General principles

    A. A pathologic process at L7–S1 vertebral space causes clinical signs in both dogs and cats.

    B. Clinical presentation

      1) Usually affects older dogs, Manx kittens, English bulldog puppies, and young adult cats

      2) Occurs in either sex

    C. Primary complaints

      1) Pain—may bite tail, chase flank

      2) Inability to lift tail

      3) Soiled tail

      4) Urinary or fecal incontinence

      5) Usually a slow, progressive disease

    D. Physical examination

      1) Inability to lift tail

      2) Atrophy of semimembranous or semitendinous muscles as a result of partial sciatic involvement

    E. Neural examination

      1) Decreased anal tone

      2) Decreased flexor reflex

      3) Proprioceptive deficit in rear limbs

      4) Pain at L7–S1 vertebral interspace in animals with acquired conditions

  2. Diagnostic considerations

    A. Vertebral or peripheral nerve neoplasia

    B. Discospondylitis (intradiscal osteomyelitis)

    C. Ligamentous hypertrophy

    D. Malformations

    E. Fungal infections in cats

    F. LSA in cats

    G. Trauma

    H. Lumbosacral stenosis

    I. Intervertebral disk disease

  3. Diagnostic approach

    A. EMG

      1) Often yields normal results

      2) May show decreased or absent coccygeal nerve conduction

      3) May reveal denervation of the perineum

    B. Roentgenograms

      1) Plain films show the following:

        a) Intradiscal osteomyelitis

        b) Tumors

        c) Fractures or avulsions

      2) Contrast studies

        a) Epidural myelograms

        b) Venous sinography (This is a

difficult area in which to perform valid contrast roentgenograms.)

4. Treatment

A. Surgical decompression is the treatment of choice for compressive lesions.

B. Infections may be treated medically. This may not alleviate the signs, however, and surgery may be required in these cases as well.

5. Prognosis

A. Determined by the etiology

B. Animals with compressive lesions (lumbosacral stenosis) may have a very good prognosis if diagnosed and treated early. Neoplasia carries a poor prognosis.

Brachial Plexus Nerve Root Avulsion

1. Traumatic injury to the nerve roots that form the brachial plexus. The injury may involve any combination of roots (both dorsal and ventral) and so affected animals have variable signs. The pathology may include tearing or shearing of nerve roots, compression of roots from fractures or hematomas, and stretching of roots.

2. Clinical presentation

A. History of major trauma with subsequent forelimb monoparesis

B. Clinical signs usually are referable primarily to the radial nerve, and include an inability to bear weight, loss of proprioception, and variable loss of pain perception.

C. If the nerve roots of T-1 and T-2 are involved, the animal may have an ipsilateral Horner's syndrome.

1) Miosis

2) Protrusion of third eyelid

3) Enophthalmos

3. Diagnostic approach

A. EMG—Needle EMG reveals positive sharp waves, fibrillation potentials, and bizarre high-frequency discharges in denervated muscles.

B. Nerve conduction—There may be no response or slowed nerve conduction, depending on the severity of the injury.

4. Treatment

A. Surgical

1) Exploration and repair of torn nerves if the lesion is in the plexus

2) Removal of hematomas or compressive lesions in the plexus

B. Medical

1) Physical therapy to prevent tendon contractions

2) Bandaging or covering of the feet to prevent self-trauma

5. Prognosis

A. The prognosis in most traumatic nerve injuries (e.g., brachial plexus injuries) is guarded.

B. If, after an appropriate time (two to six months), there is no evidence of return of function, amputation of the limb may be advised.

C. During recovery, abnormal sensation (paresthesias) may result in lick granuloma formation.

Diffuse Motor Unit Disorders

Diffuse motor unit disorders are those diseases that may affect any or all motor units in the animal (Figure 17-8). The selectivity in these diseases depends on which portion of the motor unit they affect. Focal lesions tend to cause total loss of function; diffuse motor unit diseases tend to create weakness rather than paralysis. The latter cause loss of muscle tone and muscle mass, and so are characterized by atrophy. Most of these diseases are not painful. The primary sign of diffuse motor unit disease is weakness. In the early stages, this may be manifested as lameness. In severe cases, the animal may be recumbent.

The animal's disease must be differentiated from other causes of tetraparesis—namely, brain or spinal cord disorders—by performing a reflex examination. Animals with diffuse motor unit disease usually have hyporeflexia. Table 17-9 offers some guidelines for localizing these lesions.

Disorders of the Ventral Horn Cell

1. Inflammatory disease or diffuse myelitis

A. Inflammatory diseases, such as toxoplasmosis, canine distemper, and feline infectious peritonitis (FIP), may diffusely affect the ventral horn cell.

B. Clinical presentation

1) Signs are usually acute.

2) Signs are usually multifocal and

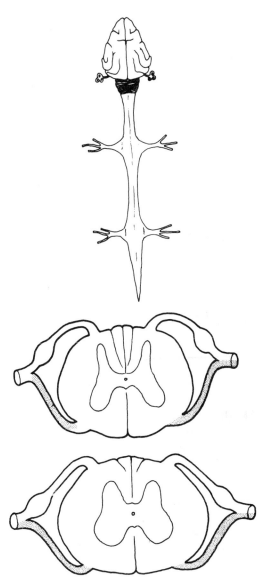

Figure 17-8. *Motor unit disorders may cause disorders of gait with weakness alone. Symptoms include severe weakness, slow reflexes, and decreased muscle tone. These disorders may be brought about by myasthenia gravis, coonhound paralysis, polymyositis, tick paralysis, or botulism.*

spotty, sparing some nerves and affecting others.

     3) Affected animals often appear painful.

     4) Often, there is no other significant history.

     5) Neurologic examination

          a) Combination of UMN and LMN signs

          b) Sensory deficits

  C. Diagnostic approach

     1) Abnormal results on CSF evaluation

          a) Increased protein

          b) Increased cell count

     2) Abnormal EMG

  D. Prognosis—grave; treatment is merely supportive.

  2. Metabolic disease, such as spinal muscular atrophy of Brittany spaniels

  A. Progressive disease of Brittany spaniels (or other purebred dogs)

  B. Seen in animals of less than one year of age (and as early as six months)

  C. Clinical presentation—progressive atrophy of the spinal muscles secondary to motor neuron disease

     1) Rear limb weakness progressing to forelimbs

     2) Severe muscle atrophy in affected muscles

     3) Occasional cranial nerve involvement

     4) Proprioception is often normal.

     5) Reflexes are depressed.

  D. Diagnosis

     1) EMG, denervation potentials

     2) Normal results are obtained from nerve conduction studies.

     3) Muscle biopsies reveal a characteristic pattern.

  E. There is no treatment.

  F. Similar disorders are reported in other breeds and species.

Polyneuropathy and Polyradiculopathy

  1. Diffuse involvement of either peripheral nerves or nerve roots by any disease causing wallerian degeneration or demyelination may produce LMN weakness.

  A. Toxicity, from lead and other drugs

  B. Metabolic disorder, from diabetes mellitus, hypothyroidism, uremia, or cancer

  C. Nutritional disorder, from thiamine deficiency

  D. Immunologic disorder, from coon-

Table 17-9. **Principles of localizing diffuse motor unit disorders**

	Radiculoneuropathies	Neuromuscular Junction	Muscle
Distribution of weakness	Diffuse	Diffuse	Diffuse
Muscle tone	Decreased	Normal	Normal
Atrophy	Widespread, acute	None	None early, moderate late
Reflexes	Decreased or absent	Normal to decreased	Normal
EMG changes	+	Normal	+
Nerve conduction velocity	Normal or decreased	Normal	Normal
Evoked potentials	Polyphasic, giant	Normal to decreased amplitude	Normal to polyphasic (decreased amplitude)
Repetitive nerve stimulation	Normal	Myasthenia Decremental	Normal
		Botulism Incremental	

hound paralysis or acute idiopathic polyneuritis (see Chapter 7 on intermittent weakness)

2. Chronic polyneuropathy

A. A chronic, progressive disease of the peripheral nerves that is possibly attributable to immunologic, metabolic, toxic, or nutritional causes. Many times, the actual cause is unknown.

B. Clinical presentation

1) Any age, breed, or sex of dog may be affected.

2) Slow, progressive weakness progressing over a period of several weeks to months

3) Severe muscle atrophy in all four limbs and paraspinal muscles

4) Loss of muscle tone

5) May have intercostal and phrenic nerve paresis (dyspnea)

6) May have cranial nerve signs

C. Differential diagnosis

1) Lysosomal storage diseases

2) Metabolic disorder, from Cushing's syndrome, hypothyroidism, insulinomas, uremia, thiamine deficiency

3) Toxicity, from lead, organophosphates

D. Diagnostic approach

1) EMG reveals trains of positive sharp waves and fibrillations in all paraspinal and limb muscles.

2) Slowed nerve conduction velocity (NCV)

3) Nerve biopsy of a superficial radial or lateral plantar nerve reveals axonal degeneration/demyelination.

4) CSF findings are usually normal.

E. Treatment—Diagnose and treat the underlying causes.

F. Prognosis

1) Depends on cause

2) Often, the underlying cause is not determined, and the signs continue to progress.

3. Inherited canine hypertrophic neuropathy—an inherited, progressive, demyelinating disease of Tibetan mastiffs. The underlying problem appears to be in the Schwann cell.

A. Clinical presentation

1) Progressive weakness first appears in affected animals at 7 to 12 weeks of age. There is progressive atrophy of the limbs with contractures of the joints.

2) During the early stages of the disease, the tibial nerve appears to be the most affected, so animals have a plantigrade stance.

B. Diagnostic approach

1) Electrodiagnostic testing reveals mild denervation with severe slowing of NCV.

2) Some affected patients have an

albuminocytologic dissociation on CSF analysis.

    3) The definitive diagnosis rests on biopsy of the peripheral nerve.

    C. Treatment—There is no effective therapy.

    D. Prognosis—This is an invariably fatal disease.

    4. Canine sensory neuropathy—This neuropathy is unique in that it is characterized by loss of nociceptive ability without proprioceptive or motor deficits. As a result of the sensory deficits, the animals self-mutilate their feet. The condition has been reported in short-haired pointers, English pointers, and long-haired dachshunds.

    A. Clinical presentation

    1) Affected animals often appear smaller than their littermates.

    2) Lack of pain perception is seen as early as 11 weeks of age.

    3) Animals chew and bite at their extremities causing severe self-mutilations. Despite severe inflammation and ulceration of the feet, the animals walk on them normally since they cannot feel.

    4) Tendon reflexes are preserved, but flexor reflexes are diminished.

    B. Diagnostic approach—With the exception of histopathologic results, all diagnostic tests are normal. The only histopathologic changes are in the dorsal root ganglia and in Lissauer's tract of the spinal cord.

    C. Treatment—No therapy is currently available.

    D. Prognosis—This condition invariably results in euthanasia because of the disfiguring mutilation and pododermatitis.

    5. Progressive axonopathy of boxers—This is an inherited axonal disease of boxers that affects both the CNS and the PNS. Clinically, the predominant signs are referable to the PNS. The pathologic process appears to be demyelination and remyelination, but the underlying mechanism of injury remains to be determined.

    A. Clinical presentation

    1) The signs usually appear at around six months of age and begin with ataxia that progresses to weakness. The pelvic limb is affected first, then the thoracic limbs.

    2) The tendon reflexes are diminished, as is muscle tone.

    3) Pain perception is normal.

    B. Diagnostic approach

    1) There is moderate slowing of nerve conduction with decreased amplitude of the evoked response. Otherwise, the electrodiagnostic examination is normal.

    2) Nerve biopsy shows fairly characteristic changes.

    C. Treatment—None is currently available.

    D. Prognosis—This condition invariably progresses to complete paralysis.

    6. Giant axonal neuropathy—This is an inherited disease of young German shepherds. The disease appears to be caused by an inherited defect in axon transport. As a result, there is inadequate maintenance of myelin and giant axons form.

    A. Clinical presentation

    1) The onset of signs usually occurs at about 15 months of age.

    2) Affected animals often have abnormally curly hair, there is pelvic limb ataxia and weakness, the tendon reflexes in the pelvic limbs are diminished, and the limbs are hypotonic. There is megaesophagus with subsequent regurgitation. The animals usually have decreased pain perception in the pelvic limbs and fecal incontinence.

    3) The thoracic limbs are usually only mildly involved.

    B. Diagnostic approach

    1) NCVs are slowed and the amplitudes are generally diminished.

    2) Nerve biopsy reveals onion-bulb formation with nodal and paranodal axonal swelling.

    3) There are characteristic filamentous accumulations in nonmyelinated fibers, Schwann cells, astrocytes, and endothelial cells.

    C. Treatment—None is currently available.

    D. Prognosis—This condition invariably results in euthanasia.

    7. Delayed organophosphate neuropathy—Certain organophosphates not only affect acetylcholinesterase, but also phosphorylate a protein esterase in the nervous system that is essential for axon transport. Exposure to a member of this family or organophosphates can lead to a delayed polyneuropathy. The half-life of this phosphorylation can be months, so recovery may be delayed.

A. Clinical presentation

1) Symptoms begin one to three weeks following exposure to the organophosphates. A progressive symmetrical, primarily motor, neuropathy develops.

2) Many affected animals will be tremulous, with very fine oscillatory movement of the head and limbs.

3) Cats appear to be highly susceptible to the disorder.

B. Diagnostic approach—Electrodiagnostic examination reveals evidence of distal denervation, the evoked response is often decreased in amplitude, there are delayed terminal motor latencies, but motor NCV is normal.

C. Treatment—None is currently available.

D. Prognosis—This condition may spontaneously go into remission, but the recovery period is quite protracted.

8. Ganglioradiculoneuritis—an inflammatory disease of dorsal root and cranial nerve ganglia that produces a progressive ataxia. The cause of the inflammation is unknown. To date, the condition has been reported in Brittany spaniels, Siberian huskies, and Welsh corgis.

A. Clinical presentation

1) Affected animals all have megaesophagus and regurgitation. There is atrophy of the masticatory muscles, loss of facial pain perception, loss of limb proprioception, limb ataxia, and decreased tendon reflexes.

2) The condition is seen only in adult animals, but no precipitating event has been detected.

B. Diagnostic approach

1) Decreased sensory NCVs occur, but otherwise, the electrodiagnostic examination is normal.

2) Nerve biopsy reveals axonal degeneration. Biopsy of a dorsal ganglion reveals nonsuppurative inflammation.

C. Treatment—None is currently avail-

able, although the use of steroids is being investigated.

D. Prognosis—This condition invariably results in euthanasia.

Neuromuscular Junction Disorders

1. Neuromuscular junction disorders (see Chapter 7 on intermittent weakness) are toxic or immunologic processes that affect the normal transmission of acetylcholine across the neuromuscular junction.

A. Tick paralysis

B. Botulism

C. Myasthenia gravis

Polymyopathies

1. Inflammatory and degenerative processes of muscles caused by many conditions

A. Nutritional disorders, vitamin-E deficiency

B. Metabolic disorders, Cushing's syndrome, hypothyroidism

C. Toxicity

D. Inflammatory disorders, either immune-mediated or infectious

E. Inherited disorders, as in Irish terriers and golden retrievers. Golden retrievers appear to have a true muscular dystrophy.

Polymyositis

1. A generalized inflammatory condition of the skeletal muscles affecting dogs of any breed or sex. There have also been cases reported in cats.

2. Clinical presentation

A. Chronic progressive weakness in all four limbs which worsens with exercise

B. Vomiting may occur as a result of megaesophagus (documented by roentgenography).

C. Muscle atrophy

D. Spinal reflexes are often normal.

E. Possible muscle pain

3. Differential diagnoses

A. Idiopathic

B. Collagen vascular

1) Systemic lupus erythematosus (SLE)

2) Rheumatoid disorders

C. Infectious

1) Toxoplasmosis

2) Trichinosis

3) Viral

D. Eosinophilic myositis

4. Diagnostic approach

A. An EMG reveals trains of positive waves and fibrillations with low-amplitude motor unit action potentials in all limb muscles.

B. Serum muscle enzymes—increased creatine phosphokinase (CPK), lactic dehydrogenase (LDH), and serum aspartate transferase (AST)

C. Muscle biopsy—infiltration of muscle fibers by lymphocytes and plasma cells in immune disorders, and by neutrophils in infectious disorders

D. Perform immunologic tests (lupus erythematosus [LE] prep and ANA)

5. Criteria for diagnosis

A. Primary myopathy

1) Clinically progressive

2) Diffuse muscle involvement

3) Muscle pain

4) Laboratory confirmation—biopsy results and CPK levels

B. Systemic disease

1) Abnormal immunologic work-up

2) Endocrine dysfunction

6. Treatment—Corticosteroids if the disorder is immunologic in origin; antibiotics, if it is infectious

7. Prognosis—Poor. Condition may be controlled for a period of time, but may eventually progress in some cases.

Metabolic Myopathies

1. Metabolic myopathies are degenerative diseases of the muscle that occur in any animal species secondary to some other primary metabolic disease, especially cancer, hypothyroidism, or Cushing's disease.

2. Clinical presentation—Animals may present with generalized debility or complaints centering around a specific problem

(skin disease, polydipsia) that is related to the underlying etiology.

3. Diagnosis—The diagnosis of the myopathy is incidental.

4. Treatment—Therapy consists of treating the underlying disease process.

Feline Hypokalemic Polymyopathy

Feline hypokalemic polymyopathy is an inflammatory polymyositis that develops secondary to profound (<2.8 mEq/L) hypokalemia. The cause of the hypokalemia remains controversial. Some investigators believe that it is nutritional (related to diets formulated to acidify urine, which promote excess urine potassium excretion), whereas others believe that it is secondary to renal disease. Regardless of the initiating event, the hypokalemia results in a necrotizing polymyopathy/polymyositis.

1. Clinical presentation

A. There appears to be no age, breed, or sex predilection.

B. Affected animals are weak, have a characteristic ventroflexion of the head, and experience weight loss, anorexia, dysphagia, dyspnea, and muscle pain. The signs are generally rapid in onset, developing over a period of five or fewer days.

2. Diagnostic approach

A. Affected animals have pronounced serum hypokalemia and elevations in muscle enzymes.

B. The electrodiagnostic examination is generally abnormal, especially the EMG.

C. Muscle biopsy reveals variations in fiber size and lymphocytic inflammation of the affected muscles.

3. Treatment

A. The essential feature of therapy is correction of the hypokalemia. How to do this remains controversial.

1) Some advocate intravenous (IV) correction of the potassium depletion over a period of two to three days. The disadvantage of this is that it does not appear to correct the anorexia.

2) Others prefer oral hyperalimentation, which provides a more gradual correction. This appears to correct the anorexia, but the animals remain ill longer.

    3) In addition to the correction of the potassium depletion, some clinicians advocate the use of immunosuppressive doses of steroids to correct the myositis. However, this therapy is falling out of favor now that the disease is better understood.

  4. Prognosis—Early reports indicated that 75% of affected animals would improve, but 42% would have relapses. With improved modes of therapy, the prognosis appears to be improving. Relapse rates are declining and the percentage of cases recovering at the author's institution exceeds 90%.

Myotonia

Myotonia is a disorder of electrolyte transport across the muscle cell membrane. The primary defect appears to be one of chloride transport. As a result of the disorder, muscle contraction persists after stimulation. In short, myotonia is a condition in which there is either failure of or delay in muscle relaxation. Myotonia has been reported in chows, King Charles spaniels, Irish terriers, Staffordshire terriers, Samoyeds, and dachshunds as a congenital disorder. It may also occur in association with Cushing's disease, whether spontaneous or iatrogenic.

  1. Clinical presentation

    A. As a result of delayed muscle relaxation, affected animals appear to be stiff or spastic. They may be unable to initiate movement in severe cases, and they appear to develop muscle spasms. The stiffness is at its worst in the morning or after a period of rest. Most affected animals will "warm out" of their signs.

    B. Aside from the abnormal muscle tone and gait, the affected muscle may dimple when it is percussed.

    C. Otherwise, the physical examination is normal.

  2. Diagnosis

    A. On EMG, there are very characteristic changes. These changes consist of waxing

and waning trains of high-frequency discharges, known as myotonic discharges.

    B. The rest of the electrodiagnostic examination is usually normal.

    C. In some patients, there may be elevation of the creatinine kinase (CK) levels. These elevations are generally mild.

  3. Treatment—There is no effective therapy at present. Membrane stabilizing agents, such as procainamide may be beneficial, but no long-term studies on its use are yet available.

  4. Prognosis

    A. Although not a fatal, or even disabling disease, this condition is disconcerting to most owners. The affected animals will never recover and will always be symptomatic.

    B. As all evidence suggests that the congenital form of the disorder is hereditary, it is advised that affected animals be neutered and the breeder counseled against using the same genetic pool for breeding in the future.

Muscular Dystrophy

Several breeds of dogs appear to have distinct, probably inherited, myopathies that bear clinical and pathologic features that are similar to the muscular dystrophies. These include the Labrador retriever, golden retriever, Irish terrier, and Alaskan malamute.

  1. Clinical presentation

    A. There may be either muscle hypertrophy or atrophy, depending on the stage of the disease. Most affected animals become symptomatic by eight weeks of age.

    B. There is progressive restriction of limb movement, dysphagia, and abduction of limbs.

  2. Diagnosis

    A. There is marked elevation of CK levels, both at rest and following exercise.

    B. Bizarre, high-frequency discharges are noted on EMG.

    C. Muscle biopsy is abnormal and reveals necrotic fibers and various stages of phagocytosis of muscles. There is also evidence of muscle regeneration.

  3. Treatment—No treatment is effective in these disorders.

4. Prognosis—The prognosis is quite poor, and most of these dogs die of respiratory failure or aspiration pneumonia.

Exertional Myopathies

Exertional myopathy is a condition seen in racing greyhounds. It is an acute necrosis of muscle that occurs when a period of exercise follows a period of rest. The disease is believed to be related to glycogen depletion in the muscles, with resultant lactic acid accumulation in the muscle. This damages muscle cell membranes and causes release of myoglobin, which is nephrotoxic. The end result may be renal failure.

1. Clinical presentation

    A. Affected animals will have marked muscle stiffness and pain during vigorous exercise. If the exercise is continued, severe muscle spasms ("tying up") may develop.

    B. There is profuse sweating, and the involved muscles become painful and tense.

    C. Within 24 hours, the urine becomes dark brown from myoglobin pigment.

    D. After a severe attack or after repeated mild attacks, the affected muscle—usually, the gluteals and pelvic limb muscle—may atrophy.

2. Diagnosis

    A. Marked elevation of muscle enzymes in association with lactic acidosis.

    B. Urinalysis demonstrates myoglobinuria.

3. Treatment

    A. The principle treatment is rest.

    B. Correct any electrolyte and acid–base abnormalities that are detected. Provide supportive therapy, especially fluids.

    C. Corticosteroids appear to be contraindicated. Muscle relaxants may be beneficial, as are nonsteroidal anti-inflammatory drugs, such as aspirin or phenylbutazone.

4. Prevention—Regular conditioning exercise, proper diet, and proper cool-down periods can help to prevent the occurrence of myoglobinuria.

5. Prognosis—In most cases, the prognosis appears to be good.

Type II Myopathy of Labrador Retrievers

1. Hereditary disease of Labrador retrievers

2. Clinical presentation

    A. Generalized muscle weakness

    B. Generalized atrophy of muscles

        1) Exercise intolerance

        2) Cold intolerance

    C. Signs begin at three to five months of age; they are slowly progressive, peak, and then stabilize at about maturity.

3. Diagnosis

    A. An EMG reveals myotonic discharges.

    B. CPK levels are normal, but there are increased urinary creatine levels with decreased urinary creatine to creatinine ratios.

    C. Pathologic examination reveals variations in fiber size; changes in the fiber nuclei, especially changes in position; and generalized atrophy and reduction in the number of type II fibers.

Scotty Cramps

1. A hereditary disorder of movement

2. When stimulated, affected animals initially can move normally, but they become progressively more hypertonic, leading to:

    A. Arched back

    B. Stiff-legged gait

    C. Total inability to move

3. When the stimulus is removed, all signs abate.

    A. Nonpainful

    B. No abnormalities at rest

    C. Normal neural examination

4. Valium improves the clinical signs.

5. No pathologic changes are seen. The disorder is believed to be related to abnormalities in serotonin levels.

Summary

1. Focal motor unit diseases tend to:

    A. Be unilateral

    B. Have associated signs limited to a single (or a few) nerve(s)

    C. Be accompanied by both motor and sensory signs

2. Diffuse motor unit diseases tend to:

A. Involve all spinal and some cranial nerves

B. Be characterized by motor signs only

3. Both groups are characterized by:

A. Absence of function

B. Absence of reflexes

C. Absence of tone

D. Atrophy

4. Abnormal EMG findings in motor unit diseases may be summarized as follows:

A. Increased insertional activity may be seen in:

1) Neuropathies

2) Myopathies

3) Myotonia

4) Cramps

B. Spontaneous activity may be seen in:

1) Myopathies

2) Neuropathies

C. Alteration in evoked potentials

1) Decreased size is seen in myopathies.

2) Increased size is characteristic of reinnervation.

D. Decreased numbers of evoked potentials are seen in neuropathies.

E. Special phenomena (i.e., myotonic discharges) are seen in myotonia, some normal animals, and some endocrine myopathies.

Spinal Cord Disorders

General Approach

Location and Severity of Lesion

In spinal cord disease, the clinical signs reflect both the anatomic location and the severity of the lesion (Figs. 17-9 to 17-12 and Table 17-10). Anatomically three factors need to be considered: longitudinal location (spinal cord segment injured); circumferential location of the injury (left side versus right side); and grey matter injury versus white matter injury. A grey matter injury causes LMN dysfunction in those muscles innervated by the cell bodies at the site of the injury. A white matter injury causes both ataxia from

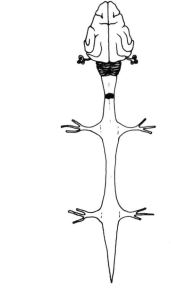

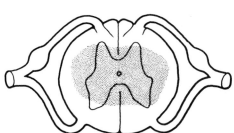

Figure 17-9. *A bilateral cervical spinal injury may create disorders of gait with ataxia and weakness combined. The associated signs of this condition are a normal cranial nerve examination (except possible Horner's syndrome), tetraparesis, and pain. The disease processes include disk disease, external trauma, cervical instability, atlantoaxial (AA) luxation, neoplasia, inflammations, and vascular disease, such as fibrocartilaginous infarct and LSA.*

interruption of proprioceptive pathways, and UMN weakness in the limbs at or caudal to the site of the white matter injury.

The circumferential location is important because most fiber tracts in the spinal cord run ipsilaterally. Thus, an injury to the left side of the spinal cord causes predominantly left-sided clinical signs; an injury to the right side of the spinal cord causes predominantly right-sided clinical signs. The longitudinal location of the lesion is important because it determines the location of any grey matter injury. Grey matter injury to the spinal segment of a limb causes LMN dysfunction in that limb, which often carries a graver prognosis than a similar UMN spinal cord injury.

The severity of injury helps determine clinical signs because of the difference in

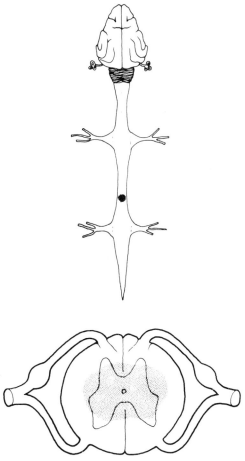

Figure 17-11. *Bilateral thoracic or lumbar spinal cord injury may cause disorders of gait with ataxia and weakness combined, with associated signs of only rear limb involvement and pain. The disease processes from trauma include intervertebral (IV) disk disease or external trauma. Diseases also involve discospondylitis; degenerative processes, such as Afghan myelopathy and degenerative myelopathy; vascular disease; neoplasia; inflammation; and malformations.*

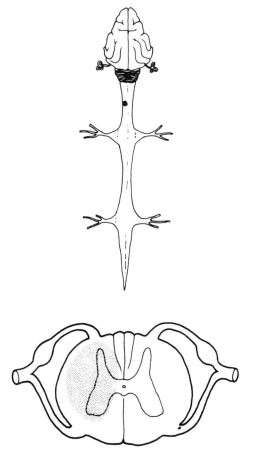

Figure 17-10. *Unilateral cervical spinal injury may cause disorders of gait with ataxia and weakness combined. It is associated with the following signs: hemiparesis, normal cranial nerve examination, and pain. The disease processes include disk disease, external trauma, cervical instability, AA luxation, neoplasia, and inflammations; in cases of vascular injury, the signs are fibrocartilaginous infarct and LSA.*

susceptibility to injury among fiber types in the spinal cord. The larger a fiber and the more myelin it contains, the more susceptible it is to injury. The proprioceptive fibers are the most susceptible to injury, the motor fibers are second in susceptibility, and pain fibers are the least susceptible to injury.

Animals only exhibiting ataxia or signs referable to proprioceptive injury may be

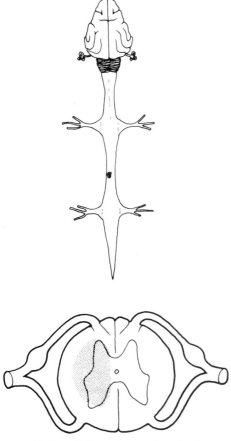

Figure 17-12. *Unilateral thoracic or lumbar spinal disease causes disorders of gait with ataxia and weakness, and is associated with signs of monoparesis of a rear limb and pain. The disease processes include intervertebral (IV) disk disease or external trauma, discospondylitis, vascular injury, neoplasia, inflammation, and malformations.*

classified as having a mild spinal cord deficit. Animals with a combination of ataxia and weakness (both proprioceptive loss and motor loss) may be described as having a moderate spinal cord injury. Finally, animals with loss of all three types of function (proprioceptive, motor, and pain perception) may be defined as having a severe spinal cord injury.

Prognosis

In addition to the general concepts underlying diagnosis of spinal cord disease, some gen-

eral concepts regarding the prognosis for animals with spinal cord disease should be considered. The prognosis in neurologic disease requires both a knowledge of the neurologic signs and a knowledge of their etiology (Table 17-11). The less severe the spinal cord disease is, the more likely is recovery. The progression of signs indicates an increase in severity of disease. As each of these signs becomes apparent, it implies a longer time period to recovery and a worse prognosis for total recovery.

The first sign seen in spinal cord dysfunction is loss of proprioception. Because the conscious and unconscious proprioceptive fibers are closely related, loss of both conscious and unconscious proprioception is common in spinal cord disease. This helps to differentiate high cervical cord diseases from cerebellar diseases (which would be characterized by pure loss of unconscious proprioception) or cerebral diseases (which would be associated with pure loss of conscious proprioception). Thus, proprioceptive deficits of spinal cord origin with no other signs imply mild spinal cord disease and a good prognosis if the disease can be reversed. Proprioceptive deficits are followed by paresis in order of severity. Paresis implies motor tract involvement and is characterized by weakness. In addition, with paresis, there may be reflex changes. Next in order of severity is paralysis, or total loss of voluntary movement. This implies severe spinal cord dysfunction and is associated with spinal cord reflex changes. Last in order of severity is loss of pain perception. Loss of pain perception implies severe bilateral spinal cord dysfunction and is a grave prognostic sign. Many clinicians believe that, in an acute spinal cord injury, the absence of pain perception for more than 48 hours indicates total, irreversible cord dysfunction. If the animal has a treatable disease, proprioceptive loss implies mild dysfunction and is a reversible lesion associated with a short recovery time; paresis implies moderate dysfunction and is a reversible lesion associated with a moderate recovery time, paralysis implies moderate to severe spinal cord dysfunction and is a reversible lesion characterized by a prolonged recovery time; anesthesia implies bilateral

Table 17-10. *Localization of spinal cord disease*

Both Forelimbs and Rear Limbs Involved	Only Rear Limbs Involved
Forelimb reflexes	Rear limb reflexes
UMN	*UMN*
Lesion is either C1–C5 or a white matter injury	Lesion is T2–L3
LMN	*LMN*
Rear limb reflexes—UMN: lesion is C6–T2	Lesion is L4–S3
Rear limb reflexes—LMN: multifocal disease, involving either spinal cord or peripheral nerve	
Normal findings, but apparent increased tone	
Possible Schiff-Sherrington syndrome; lesion is T2–L7	

spinal cord destruction and is an irreversible lesion with a very grave prognosis.

Another factor to be considered in the prognosis of spinal cord disease is that grey matter injuries tend to be more permanent than white matter injuries. White matter injuries often reflect demyelination rather than severing of axons. Grey matter lesions generally imply loss of neurons with irreversible dysfunction. With focal spinal cord disease, the presence of LMN signs implies a worse prognosis than the same degree of clinical signs with a purely UMN lesion.

Treatment Principles

Some general statements should be made regarding the treatment of the animals with spinal cord dysfunction. Regardless of the cause of spinal cord disease and its reversibility, the long-term outcome is often determined by nursing care. Animals with spinal cord disease have a high incidence of both

Table 17-11. *Etiology of spinal cord disease*

Focal		Diffuse	
Intramedullary	*Extramedullary*	*Intramedullary*	*Extramedullary*
Vascular disease	Neoplasia	Degeneration	Inflammations/infections
Fibrocartilaginous infarct	Meningioma	German shepherd myelopathy	FIP
Trauma	Lymphosarcoma	Afghan myelopathy	Distemper
Neoplasia	Neurofibroma	Lysosomal storage disorders	Systemic fungal disease
Astrocytoma	Bone tumors	Spinal muscular atrophy of Brittany spaniels	Meningitis
Oligodendroglioma	Disk disease	Neoplasia	Trauma
	Trauma	Inflammations/infections	
	Infections	FIP	
	Intradiscal osteomyelitis	Canine distemper	
	Malformations or malarticulations	Fungal disease	
	Cervical spondylopathy	Toxoplasmosis	
	AA luxation	Malformations	
	Hemivertebrae	Spinal dysraphism	
	Spina bifida		

urinary and fecal retention. The fecal retention leads to constipation or obstipation. Animals that are recumbent should be watched to be certain that they are eliminating stool properly. Urinary tract disease is more complicated. Animals with spinal cord disease may have either an inability to retain urine or an inability to expel urine, depending on the location of the disease. If the animal is unable to retain urine, it constantly dribbles on itself, becomes urine-soaked, and develops urine scalding. Because of the lack of sphincter function, this animal also frequently has cystitis and, potentially, pyelonephritis. Urinary retention may lead to overdistention of the bladder and permanent bladder dysfunction, even if spinal cord function is improved. These animals must have their bladders emptied, either by expression or by sterile, intermittent catheterization. All animals that are recumbent should be cared for carefully to prevent decubital ulcers, bathed frequently to prevent urinary and fecal scalding, and afforded physical therapy to prevent disuse atrophy of muscles.

Diagnostic Principles

The primary diagnostic aid in spinal cord disease is roentgenography. The spinal cord is enclosed completely in a bony structure, the spinal vertebrae. The vertebrae have multiple articulations and special supportive devices (the intervertebral disks), both of which are prone to disease. Most cases of spinal cord dysfunction in veterinary medicine relate to external compressive injury from the spinal vertebrae or their supporting structures. Roentgenography is the first and principle diagnostic aid in spinal vertebral diseases. CSF collection is essential in the diagnosis of inflammatory or neoplastic diseases.

Another diagnostic aid that is used in spinal cord diseases is the EMG. Although some people value the EMG highly in the diagnosis of spinal cord diseases, in the author's experience, it has been of limited usefulness in focal spinal cord disease. However, it is of inestimable value in diffuse spinal cord and motor unit diseases.

Clinical Signs

Clinical signs seen in spinal cord disease include weakness, pain, ataxia, loss of proprioceptive function, and urinary or fecal incontinence.

The combination of limbs involved in the disease and the reflex changes in those limbs allows further localization of the lesion.

Pathoanatomic Localization of Signs

1. Injuries of the cervical spine may cause tetraparesis (weakness in all four limbs) or hemiparesis (weakness in one front limb and one rear limb on the same side as the spinal cord injury). (See Figs. 17-9 and 17-10.)

A. Caudal cervical—If the injury is in the caudal cervical spine, the animal has LMN reflex changes in the front limb and may have signs of Horner's syndrome in the ipsilateral eye.

B. Cranial cervical—If the injury is in the cranial cervical spine, the animal should have UMN signs in both the front and rear limbs.

2. Animals with thoracolumbar disease present with either caudal paresis (weakness of both rear legs) or monoparesis (weakness of one rear leg). (See Figs. 17-11 and 17-12).

A. Disease of the thoracic and cranial lumbar spine presents with UMN signs in the limbs involved.

B. Disease of the lumbosacral spine presents with signs of LMN disease in the limbs affected.

C. Other signs commonly seen with thoracic and lumbar spinal cord disease include urinary incontinence, fecal incontinence, and decreased tail function. If the lesion is in the thoracic or cranial lumbar spine, the incontinence is associated with a normal anal reflex. If the disease is in the caudal lumbar or sacral spine, the incontinence is associated with loss of anal tone and reflex.

Focal Injuries to the Spinal Cord

Vertebral Malformations

1. Vertebral malformations include hemivertebrae, spina bifida, and atlantoaxial (AA) malformations with subluxations.

2. Occur generally in young animals, and frequently in toy breeds or Manx cats. Clinical signs are usually typical of slowly progressive, focal, neurologic disease.

A. AA luxation, UMN tetraparesis; usually symmetrical; may be acute in onset

B. Spina bifida frequently involves the sacrum; clinical signs usually are urinary and fecal incontinence.

C. Hemivertebrae may occur at any site in the vertebrae, but most frequently involves the thoracic or lumbar vertebrae (generally UMN caudal paresis).

3. Diagnosis is based on roentgenographic confirmation of vertebral malformation.

A. Myelographic studies are often needed to confirm that the vertebral malformation is associated with clinical signs.

B. In older animals with no history of neurologic disease, the finding of a vertebral malformation is usually incidental and not associated with clinical signs.

4. Treatment

A. If there is roentgenographic documentation that the lesion is the cause of neurologic disease, therapy consists of surgical decompression and stabilization.

B. If surgery cannot be performed, treatment with corticosteroids is recommended.

5. Prognosis is dependent on the surgical response to therapy and the duration of signs prior to diagnosis. The longer the signs have been present, the slower the recovery will be.

Intervertebral Disk Diseases

1. Cervical intervertebral disk diseases

A. Clinical presentation

1) Predominant signs usually include neck pain and paresis.

2) Generally affects middle-aged, obese, chondrodystrophic animals (beagles, dachshunds, poodles)

3) Occasionally affects mature, large breed dogs with cervical vertebral instability

4) The history generally reveals an acute onset, possibly with waxing and waning signs

B. Diagnosis requires roentgenography; myelography may be needed to confirm localization of the lesion.

C. Treatment

1) Medical therapy consists of cage rest and anti-inflammatory drugs. This mode of therapy is reserved for dogs having pain without evidence of paralysis or paresis.

2) Surgical treatment consists of decompression, and is generally indicated in animals with evidence of paresis or paralysis.

D. Prognosis—With rapid therapy, the prognosis is generally good.

2. Thoracolumbar disk disease

A. Clinical presentation

1) The most common sign is rear limb weakness, with or without pain.

2) Generally affects middle-aged, chondrodystrophic, or toy-breed dogs (dachshunds, Pekingese, Lhasa apso, poodles)

3) Initial complaints generally include a reluctance to go up and down stairs, pain on being lifted, and weakness or paralysis.

4) The history generally reveals a fairly acute onset of signs; the signs may wax and wane with slow protrusion of disk.

B. Diagnosis requires spinal roentgenograms, often with myelography to confirm localization of the lesion.

C. Treatment consists of medical therapy for animals without evidence of paralysis, and surgical therapy for those with paralysis.

D. Prognosis is dependent upon the severity of signs and the duration of signs prior to instituting therapy. Animals with paralysis have a worse prognosis than do those with pain and an abnormal gait. Animals that have lost deep pain sensation have a guarded to poor prognosis, and may never regain function.

Cervical Vertebral Malformation/Malarticulation Complex

1. Also known as cervical vertebral instability and wobbler syndrome

2. The disease affects large breed dogs and is seen in two age groups: animals younger than 18 months of age (Great Danes), and middle-aged or older animals about four to six years of age (Doberman pinschers, rottweilers, mastiffs).

3. The lesion is caused by malarticulation

of the cervical vertebrae and associated vertebral malformation. Changes include:

A. Vertebral malformation with a stenotic
vertebral canal

B. Malarticulation of articular facets with
secondary vertebral degeneration

C. Subluxation of the vertebrae upon
movement of the neck, secondary to malarticulation of facets

D. Intervertebral disk degeneration and
protrusion

E. Hypertrophy of ligaments, with spinal
cord compression

4. Clinical presentation

A. Slowly progressive, usually symmetrical ataxia, with rear limbs generally worse
than front limbs

B. The clinical signs generally reflect
UMN disease in the rear limbs.

C. There may be LMN involvement in the
front limbs, especially of the musculocutaneous nerve.

5. Diagnosis

A. Roentgenography is required.

B. Generally, myelography is also required to confirm that the spinal cord injury
is secondary to the malarticulation. Surgery
should not be performed without first obtaining a myelogram. In most animals, flexed and
extended views of the neck will be necessary.

6. Treatment

A. At present, treatment consists primarily of neck immobilization, rest, and corticosteroids. This is only symptomatic, palliative
therapy.

B. Surgical success is limited in many
cases.

7. The long-term prognosis in these animals
is guarded, but with medical therapy, they
may do well for years. In selected cases,
surgery may be of great benefit.

Vascular Disease of the Spinal Cord

Vascular disease of the spinal cord may occur in any animal species. It is characterized
by an acute onset of focal neurologic disease.
Often, there is no associated history of back
or neck pain. The causes, by species, include
bleeding disorders, hypothyroidism, and fibro-

cartilaginous infarcts in dogs, and lymphosarcoma and fibrocartilaginous infarcts in cats.
Fibrocartilaginous infarcts are discussed here
as being representative of the syndrome.

1. Clinical presentation

A. History of peracute onset of tetraparesis or caudal paresis

B. Frequent LMN limb involvement, especially in giant breed dogs

C. In cervical infarction, there is frequently an ipsilateral Horner's syndrome
noted.

D. Affected animals generally do not
appear to be in pain.

2. Diagnostic approach

A. Diagnosis of exclusion

B. Normal roentgenographic results

C. CSF analysis may reveal mildly elevated protein levels.

D. Myelographic results are generally
normal, although there may be intramedullary
swelling of the spinal cord at the level of the
infarct.

3. Treatment—consists of physical therapy
and short-term administration of corticosteroids

4. The prognosis is guarded in animals that
have LMN involvement of the limbs. When all
limb involvement is UMN, the prognosis is
fair to good.

Neoplasia

1. Clinical presentation

A. Dogs

1) Generally affects middle-aged or
older animals

2) Extramedullary tumors

a) Slowly progressive

b) Asymmetrical ataxia and
weakness

c) Frequently painful

3) Intramedullary tumors

a) More rapidly progressive

b) Nonpainful

c) Initially asymmetrical, but becomes symmetrical as disease progresses

B. Cats

1) Usually affects cats that are two to
three years of age

2) LSA is the most common tumor of the spinal cord

    a) Variable onset of caudal paresis

    b) May have one limb involved initially, secondary to nerve root disease. LMN monoparesis occurs.

2. Diagnostic approach

    A. Diagnosis depends on myelography and CSF analysis.

    B. Roentgenography

        1) Plain films may show bony defects in animals with metastatic tumors.

        2) Sublumbar masses are often seen in animals with LSA and metastatic tumors.

        3) Myelograms are required in most cases.

    C. CSF analysis

        1) Elevated pressure (rarely)

        2) Elevated protein values in some cases

3. Treatment

    A. The treatment for extramedullary tumors is surgical removal. Because they usually can be only partially excised, irradiation is indicated after surgery.

    B. For intramedullary tumors, radiation therapy and/or chemotherapy may cause temporary clinical improvement.

4. The prognosis in all spinal cord tumors is guarded; however, animals with extramedullary tumors that undergo surgical excision may experience a clinical remission for months.

Intradiscal Osteomyelitis (Discospondylitis)

1. A bacterial or fungal infection of an intervertebral disk and the adjacent vertebrae. This condition is rare in cats. If seen, it is evaluated the same as in dogs.

2. Clinical presentation

    A. Pain is the most common sign secondary to periosteal, nerve root, and meningeal inflammation.

    B. Paresis or paralysis may occur as a result of bony proliferation or pathologic fractures of the vertebrae.

    C. Fever, depression, and other signs of systemic illness may occur.

    D. If the disease is secondary to infection with *Brucella canis*, a past history of orchitis in males or infertility and abortions in females may be elicited.

3. Diagnostic approach

    A. Spinal roentgenograms reveal lysis and associated proliferation of the bony endplates of vertebrae.

    B. There may be multiple disk spaces involved.

4. Microbiologic examination

    A. Blood and urine cultures should routinely be performed in dogs with intradiscal osteomyelitis.

    B. If surgical therapy is indicated, the lesion is cultured also.

    C. Perform serologic tests for *B. canis*.

    D. CSF taps are generally of little benefit.

5. Treatment

    A. In animals without paresis, appropriate antibiotic therapy may be all that is required.

    B. In animals with paresis, consider surgical decompression followed by an appropriate antibiotic regimen.

6. Prognosis is fair to good in dogs that are diagnosed early and treated appropriately.

Traumatic Injury

Traumatic injury to the spinal cord will be discussed in a separate section on head and spinal trauma later in this chapter.

Diffuse Spinal Disorders

Inflammations

1. General principles

    A. Inflammatory diseases cause multifocal CNS signs.

    B. Inflammatory processes may affect the meninges and dorsal roots, causing pain.

    C. Grey matter and ventral nerve roots may be affected (causing LMN dysfunction), as may white matter (causing UMN dysfunction). Frequently, inflammations affect the brain as well as the spinal cord.

2. Clinical presentation

    A. Rapid onset of multifocal neurologic disease

    B. May be seen in animals of any age

C. Progressive in nature

D. Signs are usually asymmetrical.

3. Differential diagnosis

A. Dogs

1) Canine distemper

2) Systemic fungal disease

3) Toxoplasmosis/*Neosporum caninum*

4) Granulomatous meningo-encephalitis

5) Parasite migration

B. Cats

1) FIP

2) Toxoplasmosis

3) Systemic fungal infections

4) Parasite migration

4. Diagnostic approach

A. Opthalmic exam

1) Chorioretinitis may be seen in all of the inflammatory disorders.

2) Corneal keratic precipitates are seen in animals with FIP

3) Granulomatous uveitis

a) Fungal diseases

b) Protozoal diseases

B. CSF analysis—Elevations may be seen in pressure (rarely), protein, and cells.

1) Protein

a) Highest elevations are seen with FIP in cats and granulomatous diseases in dogs.

b) Lowest elevated levels occur in canine distemper.

2) Cells

a) Mixed neutrophils and lymphocytes are noted in cases of FIP.

b) Eosinophils may be present in animals with fungal and parasitic diseases.

c) Often normal in canine distemper

C. Normal findings on roentgenography

D. Serologic tests for fungal, protozoal, rickettsial, and viral diseases

E. Rule out bacterial disease by CSF cytology and culture.

5. Therapeutic considerations

A. If the disease is bacterial in origin, treat with antibiotics.

B. Treat fungal diseases with amphotericin B and ketaconazole.

C. Toxoplasmosis may be treated with sulfa drugs and folic acid inhibitors (pyrimethamine).

6. The prognosis for all nonbacterial inflammatory diseases affecting the CNS is guarded to grave.

Degenerative Processes

1. Degenerative myelopathy of older dogs

A. A slowly progressive disorder of the myelinated fibers in older, large breed dogs, especially German shepherds

B. Clinical presentation

1) The primary sign is ataxia that progresses to weakness.

2) Patients rarely appear to be in pain.

3) Affected animals generally maintain urinary and fecal continence.

4) Patients may have weak or absent patellar reflexes (a sign of LMN dysfunction) with positive crossed extensor reflexes (a sign of UMN dysfunction) in the same limb.

5) Owners often think the dog has hip dysplasia.

C. Diagnostic considerations

1) Diagnosis of exclusion

2) Normal results on roentgenography, including myelography

3) Normal CSF results

4) Normal findings on EMG

5) Normal ophthalmoscopic examination

D. Treatment—No treatment for this condition has been documented to be effective. The use of multivitamin therapy and aminocaproic acid is currently being investigated.

E. Prognosis

1) A slowly progressive, eventually incapacitating disease

2) Affected animals can make acceptable pets for many weeks or months.

2. Demyelinating myelopathy of Afghans

A. An apparently inherited, progressive, and fatal demyelinating disease affecting young Afghans

B. Clinical presentation

1) Rapidly progressive ataxia leading to rear limb paralysis in young, purebred Afghans

2) Forelimbs may become involved as the disease progresses.

3) Usually seen in animals 2 to 13 months of age

4) Animals die of respiratory paralysis.

   C. Diagnostic considerations

      1) A diagnosis of exclusion

      2) All diagnostic tests are reported to be normal.

   D. Treatment—There is no known therapy.

   E. Prognosis—grave

3. Lysosomal storage disorders

   A. Autosomal recessively inherited degenerative diseases affecting both dogs and cats

   B. Clinical presentation

      1) Steady, progressive, multifocal disease of young, purebred animals

      2) All parts of the CNS may be involved; affected animals may have any combination of signs, including:

         a) Ataxia

         b) Personality changes

         c) Urinary incontinence

         d) Paralysis

      3) The disorder is always fatal.

   C. Diagnostic approach

      1) Generally, laboratory tests yield normal results.

      2) In selected disorders, storage products may be observed on testing in WBCs, and on skin biopsy and liver biopsy.

      3) Diagnosis is confirmed at necropsy.

   D. Treatment—None is currently available.

   E. Prognosis—grave

Disorders Affecting the Brain Stem

1. Pathologic processes that affect the brain stem may cause a variety of clinical signs (Fig. 17-13).

   A. Cranial nerve deficits

      1) Cranial nerves III through XII arise from the brain stem.

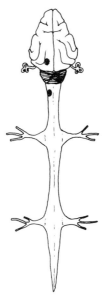

Figure 17-13. *Brain stem disorders may bring about gait disorders with ataxia and weakness combined. The associated signs include vestibular dysfunction, altered consciousness, and cranial nerve disorders. With focal disorders, the causes may include neoplasia, trauma, or vascular disease. Diffuse disorders may be caused by inflammations, such as FIP, canine distemper, toxoplasmosis, systemic fungal disorders, or granulomatous meningoencephalitis, or by degenerative processes, such as lysosomal storage disorders and thiamine deficiency.*

      2) Usually, several nerves are involved with brain stem lesions.

   B. Vestibular signs

   C. Ataxia

      1) From involvement of the proprioceptive pathway

      2) From vestibular involvement

   D. Weakness secondary to injury of the motor pathways

   E. Abnormal consciousness from injury to the ascending reticular activating system (ARAS)

   F. With severe injury, the following may be seen:

      1) Altered heart rate and rhythm

      2) Altered respiratory pattern

   G. The principle disorders that may affect the brain stem, and the unifying features of brain stem illness, are as follows:

   1) Vestibular signs
      a) Pathologic positional nystagmus
      b) Abnormal doll's eye
      c) Circling
      d) Head tilt
      e) Ataxia
   2) Other neurologic cranial nerve signs
      a) Strabismus
      b) Abnormalities of CNs V, VI, VII, IX, X, and XII
      c) Paresis or paralysis of limbs with UMN reflex changes
      d) Proprioceptive deficits in limbs
   2. Disorders that affect the brain stem may be divided into two major groups: focal and diffuse.

Focal Brain Stem Diseases

Neoplasia

   1. Clinical presentation
      A. Most commonly seen in middle-aged and older animals
      B. Vestibular signs have an acute onset; there is slow progression of other signs.
      C. Paresis may be a late finding.
   2. Differential diagnosis
      A. Cats
         1) Meningioma
         2) LSA
         3) Bony tumors
      B. Dogs
         1) Choroid plexus tumors
         2) Meningiomas
         3) Reticulosis (primary CNS lymphoma)
         4) Astrocytoma
         5) Oligodendroglioma
         6) Metastatic tumors
   3. Clinical course
      A. Slow, relentless disorder with orderly progression of cranial nerve deficits and paresis
      B. The late stages of the disease are frequently characterized by stupor or coma.
      C. Disease may be steroid-responsive initially.
      D. Sudden death from respiratory paralysis may occur.
   4. Diagnostic approach
      A. A CSF tap is the test of choice.
         1) Elevated pressure
         2) Elevated protein level, especially in animals with choroid plexus tumors and reticulosis, the latter of which is associated with protein that is primarily globulin.
         3) May see elevated WBC counts (lymphocytes and macrophages) with reticulosis
         4) Polymorphonuclear neutrophil lymphocytes (PMNs) may be observed in cases of meningioma if necrosis is present.
      B. Skull films may be beneficial in cases of meningioma or bony tumors.
      C. Ophthalmoscopic examination may reveal an optic nerve lesion in animals with reticulosis or astrocytoma.
      D. Computed tomography (CT scan) or magnetic resonance imaging (MRI), will confirm the presence of a mass and allow biopsy in some cases.
   5. Treatment
      A. Palliative therapy is the basic therapy at present.
      B. Corticosteroids
         1) Decrease edema
         2) Reduce intracranial pressure
      C. Radiation therapy will shrink tumors and improve signs.
      D. Chemotherapy may be beneficial in cases of reticulosis or feline LSA.
   6. Prognosis—grave. Therapy may result in satisfactory improvement for a few weeks or months. Sudden decreases in steroid dose could precipitate edema and death.

Vascular Disease

   1. Clinical presentation
      A. Acute onset of severe focal brain stem signs
      B. The signs stabilize rapidly and then slowly improve.
      C. Often associated with a systemic bleeding disorder, sepsis, or other systemic

metabolic illness, especially disseminated intravascular coagulation (DIC)

D. May be seen in dogs of any age, but is rare in cats

2. Diagnostic approach

A. Diagnosis of exclusion

B. CSF analysis may be normal.

C. Occasionally, the following CSF changes are observed:

1) Increased protein (mild)

2) Increased cell count

3) Nonsuppurative inflammation and erythrophagocytosis

D. A CT scan or MRI will reveal an area of decreased blood flow and a mass effect if thrombosis is present.

3. Treatment

A. Corticosteroids for edema and inflammation

B. Treat any underlying systemic disorder.

4. Prognosis—These animals have a fair to good prognosis if the disorder is idiopathic. In other cases, the prognosis is determined by the underlying disorder.

Brain Abscess

Brain abscesses are focal accumulations of pus in the CNS with clinical signs of a rapidly progressive mass lesion. They have been seen in all animal species.

1. Clinical presentation

A. A rapid onset of focal neurologic disease. The signs are referable to the part of the nervous system involved.

B. There may be a prior history of respiratory or oral infection.

C. There is often an antecedent middle ear infection.

D. These conditions are usually rapidly progressive.

2. Diagnosis

A. A rapidly progressive focal CNS disorder that is closely associated with an antecedent illness

B. CSF analysis

1) Increased protein

2) Increased cell count—usually PMNs

C. A CT scan or MRI will confirm the presence of a mass lesion.

3. Treatment

A. High-dose antibiotics

B. In small animals, surgical drainage may become feasible.

4. Prognosis—very grave

Trauma

1. Clinical presentation

A. Acute onset of vestibular signs associated with an objective history of trauma

B. If the brain stem is involved, the injury is usually quite severe and the prognosis is guarded.

2. Diagnostic approach

A. Skull roentgenograms are obtained to rule out or confirm fracture(s).

B. CSF taps are usually not required, and may, in fact, hurt the posttraumatic patient.

3. Treatment

A. Rest and supportive therapy

B. May require sedation to prevent self-injury

C. Corticosteroids

4. The prognosis for any animal sustaining brain stem trauma is guarded.

Diffuse Brain Stem Diseases

Inflammation

1. Clinical presentation

A. Subacute onset of multifocal nervous system disease in animals of any age

B. Signs are usually progressive, but are not logical or systematic in their progression.

2. Differential diagnosis

A. Cats

1) FIP

2) Toxoplasmosis

3) Systemic fungal diseases, especially cryptococcosis

4) Aberrant parasite migration

B. Dogs

1) Canine distemper

2) Granulomatous meningoencephalitis

3) Toxoplasmosis/*Neosporum caninum*

4) Systemic fungal diseases

5) Rocky Mountain spotted fever

6) Aberrant parasite migration

3. Diagnostic approach

   A. CSF tap

   1) Elevation in WBC count

   2) Encephalitis

   a) Highest WBC count is seen in cats with FIP

   b) Highest WBC count is seen in dogs with granulomatous meningoencephalitis

   c) Organisms or eosinophils may be noted in animals with systemic fungal infections

   d) The protein elevation is often minimal in canine distemper.

   B. Ophthalmoscopic examination

   1) Chorioretinitis

   a) Fungal disease

   b) Toxoplasmosis

   c) FIP

   d) Canine distemper

   2) Keratic precipitates in the cornea of cats with FIP

   3) Granulomatous uveitis occurs with fungal diseases.

   C. Perform serologic tests on blood or CSF if such tests are available.

   D. A CT scan or MRI will identify any granulomas or other mass effects.

4. Treatment

   A. General supportive therapy

   B. Fungal diseases—amphotericin B and ketaconazole

   C. Toxoplasmosis—First, consider the public health hazard if diagnosed in a cat; then prescribe sulfisoxazole and folic acid inhibitors.

Granulomatous Meningoencephalitis

Granulomatous meningoencephalitis, a disease of the CNS of dogs, is associated with marked perivascular proliferation of reticuloendothelial (RE) cells. It has also been reported in cats.

1. Clinical presentation

   A. May occur in any portion of the CNS; presents as a focal or multifocal mass

   B. Reported predilection for the cerebrum or cerebellopontine angle

   C. Lymphocytes, plasma cells, and neutrophils, with no mitotic activity, constitute the major lesion.

   D. No breed or sex predilection; affects animals of any age older than one year

   E. Signs are referable to the area of involvement.

   1) Predominantly cerebral or cerebellar

   2) Visual (optic neuritis)

2. Diagnosis

   A. CSF analysis—elevated cell count; predominantly mononuclear

   1) Increased protein (mild to moderate), especially globulins

   2) May reveal anaplastic reticular cells

   B. A CT scan or MRI will identify any mass lesions.

3. Treatment—may be responsive to treatment with steroids or irradiation

4. Prognosis—grave

Disorders of the Vestibular System

The vestibular system maintains posture, regulates tone in antigravity muscles, and corrects for changes in body posture. The vestibular system also is responsible for control of involuntary eye movements and eye movements that correct for changes in head position. The vestibular system includes the inner ear, the peripheral eighth cranial nerve (which connects the inner ear to the brain stem), the brain stem vestibular nuclei, and the cerebellar nuclei that coordinate vestibular motor responses. An injury to any of these parts is capable of causing vestibular signs that are manifested primarily as loss of balance.

Clinical Presentation

Animals with vestibular disorders tend to have certain similar signs, regardless of the location of the pathologic process. A list of these unifying clinical signs follows. For additional signs, see section on loss of balance.

Circling

Animals with vestibular dysfunction walk in tight circles, usually toward the affected side.

Head Tilt

Vestibular dysfunction causes the head to be tilted, generally with the affected side held lower than the normal side.

Rolling or Falling

Vestibular dysfunction causes animals to fall toward the affected side. Often, these animals cannot stop themselves after falling, and they continue to roll.

Dizziness (Vertigo)

Animals with loss of balance may appear to be disoriented, confused, excited, or restless as a result of vestibular dysfunction.

Limb Hypotonia

Animals with vestibular injury will have decreased extensor muscle tone on the side of the injury. This causes them to lean to that side, and may also make the animals appear to be weak.

Nystagmus

Affected animals may exhibit an involuntary, rhythmic, oscillating eye movement that results from an imbalance in the resting muscle tone in the extraocular muscles. The resting tone is determined by the vestibular apparatus. Thus, in most clinical cases, nystagmus is a sign of vestibular dysfunction. Nystagmus is classified according to both the direction of eye movement and the the time during which the nystagmus is present.

General Diagnostic Approach

Loss of balance is generally a sign of vestibular injury. The first step in diagnosis is to decide whether the lesion is in the inner ear, peripheral nerve, brain stem, or cerebellum. Because the vestibular signs are the same regardless of the location of the disease, the associated signs are used to localize the lesion (Table 17-12).

After you have localized the injury, appropriate diagnostic aids must be selected. Specific tests for animals with vestibular dysfunction include the following:

1. Ophthalmoscopic examination
2. Skull roentgenograms
3. CSF taps if brain stem or cerebellar injury is suspected
4. CT scan or MRI if a mass lesion is suspected

Table 17-12. **Vestibular disease**

Peripheral		Central	
Inner ear	**CN VIII**	**Brain stem**	**Cerebellum**
CN VIII deficit	No other signs	Multiple cranial nerve deficits	Dysmetria
Horner's syndrome	Horizontal nystagmus	Altered consciousness	Tremor
Possible inflamed tympanic membrane		Reflex changes—UMN	Absent menace reflex
Horizontal nystagmus		Loss of proprioception	Positional vertical nystagmus
		Positional vertical nystagmus	Normal strength
			Normal reflexes

Common Diseases (Peripheral Lesions) by Location

*Inner or Middle Ear**

1. Infection (Tables 17-13 and 17-14, Fig. 17-14)
    A. Clinical presentation
        1) Affects all species at any age
        2) Slow, progressive signs
        3) Most common vestibular disease in dogs
    B. Physical examination
        1) CN VII abnormality and Horner's syndrome may be present.
        2) Otherwise, the results of physical examination are normal.
    C. Diagnostic approach
        1) Abnormal results may be obtained on otoscopic examination.
        2) Skull roentgenograms of the tympanic bulla may reveal a lesion.
    D. Treatment
        1) Systemic antibiotics
        2) May require surgery if there is a poor response to antibiotic therapy
    E. Prognosis
        1) Fair, if diagnosed early. Head tilt and dry eye may be permanent sequelae.
        2) If left untreated, the infection may migrate to the brain stem, causing fatal suppurative encephalitis.
2. Trauma—all species, any age; one of most common sequelae of head trauma
    A. History—significant trauma with acute onset of signs
    B. Physical examination—Signs of vestibular disease may be masked initially by central disease; they may appear subsequently as the level of consciousness improves.
    C. Diagnostic approach
        1) Skull films may show fractures.
        2) Otoscopic examination may reveal hemorrhage in the middle ear.
    D. Treatment
        1) Sedative drugs (phenothiazine tranquilizers or diazepam), if needed, to prevent self-injury

* See Tables 17-13 and 17-14, and Figure 17-14.

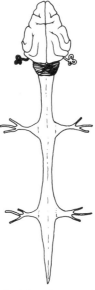

Figure 17-14. *Peripheral vestibular lesions may cause disorders of gait (ataxia alone). The associated signs are head tilt, nystagmus, circling, disorientation, seventh cranial nerve paralysis, and Horner's syndrome. These lesions may result from infections (e.g., suppurative otitis) or trauma involving the inner ear, or from vesticular neuronitis, neoplasia, or metabolic neuropathies of the eighth cranial nerve.*

        2) Steroids, low doses
    E. The prognosis, if the lesion is an isolated CN VIII injury, is good.
3. Tumor of petrous bone
    A. Clinical presentation
        1) Slow, progressive illness
        2) Affects older dogs and cats
    B. Physical examination—CN VII paralysis and Horner's syndrome after onset of vestibular signs
    C. Diagnostic approach—Skull films may be normal.
    D. A CT scan may identify the mass.
    E. Treatment
        1) No adequate treatment is available.
        2) Surgery may be attempted.
    F. Prognosis—guarded to grave

Peripheral Nerve

1. Neoplasm (see Tables 17-13 and 17-14, and Fig. 17-14)

Table 17-13. Disorders affecting the vestibular system

Cause	Inner Ear	Cranial Nerve VIII	Brain Stem	Cerebellum
Inflammation	Otitis interna	Idiopathic vestibular disorder	Granulomatous meningoencephalitis	Same as for brain stem
			Systemic fungal infections	
			Viral encephalitis	
Vascular disease			Secondary to hypothyroidism	Same as for brain stem
			Secondary to bleeding disorders	
			Spontaneous bleeding	
Neoplasia	Bony tumors	Bony tumors	Meningioma	Same as for brain stem
		Meningioma	Neuroectodermal tumors	
		Neurofibroma		
Trauma	Fractured bones	Fractures	Contusion	Contusion
	Rupture of tympanic bulla			
	Hemorrhage			
Metabolic disorder		Endocrine disorders	Thiamine deficiency	

Adapted from Baloh RH, Honrubia V: Clinical Neurophysiology of the Vestibular System. Contemporary Neurology Series 18: 1–230. Philadelphia, FA Davis, 1979

Table 17-14. Clinical findings in vestibular disease

Parameter Tested	End-Organ Inner Ear	Peripheral Nerve	Cerebello-pontine Angle	Brain Stem	Cerebellum
Ear examination	May be abnormal	Normal	Normal	Normal	Normal
Other cranial nerves	Horner's syndrome, CN VII	VII	V, VI, VII	V, VI, VII, IX, X	None
Equilibrium	Abnormal	Abnormal	Abnormal	May be normal	May be normal
Ataxia	Yes	Yes	Yes	Yes	Yes
Pathologic nystagmus	Horizontal or rotary	Horizontal or rotary	Horizontal or rotary	Vertical or rotary	Vertical or rotary
	Constant	Constant	Constant	Positional	Positional
Doll's eye	Normal	Normal	Abnormal	Abnormal	Normal or ataxic
Paresis	No	No	No/yes	Yes	No
Proprioceptive loss	No	No	No/yes	Yes	No
Tremor	No	No	No/yes	No	Yes

Adapted from Baloh RH, Honrubia V: Clinical Neurophysiology of the Vestibular System. Contemporary Neurology Series 18: 1–230. Philadelphia, FA Davis, 1979

A. Clinical presentation—usually affects aged animals

B. Physical examination

   1) Frequently, other cranial nerve deficits, especially involving CN VII and occasionally CN V or VI, are present.

   2) Usually progresses to involve the brain stem, with subsequent paresis and weakness

C. Diagnosis—based on a history of progressive peripheral vestibular disease

   1) Skull films may be helpful.

   2) Otoscopic examination is normal.

   3) CSF analysis is normal early in the course of the disease. In the late stages, increased pressure and increased protein levels may be noted.

   4) A CT scan may help to identify the mass.

D. Treatment—Consider surgery and/or radiation therapy.

E. Prognosis—poor

2. Trauma

A. History—Usually, there is an objective history of head trauma.

B. Physical examination—CN VII paralysis or Horner's syndrome are common complications.

C. Diagnostic approach—skull films in cases of cranial fracture

D. Treatment—Affected animals may require sedation to prevent them from injuring themselves.

E. Prognosis—If there are no other neural injuries, the prognosis is favorable.

3. Metabolic disease—endocrine neuropathies

A. May be seen with hypothyroidism, Cushing's disease, and possibly other endocrine diseases

B. Clinical presentation

   1) Usually acute onset of signs

   2) Usually evidence of a long-standing endocrine disorder (e.g., skin disease)

C. Physical examination

   1) May have associated CN VII paralysis

   2) Diagnosis depends on eliminating other causes for signs and on positive diagnosis of endocrine disease.

D. Diagnostic approach—specific biochemical testing for endocrinopathies

E. Treatment—Treat the underlying condition.

F. Prognosis—variable recovery

4. Idiopathic vestibular disease

A. Clinical presentation

   1) Seen in all species

   2) Most common vestibular disease in cats; second most common in dogs

   3) Acute onset; spring, summer, early fall

   4) May occur in cats of all ages; usually affects middle-aged or older dogs.

B. Physical examination—No other signs are seen.

C. Diagnostic tests—all normal

D. Treatment—none

E. Prognosis—good, in that it is a self-limiting disease. The animal may have a residual head tilt.

Cerebellar Vestibular Dysfunction

1. Physical examination (Fig. 17-15, see Tables 17-13 and 17-14)

A. Vestibular signs

   1) Positional pathologic nystagmus

   2) Normal doll's eye

   3) Head tilt

   4) Circling

   5) Ataxia

B. Other neurologic signs

   1) Tremor of head and trunk

   2) Absent menace reflex (occasionally)

   3) Normal reflexes

   4) Normal strength

2. See the section on Disorders of the Cerebellum that follows for a discussion of individual disorders.

Brain Stem Vestibular Disorders

1. Physical examination (see Tables 17-13 and 17-14, and Fig. 17-13)

A. Vestibular signs

   1) Pathologic positional nystagmus

   2) Abnormal doll's eye

   3) Circling

4) Head tilt
5) Ataxia
B. Other neurologic signs
    1) Other cranial nerve signs
        a) Strabismus
        b) CNs V, VI, VII, IX, X, and XII abnormalities
    2) Paresis or paralysis of the ipsilateral limbs accompanied by UMN reflex changes
    3) Proprioceptive deficits in limbs
  2. See the immediately preceding section on Disorders Affecting the Brain Stem for a discussion of individual diseases.

Disorders of the Cerebellum

The cerebellum is that portion of the nervous system concerned with integration and coordination of movement. For that reason, ataxia, incoordination, and tremors are the primary signs seen in cerebellar disease.

General Clinical Presentation

1. Clinical abnormalities of gait (see Fig. 17-15) characterized by:
  A. A wide base
  B. Irregular, deviating, clumsy limb movements
  C. Ataxia accentuated by circling or turning
  D. Veering when attempting to walk a straight line
  E. Hypermetria
2. Ataxia of head and trunk
3. Normal strength and normal reflexes
4. Normal postural reactions
5. Possible associated vestibular signs (head tilt, pathologic nystagmus, circling)
6. Possible menace reflex deficit, with normal vision and normal seventh cranial (facial) nerve function
7. Intention tremor—When the animal decides to make a move, a brief, fine tremor may develop in the portion that is moving; this is called an *intention tremor*. This is

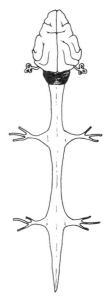

Figure 17-15. *Cerebellar lesions may cause disorders of gait (ataxia alone) with associated signs of circling, head tilt, nystagmus, tremor, and normal strength. They may involve focal diseases, such as neoplasia; vascular or trauma-induced diseases; cerebellar hypoplasia; or cerebellar abiotrophy. These lesions may also result from diffuse diseases—either inflammations, such as FIP, canine distemper, granulomatous meningoencephalitis, toxoplasmosis, neosporum canis and systemic mycoses, or lysosomal degenerations.*

especially prominent in highly controlled movements, such as those involved in eating.

Diagnostic Approach

1. CSF tap
2. Ophthalmoscopic examination
3. Skull roentgenography
4. MRI or CT scan

Specific Disorders

Disorders of the Neonate

1. Cerebellar hypoplasia
  A. Associated with lack of development or in utero injury to the cerebellum

1) May be genetic

2) May be the result of an in utero viral or toxic injury

B. Clinical presentation

1) Not all animals in the litter are necessarily affected.

2) Clinical signs are present at birth.

3) Static, nonprogressive disease

4) Affects both dogs and cats

C. Diagnostic approach

1) Diagnosis of exclusion

2) Most diagnostic tests yield normal results.

3) MRI or a CT scan reveals reduced cerebellar size.

D. Treatment—none

E. Prognosis

1) Many affected animals make functional pets.

2) Generally, there is no marked clinical improvement.

2. Cerebellar abiotrophy

A. Generally an inherited, slowly progressive, degenerative disease of the cerebellum. It has been reported in many breeds of dogs, including Kerry blue terriers, Gordon setters, Labrador retrievers, golden retrievers, cocker spaniels, cairn terriers, Great Danes, Airdales, Finnish harriers, and Bern running dogs.

B. Clinical presentation

1) Signs usually begin at two months of age or older.

2) Generally, affected animals show only cerebellar signs.

3) Signs are usually slowly progressive.

C. Diagnostic approach

1) A diagnosis of exclusion

2) Diagnostic test results are normal.

D. Treatment—No known therapy exists at present.

E. Prognosis—These are not usually fatal diseases, but the animal's disability may become great enough to require euthanasia.

3. Lysosomal storage disease (lipid storage disease, leukodystrophy)

A. Autosomal recessive inherited disease causing enzymatic defects

B. Clinical presentation

1) Disease affecting purebred young animals

2) Relentlessly progressive, multifocal, always fatal disease; therefore, they are not characterized by purely cerebellar signs

3) Reported in both dogs and cats

4) Signs usually begin at about four to six months of age. Death occurs within one year of onset of signs.

C. Diagnostic approach

1) Diagnostic tests usually are normal.

2) Some animals may have inclusion bodies in neutrophils, skin, or liver.

D. Treatment—There is no known therapy at present.

E. Prognosis—always fatal

4. Hypomyelinogenesis (dysmyelinogenesis)

A. A group of diffuse disorders that preferentially affect the fiber tracts of the general proprioceptive system. As a result, the clinical signs mimic those of cerebellar disease. These conditions usually occur in neonates.

B. Clinical presentation

1) At birth or when the animals first walk, tremors (myoclonus) of the limbs and head appear.

2) Neurologic signs include wide-based stance and a rocking horse gait.

3) Ataxia is pronounced, but there is no weakness.

4) The tremors are enhanced with excitement and movement, but usually abate with rest and sleep.

5) Some animals in the litter appear more ataxic than others.

6) Unlike cerebellar hypoplasia, this disease usually affects multiple animals in a given litter.

7) The signs are not usually progressive. In fact, many patients improve over a period of several weeks to months, even returning to normal in some cases.

8) Unless the neonate cannot nurse, the physical examination is usually normal. If they cannot nurse, cachexia is observed.

C. In dogs, the condition appears to be inherited. So far, it has been reported in chow chows, schnauzers, Australian silky terrier, and dalmatians.

D. Diagnosis

1) The diagnosis can only be confirmed at necropsy.

2) Clinical diagnosis, then, rests on the animal's history, with confirmation by histologic and histochemical examination demonstrating abnormal myelin composition.

E. Treatment—No therapy is currently available, but many patients spontaneously improve.

F. Prognosis—Many animals recover with time.

Diseases of Adult Onset

1. Inflammatory disease

A. Many inflammatory diseases are reported to affect the cerebellum; these include canine distemper virus, FIP virus, toxoplasmosis, systemic fungal diseases, and *Neosporum caninum.*

B. Clinical presentation

1) Inflammatory diseases are characterized by a subacute onset, and are generally progressive.

2) Signs are usually multifocal and thus do not reflect purely cerebellar involvement.

3) Affected animals may have signs of systemic illness and ophthalmic changes.

4) May occur at any age

C. Diagnostic approach

1) The diagnostic test of choice is CSF analysis.

    a) Elevated protein levels

    b) Increased CSF leukocyte count

    c) Possible positive results on culture

    d) Fungal organisms may be seen.

2) Ophthalmic abnormalities may be noted.

D. Treatment

1) Antibiotics

2) If culture results are negative and there is evidence of viral disease, use of steroids should be considered.

3) Valium is a centrally acting muscle relaxant; it may relieve tremors.

E. Prognosis—The prognosis in most inflammatory diseases is guarded.

2. Neoplastic disease

A. Mass lesions cause clinical signs by replacement and compression of neural tissue. Many of the clinical signs are secondary to edema.

B. Clinical presentation

1) Generally affects elderly animals

2) Signs are slowly progressive.

3) Initially, signs are purely cerebellar; however, as the mass enlarges, secondary brain stem signs (cranial nerve deficits, alterations in consciousness, alterations in respiration) may become evident.

4) Death is usually caused by brain stem compression secondary to herniation.

C. Diagnostic approach

1) CSF tap

    a) Elevated CSF pressure

    b) Elevated CSF protein levels

    c) Generally, no abnormal cells

2) Skull roentgenograms are usually normal, except in animals with calcifying tumors (e.g., meningioma of cats)

3) A CT scan or MRI will identify a mass lesion.

4) Brain biopsy is feasible in the cerebellum.

D. Treatment

1) Corticosteroid administration is only palliative therapy.

    a) Decreases edema

    b) Reduces inflammation

2) Surgery—If the mass can be localized, and it is an extramedullary tumor, surgical excision may be considered.

3) Radiation therapy has shown promise in improving the length and quality of affected animals' lives.

E. The prognosis in these animals is guarded to grave.

3. Traumatic cerebellar injury

A. Head injury may result in CNS signs as a result of direct injury to neural tissue, fractures, or vascular injury.

B. Traumatic injury to the cerebellum is a common sequela of head trauma.

C. Clinical presentation

1) There is usually an objective history of trauma.

2) Most affected animals have multifocal disease.

3) Many animals develop clinical signs of cerebellar ataxia several days after the injury when their other problems have improved enough to allow the cerebellar signs to appear.

    D. Diagnostic approach

        1) Skull roentgenograms are performed to rule out fractures.

        2) MRI or a CT scan may be useful in detecting hemorrhage.

    E. Treatment—cage rest, avoidance of sedative drugs, administration of corticosteroids

    F. Prognosis

        1) In terms of recovery from cerebellar injury, the prognosis is generally good.

        2) The animal's prognosis is determined by the extent of other neural injuries.

  4. Cerebellitis (white dog shaker syndrome)

    A. A disease of acute onset seen primarily in dogs

    B. Etiology unknown

    C. Affects young to middle-aged dogs, especially those with white hair coats

    D. Clinical presentation—peracute onset of diffuse tremor; no other history of note

    E. Physical examination—Affected animals are often hyperthermic from tremors.

    F. Neurologic examination—chaotic, random eye movement; severe, disabling tremors

    G. Diagnostic test results are all normal.

    H. Treatment—steroids, valium

    I. Prognosis—Almost all dogs recover completely if treated early.

Disorders of the Cerebrum

Cerebral disease of any etiologic origin tends to cause similar signs (Fig. 17-16). These include the following:

  1. Seizures
  2. Personality changes
  3. Abnormal mentation
  4. Visual abnormalities with normal PLRs
  5. Circling
  6. Proprioceptive loss
  7. Occasional cranial nerve weakness, especially of CN VII
  8. Sensory deficits

These signs may occur in any combination, and not all of the signs listed must be present

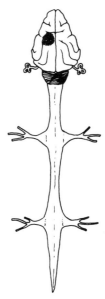

Figure 17-16. *Cerebral disorders may rarely cause gait disorders with ataxia and weakness. The usual signs are seizures, dementia, circling, hemiparesis, and visual deficits. Focal disorders are caused by neoplasia, vascular disease, trauma, and malformations. Diffuse disorders include metabolic diseases, inflammations, such as FIP, canine distemper, toxoplasmosis, systemic fungal disorders, and granulomatous meningoencephalitis; degenerative processes; and intoxications.*

in all cases of cerebral disease. An etiologic classification system for cerebral diseases, which may assist in further clinical evaluation of these patients, follows.

Cerebral Diseases of Extracranial Origin

  1. Cerebral diseases of extracranial origin result from systemic metabolic and toxic processes that cause secondary cerebral signs.

  2. The predominant clinical signs are personality changes, waxing and waning dementia, and seizures.

  3. The general physical examination (not including the neural examination) is often abnormal in these patients.

  4. The neurologic examination of these patients is frequently normal.

5. These disease processes are diagnosed on the basis of laboratory evaluation of blood, urine, or body tissue, as well as roentgenography.

Cerebral Diseases of Intracranial Origin

Cerebral diseases of intracranial origin are neurologic disorders that result from CNS dysfunction and that may be further subdivided as follows:

1. Structural (organic) disorders

    A. Affected animals have an actual anatomic lesion involving the CNS.

    B. Predominant clinical signs include seizures, visual loss, circling, weakness, personality changes, and other neural deficits.

    C. The general physical examination in these patients is usually normal.

    D. The neurologic examination usually reveals abnormalities, even between seizures.

    E. The diagnosis in these cases requires specific neurologic diagnostic aids, such as CSF analysis, EEG, skull radiography, CT scans, MRI, and so forth.

2. Functional cerebral disorders (idiopathic epilepsy)—In idiopathic epilepsy, seizures are the only clinical abnormality. (This disorder is covered separately in this chapter.)

    A. Except during the seizure (and postictal period), the animal is normal.

    B. All laboratory test results are normal.

    C. This is a diagnosis of exclusion.

Extracranial Disorders

Hypoglycemia

The cerebrum functions principally by aerobic metabolism. Glucose deprivation causes neuronal energy depletion and CSF lactic acidosis, which cause neurologic symptoms (see Chapter 22).

1. Clinical presentation

    A. Hypoglycemic animals may exhibit any combination of neurologic signs, including:

      1) Blindness

      2) Weakness

      3) Ataxia

      4) Seizures

      5) Coma

    B. Hypoglycemia should be one of the first disease processes considered in neurologic disease affecting:

      1) Young puppies

        a) Toy breeds

        b) Unhealthy or thin puppies

      2) Hunting dogs that only show signs when working

      3) Middle-aged and older dogs with seizures of recent onset

      4) Diabetic animals with a history of acute onset of neurologic signs (insulin overdose)

2. Diagnostic approach

    A. Blood glucose testing should be performed prior to treating the dog.

    B. In adult dogs, 48-hour fasting glucose levels of less than 60 mg/dL are highly suggestive of an insulin-secreting tumor.

    C. If concerned that the dog may have an insulin-secreting tumor, determine the insulin : glucose ratio.

    D. Simultaneously evaluate young puppies with hypoglycemia for parasites, distemper, glycogen storage disorders, hydrocephalus, lead poisoning, and hepatoencephalopathy.

3. Treatment

    A. Puppies

      1) Treat any associated conditions.

      2) Administer thiamine, followed by dextrose, 1 g/kg, if the animal is having active seizures.

      3) Provide good nursing care.

    B. Insulin-secreting tumors

      1) Administer 1 g/kg of dextrose intravenously (IV) if the animal is having active seizures; maintain dextrose supplementation.

      2) Surgically excise the tumor, if possible.

        a) Most are carcinomas.

        b) Many are not grossly visible at surgery.

        c) Most have metastasized by the time of diagnosis.

      3) Oral hyperglycemic agents, such as diazoxide, may be helpful.

4. Prognosis

A. Good, if the disorder represents an isolated, stress-related event

B. Guarded

1) In dogs with insulin-secreting tumors

2) In puppies with distemper or hydrocephalus

Thiamine Deficiency

1. Thiamine deficiency is a clinical syndrome associated with vascular injury and neuronal damage of the grey matter caused by vitamin B_1 deficiency.

A. In dogs, it causes a diffuse cerebrocortical necrosis.

B. In cats, it causes midbrain microhemorrhages and necrosis.

2. Thiamine is essential in the normal oxidative energy pathways of the CNS.

3. Clinical presentation

A. In dogs, progressive seizures and dementia are noted, often with an associated blindness (but normal pupils).

B. In cats, the stereotypic signs include:

1) Fixed, dilated pupils

2) Paralysis of the extraocular muscles

3) Stress-induced "seizures" that involve rigid extension of all four limbs with the head and neck ventroflexed between the front limbs. These seizures may actually be a manifestation of vestibular dysfunction, rather than true seizures.

4) Acute onset of signs

5) Frequently, there is a history of a raw fish diet or a period of total anorexia in the immediate past

4. Diagnostic approach

A. The diagnosis is based on clinical signs and history.

B. All routine laboratory test results are normal.

5. Treatment

A. Administer injectable thiamine hydrochloride initially.

B. Maintenance therapy with thiamine hydrochloride for one to three weeks may be beneficial.

C. A proper diet is essential.

D. Administering IV dextrose prior to the use of thiamine may cause an exacerbation of signs.

6. Prognosis—excellent if the disease is treated early and the diet is improved

Hepatoencephalopathy

Hepatoencephalopathy is a neurologic condition associated either with shunting of portal blood directly into the systemic circulation, or with failure of the liver to remove toxins and by-products of digestion. Current explanations for the clinical signs include hyperammonemia, altered permeability of the blood–brain barrier, and abnormal (or false) neurotransmitters in the circulation. False neurotransmitters are chemical molecules that resemble biogenic amines. They cause signs by occupying neurotransmitter sites.

1. Clinical presentation

A. Animals with hepatoencephalopathy generally have waxing and waning alterations of consciousness and seizures. Other neural signs include visual deficits, circling, ataxia, and weakness.

B. Signs are often associated with eating.

C. The animal may have overt signs of liver failure.

1) Cachexia

2) Ascites

3) Hypoalbuminemia

D. There may be a history of polydipsia or polyuria.

E. Dogs with congenital portosystemic shunts frequently have chronic diarrhea.

F. The CNS signs may be precipitated by use of drugs, such as tranquilizers and diuretics.

2. Diagnostic considerations

A. Young dogs—congenital portosystemic anomalies, especially in German shepherds, schnauzers

B. Old dogs—secondary to cirrhosis

C. Urea cycle enzyme deficiency

D. Consider this diagnosis in any dog that has general systemic illness and neurologic signs, as well as in dogs that have idiosyncratic reactions to drugs or that seem to be unable to metabolize drugs.

3. Diagnostic approach

A. Biochemical evaluation

1) Serum bile acid levels are the test of choice. Postprandial bile acids will be markedly elevated in hepatoencephalopathy.

2) Liver enzyme levels may be normal (i.e., SGOT, SGPT).

3) A bromsulphalein (BSP) dye excretion test shows increased retention.

4) Elevated ammonia tolerance test results

5) Low albumin levels

B. Urinalysis—Check for ammonium biurate crystals. (These are considered to be normal in some dogs.)

C. Roentgenography

1) Small liver size on plain films

2) Splenoportography or mesenteric angiography may demonstrate shunts.

D. Liver biopsy in cirrhotic dogs

4. Treatment

A. Medical

1) Dietary

a) Low-protein, high-carbohydrate diet

b) Portions should be divided into several feedings per day.

2) Antibiotics—Oral enteric antibiotics (neomycin or kanamycin) may decrease the number of ammonia-splitting bacteria.

3) Lactulose alters gut pH to decrease production of ammonia.

4) Avoid anticonvulsants if at all possible.

5) Avoid other drugs, especially tranquilizers.

6) Provide general supportive therapy (i.e., fluids, dextrose, etc.)

B. Surgical—If a single shunt can be identified, it can be surgically ligated.

C. If the animal is comatose, manage appropriately (as for any comatose patient).

5. Prognosis

A. Many animals may be clinically improved for a period of weeks or months; however, unless the animal has a surgically correctable shunt, its long-term prognosis is grave.

B. Affected animals may experience sudden gastrointestinal (GI) bleeding that can precipitate coma.

C. Some dogs appear to develop intractable seizures following shunt ligation.

Lead Intoxication

Intoxication with lead alters cerebral metabolism and leads to edema, hypoxic changes, and eventually (if untreated), cerebrocortical necrosis.

1. Clinical presentation

A. Usually affects young animals

B. Often, an objective history of lead exposure is elicited, which may include exposure to:

1) Caulking material

2) Batteries, crankcase oil, grease

3) Dry wall, plasterboard, or sheetrock

4) Old buildings with lead paint

C. Acute onset of signs

1) GI signs

a) Diarrhea or, occasionally, constipation

b) Colic

2) CNS signs

a) Dementia

b) Blindness

c) Hysteria

d) Seizures

2. Diagnostic approach—Canine distemper in dogs is a principal differential diagnosis to be considered.

A. Hematologic examination—Many nucleated RBCs are noted in peripheral blood, with mild anemia.

B. Roentgenography—Metal or dense material is visible in the GI tract.

C. Blood lead levels

1) Use unclotted blood

2) Do not use an EDTA tube because it chelates lead and gives falsely low readings.

3) Blood lead levels of greater than 40 μg/dL in the presence of clinical signs are highly suggestive of intoxication; levels greater than 60 μg/dL are diagnostic.

3. Treatment

A. Treat with calcium EDTA, 100 mg/kg/d.

1) Divide into four daily doses.

2) Dilute to a 10% solution in $2\frac{1}{2}$% dextrose in water.

   3) Administer subcutaneously (SQ).

   4) Continue therapy for five days (20 total treatments).

   B. Prior to initiating therapy, obtain roentgenograms of the abdomen. If there is lead in the GI tract, remove it with cathartics or enemas prior to EDTA therapy.

   C. If the seizures persist during therapy, begin treatment with appropriate anticonvulsants.

   D. If the animal shows progressive decreases in the level of consciousness after therapy is started, maintenance dexamethasone, 0.1 mg/lb/d, may be administered to decrease cerebral edema.

   4. Prognosis—good, if the condition is diagnosed early and treated adequately

Hypocalcemia

Calcium is essential for normal cell membrane and neuromuscular function (see Chapter 25). Decreases in calcium are capable of causing profound neurologic symptoms.

   1. Clinical presentation

   A. Generally seen in postparturient toy breeds of dogs

   B. May occur in association with hypoparathyroidism (affecting any age or breed)

   C. Principle signs include:

      1) Restlessness and apprehension

      2) Muscle tremors and fasciculations

      3) Hyperthermia secondary to muscular activity

      4) Mild cases may simply be accompanied by weakness.

      5) Severe cases may be associated with generalized seizures.

   2. Diagnostic approach

   A. With postparturient females, try administering calcium gluconate IV empirically and monitor the response.

   B. Serum Ca^{++} levels—Hypoalbuminemia may falsely lower Ca^{++}.

   C. Measure serum parathyroid hormone levels.

   D. Parathyroid biopsy

   3. Treatment

   A. Calcium gluconate IV for seizures or severe tremors

   B. In postparturient dogs, remove the mother from pups to stop lactation.

   C. For hypoparathyroid dogs, administer:

      1) Oral Ca^{++} lactate

      2) Oral vitamin D_3 (dihydrotachysterol)

   4. Prognosis

   A. Excellent for postparturient female dogs

   B. Good for hypoparathyroid dogs if Ca^{++} levels are carefully monitored and maintained.

Intoxications

Intoxication with ethylene glycol, organophosphates, strychnine, amphetamines, or metaldehyde causes seizures, which sign is the primary manifestation of intoxication. For more detailed information, see Chapter 28.

Intracranial Disorders

Structural Cerebral Disorders

Focal Disorders

   1. Neoplasia

   A. Most common types

      1) Cat

         a) Meningioma

         b) Lymphosarcoma

         c) Bony tumors

      2) Dog

         a) Astrocytoma

         b) Oligodendroglioma

         c) Meningioma

         d) Lymphoma

         e) Metastatic tumors

         f) Pituitary tumor

   B. Clinical picture

      1) The onset of signs is often sudden and dramatic in the owner's mind because of associated seizures.

      2) History of personality changes, learning disabilities, and so on

      3) General signs of cerebral dysfunction

      4) Usually affects older animals

      5) Clinical signs are often transiently

steroid-responsive, but the disease is otherwise constantly progressive.

    6) Animals may demonstrate endocrine signs.

      a) Polydipsia or polyuria

      b) Marked gonadal atrophy

      c) Unexplained obesity

      d) Abnormal hair coat

  C. Diagnostic approach

    1) CSF Tap

      a) Elevated pressure

      b) Elevated protein level—not a consistent finding

      c) Normal to mild increase in cell count

    2) EEG

      a) Focal spikes, sharp waves, or slow waves may be evident.

      b) Generalized slow-wave activity secondary to edema may be noted.

    3) Ophthalmoscopic examination—Optic nerve edema may be present.

    4) Roentgenograms—usually normal except in the following:

      a) Bony tumors

      b) Meningiomas

    5) A CT scan or MRI will identify mass lesions.

    6) Brain biopsy will identify tumor type.

  D. Treatment

    1) Anticonvulsant therapy if the animal has seizures

    2) Steroids

      a) To reduce elevated intracranial pressure

      b) To decrease CNS edema

    3) Chemotherapeutic agents have proved beneficial in cases of LSA; for other tumor types, chemotherapy is less effective.

    4) Surgical therapy has been successful in animals with bony tumors or meningiomas. With improved techniques, surgical debulking of intramedullary tumors is becoming practical, as well.

    5) Radiation therapy significantly prolongs life in most cases of cerebral neoplasia.

  E. Prognosis

    1) Fair for clinical improvement lasting up to one year.

    2) Guarded in terms of cure or protracted improvement.

2. Vascular disease

  A. Usually associated with systemic illness, such as hypothyroidism, bleeding disorders, or septicemia

  B. May be unrelated to any known disorders, such as feline ischemic encephalopathy

  C. Clinical presentation

    1) The onset of signs is acute to peracute, with the greatest severity of signs occurring at the onset of the disease.

    2) Feline ischemic encephalopathy occurs seasonally, and is especially prevalent in late summer.

    3) The signs are those of focal cerebral disease.

      a) Seizures

      b) Personality changes

      c) Dementia

      d) Paresis

      e) Visual deficits

  D. Diagnostic considerations

    1) In dogs, careful screening for endocrine dysfunction, especially hypothyroidism, is warranted.

    2) Other causes of neurovascular disease include:

      a) Polycythemia

      b) Hyperviscosity syndromes

        i. Plasma cell neoplasms (multiple myeloma)

        ii. Macroglobulinemia

      c) Bleeding disorders

      d) Vasculitis

        i. Immune disease

        ii. Uremia

        iii. Sepsis

        iv. Rocky Mountain spotted fever

      e) Arteriovenous (AV) malformations

      f) DIC

      g) Vascular tumors

      h) Cardiomyopathy

  E. Diagnostic approach

    1) Triiodothyronine (T_3) and thyroxine (T_4) levels

    2) Screen for FeLV-related disease in cats.

    3) Bleeding disorder evaluation

4) Serum protein evaluation (electrophoresis)

5) ECG to detect myocardial disease

6) Ophthalmic examination

    a) Chorioretinitis

    b) Hemorrhage

    c) Vascular changes

7) CSF tap

    a) Mild increase in pressure

    b) Possible increase in CSF protein levels

    c) Occasionally, cells are noted—erythrophagocytosis

8) A CT scan or MRI will distinguish between hemorrhage and infarct.

F. Treatment

1) If an underlying disease is detected, it should be treated appropriately.

2) Corticosteroids decrease inflammation and edema.

3) Anticonvulsants are administered if the animal is having active or frequent seizures.

G. Prognosis

1) Determined by etiology

2) If the disorder is idiopathic, the prognosis is usually fair to good for return of function.

3) Affected animals may have permanent residual deficits.

3. Hydrocephalus

A. A pathologic accumulation of fluid within the ventricular system of the brain. It may be a primary or a secondary condition, and it may or may not be associated with clinical signs.

B. Clinical presentation—primary (congenital) hydrocephalus

1) Seizures, visual deficits, and dementia are all common complaints in animals with hydrocephalus.

    a) Some animals have an open fontanelle; however, this is not diagnostic of hydrocephalus because it may occur as a normal variant in otherwise healthy dogs.

    b) Affected animals may have a dome-shaped, prominent calvarium.

    c) A bilateral divergent strabismus ("setting sun sign") may be present.

2) Secondary hydrocephalus results from obstruction of the ventricular system. Frequently, these animals have a recent history of inflammatory CNS disease or traumatic head injury. Secondary hydrocephalus is often rapidly progressive.

C. Diagnostic approach

1) Skull films

    a) Reveal thinning of the calvarium

    b) Often demonstrate a loss of roentgenographic bony gyral pattern

    c) Contrast ventriculography is diagnostic.

2) Ultrasonography—If the fontanelle is open, ultrasonography of the brain is feasible.

3) CSF tap—Increased pressure is an inconsistent finding.

4) Serum biochemical studies—Many hydrocephalic dogs are marginally hypoglycemic. If continued abnormalities exist in a dog, treat it for hypoglycemia, but consider hydrocephalus.

5) A CT scan or MRI will confirm the diagnosis.

D. Treatment

1) Steroids

    a) Some success has been achieved with long-term maintenance therapy with prednisone.

    b) The mechanism for this appears to be decreased production of CSF.

2) Long-term, low-dose furosemide decreases CSF production.

3) Surgical drainage

    a) Surgical drainage has been of benefit in some cases.

    b) This requires permanent placement of a ventriculovenous shunt.

E. Prognosis

1) Fair if the condition is diagnosed early and treated

2) Affected animals may always be dull and have a limited ability to learn.

Diffuse Disorders

1. Inflammation

A. Multifocal processes that affect all areas of the nervous system. Although the animal may present with historical signs referable to one area of the nervous system (e.g., seizures), a careful neurologic examination may reveal symptoms related to other areas of the nervous system.

 B. Clinical presentation

  1) Subacute onset of multifocal neurologic disease

   a) Cerebral signs

    i. Seizures

    ii. Dementia

    iii. Visual deficit

    iv. Paresis

   b) Signs of vestibular, cerebellar, brain stem, or spinal cord disease may be present as well.

  2) Inflammation may occur in any age, breed, or sex of animal.

  3) There is often an associated systemic illness, especially respiratory disease.

  4) The clinical signs are generally progressive.

 C. Diagnostic considerations

  1) Dogs

   a) Canine distemper

   b) Granulomatous meningoencephalitis

   c) Toxoplasmosis/*Neosporum caninum*

   d) Systemic fungal infection

   e) Pseudorabies

   f) Rabies

   g) Parasite migration

  2) Cats

   a) FIP

   b) Toxoplasmosis

   c) Systemic fungal infection

   d) Rabies

   e) Parasite migration

 D. Diagnostic approach

  1) Ophthalmic examination

   a) Chorioretinitis may be seen in any of these disorders.

   b) Granulomatous uveitis may accompany fungal and protozoal disorders.

   c) Retinal vascular changes are seen in FIP.

  2) CSF tap

   a) Elevated protein levels (especially globulins) may be associated with any of these disorders.

    i. In granulomatous disorders, it is often quite marked.

    ii. In cases of distemper, it is often minimal.

   b) Cytologic examination

    i. FIP—increased numbers of mixed neutrophils and mononuclear cells

    ii. Protozoal and fungal diseases—may see eosinophils; predominantly non-suppurative cell picture, regardless of specific etiology

  3) Hematologic evaluation

   a) Canine distemper—Neutrophils with inclusion bodies may be seen.

   b) A marked polyclonal elevation of serum protein level occurs in some cases of FIP.

   c) Perform serologic studies to confirm a specific diagnosis.

 E. Treatment

  1) For viral diseases

   a) Supportive therapy

   b) Anticonvulsants

  2) For fungal diseases

   a) Anticonvulsants

   b) Combination of amphotericin B and ketoconazole

 F. Prognosis—In all of these cases, the prognosis is quite guarded.

 2. Granulomatous meningoencephalitis

 A. A granulomatous disease of unknown etiology involving the CNS of dogs.

 B. Clinical presentation

  1) Disease of acute onset in adult dogs

  2) Cerebral signs

   a) Seizures

   b) Dementia

   c) Personality changes

  3) Brain stem signs

   a) Loss of balance

   b) Cranial nerve paralysis

   c) Hemiparesis or tetraparesis

   d) Altered consciousness

  4) The disease is progressive in nature.

  5) Some affected animals are reported to have intermittent fever.

 C. Diagnostic approach

  1) CSF tap

a) Elevated WBC count—predominantly mononuclear cells

b) Elevated protein level

2) EEG—consistent with diffuse cortical disease

D. Treatment—No known therapy is successful, but steroids may cause a temporary improvement.

E. Prognosis—grave

3. Rabies encephalitis

A. An invariably fatal viral infection of the CNS of warm-blooded animals. The disease is transmissible to humans.

B. Clinical presentation—A variable incubation period follows either aerosol exposure or inoculation from the bite of a rabid animal.

1) Initial excitatory phase

a) Restlessness

b) Aggressiveness

c) Personality changes

2) Clinical phase

a) Rapidly progressive personality changes

b) Marked aggressiveness

3) Paralytic form—progressive brain stem paralysis and respiratory paralysis. Death occurs within two weeks of onset of either form.

C. Diagnostic considerations—postmortem diagnosis

1) Fluorescent antibody test on brain

2) Mouse inoculation test

D. Treatment—none available

E. Prognosis—grave. Most affected animals do not survive. The virus may be present in the saliva three days before clinical signs are observed.

4. Postvaccinal rabies

A. A disease beginning 12 to 14 days after rabies inoculation

B. The signs usually include LMN paralysis of the vaccinated limb.

C. The signs may progress or may be confined to the affected limb.

5. Pseudorabies (Aujeszky's disease)

A. A herpesvirus disease

B. Clinical presentation

1) Sudden death

2) Profound dementia, pain, seizures, self-mutilation, and so on, progressing rapidly to death

C. Diagnostic approach

1) CSF analysis—increased cells (mononuclear)

2) Mouse inoculation

D. Treatment—No therapy is available.

E. Prognosis—The disease is always fatal.

6. Lissencephaly

A. A disorder that has been reported in Lhasa apso dogs and one cat; possibly inherited

B. Signs begin at two to three months of age, and consist of mild motor signs, mild proprioceptive signs, severe behavioral changes, visual deficits, and seizures.

C. Diagnosis

1) EEG—high-voltage, low-frequency—asynchronous

2) Pathologic examination—absence of gyri and sulci in the neocortex; very thin periventricular white matter

D. Treatment—No known treatment halts the progress of this disease.

Functional Cerebral Disorders

1. Epilepsy (see the section on Seizures, later in this chapter)

2. Narcolepsy—cataplexy

Sleep disorders have been described in both dogs and cats. Many purebred breeds of dogs are now reported to have narcolepsy, including the beagle, cocker spaniel, dachshund, Doberman, Irish setter, Labrador, and poodle. Genetic studies of Labradors and Dobermans support a recessive inheritance with complete penetrance. With the hereditary form of the disease, the signs generally appear between one and six months of age. There are also acquired forms of sleep disorders in which the signs may not appear until the animals are seven years of age.

3. Pathophysiology—Both narcolepsy and cataplexy are believed to represent abnormalities of neurotransmitter balance. Abnormalities in the ability to release or turn over serotonin could produce the signs seen in both conditions.

4. Clinical presentation

A. Cataplexy—a disorder characterized by brief episodes of muscle paralysis with loss of tendon reflexes secondary to motor inhibition. The animal may not be asleep during these episodes, and will appear alert and able to follow objects with its eyes. The signs are short in duration and completely reversible. The episodes are initiated by periods of excitement, such as may occur with eating, playing, sexual arousal, and the like.

B. Narcolepsy—a disorder characterized by excessive daytime sleepiness. Unless associated with cataplectic attacks, this disorder may be difficult to diagnose.

C. Clinical signs—The physical examination, including the neurologic examination, is usually normal except during the actual attacks. The onset of signs is rapid, and the signs may last seconds to 30 minutes. During attacks, the muscles are hypotonic. Partial attacks may only involve the pelvic or thoracic limbs. The signs are usually induced by excitement, activity, or arousal. Animals can usually be aroused from the episode by loud noises, petting, or other external stimuli. Frequently, the observer will see behavior associated with rapid eye movement (REM) sleep during episodes (i.e., ocular motility, twitching of the facial muscles, whining). Affected animals may have many episodes during the course of a day.

5. Differential diagnosis—A variety of other conditions, both neurologic and nonneurologic, must be considered among the differential diagnosis for sleep disorders.

A. Cataplexy—myasthenia gravis, hypoglycemia, hypocalcemia, hypokalemia, adrenal insufficiency, polymyositis, nonmotor epilepsy (lapse attacks/drop attacks), syncope

B. Narcolepsy—hypothyroidism, chronic hypoxia, obesity, other metabolic illnesses

6. Diagnostic approach

A. Food-elicited cataplexy test—Place 10 pieces of food, each 1 cm³, in a row. Leave 30.5 cm between each piece. Record the time required to eat all pieces, as well as the number, type, and duration of any cataplectic attacks that occur. A complete attack is considered to be one in which the patient drops completely to the ground with its head resting on the floor. A partial attack is when the patient drops its hindquarters, forequarters, or both to the ground, but does not drop its head.

1) A normal dog will eat all of the food in less than 45 seconds and will have no attacks.

2) A cataplectic dog will require more than two minutes to eat the food and will have between 2 and 20 attacks.

B. Pharmacologic testing

1) Physostigmine challenge—First, administer 0.025 mg/kg of physostigmine salicylate IV; then, repeat the food-elicited cataplexy test 5 to 15 minutes after each injection. The test may be repeated using increasing doses of physostigmine (0.05 mg/kg, then 0.075 mg/kg, and finally, 0.10 mg/kg). This test will consistently produce signs in affected patients, causing up to a 300% increase in the number and duration of episodes. The signs will increase in severity and frequency in a dose-dependent manner. The effects of each dose will last 15 to 45 minutes.

2) Arecoline challenge—For this test, 0.15 mg/kg of arecoline hydrochloride are administered SQ; the food-elicited cataplexy test is then repeated, as in the physostigmine challenge test. The results should be similar to those derived from the physostigmine challenge test, with the effects lasting about one hour.

3) Atropine response—Administer 0.1 mg/kg of atropine sulfate IV, then repeat the food-elicited cataplexy test, as in the physostigmine challenge test. A marked decrease in the number of cataplectic attacks should be noted.

7. Treatment—The primary goal of therapy in dogs is to decrease the severity and frequency of the cataplectic attacks. The increased drowsiness is usually of lower concern to the client, and so its treatment is not a primary therapeutic goal.

A. Client education—Explain that this is not a fatal disease. Also, inform clients that choking on food and airway obstruction have not been reported. Try to avoid situations in which the attacks could endanger the patient (i.e., avoid hunting or swimming, and walk the animal only when restrained by a leash or fenced yard).

B. Drug therapy—Administer drugs that block serotonin uptake, decrease concentrations of dopamine, decrease turnover of nor-

epinephrine, or have anticholinergic properties. In addition, the drug selected must
be able to cross the blood–brain barrier.
Monoamine oxidase inhibitors (MAOI) are
relatively contraindicated in dogs, as they appear to have toxic cardiovascular side effects.

1) Imipramine—an anticataplectic
drug. Administer 0.5 to 1.0 mg/kg t.i.d. by
mouth and titrate the dose based on clinical
effect.

2) Methylphenidate (Ritalin)—Administer 5 to 10 mg orally on a daily basis and
then titrate the dose. This drug is primarily
used as a supplement to imipramine.

3) Dextroamphetamine—Administer 5
to 10 mg/day orally; then, titrate the dose
based on clinical efficacy. This drug is also
used as a supplement to imipramine.

8. Prognosis

A. The disease is not fatal, so the prognosis is good for life. Many of the animals
(Dobermans and Labradors) that are afflicted
with the inherited form will improve with
increasing age.

B. The prognosis is more variable in
terms of client satisfaction, as the disease is
not curable and, even with rigorous therapy,
many patients remain symptomatic. In addition, many patients will develop drug tolerance, so the therapeutic regimen will
need to be changed or it will become ineffective. A final concern expressed by many
clients is the fact that therapy may be expensive.

Disorders That Affect
the CNS Diffusely

There are groups of diseases that may affect
all parts of the CNS and may also involve the
PNS. Although the affected animal's history
may appear to reflect a focal disease (e.g.,
seizures, head tilts, ataxia), careful neurologic
examination may reveal signs that cannot be
explained by a focal lesion (Fig. 17-17). There
are two major groups of diffuse disorders that
affect the CNS: inflammatory disorders and
degenerative disorders.

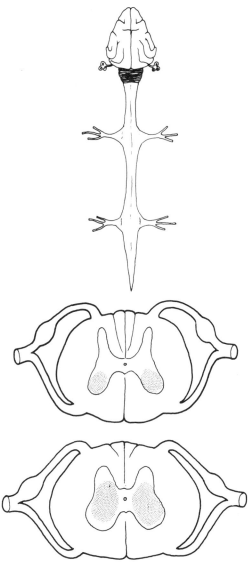

Figure 17-17. *Diffuse disorders involve all parts
of the nervous system and may bring about disorders of gait, with ataxia and weakness combined.
In addition, signs referable to other focal regions
of the nervous system may be noted.*

Inflammatory Disorders

Infections

1. Infections of the brain with resulting
cerebral signs may be attributable to viruses,

bacteria, protozoa, or fungi. The most frequently seen disorders are:

    A. Viral—canine distemper, rabies, canine herpes, infectious canine hepatitis (ICH), pseudorabies, FIP, parainfluenza, postvaccinal rabies, and postvaccinal distemper

        1) Distemper in dogs

        2) FIP in cats

        3) Toxoplasmosis in cats and dogs

        4) Pseudorabies in dogs and cats

        5) Rabies in dogs and cats

    B. Protozoal—any protozoa may affect the CNS

    C. Bacterial—any bacteria may affect the CNS

    D. Actinomycetes; Nocardia species—any

    E. Mycotic—*Cryptococcus neoformans, Coccidioides immitis, Blastomyces dermatitidis, histoplasma capsulatum,* Paecilomyces species

    F. Parasitic—nematodiasis, cuterebriasis, aberrant heartworms

Infectious Canine Distemper

1. A paramyxovirus infection. It is among the most common causes of CNS signs in the dog. The disease may be systemic in puppies, producing respiratory, GI, and other signs, in addition to neurologic signs. The disease involves the meninges as well as the neuraxis; lesions involve both grey and white matter.

2. Any age, breed, or sex of dog may be affected. The disease tends to be manifested in different patterns in different age groups.

3. Immature animals

    A. Systemic illness

        1) GI signs; respiratory illness

        2) Retinal lesions

    B. The neurologic signs are multifocal; often, cerebellar signs appear first.

        1) Myoclonus primarily involves limb flexion, but may be seen in any muscle group. This is involuntary and present during sleep.

        2) The results of CSF analysis are often normal.

            a) The cell count may be mildly increased; 15 to 60 mononuclear cells.

            b) The protein level may be slightly increased.

        3) CNS pathologic changes—mononuclear perivascular cuffing, gliosis, microglial proliferation, inflammatory cell infiltration of the pia

            a) Often, lesions are most severe in the periventricular grey matter.

            b) Intranuclear or intracytoplasmic inclusion bodies may be present.

            c) Severe demyelination of the white matter may occur.

4. Mature dogs

    A. Multifocal encephalitis

        1) Chronic, progressive, multifocal neurologic disease that is not associated with any systemic illness

        2) May be seen in vaccinated animals; lesions predominantly involve the brain stem and cerebellum, and so the signs are typical of these anatomic locations.

            a) CSF analysis yield findings similar to those in young dogs.

            b) Pathologic changes—multifocal necrosis and perivascular cuffing

            c) Rarely see inclusions

            d) Rarely see cerebral lesions

    B. Old dog encephalitis

        1) Affects mature dogs

        2) No systemic signs

        3) Visual and cerebral signs predominate

        4) CSF analysis—normal

        5) EEG—encephalitic

        6) Pathology—CNS perivascular cuffs and demyelination

5. Postvaccinal distemper encephalitis

    A. Seen only in young animals (generally younger than six months of age)

    B. Signs occur one to two weeks after onset of illness

    C. No systemic illness

    D. Often accompanied by severe personality changes

6. Physical examination

    A. Enamel hypoplasia, all forms

    B. Pyoderma, juvenile form

    C. Conjunctivitis with ocular discharge, juvenile form

    D. Chronic cough with nasal discharge, juvenile form

E. Harsh lung sounds, juvenile form

F. An ocular fundus examination may reveal chorioretinitis (any form)

7. Neurologic examination—multifocal disease with the cord, brain stem, cerebellum, and cerebrum all involved

A. Spinal cord—paresis. May have myoclonus (rhythmic contraction of a group of muscles)

B. Brain stem—cranial nerve deficits

C. Cerebellum—dysmetria, tremors (both intentional and postural)

D. Cerebrum—seizures, dementia, circling, blindness

8. Diagnosis

A. Based on the history, physical, and neurologic examination findings

B. An EEG may suggest encephalitis; this study not valid, however, in dogs younger than five months old

C. CSF analysis—increased cells, usually lymphocytes (occasionally, neutrophils), with increased protein levels. CSF analysis may also be normal. Serologic testing of the CSF may prove to be diagnostic.

D. Conjunctival, prepucial, or vaginal cytology may show intracytoplasmic inclusion bodies.

E. Fluorescent antibody staining of cytologic preparations may also be performed in cases of the juvenile form.

9. Treatment

A. Corticosteroids and antibiotics

B. If pneumonia is a factor, corticosteroids are contraindicated.

C. Supportive therapy

D. Anticonvulsants are administered if seizures occur.

10. Prognosis

A. Guarded; the myoclonus is usually permanent.

B. The seizures may be controlled in some patients.

C. The other neural deficits may improve as the inflammation resolves. However, some animals deteriorate regardless of therapy. At present, there are no specific, effective antiviral agents for this disease.

Herpes Canis

1. Herpes canis is a viral encephalitis that is seen occasionally in nursing puppies and is often fatal.

2. It also has been incriminated as producing a nonsuppurative meningoencephalitis in adult dogs.

Feline Infectious Peritonitis

1. FIP is a coronavirus disorder of cats that causes polyserositis and peritoneal and pleural effusions. The virus also produces a nonsuppurative meningoencephalitis in about 63% of affected animals.

2. Clinical presentation

A. Cats of any breed, age, or sex may be affected.

B. History

1) Acute onset of neurologic signs that are multifocal and slowly progressive

2) The animal may be anorexic, febrile, anemic, depressed, and so forth.

C. Physical examination

1) Fever

2) Ocular lesions, chorioretinitis, keratic precipitates, anterior uveitis

3) Usually, there are no pleural or peritoneal effusions in animals with CNS signs.

4) Possible irregular kidney size

D. Neurologic examination—multifocal disease

1) Ataxia, paresis, or paralysis of the rear limbs and, possibly, the forelimbs

2) Seizures

3) Dementia, blindness, circling, pacing

4) Vestibular signs are common.

3. Diagnosis

A. Clinical presentation

B. EEG—diffuse, high-amplitude, slow-wave

C. CSF analysis usually reveals increased lymphocytes or neutrophils and increased protein levels.

D. Elevated serum globulin levels

E. Serologic studies are of limited benefit.

4. Treatment

A. No treatment is currently available.

B. Corticosteroids and antibiotics have been used without success.

5. Prognosis—poor

Toxoplasmosis

1. Infections with the coccidian protozoa *Toxoplasma gondii* and *Neosporum caninum* may occasionally produce neurologic signs. Most cases are subclinical, but toxoplasmosis may cause respiratory disease, GI disorders, ocular disease, and abortions, in addition to neurologic disease.

2. Clinical presentation

    A. Any age, breed, or sex may be involved; toxoplasmosis occurs in all species, but Neosporum infections have only been documented in dogs.

    B. History

        1) The animal may have had a prior respiratory disease or be chronically ill.

        2) There may be a concurrent immunosuppressive illness (i.e., cancer, viral infections, etc.).

    C. Physical examination

        1) Respiratory illness—radiographic documentation of granulomatous pneumonia

        2) Icterus as a result of liver involvement

        3) Muscle pain if myositis is present

        4) Uveitis and chorioretinitis

    D. Neurologic examination—multifocal disease

        1) Dementia, seizures, and other cerebral signs

        2) Ataxia or paresis

        3) Vestibular signs

        4) Tremor and other cerebellar signs

        5) Dogs younger than six months of age exhibit a radiculitis/myositis. Extreme limb rigidity is seen in puppies.

3. Diagnosis

    A. Clinical presentation

    B. Fecal examination in cats

    C. CSF analysis—increased cells and increased protein levels if an active inflammation is present

    D. Serologic tests—Those available for toxoplasmosis include Sabin-Feldman dye test, indirect fluorescent antibody test, indirect hemagglutination, and complement fixation. None are currently available for Neosporum.

    E. Changing titers, especially rising titers, are more significant than one isolated titer. Rising titers are indicative of active infection, but this is not always synonymous with clinical disease.

4. Treatment

    A. Sulfonamides and pyrimethamine may be used.

    B. Clindamycin is effective in treating *Toxoplasma polymyositis.*

    C. Control may be achieved without cure.

    D. Toxoplasmosis is a public health hazard caused by cats that shed oocysts in the feces.

Mycotic Encephalitis

1. Fungal encephalomyelitis may occur in animals. Fungal organisms reported in the nervous system include:

    A. Cryptococcosis is the most common cause.

    B. Coccidioidomycosis

    C. Histoplasmosis

    D. Blastomycosis

    E. Aspergillosis

    F. Mucor

2. Cryptococcosis is the most frequent mycotic encephalitis. It may occur at any age. There is no breed predilection.

    A. Chronic rhinitis is common. The organism may be seen on cytologic examination of nasal exudate.

    B. Neurologic signs include depression, dementia, ataxia, weakness, cranial nerve deficits, and LMN paralysis of the limbs.

    C. CSF analysis—The organism may be seen on cytologic examination. Increased cells and increased protein levels may be noted.

    D. Treatment—Amphotericin B and ketoconazole (in combination) are used to treat most systemic mycotic infections. The success of the therapy is limited.

    E. Prognosis—usually grave

Postvaccinal Distemper

1. Seen one to two weeks after vaccination

2. Anorexia and fever

    A. Direct to neural signs

    B. No other evidence of systemic illness

    C. Primarily cerebral and postural signs

    D. Rapidly progressive

Postvaccinal Rabies

1. Signs appear 12 to 14 days after vaccination.
2. Usually associated with ascending LMN paresis
3. Affected animals usually recover within one to two months

Noninfectious Inflammation

Granulomatous Meningoencephalitis

1. Granulomatous meningoencephalitis is a proliferation of the adventitial cells of the blood vessels of the brain with accumulation of lymphoid, mononuclear, plasma, polymorphonuclear, and giant cells.
2. Clinical presentation
   A. Primarily brain stem and cerebellar signs
   B. Cerebral, meningeal, and spinal cord signs may be evident as well.
   C. Acute onset; intermittent fever (and often, severe neck pain) is the first sign. The disease is invariably progressive.
3. Diagnosis
   A. CSF—100+ WBCs (as high as 1000/mm³), primarily mononuclear cells. Protein levels are elevated from mild to 1 g/dL.
   B. EEG—consistent with encephalitis
   C. Brain biopsy—perivascular infiltrates of mononuclear cells, lymphoid, plasma, and reticuloendothelial cells. Necrosis and hemorrhage, secondary to inflammation, may also be evident.
4. Treatment—This condition may be transiently steroid-responsive. Early reports suggest that combination chemotherapy and/or radiation therapy may reverse this disease.

Polioencephalomyelitis of Cats

1. Slowly progressive, chronic disease of cats
2. No age predilection
3. Spinal cord, cerebellar, and rarely, brain stem or cerebral signs
4. Affected animals have nonregenerative anemia.
5. Nonspecific inflammatory disease
6. Is not associated with meningitis or ependymitis, which distinguishes it from FIP

Degenerative Disorders

Lysosomal Storage Disorders

1. Lysosomal storage disease
   A. Lysosomes are single-membrane–bound, cytoplasmic particles that are present in all cells containing hydrolytic enzymes. They are responsible for degradation of protein, polysaccharides, and nucleic acids. They require an acid pH environment. Their functions are twofold:
      1) Intracellular—They fuse with vacuoles containing cellular material to be degraded, or engulfed foreign material. These are secondary lysosomes, and enzymatic digestion occurs here.
      2) Extracellular—They fuse with cell membrane to release enzymes. Genetic defects causing lysosomal deficiency lead to secondary lysosomal engorgement with undegraded material; cell function is compromised because of lysosomal hypertrophy. Sphingolipids, mucopolysaccharides, and glycoproteins constitute the bulk of the substrates that accumulate. Similar cells are distended with storage material that may or may not be demonstrable, depending upon its solubility in the solution used during preparation of the material. Ultrastructurally, the material is contained within membrane-bound structures.
   B. Clinical presentation
      1) All forms of lysosomal storage disease are rare.
      2) Affected animals are normal at birth.
      3) All fail to develop concomitantly with littermates.
      4) Usually only a single member of the litter is affected.
      5) Usually occurs in certain breeds
      6) History of in-breeding
      7) Always fatal, always progressive
      8) Age of onset and speed of progression vary.
      9) More than one body system may be affected.
   C. Diagnosis
      1) Biopsy—blood, bone marrow, CSF, lymph node, nerve, rectal smooth muscle, brain

2) Certain breeds and the animal's clinical history raise the index of suspicion.

3) Necropsy results

D. Prevention and control—test at necropsy; institute breeding controls

2. Gangliosidosis

  A. Ganglioside GM_1

    1) Feline GM_1—Siamese, Korat, mixed breeds

    2) Canine GM_1—beagles, mixed breeds

  B. Ganglioside GM_2

    1) Canine GM_2—German short-haired pointers

    2) Feline GM_2—mixed breeds

  C. All forms of the disease involve abnormalities of the lysosomal system. The lysosomal system is the principle site of intracellular digestion. Blockage of lympholytic activity leads to decreased catabolic activity, with resulting intralysosomal accumulation of complex macromolecules (e.g., glycolipids, proteoglycans). This results in eventual metabolic failure (probably secondary to crowding) and cell death.

  D. All forms of the disease are characterized by:

    1) Progressive CNS deterioration that begins in early life and proceeds to death

    2) Autosomal recessive pattern of inheritance

    3) Lysosomal hypertrophy in neurons

    4) Deposition of complex macromolecules with lysosomes of hepatocytes, macrophages, and other cells

    5) Specific enzyme deficits

  E. GM_1

    1) Cats—Signs start at four to six months of age and progress over a period of six to ten months.

      a) Ataxia, tremors, paresis, visual loss, seizures, behavioral changes

      b) Occasionally, corneal lesions and retinal lesions

      c) Cells in the CNS and liver, and pancreatic acinar cells are involved.

    2) Dogs—Signs appear at two to four months of age and progress to death by eight months of age.

      a) Visual signs, tremors, dysmetria, paresis, behavioral changes

      b) Pathologic lesions in the nervous system, liver, kidney, spleen, and lymph nodes

  F. GM_2

    1) Cats—Signs begin at four to ten weeks of age.

      a) Tremors, dysmetria, ataxia, paresis

      b) Dwarphism

      c) Corneal opacity

      d) Lesions may involve the nervous system, liver, endothelium, bone marrow, spleen, and kidney

    2) Dogs—Signs begin at six months of age, with death ensuing by two years of age.

      a) Behavioral changes, seizures, ataxia, weakness, visual signs, coma

      b) Lesions involve only the nervous system

  G. Sphingomyelin lipidosis—Affects cats (Siamese and domestic short-hair breeds)

    1) Onset of signs at three to six months of age

    2) Death by nine months of age

    3) Stunted growth, ataxia, dysmetria, tremors

    4) Lesions involve the nervous system, liver, lung, spleen, lymph nodes, kidney, bone marrow, adrenal gland

  H. Glucocerebrosidosis

    1) Dogs—Silky terrier

      a) Signs start at seven months of age.

      b) The animal is dead within one month after the onset of signs.

      c) Signs are not reported in the one available research article.

      d) Lesions may involve the nervous system and liver.

  I. Neuronal ceroid lipofuscinosis

    1) Dogs—English setters

    2) Cats

    3) Signs begin at 14 to 18 months of age and may include visual changes, mental changes, behavioral changes, cerebellar signs, and seizures; death ensues by 24 to 26 months of age.

    4) Lesions involve the nervous system, lymph nodes, salivary gland, prostate, kidney, and others.

3. Leukodystrophy
  A. Characterized by disturbed myelin formation or maintenance
  B. Lesions are often predominant in cerebral and cerebellar white matter.
  C. The signs are usually symmetrical in all other respects.
  D. Globoid cell
    1) Dogs—cairns and West Highland white terriers
    2) Tremor, dysmetria, paresis, muscle atrophy, visual changes, mental changes
    3) Onset at 11 to 30 weeks of age
    4) The average duration of disease is two to three months.
    5) Lesions involve only the nervous system.
    6) Also rarely seen in beagles, blue tick hounds, poodles, and cats

Disorders Causing Abnormal Consciousness

1. *Stupor* is a state of extreme depression or drowsiness from which an animal can be aroused only by a strong noxious or painful stimulus. When the stimulus is removed, the animal returns to the nonresponsive state.
2. *Coma* is a condition of persistent unresponsiveness from which the animal cannot be aroused.

General Principles

1. Normal consciousness comprises both appropriate content of consciousness and level of arousal.
  A. Disorders in content of consciousness are concerned with functions, such as an animal's mentation, ability to remember commands, and personality, which are under cerebral control.
    1) Abnormalities in mentation (content of consciousness)
      a) Result in dementia
      b) Imply a cerebral disorder
      c) May result from any of the disease processes that affect the cerebrum

    2) Examples of disorders causing dementia
      a) Functional cerebral disorders (e.g., idiopathic epilepsy)
        i. The dementia is a manifestation of postictal behavior.
        ii. It is seen only in association with, or immediately following, a seizure.
      b) Metabolic disorders affecting the cerebrum
        i. Dementia may be the only clinical abnormality seen.
        ii. Dementia in metabolic disease generally waxes and wanes.
        iii. In liver disease, dementia often occurs in relation to meals.
      c) Structural cerebral disease
        i. Dementia is generally a constant finding.
        ii. There are usually other neurologic deficits seen in addition to the dementia.
    3) Clinical manifestations of dementia
      a) Unusual or aggressive behavior
      b) Bumping into objects
      c) Loss of continence
      d) Failure to recognize people
      e) Abnormal performance of any learned or voluntary activity may be a manifestation of dementia resulting from cerebral disease.
  B. Disorders affecting arousal produce a progressively sleeplike state.
    1) At its mildest, this produces depression or lethargy; an animal in this condition can be aroused easily.
    2) When an animal requires a painful or noxious stimulus to produce arousal, it is described as being stuporous.
    3) When the animal can no longer be aroused, the clinical condition is described as coma.
  C. Alterations in the level of arousal may rise from lesions in two parts of the nervous system.
    1) Sleep–wake cycles are controlled by the ascending RAS.

a) The RAS is located in the rostral brain stem.

b) Focal injury to the rostral brain stem may abolish the RAS and result in a disease process characterized by coma.

    2) The RAS is responsible for arousing or activating the cerebrum. Any diffuse process that affects the cerebrum may have the following effects:

a) An inability to respond to activation by the RAS

b) Stupor or coma

    2. Diseases that may cause alterations in consciousness maybe subdivided into three basic groups: structural mass lesions, structural generalized lesions, and metabolic diseases. Each of these tends to have certain features that allow you to arrive at a tentative diagnosis based on your clinical examination (Table 17-15).

Principles of Diagnosis

    1. Examine the patient for asymmetrical neurologic deficits.

    A. Asymmetrical deficits are called *lateralizing signs*.

    B. They usually imply structural and focal neurologic disease.

    2. Evaluate the PLR and pupillary size. Pupil size and pupil response is controlled in the midbrain.

    3. Consider the animal's eye movements, both voluntary and involuntary. The vestibular apparatus is responsible for control of eye movement and is located in the brain stem.

    4. Evaluate the animal's posture and tone of limbs.

    5. Evaluate respiratory patterns.

Lateralizing Signs

    1. Animals with lateralizing signs almost always have structural disease.

    2. Lateralizing signs may be manifested as:

    A. Asymmetry in reflex activity from one side to another

    B. Changes in pain perception from one side to another

    C. Presence or absence of voluntary

movement on one side as opposed to the other

    3. In metabolic disorders (especially hypoglycemia and renal disease), asymmetry does occasionally occur; however, the asymmetry usually changes constantly and frequently.

Pupillary Light Responses and Pupil Size

    1. The sympathetic innervation of the eyes arises in the diencephalon, immediately rostral to the midbrain. A lesion at this level leaves the patient with a small reactive pupil.

    2. Lesions in the midbrain cause loss of both sympathetic and parasympathetic fibers. Findings would include midrange and unresponsive pupils.

    3. A lesion arising outside the brain stem at the level of the third nerve involves only the parasympathetic innervation to the eye. A fixed and dilated pupil results from such a lesion.

    4. Lesions in the pons are often associated with small or pinpoint pupils that are fixed and unresponsive to light.

    5. Metabolic disorders are generally associated with midrange or small pupils that are reactive to light.

Eye Movements

    1. Eye movement in dogs and cats is primarily under vestibular control.

    A. Check for the presence of physiologic nystagmus (the doll's eye response).

    B. Check for pathologic or spontaneous nystagmus.

    2. In all animals with cerebral disease:

    A. The doll's eye response is normal.

    B. No pathologic nystagmus is present.

    3. In an animal with structural disease involving the diencephalon or midbrain, there is:

    A. Possible abnormal or absent physiologic nystagmus

    B. Possible positional pathologic nystagmus

    C. Generally no abnormal spontaneous eye movements

Table 17-15. **Classification of coma**

Focal or Lateralizing Neurologic Signs*

Neurologic findings	Etiologic considerations
Asymmetrical motor signs	CNS hemorrhage secondary to systemic bleeding disorders
Abnormal pupils	CNS infarction secondary to thrombosis or embolism (hypothyroidism,
Abnormal eye movements	feline ischemic encephalopathy)
Signs progress in an orderly fashion	Epidural and subdural hemorrhage secondary to brain trauma
CSF often abnormal	CNS neoplasia
	Focal encephalomyelitis
	Granulomatous disease (granulomatous meningoencephalitis, fungal infections, parasite migration)

Meningeal Irritation†

Neurologic findings	Etiologic considerations
Neck pain	Encephalitis
Abnormal CSF	Toxoplasmosis
Abnormal reflexes	Cryptococcosis
	FIP
	Canine distemper
	Other infections
	Meningitis
	Subarachnoid hemorrhage

No Focal or Lateralizing Neurologic Signs‡

Neurologic findings	Etiologic considerations
Usually normal reflexes	Intoxication
Normal pupils	Metabolic disturbances (diabetic acidosis, uremia, addisonian crisis,
Normal CSF	hepatic coma, hypoglycemia, hypoxia)
	Severe systemic infections
	Circulatory collapse (shock) from any cause
	Epilepsy (postictal behavior)
	Hyperthermia or hypothermia
	Concussion

* With or without changes in the CSF

† With blood or an excess of WBCs in the CSF; usually without focal or lateralizing signs

‡ No alteration of cellular count of CSF

Adapted from Adams, RD: in Harrison's Principles of Internal Medicine, Wintrube, MM (ed), 7th ed. NY, McGraw-Hill.

D. Possible external ophthalmoplegia (paralysis of eye movement in all directions)

4. Animals with disease involving the pons exhibit:

    A. Spontaneous pathologic nystagmus

    B. Positional pathologic nystagmus

    C. Abnormal physiologic nystagmus

Posture and Muscle Tone

1. Coma is generally associated with increased muscle tone as a result of UMN disease.

2. With disease involving the rostral midbrain, the following may be seen:

A. Decerebrate posture characterized by opisthotonos

    1) The head is extended.

    2) Severe extensor rigidity is present in all four limbs.

B. Lesions are associated with normal posture until the animal is stimulated. On stimulation, transient decerebrate posturing occurs.

3. Animals with selective lesions involving the pons and destruction of the vestibular apparatus may have:

    A. Flaccid or hypotonic muscle tone

    B. Normal or exaggerated reflexes

Respiratory Pattern

1. Respiratory patterns do not appear to be of great significance in the diagnosis of coma in veterinary medicine, except for metabolic causes (Table 17-16).

2. Animals with cerebral disease generally have normal respirations.

Table 17-16. *Respiratory changes and acid–base status in metabolic coma*

Hyperventilation	
Metabolic acidosis	*Respiratory alkalosis*
Ethylene glycol	Hepatic coma
Diabetic coma	Pulmonary thrombosis
End-stage renal disease	Heartworms
	Nephrotic syndrome
Postictal lactic acidosis	Pulmonary disease
	Pneumonia
Toxins	Pulmonary edema
	Sepsis
	Aspirin intoxication

Hypoventilation	
Respiratory acidosis	*Metabolic alkalosis*
Respiratory paralysis	Rare
Coonhound paralysis	Persistent hypokalemic states (e.g., diuretic excess, Cushing's disease)
Myasthenia gravis	
Drug intoxication	

Adapted from Plum F, Posner JB: The Diagnosis of Stupor and Coma, 3rd ed. Philadelphia, FA Davis, 1980

3. Animals with brain stem diseases may have ataxic or irregular respirations.

Diagnostic Approach

First, when presented with a patient with coma, stabilize the patient. This includes ensuring a patent airway, making certain that there are no cardiac arrhythmias or respiratory paralysis, establishing an IV fluid line, and instituting general supportive therapy. When this is accomplished, diagnostic procedures may be performed.

1. Diagnosis requires:

    A. An adequate history

    B. An adequate physical and neurologic examination

    C. Use of appropriate laboratory tests

2. History

    A. An acute onset may imply traumatic, vascular, or infectious diseases.

    B. A slow, progressive onset implies degenerative, metabolic, or neoplastic disease.

    C. Question the owner about possible asymmetry of signs, which would be suggestive of focal neurologic disease.

    D. Question the owner about any possible relationship of signs to meals or toxin exposure; this may suggest a metabolic or a toxic disease process.

3. The neurologic examination must be complete, with special emphasis on:

    A. Asymmetry of signs

    B. PLR

    C. Eye movements

    D. Posture and muscle tone

    E. Respiratory patterns

Laboratory Diagnosis

1. Serum biochemical studies are performed to rule out metabolic disease.

2. CSF analysis will rule out primary disease of the CNS.

Differential Diagnosis

1. Structural mass lesions that cause coma (see Table 17-15)

A. Create asymmetrical motor signs

B. Generally cause abnormal pupils

C. Generally cause abnormal eye movements

D. The signs generally are progressive and proceed in an orderly fashion.

E. The animals often have abnormalities noted on CSF analysis.

F. Diseases

    1) CNS neoplasia

        a) Slowly progressive

        b) Affects middle-aged or older animals

        c) Increased CSF pressure

        d) Elevated CSF protein levels

        e) Possibly abnormal findings on fundic examination

        f) Frequently responsive to steroids

    2) CNS vascular disease

        a) Acute onset

        b) Stabilizes rapidly

        c) Elevated CSF pressure and protein levels

        d) May have an increased number of cells in the CSF

        e) Responsive to steroids

    3) CNS trauma

        a) Acute onset

        b) The history is usually diagnostic.

        c) CSF taps are contraindicated in head trauma.

    4) Focal inflammatory diseases (e.g., granulomatous encephalomyelitis)

        a) Slowly to rapidly progressive disease

        b) Elevated CSF protein level and cell count

        c) Often, there is multifocal CNS involvement (cerebellum, spinal cord, peripheral nerve, as well as brain stem and cerebrum).

        d) Fundic examination may be normal.

    5) Granulomatous encephalomyelitis

        a) Acute, rapidly progressive onset

        b) Elevated CSF protein level

        c) Elevated CSF cell count

        d) With recurrent disease, affected animals are initially responsive to steroids.

        e) Frequently multifocal signs

2. Structural nonmass lesions that cause coma

  A. Generally indicate diffuse disease

  B. Symmetrical motor signs

  C. Normal PLR

  D. Possibly abnormal eye movements

  E. Signs are frequently progressive.

  F. Possible neck pain

  G. Generally abnormal findings on CSF analysis

  H. Diseases

    1) Encephalitis (toxoplasmosis, *Neosporum caninum*, cryptococcosis, other systemic fungal diseases, FIP, canine distemper virus encephalitis, other infectious and inflammatory diseases)

        a) Generally acute onset of signs

        b) Progressive course of disease

        c) Possible evidence of general systemic illness

        d) Specific diagnosis requires serologic and other specific laboratory diagnostic tests.

        e) The results of a fundic examination are frequently abnormal.

        f) Increase in CSF protein level and cell count

    2) Meningitis

        a) Generally associated with severe neck pain

        b) Uncommon disease in veterinary medicine

        c) Marked elevation in CSF cell count

    3) Subarachnoid hemorrhage

        a) Generally associated with severe neck pain

        b) History of trauma

        c) Possibly associated with systemic bleeding disorder

3. Metabolic diseases causing coma

  A. Usually associated with a normal neurologic examination

  B. Normal findings on CSF analysis

  C. Consider the following:

    1) Hypoxic disease

    2) Hypoglycemia

    3) Thiamine deficiency disorders

    4) Liver disorders

    5) Toxins

6) Drug intoxication

7) Acid–base disorders

D. Diagnosis requires serum biochemical analysis.

Management of the Comatose Patient

The long-term management of the comatose patient primarily involves good nursing care.

1. Maintenance of an airway and adequate oxygenation. If paralysis of the respiratory muscles occurs, maintain the animal on a respirator.

2. Animals with abnormal consciousness may have an abnormal thermal regulatory center.

A. May manifest all extremes of body temperature

B. Monitor the animal's temperature regularly and attempt to stabilize the body temperature.

3. Careful maintenance of bladder and bowel functions

4. Prevention of secondary infections

A. Comatose animals may aspirate

Summary of the Management of Comatose Patients

1. Stabilization

Ensure an adequate airway.

Monitor the animal's cardiac status.

Establish an IV fluid line.

2. Diagnosis

Neural examination

Laboratory work-up

Blood tests

Glucose, acid–base balance, electrolyte determinations

Liver function

CSF analysis

Roentgenography

3. Treatment

Provide supportive nursing care.

Prevent injury if the animal is delerious.

Turn the animal frequently.

Prevent urine scalding.

Keep the animal's bladder and colon empty.

Maintain respirations.

Preserve adequate electrolyte supplementation.

Administer fluid therapy.

Provide nutrient supplementation.

Prevent aspiration pneumonia which may result from normal oral and pharyngeal secretions, as well as vomitus.

A. Monitor the animal carefully for aspiration pneumonia.

4. Turn the animal frequently to prevent decubital ulcers.

5. Bathe the animal frequently and keep it dry to prevent development of urine scalding.

6. If the animal is delirious or thrashing wildly, restrain it either physically or chemically to prevent self-injury.

7. Many disorders associated with coma also cause epilepsy; if seizures occur, treat them appropriately.

8. Animals with disease involving the CNS and causing coma frequently have significant acid–base or electrolyte disturbances, especially abnormalities of water balance and sodium balance. Test the animal's electrolytes regularly and make a vigorous effort to maintain adequate electrolyte balance. If this is not done, the secondary complications may prove fatal in an otherwise treatable disease.

Seizures

A seizure is a clinical period of abnormal behavior that is caused by a sudden, abnormal, excess electrical discharge from the brain. Any condition in which the seizures recur is called epilepsy, and any condition that alters cerebral function may potentially cause epilepsy.

Clinical Presentation

The clinical findings in epilepsy reflect the discharging area of the brain, not the cause of the discharge.

1. Motor seizures—The clinical seizure is manifested as an involuntary, uncontrolled, motor activity.

A. Generalized motor seizures
    1) Classic grand mal seizures
    2) No localizing origin
    3) Usually accompanied by loss of consciousness
    4) Involve entire body
B. Partial motor seizures (simple)
    1) Focal motor seizures
    2) Involve only isolated groups of muscles
    3) Rarely associated with loss of consciousness
    4) Indicate focal brain injury
C. Partial motor seizures (complex)
    1) Focal seizures that generalize
    2) Often involve behavioral abnormalities (fly chasing, floor licking, tail chasing)
    3) Often called psychomotor or temporal lobe seizures
    4) Possible loss of consciousness
2. Nonmotor seizures—These seizures are associated with loss of consciousness and transient collapse, but not with involuntary movement. They are called lapse attacks or petit mal seizures. These seizures must be differentiated from syncope (see Chapter 9) and narcolepsy.

Etiologic Classification

1. Extracranial (Table 17-17)
  A. Include disease processes (such as hypoglycemia, lead poisoning, hepatoencephalopathy) causing systemic or metabolic abnormalities that lead to seizures
  B. May cause any clinical type of seizure
  C. Often associated with waxing and waning dementia between seizures
  D. Usually characterized by normal neurologic examinations between seizures except for the dementia
  E. Findings on physical examination are often abnormal.
2. Intracranial
  A. Structural diseases—The disease process is associated with primary injury to the brain and damage to, or destruction of, the tissue (e.g., encephalitis or tumors)
    1) Normal physical examination except for the neurologic examination
    2) May cause any type of epilepsy; primarily associated with partial or focal seizures
    3) Neurologic deficits often persist between seizures.

Table 17-17. *Epilepsy**

Functional Epilepsy	*Structural Epilepsy*		*Metabolic Epilepsy*
Normal physical examination	Normal physical examination		Abnormal physical examination
Normal neural examination	Abnormal neural examination		Normal neural examination (may have dementia)
Normal blood studies	Normal blood studies		Abnormal blood studies
Normal CSF analysis	Abnormal CSF analysis (not always present)		Normal CSF analysis
	Focal	*Diffuse*	Hypoglycemia
	Vascular	Degenerations	Lead
	Hypothyroidism	Lysosomal storage	Hepatoencephalopathy
	Bleeding	disorders	Ethylene glycol
	disorders	Hydrocephalus	Thiamine deficiency
	Arteriovenous	Inflammations	Other toxins
	malformation	Canine distemper	Hypocalcemia
	Neoplasia	FIP	Acid–base disorders
	Trauma	Granulomatous	Uremia
	Focal inflammations	encephalomyelitis	

* Spontaneous, paroxysmal events of cerebral origin characterized by a period of clinical abnormality

4) Frequently abnormal CSF and EEG findings

5) Possibly abnormal ophthalmoscopic examination

B. Functional epilepsy

1) Primary functional disorder of the cerebrum (idiopathic epilepsy)

2) No pathological cause for the process can be detected.

3) Normal examination between seizures

4) Normal physical examination

Diagnostic Approach

History and Type

1. Age (Fig. 17-18)

A. In young animals, it is usually an inherited or congenital disorder.

B. In older animals, neoplastic disorders or degenerative disorders are usually involved.

2. Environment (toxins such as lead)

3. Diet (fish diet in cats for thiamine deficiency)

4. Chronology of problem—The longer the animal has epilepsy, the more likely the etiology is to be "benign," or functional, epilepsy.

Physical and Neurologic Examination

1. Abnormal general physical examination—Look for metabolic and toxic causes.

2. Abnormal neurologic examination—Look for structural intracranial causes.

3. When both physical and neurologic examinations are normal, look for functional causes.

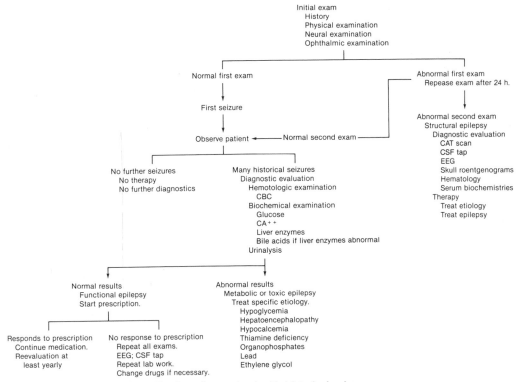

Figure 17-18. *Diagnostic evaluation of an animal with historical seizures. (Adapted from Fenner WR: Seizures and head trauma. Vet Clin North Am 11:31, 1981)*

Diagnostic Aids

1. Nucleated RBS detected on CBC may suggest lead intoxication. Confirm this by testing blood lead levels.

2. Serum biochemical studies are important in the diagnosis of metabolic diseases and in the evaluation of liver injury secondary to anticonvulsant medication. Blood glucose, liver enzyme, and serum calcium tests encompass the basic information needed for diagnosis of an animal with seizures.

3. CSF analysis

    A. An increase in pressure is suggestive of a mass effect ($>$170 mm H_2O in the dog; $>$100 mm H_2O in the cat).

        1) Neoplasia

        2) CNS edema

        3) Vascular lesions

        4) Encephalitis (rarely)

    B. WBC count as an indicator of inflammation ($>$10 WBC/mm^3)

        1) Encephalitis

        2) Vascular disorder

        3) Granulomatous disorder

        4) Rarely, neoplasia

    C. RBC count ($>$5 RBC/mm^3)

        1) Vascular disorder

        2) Neoplasia (rarely)

        3) Trauma

    D. Elevation in protein level ($>$25 mg/dL)

        1) Inflammatory disorders

        2) Vascular disorders

        3) Neoplastic disorders

        4) Trauma

4. Ophthalmoscopy is of great value in the diagnosis of inflammatory disorders affecting the CNS.

5. Skull films are of little value except in cases of head trauma and hydrocephalus, and occasionally, in neoplasia.

6. Electroencephalography, if available, often provides valuable information. It is of greatest value in the diagnosis of structural diseases of the CNS.

7. MRI or a CT scan should be performed in all patients with focal seizures or an abnormal neurologic examination.

Treatment

1. If an underlying condition is present, treat that condition.

2. If this does not resolve the epilepsy, then consider specific anticonvulsant therapy.

    3. Drugs available

        A. Phenobarbital

            1) This drug is safe in all animals.

            2) Start at a dosage of 2 to 4 mg/kg/d in divided doses.

            3) This is the drug of choice for initial treatment.

            4) Therapeutic serum level is 15 to 45 mg/L.

        B. Potassium bromide

            1) Not licensed for use

            2) The initial dosage is 20 mg/kg/d.

            3) Prominent sedation

            4) Usually effective only if combined with phenobarbital

        C. Diazepam

            1) Safe in all animals

            2) Start at a dosage of 1 to 2 mg/kg t.i.d.

            3) Rapid tolerance develops in dogs.

            4) Often the best drug in cats

        D. Clorazepate

            1) A benzodiazepine

            2) Start at a dosage of 2 mg/kg/d

            3) Usually not effective unless combined with phenobarbital

            4) Quite expensive

        E. Primidone

            1) This drug is only approved for use in dogs, but is often used in cats.

            2) Administer 50 mg/kg/d in divided doses for dogs; 40 mg/kg/d in cats.

            3) Personality changes are seen in some animals receiving this medication.

            4) Hepatotoxic in dogs

            5) The therapeutic serum level is the same as that for phenobarbital.

        F. Dilantin

            1) Not indicated for use in cats

            2) Administer 35 mg/kg t.i.d.

            3) Do not use in animals receiving chloramphenicol.

            4) Hepatotoxic in dogs

Goals of Therapy

1. Decreased severity of the seizures
2. Decreased frequency of the seizures
3. Decreased severity of the postictal behavior
4. Attempt to accomplish these goals by using the lowest possible dose of medication and the fewest number of medications with the fewest side effects.

Maintenance Therapy

1. Begin with one drug and allow an adequate time for the drug to work before changing the therapeutic regimen. Monitor serum levels before adjusting therapy.
2. Start treatment in any animal that is having seizures more than once per month or in any animal having severe or protracted seizures. The following chart outlines a protocol for long-term maintenance anticonvulsant therapy (Fig. 17-19).
3. Never change drugs without monitoring serum levels.
4. Among the major causes of failure of therapy is impatience on the part of the clinician. Most epileptics can be controlled given proper time, patience, good client communication, and appropriate use of serum drug monitoring.

Therapy for Active Seizures

Stop the seizures (without harming the patient); then diagnose the problem.
Confirm the presence of seizures. Rule out:
    Acute vestibular disease

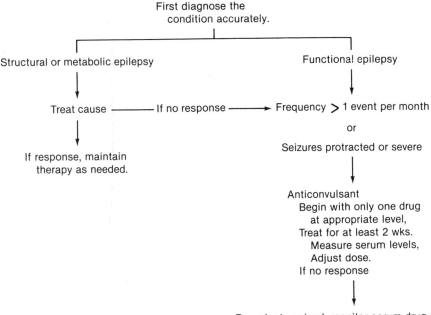

Figure 17-19. *Long-term medical treatment of epilepsy. (Adapted from Fenner WR: Seizures and head trauma. Vet Clin North Am 11:31, 1981)*

Narcolepsy
Tetanus
Hypocalcemia
Then:
Establish an IV line
Conduct blood studies:
Glucose determinations in all dogs
Ca^{++} levels in postparturient females
Acid–base determinations if seizures
have been prolonged
Then:
Administer IV thiamine, followed by dextrose, 1 g/kg, administered by slow IV drip.
If the animal responds, maintain a 5% dextrose drip and complete the evaluation.
If there is no response, then:
Maintain an airway and administer IV anticonvulsants. Begin with valium, administered by slow IV drip to effect, 0.7 to 2.0 mg/kg, plus a loading dose of phenobarbital. If treating a patient that is not on anticonvulsants administer 20 mg/kg slowly.
If the animal responds:
Maintain IV supportive therapy (fluids). Complete the diagnostic evaluation.
If there is no response within 15 minutes:
Repeat administration of valium (may be done up to a total of three doses).
If no effect is achieved:
Anesthetize the animal using pentobarbital.
After the animal has recovered from the effects of the seizures and the drugs, complete the diagnostic examination.

The patient that is actively having seizures presents a true medical emergency. If the seizures are not stopped, the combination of cerebral, CSF, and systemic metabolic alterations that accompany them may be fatal. Treatment in such cases is to administer enough IV anticonvulsant to stop the seizures rapidly without harming the patient. The treatment protocol may be summarized as follows:

1. Administer all medications IV.
2. Treat potentially reversible metabolic diseases first.

Hypoglycemia
Hypocalcemia
3. Always go from the shortest-acting to the longest-acting anticonvulsant, reserving general anesthesia as a last resort.
4. Use the fewest combinations of drugs possible.
5. Maintain an airway and provide supportive therapy as needed.

Prognosis

The prognosis for animals who present in status epilepticus is guarded. These animals always warrant a complete neurologic evaluation when the seizures have been controlled and they have recovered from the effects of the anticonvulsant medication.

Summary

1. Any disorder that affects the cerebrum may cause epilepsy.
2. A logical etiologic classification is:
  A. Extracranial epilepsy
    1) Metabolic
    2) Toxic
    3) Diagnosis rests on laboratory evaluation.
  B. Intracranial epilepsy
    1) Structural
      a) Focal mass
      b) Diffuse
        i. Encephalitis
        ii. Degenerative processes
    2) Functional
3. Therapeutic guidelines
  A. Establish an adequate diagnosis for extracranial causes and structural intracranial causes. Treat the animal on the basis of the etiology. If that fails, treat the seizures themselves.
  B. For intracranial functional epilepsy, treat the seizures.

Nervous System Injury

Head Injury

Definitions and Etiology

1. Craniocerebral trauma—Many traumatized patients injure their head, but the vast majority of them never suffer any CNS damage. Those patients that do sustain damage to their CNS are defined as having incurred craniocerebral trauma (CCT), regardless of the precise location of the injury.

2. Etiology—The most common cause of CCT is a motor vehicle accident, also known as an HBC (Hit By Car). Other causes in animals include blunt trauma (such as from being hit by bats, swings, children falling on them, etc.), animal fights, falls, and gunshot wounds.

Pathogenesis

Traumatic injury to the nervous system not only results in immediate and direct injury to the tissues of the nervous system, it initiates a cascade of secondary, metabolic events that result in worsening of the neurologic disease as well as in systemic and metabolic derangements (Fig. 17-20). The result may be increased intracranial pressure, systemic hypertension, myocardial necrosis, cardiac arrhythmias, pulmonary edema, and increased nutritional requirements.

1. Secondary events

A. Pressure changes—Most patients with CNS trauma have a rise in intracranial pressure, usually as a result of edema and hemorrhage.

B. Edema—Edema is both intracellular and extracellular. Intracellular edema results from hypoxia, which produces CNS acidosis. Extracellular edema results from leakage of fluid across the blood–brain barrier.

C. Hypoxia—Hypoxia results from decreased tissue perfusion.

D. Hypercarbia (increased CO_2 levels)—Systemic hypercarbia results in venodilation, which decreases cerebral perfusion pressure and cerebral oxygenation and further exacerbates cerebral edema.

E. Vascular changes—The venodilation that results from hypercarbia has already been mentioned. In addition, some patients develop arterial spasm.

2. Direct events

A. Necrosis/lacerations—The primary events, which occur at the time of injury, are largely mechanical in nature. They produce mechanical disruption of fiber tracts and mechanical injury to the cell membranes. These mechanical disruptions may not be reparable. This immediate injury is called a *contusion*.

B. Transient neuronal dysfunction—At the time of injury, some cells will undergo physiologic disruption of function. This may

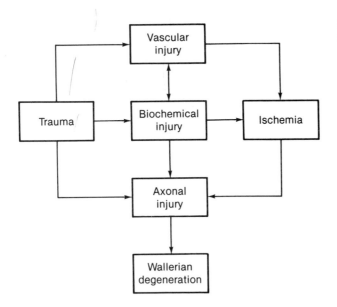

Figure 17-20. *Pathogenesis of injury in CNS trauma*

be from hypoxia, acidosis, or from an unknown cause. This dysfunction is not based on an anatomic injury, and is completely reversible. Such an injury is known as a *concussion*, which is the term used to describe a transient loss of CNS function secondary to trauma, without structural injury.

3. Seizures

A. Seizures may occur at the time of the injury or any time afterward. They potentiate all of the harmful events that can occur in the cranial vault, including elevation of intracranial pressure, hypoxia, acidosis, edema, and the like.

B. Because of this fact, seizures should be treated in head trauma patients. Short-acting drugs should be the first choice, if possible (i.e., diazepam).

Clinical Approach

1. Treat all life-threatening nonneural injuries first (Figs. 17-21 to 17-24).

A. Stop any hemorrhage.

B. Ensure a patent airway.

1) Intubate the animal if necessary.

2) Evaluate for hemothorax or pneumothorax.

C. Treat shock.

2. Evaluate the nervous system.

3. Localize the lesion(s).

A. Importance of localization

1) Difference in therapeutic approach

a) PNS injuries usually do not require therapy.

b) CNS injuries frequently require vigorous therapy.

2) Difference in prognosis

a) PNS injury—Usually, the patient survives with no serious sequellae and some isolated cranial nerve deficits.

b) CNS injury—Many patients do not survive, and those that do may have serious sequellae, including epilepsy, personality changes, and paralysis.

B. CNS versus PNS lesion

1) Neurologic examination

a) Mental status examination—The evaluation of consciousness is one of the best tools available for localizing a lesion and establishing a prognosis for a patient with CCT. Immediate and sustained loss of consciousness generally indicates a brain stem injury. Immediate and persistent dementia generally reflects a cerebral injury. Patients who have a normal level of consciousness immediately following the trauma, but who later begin to deteriorate, are often developing brain herniation, either from brain edema or intracranial hemorrhage. These patients require immediate intervention if they are to be saved.

Figure 17-21. *Flow chart for treatment of head trauma. (Adapted from Fenner WR: Seizures and head trauma. Vet Clin North Am 11:31, 1981)*

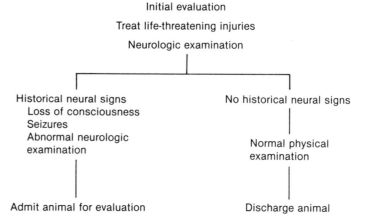

Head Trauma

Initial evaluation

Treat life-threatening injuries

Neurologic examination

Historical neural signs
Loss of consciousness
Seizures
Abnormal neurologic
examination

No historical neural signs

Normal physical
examination

Admit animal for evaluation

Discharge animal

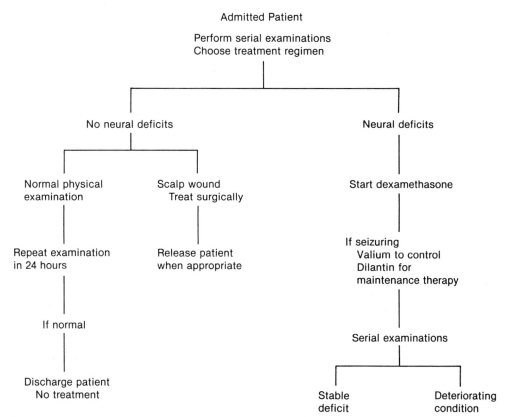

Figure 17-22. *Flow chart for an admitted patient. (Adapted from Fenner WR: Seizures and head trauma. Vet Clin North Am 11:31, 1981)*

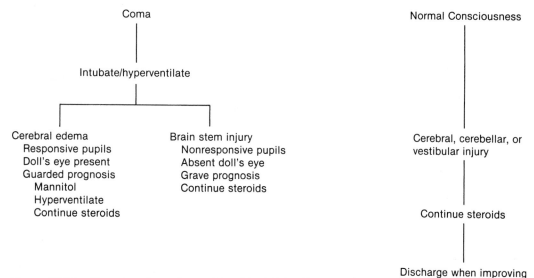

Figure 17-23. *Flow chart for patients with stable deficits. (Adapted from Fenner WR: Seizures and head trauma. Vet Clin North Am 11:31, 1981)*

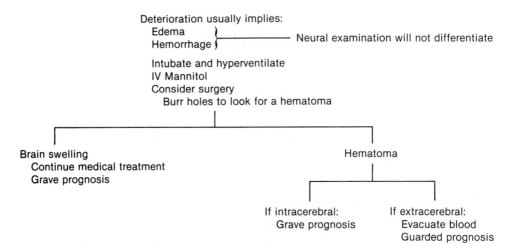

Figure 17-24. *Flow chart for a deteriorating patient. (Adapted from Fenner WR: Seizures and head trauma. Vet Clin North Am 11:31, 1981)*

i. Normal consciousness— PNS or cerebellar lesion

ii. Stupor/coma—diffuse cerebral injury or brain stem injury

    A. Normal PLR—diffuse cerebral injury

    B. Normal doll's eye— diffuse cerebral injury

    C. Abnormal PLR—brain stem injury

    D. Abnormal doll's eye— brain stem injury

iii. Dementia—cerebral injury

2) Head posture

  a) Opisthotonus—cerebellar or brain stem injury

    i. Normal mentation—cerebellar injury

    ii. Normal PLR—cerebellar injury

    iii. Stupor/coma—midbrain injury

    iv. Abnormal PLR—midbrain injury

3) Cranial nerve examination

  a) Small reactive pupils—cerebral, ophthalmic, or middle ear injury

  b) Small nonreactive pupils— pontine (brain stem) injury

  c) Large reactive pupils—fear/ stress

  d) Large nonreactive pupils— midbrain (brain stem) injury, bilateral CN II or CN III injury

4) Doll's eye response (oculocephalic response)

  a) Evaluates the vestibular input and brain stem connections for involuntary eye movement.

  b) Of greatest value in differentiating brain stem from cerebral causes of coma.

  c) A normal doll's eye indicates an intact brain stem, coma of cerebral origin, and a fair prognosis.

  d) An absent doll's eye indicates coma of brain stem origin and carries a grave prognosis.

5) Posture

  a) Animals may have generalized extensor rigidity (opisthotonos). A normal doll's eye and normal consciousness indicates cerebellar injury and a good prognosis.

  b) Decerebrate posturing, opisthotonos, and coma are associated with an absent doll's eye, brain stem injury, and a grave prognosis

6) Spinal reflexes—Absent or decreased reflexes indicate injury to the spinal cord, as well as the head. This may alter the prognosis.

Therapeutic Approach

1. Clinical presentation
    A. Historical problems only
        1) Observe the animal.
        2) No therapy
    B. Abnormal examination
        1) CNS injury
            a) Surgical therapy—Surgery is not usually needed unless the patient has depressed skull fractures that are compressing neural tissue, or an open wound that may serve as a source of infection.
            b) Medical therapy
                i. Head elevation—This facilitates passive emptying of the venous sinuses, helps to decrease intracranial pressure, enhances resorption of spinal fluid, and helps to maintain cerebral blood flow.
                ii. Oxygen supply—Oxygen will help to reverse the cerebral edema.
                iii. Steroid therapy—Steroids are thought to reduce edema. The evidence for this is mostly circumstantial in CCT, based on the known antiedematous effect of steroids in brain tumors. The initial dose of steroids should be administered IV. The author recommends dexamethasone phosphate, 1.0 mg/kg, followed by a maintenance dexamethasone dose of 0.2 to 0.4 mg/kg daily for five to seven days postinjury.
                iv. Hyperventilation—In an animal with stupor or coma, intubation and hyperventilation is the quickest way to reverse both the hypercarbia and hypoxia. In doing so, cerebral edema may be prevented or reversed.
                v. Diuretics—A number of diuretics are known to have an effect in the CNS to reverse brain edema. The author uses furosemide, 2 to 4 mg/kg t.i.d. or q.i.d. Furosemide appears to decrease the production of CSF. If the patient is deteriorating rapidly, mannitol may be added to the treatment regimen (1.25 mg/kg IV as a single dose).
                vi. Restoration of blood flow—Calcium blockers, vasodilators, narcotic antagonists, prostacyclin, and antiprostaglandins, such as aspirin, have all been advocated to prevent posttraumatic infarction. The calcium channel blockers and vasodilators appear to do this by preventing vasospasm. The mechanism of the other drugs appears to be prevention of the development of microthrombi in the arterioles of the CNS.
                vii. Relief of pain—Analgesics for relief of pain are advocated in all cases of CCT. The use of sedative drugs should be avoided, as these may alter the results of the neurologic examination.
                viii. Anticonvulsants—In patients with seizures, IV bendzodiazepines, such as diazepam or lorazepam, should be administered to control active seizures. These patients should then receive oral anticonvulsants. If the

patient remains seizure-free, the anticonvulsant therapy may be tapered and then discontinued over a period of six months.

c) Supportive therapy—Without proper supportive therapy, these patients have little or no chance of survival. This therapy should include fluids, frequent turning to prevent bed sores, and careful monitoring of electrolyte balance. Patients with CCT have a tendency to become hypernatremic, and this should be avoided. If the patient is unable to eat, hyperalimentation of some sort should be instituted as soon as is feasible.

2) PNS Injury
a) Supportive therapy

Prognosis

1. PNS injury—fairly good
2. CNS injury
A. An attempt to develop a clinical scale that can be used for prognosis is currently under way. Such a scale in humans already exists (Glasgow Coma Scale). Dr. A. Shores at Michigan State is evaluating such a scale for use in veterinary medicine (Table 17-18).
B. In general, patients with coma lasting for more than 48 hours will not recover.
C. After that generalization, the prognosis is best determined by whether the signs are stable or deteriorating, and the location of the injury in the CNS.
1. Stable injury
a) Cerebral injury—Cerebral injuries usually have a fair prognosis. The clinical features of a cerebral injury may include dementia, seizures, weakness, visual deficits, sensory deficits, and subtle cranial nerve deficits.
b) Brain stem injury—Brain stem injuries usually are associated with a poor prognosis. The clinical features of a brain stem injury may include stupor or coma, abnormal doll's eye, multiple cranial nerve deficits, tetraparesis, and abnormal pupil size and ocular position.
c) Cerebellar injury—Cerebellar injuries usually carry a fair prognosis. The clini-

cal features of a cerebellar injury may include tremor, opisthotonus, normal mentation, and, if ambulatory, an ataxic gait.
2. Deteriorating injury
a) The clinical features of deterioration in CCT include rapidly declining mentation, dilating pupils, progressive paresis, bradycardia, and/or loss of oculovestibular nystagmus. Such signs usually indicate brain herniation, which carries a grave prognosis. Very few of these patients can be saved.

Spinal Injury

Spinal cord injury may be associated with any degree of external trauma. It may occur without associated injury to supporting structures or in association with intervertebral disk disease, fractures, or vertebral luxations.

1. Edema and compression are the two immediate factors to control.
A. Edema is controlled by the use of steroids.
B. Compression is controlled by stabilization or reduction of fractures or luxations.
2. Animals with thoracic injury may have Schiff-Sherrington syndrome.
A. Release of front limbs from lumbar inhibition
1) Increased tone with rigidity in front limbs
2) Normal reflexes in front
3) Normal voluntary movement in front
B. May lead to incorrect localization of signs to the cervical spine or incorrect diagnosis of cervical, as well as thoracic, injury

Clinical Management

1. Stabilize the patient—Treat life-threatening nonneural injuries.
2. Neural evaluation (Table 17-19)
A. Spinal reflex examination to localize lesion
B. Sensory examination to establish prognosis
3. Spinal roentgenograms
A. To determine the type of injury
B. If the lumbar or sacral spine is in-

Table 17-18. *Clinical rating scale for evaluation of CCT patients**

Criteria	Score
Motor activity	
Normal gait, normal reflexes	6
Hemiparesis, tetraparesis, or decorticate activity	5
Recumbent, intermittent extensor rigidity	4
Recumbent, constant extensor rigidity	3
Recumbent, intermittent extensor rigidity/opisthotonus	2
Recumbent, hypotonia of muscles, depressed or absent spinal reflexes	1
Brain stem reflexes	
Normal PLR and oculovestibular reflexes (OVRs)	6
Slow PLR and normal to reduced OVRs	5
Bilateral/unresponsive miosis and normal to reduced OVRs	4
Pinpoint pupils and reduced to absent OVRs	3
Unilateral/unresponsive mydriasis and reduced to absent OVRs	2
Bilateral/unresponsive mydriasis and reduced to absent OVRs	1
Level of consciousness	
Occasionally alert and responsive	6
Depressed/delerious, but capable of response to stimulus	5
Obtunded/stuporous—responds to visual stimuli	4
Obtunded/stuporous—responds to auditory stimuli	3
Obtunded/stuporous—responds to noxious stimuli	2
Coma—unresponsive to noxious stimuli	1

Total Score	Likely Prognosis
3–8	Grave
9–14	Poor to guarded
15–18	Good

* Reprinted with permission from Shores A: Craniocerebral trauma: Emergency management and prognosis. Proceedings ACVIM, 6:3–5, 1988

Table 17-19. *Evaluation of spinal reflexes in spinal cord injury*

Site of Injury	Reflexes	Signs
C1–C4 vertebrae C1–C5 segments	UMN all four limbs	Tetraparesis
C5–T1 vertebrae C6–T1 spinal segments	LMN front UMN rear	Tetraparesis Possible Horner's syndrome
T2–L2 vertebrae T2–L2 spinal segments	Normal front UMN rear	Rear limb paralysis
L3–L6 vertebrae L3–S3 spinal segments	Normal front LMN rear	Rear limb paralysis Loss of anal reflex
L7–S2 vertebrae Cauda equina	Normal front Normal patella LMN sciatic LMN perineal	Can stand Decreased flexor reflex Decreased anal tone

jured, evaluate the animal for a ruptured bladder.

4. Immobilization

A. External support

B. If there is no head injury, use mild sedation if needed.

5. Anti-inflammatory therapy—Dexamethasone, 0.1 to 1 mg/lb/d

6. Hyperosmolar agents—Mannitol. Contraindicated if the dog is to undergo immediate surgery

7. Nursing care

A. Maintain bladder function.

1) Empty at least four times daily.

2) Administer urinary antibiotics.

B. Facilitate defecation.

1) Glycerin suppositories, if needed

2) Mild bulk laxatives or stool softeners

3) Soft bedding

4) Frequent turning

8. Surgical therapy—A discussion of specific surgical techniques is beyond the scope of this chapter. The general principles involved in selecting surgical versus medical management include:

A. Not exacerbating the animal's condition

B. Stabilizing any unstable lesion

C. Relieving spinal cord compression

Prognosis

1. The prognosis in spinal injury is based on both the location and the severity of the injury.

A. Location

1) Cervical cord injuries frequently respond better than lumbar cord injuries.

2) Injuries to the grey matter innervating a limb are generally more severe than injuries affecting only white matter fiber tracts to a limb.

B. Severity

1) Animal is ambulatory and has preservation of voluntary movement.

a) Mild injury

b) Good prognosis

2) Animal is nonambulatory but still has sensation and preserved voluntary movement.

a) Moderate injury

b) Fair prognosis

3) Animal is paralyzed, has no voluntary motion, but pain sensation is intact.

a) Major injury

b) Guarded prognosis

4) Animal is plegic, with loss of pain sensation.

a) Severe injury

b) Grave prognosis

One of the most common reasons for failure to establish an accurate prognosis in animals with spinal injury is the tendency to base the prognosis on roentgenograms. An adequate prognosis requires a complete neural examination and an understanding of the location and severity of injury. Therapy will also fail if spinal injuries are treated as pure orthopedic cases. Unnecessary reduction of fractures may exacerbate spinal cord injury.

Summary

1. The animal that sustains spinal trauma has two injuries.

A. Orthopedic—spinal vertebral injury

B. Neurologic—spinal cord injury

2. Proper therapy requires choosing the procedure that helps both injuries the most.

Suggested Readings

Adams RD, Victor M: Principles of Neurology. New York, McGraw-Hill, 1978

Braund KG: Clinical Syndromes in Veterinary Neurology. Baltimore, Williams and Wilkins, 1986

Chrisman CL (ed): Advances in neurology. Vet Clin North Am 10(1): 1–237, 1980

DeJong RN: The Neurologic Examination, 4th ed. Hagerstown, Harper & Row, 1979

deLahunta A: Veterinary Neuroanatomy and Clinical Neurology, 2nd ed. Philadelphia, WB Saunders, 1983

Ettinger AJ: Textbook of Veterinary Internal Medicine, 3rd ed. Philadelphia, WB Saunders, 1989

Fishman RA: Cerebrospinal fluid. In Diseases of the Nervous System. Philadelphia, WB Saunders, 1980

Greene CE: Infections of the central nervous system. In Greene CE (ed): Clinical Microbiology and Infectious Disease of the Dog and Cat. Philadelphia, WB Saunders, 1984

Kornegay JN: Cerebrospinal fluid collection, examination, and interpretation in dogs and cats. Compend Contin Educ Pract Vet 3: 85–94, 1981

Lorenz MD, Cork LC, Griffith JW et al: Hereditary spinal muscular atrophy in Brittany Spaniels: Clinical manifestations. J Am Vet Med Assoc 175: 833–839, 1979

Meric JM: Canine meningitis: A changing emphasis. J Vet Intern Med 2: 26–35, 1988

Oliver JE, Hoerlien BF, and Mayhew IG. Veterinary Neurology. Philadelphia, WB Saunders, 1987

Palmer AC: Introduction to Animal Neurology, 2nd ed. Oxford, Blackwell Scientific Publications, 1976

Pearlman AL, Collins RC: Neurologic Pathophysiology, 3rd ed. New York, Oxford University Press, 1984

Plum F, Posner JB: The Diagnosis of Stupor and Coma, 3rd ed. Philadelphia, FA Davis, 1980

CHAPTER EIGHTEEN

Ocular Disorders

Susan Winston and Keith W. Prasse

Routine Ocular Complaints

The following sections provide a diagnostic outline for common owner complaints, rather than for specific disease entities. The authors would like to acknowledge Dr. Gretchen Schmidt as the original and definitive expert on the problem-oriented approach to eye diseases. It will be apparent that there is a great deal of overlap in the presentation of diseases and diagnostic approaches in these sections. Most of these tests can be run quickly and inexpensively, and the results are immediate. If a practitioner does not own a particular piece of equipment (e.g., a tonometer), that evaluation (i.e., is the intraocular pressure elevated?) should still be part of a mental checklist. Because this is intended primarily as a diagnostic reference, little discussion is devoted to therapy. For this, the reader is referred to general ophthalmology texts.

Red Eyes

1. Differential diagnosis
   A. Conjunctivitis
   B. Anterior uveitis
   C. Acute glaucoma
   D. Ulcerative keratitis
   E. Keratoconjunctivitis sicca (KCS)
   F. Retrobulbar disease
   G. Subconjunctival hemorrhage
   H. Hyphema
   I. Third eyelid redness
   J. Corneal, conjunctival, or limbal masses
2. Diagnostic plan—The following procedures will direct the clinician to the appropriate disorder, from among those just listed, which may be associated with a red eye.
   A. Schirmer tear test
      1) This test should be done prior to the installation of a topical anesthetic or other ophthalmic solutions.
      2) Normal values are greater than 15 mm in one minute.
      3) Low values represent KCS.
   B. Fluorescein stain is used to confirm ulcerative keratitis.
   C. Tonometry
      1) Normal intraocular pressure (IOP) is 15 to 30 mmHg.
      2) By definition, increased IOP is glaucoma.
      3) Decreased IOP accompanies anterior uveitis, phthisis, or perforation of the globe.
   D. Adnexal examination
      1) Examine the eyelids for the presence of aberrant hairs—entropion, distichiasis, trichiasis, ectopic cilia, prominent nasal folds
         a) Know common breed predisposition to inherited eyelid diseases
            i. Entropion—chow chow, Chinese Shar-pei, English

ii. Lymphocytic, plasmacytic exudate can accompany viral and allergic disorders.

iii. Eosinophils are seen with eosinophilic conjunctivitis and/or keratitis (a specific syndrome in cats), allergy, and parasites.

iv. Bacteria—Small and large cocci (most commonly, staphylococcus; less frequently, streptococcus) frequently accompany neutrophilic exudate in dogs, regardless of the primary cause, and may represent opportunistic infection. Large and small rods in dogs are most likely to represent pathogenic organisms. The presence of any bacteria (rods or cocci) is considered to be clinically significant in cats.

d) Neoplasia—mast cell tumor, lymphosarcoma, squamous cell carcinoma

C. Culture—Perform a culture in previously treated, nonresponsive or severe cases. Collect the sample prior to installation of topical anesthetic.

D. Fluorescein dye—If positive results are obtained, see the section on ulcerative keratitis that follows.

E. Eyelid examination

1) Examine for aberrant hairs—distichiasis, trichiasis, entropion, ectopic cilia, nasal fold irritation, dermoid, eyelid agenesis

2) Examine for masses that could contact the cornea or conjunctiva.

F. Evaluation of the palpebral reflex for abnormal palpebral closure

1) Breed conformation for lagophthalmos, exophthalmos, ectropion

2) Facial nerve paralysis

G. Examination of the area behind the third eyelid for foreign bodies

H. Flushing of the nasolacrimal puncta— Some exudate will always accumulate, particularly with KCS. Significant flocculent exudate indicates dacryocystitis. (See the section on thick ocular discharge under Ocular Discharge.)

I. Ophthalmoscopic examination to rule out chorioretinitis or systemic disease

6. Treatment

A. Bacterial conjunctivitis in the dog is most commonly caused by Staphylococcus species, which is followed in frequency by Streptococcus species and Pseudomonas. Treatment with a commercial combination of neomycin, bacitracin, and polymyxin B is effective.

B. Feline herpes conjunctivitis, when acute, is treated with a topical, broad-spectrum antibiotic. Topical antiviral drugs are used in chronic or severe infections. The current choices are trifluridine (Viroptic), idoxuridine (Herplex, Stoxil), and adenine arabinoside (Vira-A). These drugs are not documented to be effective for the treatment of herpetic conjunctivitis as they are for herpetic ulcers.

C. Chlamydia or mycoplasma are treated by topical or oral tetracycline, or both.

D. Avoid topical steroids in feline conjunctivitis until infectious causes have been ruled out.

E. Allergic conjunctivitis is treated by topical steroids.

F. Eosinophilic conjunctivitis of cats is treated with topical steroids.

G. KCS is treated with topical 2% cyclosporine ophthalmic drops, topical artificial tears, or oral lacrimimetics (pilocarpine).

H. Treatment for secondary conjunctivitis is directed toward eliminating the underlying disorder.

Anterior Uveitis

1. Anterior uveitis refers to inflammation of the iris or ciliary body and presents as a red, painful eye.

2. Clinical findings

A. Ocular penlight examination

1) Conjunctival hyperemia is evident.

2) Ciliary flush may be present.

3) Cornea may be clear or edematous.

4) Iris may be darker, congested, swollen, and vascularized.

5) Aqueous may exhibit hyphema, hypopyon (not synonymous with infection), keratic precipitates (leukocytes adhered to corneal endothelium), lipid, flare (increase in protein content manifested as increased turbidity in anterior chamber), or fibrin.

6) Pupil will be miotic and have poor dilation with mydriatics; posterior synechiae may occur if uveitis is chronic.

7) Lens is clear or opaque (cataract may cause or result from uveitis). Pigment deposits on lens capsule can signify previous uveitis.

B. Fluorescein stain—If positive results are obtained, the anterior uveitis may be the result of severe ulcerative keratitis.

C. Tonometry—IOP is reduced unless secondary glaucoma is present.

D. Examine the lens for the presence of rapidly maturing cataracts that may precipitate lens-induced uveitis.

E. Fundus examination—This is not always possible owing to the cloudiness of ocular media and poor pupillary dilation with mydriatics. Posterior segment (vitreous, choroid, retina, optic nerve) involvement implies systemic disease. However, the lack of posterior segment involvement does not rule out systemic disease. (For findings on chorioretinitis, see the section on Acute Blindness that follows.)

F. Examine the opposite eye, including performance of an ophthalmoscopic examination, for further indication of systemic disease.

3. Disorders—The causes of anterior uveitis include ocular and systemic diseases. Diseases from the following list must be ruled out. In many instances, the cause may not be determined.

A. Infectious causes
    1) Systemic mycoses
    2) Feline leukemia virus (FeLV)
    3) Feline infectious peritonitis (FIP)
    4) Brucellosis
    5) Canine infectious hepatitis
    6) Leptospirosis
    7) Feline immunodeficiency virus (FIV)

B. Parasitic causes
    1) Rickettsial disease (Rocky Mountain spotted fever, *Ehrlichia canis* and *E. platys*)
    2) Toxoplasmosis
    3) Dirofilariasis
    4) Larval migration
    5) Leishmaniasis

C. Immune-mediated causes
    1) Hepatitis vaccine reaction (blue eye) occurs 7 to 10 days following the first vaccination using an adenovirus type 1 product.
    2) Leakage of lens protein
        a) Rapidly maturing cataract
        b) Traumatic rupture of the anterior lens capsule
        c) Sequela of cataract surgery
    3) Uveodermatological syndrome Vogt-Koyanagi-Harada syndrome (VKH) (akitas, Samoyeds, Siberian huskies)
    4) Uveal effusion syndrome
    5) Uveal changes (inciting antigen unknown)
    6) Canine infectious hepatitis producing clinical or subclinical disease

D. Trauma

E. Ulcerative keratitis and reflex oculomotor nerve irritation

F. Neoplasia

G. Prototardcosis

G. Prototardhecosis

G. Prototardhecosis

H. Ethylene glycol toxicity

I. Idiopathic

4. Diagnostic approach

A. Fever, weight loss, cough, enlarged lymph nodes, petechiae, lameness, draining skin lesions, and depigmented mucous membranes may be indicative of systemic disorders.

B. The laboratory work-up is based on the particular physical findings. Tests are selected from the following list.
    1) CBC, serum chemistry profile, urinalysis (UA)
    2) Serologic studies are available for FeLV, FIP, FIV, toxoplasmosis, rickettsial species (Rocky Mountain spotted fever, *Ehrlichia canis* and *E. platys*), systemic mycoses, brucellosis, and dirofilariasis.
    3) Ocular FIP is usually the dry form, and body cavity effusions are not available for analysis. Antemortem diagnosis is often presumptive, based on laboratory findings and

the exclusion of other diseases. A typical presentation is a young cat with bilateral anterior uveitis that is persistently febrile, FeLV-negative, and poorly responsive to uveitis therapy. There may or may not be concurrent weight loss, anemia, hyperproteinemia, and retinal vasculitis.

    4) Lymph node aspirate if nodes are enlarged.

    5) Thoracic radiographs are indicated in animals with suspected systemic mycoses or neoplasia.

    6) Aqueous centesis has limited diagnostic value except in cases of lymphosarcoma, other neoplasms, toxoplasmosis, lipid flare, and sepsis.

    7) Vitreous centesis for cytologic study and culture is recommended if there is exudate in the posterior segment.

    8) A skin biopsy for VKH is warranted if mucocutaneous depigmentation is present.

  5. Treatment

    A. Topical steroids (Cornea must be fluorescein-negative): 1% prednisolone acetate, 0.1% dexamethasone, or the equivalent. Topical hydrocortisone is usually not adequate.

    B. Subconjunctival steroids are reserved for animals that are nonresponsive to topical steroids.

    C. Systemic steroids are used only in the absence of infectious diseases. Use these agents if the response to topical and/or subconjunctival steroids is inadequate. Systemic steroids are indicated for concurrent posterior segment involvement except in cases of infectious diseases.

    D. Topical atropine is used to effect for mydriasis and cycloplegia.

    E. Topical phenylephrine can be combined with atropine for mydriasis.

    F. Systemic antiprostaglandins (not used in cats)—flunixin meglumine, 0.5 to 1 mg/kg intravenously (IV), or aspirin, 10 to 20 mg/kg b.i.d.

    G. Azathioprine can be used for animals with immune-mediated uveitis that is refractory to systemic steroids. The initial dose is 2 mg/kg b.i.d. for one week, and the maintenance dose is 1 mg/kg every other day for two weeks.

Glaucoma

  1. Glaucoma is an increase in IOP beyond that compatible with normal optic nerve function and vision.

  2. Clinical findings

    A. By definition, the IOP is elevated. Normal IOP in dogs and cats should fall within a range of 15 to 30 mmHg.

    B. The progression of glaucoma may be either insidious or acute, and the clinical signs are dictated by the course of the disease.

    C. The animal presents with a red, painful eye and reduced or absent vision.

    D. The corneal appearance varies from mild haziness to profound edema.

    E. There is episcleral congestion.

    F. The pupil is midrange to maximally dilated, and nonresponsive to light.

    G. The eye may or may not be enlarged (buphthalmic).

    H. Individual clinical signs (dilated pupil, corneal edema) are not pathognomonic for glaucoma without a concurrent increase in IOP.

    I. Consider glaucoma as the cause of a persistently red eye in breeds with a familial predisposition to inherited glaucoma. (See the list of breeds in the section on type of disorders that follows.)

  3. Diagnosis

    A. Confirmation of glaucoma requires some form of tonometry.

    1) Digital

    2) Indentation (Schiotz)

    3) Applanation

    B. Digital tonometry can help differentiate an extremely firm globe from an extremely soft one. However, the long-term management of glaucoma requires quantitation of IOP.

    C. Gonioscopy is inspection of the iridocorneal angle. Although useful to a specialist, it is not essential to the diagnosis or management of glaucoma.

    D. Evaluate the opposite eye for a predisposition to glaucoma and the need for prophylactic therapy.

  4. Type of disorders

    A. Primary glaucoma represents an inherited predisposition to glaucoma with no preceding ocular disease. Common susceptible breeds include the cocker spaniel, poodle, Norwegian elkhound, beagle, basset hound, chow, and terrier breeds.

B. Primary (inherited) glaucoma is less common in cats. Therefore, look for an underlying cause (secondary glaucoma).

C. Secondary glaucoma

1) Anterior uveitis

2) Trauma

3) Intumescent lens secondary to rapid cataract formation

4) Sequela to posterior synechia

5) Lens luxation (See the section on Ocular Emergencies for breed predispositions.)

6) Intraocular neoplasia

5. Treatment

A. The three classes of drugs used for acute primary glaucoma are osmotic diuretics, carbonic anhydrase inhibitors, and topical autonomic drugs (cholinergics, adrenergic agonists, beta-adrenergic antagonists).

B. If the onset of glaucoma is acute and there is the potential for vision, proceed as follows:

1) Initial treatment consists of 20% mannitol IV, 1 to 2 gm/kg (2–5 cc/kg) administered over a period of 15 to 20 minutes; or oral glycerin, 1 to 2 gm/kg (1–2 cc/kg). For either drug to be effective, water must be withheld from the patient for one to two hours. Either drug produces a dramatic lowering of IOP within 30 to 45 minutes.

2) Administer one of the following oral carbonic anhydrase inhibitors: dichlorphenamide, 2 mg/kg b.i.d. or t.i.d.; methazolamide, 2 mg/kg b.i.d. or t.i.d.; acetazolamide, 10 mg/kg b.i.d. or t.i.d.

a) Dichlorphenamide (Daranide) or methazolamine (Neptazane) are preferred in dogs and cats because of their efficacy and lack of systemic side effects.

b) Acetazolamide (Diamox) is more readily available, but also more likely to produce systemic side effects (vomiting, diarrhea, metabolic acidosis).

c) Do not use furosemide (Lasix). It is neither an osmotic diuretic nor a carbonic anhydrase inhibitor and does not lower IOP even though it does promote diuresis.

3) Institute topical therapy—preferably, 2% pilocarpine t.i.d. and/or a beta-adrenergic antagonist.

4) Following the emergency medical therapy just outlined, cryosurgery, laser cycloablation, or a filtering procedure is necessary for long-term glaucoma control.

5) The unaffected predisposed eye is treated with a low-dose topical prophylactic agent.

6) After this therapeutic regimen is instituted, the eye is reassessed for vision. If the eye is visual, maintain topical glaucoma therapy. If the eye is blind (allow at least four to six weeks for return of vision) and if glaucoma is still present, consider one of several surgical options: cryosurgery, laser surgery, intraocular prosthesis, enucleation, or intravitreal gentocin injection.

C. If the glaucoma is chronic and the eye is irrevocably blind on initial presentation (most instances of buphthalmia, retinal atrophy, cupped optic disk), then emergency therapy is not warranted. Carbonic anhydrase inhibitors can be used until the discomfort of the glaucoma is resolved by one of the above-mentioned surgical procedures.

Ulcerative Keratitis

1. Diagnostic plan

A. Fluorescein stain—A positive green stain is diagnostic. False-positive (nonulcerative) stain retention can occur if the corneal surface is raised, roughened, dry, or vascularized. Fluorescein may pool within a corneal depression formed by epithelialization of an earlier ulcer without full replacement of the corneal stroma. These resolved ulcers can be distinguished from active ulcers by their smooth and rounded margins. Copious irrigation may help to differentiate false from true fluorescein retention. In the case of deep ulcers that do not stain, be aware that Descemet's membrane does not retain fluorescein.

B. Eyelid examination—Examine the upper, lower, and third eyelids for sources of mechanical irritation.

C. Schirmer test—In normal animals, the result is 15 mm or greater.

D. Palpebral reflex—Breed conformation

(relative lagophthalmos) or facial nerve paralysis can predispose an animal to ulceration.

E. FA for feline herpes on conjunctival scraping

F. Bacterial or fungal culture in severe or nonresponsive cases

G. Cytologic examination—if keratomalacia is present

H. Examine the cornea for the presence of nonadherent epithelium indicative of an indolent ulcer.

1) Visualization

2) Fluorescein dye beneath redundant lip

3) Peel the edge of the ulcer with a dry Q-tip after instillation of topical anesthetic.

I. Examine the cornea for the presence of edema. Corneal epithelial loss will produce focal edema. Diffuse edema may suggest underlying endothelial disease or intraocular disease.

J. Examine the anterior chamber—Severe ulcers can cause hypopyon, miosis, or hyphema.

2. Treatment

A. Routine ulcers can be treated with a combination of neomycin, polymyxin, and bacitracin or chloramphenicol.

B. Gentamycin and tobramycin are useful for Pseudomonas infections or for other organisms that are specifically sensitive to these antibiotics. Pseudomonas should be suspected if there is marked keratomalacia.

C. Viral (feline herpes) ulcers are treated with a topical antiviral drug. The choices are trifluridine (Viroptic), idoxuridine (Stoxil), or adenine arabinoside (Vira-A).

D. Topical 7% iodine (Lugol's solution), applied by direct swab, is viricidal, bactericidal, and fungicidal. It also provides chemical debridement for indolent ulcers.

E. Administration of 10% acetylcysteine (Mucomyst) or autogenous serum is indicated for keratomalacia ("melting" ulcers).

F. Topical atropine is used to effect for mydriasis to prevent posterior synechia and to provide cycloplegia for pain. Not all superficial ulcers warrant atropine, but when in doubt, use it.

G. Systemic antiprostaglandins (flunixin meglumine, 0.5 to 1 mg/kg IV) or aspirin (10 to 20 mg/kg b.i.d.) are effective for pain.

H. Topical steroids are contraindicated in corneal ulcers.

I. Topical cyclosporine can be used except in cases of feline herpes.

J. Indolent ulcers require mechanical or surgical debridement.

K. Third eyelid flaps or conjunctival flaps are indicated for deep ulcers when perforation is imminent.

Keratoconjunctivitis Sicca

1. KCS is the lack of normal tear production or a dry eye. The name refers to the involvement of both the cornea and the conjunctiva. Thus, this disease can present with multiple manifestations, such as ulceration, redness, thick ocular discharge, ipsilateral dry nostril pain, or vision loss.

2. Disorders

A. Loss of lacrimal tissue

1) Congenital absence

2) Immune-mediated destruction of lacrimal gland

3) Senile atrophy

4) Iatrogenic (removal of gland of third eyelid)

B. Secondary to chronic conjunctivitis

C. Secondary to systemic disease (the most common of which are canine distemper and feline herpes)

D. Secondary to drug therapy

1) Atropine or similar derivatives administered topically or systemically

2) Sulfa drugs—sulfasalazine (Azulfidine), sulfadiazine (Tribrissen, Ditrim), phenazopyridine, sulfisoxazole

E. Loss of neurological innervation

1) Trauma

2) Surgery of the head

3) Secondary to otitis

4) Stroke

5) Idiopathic

F. Transient, following general anesthesia

G. Secondary to radiation therapy

3. Diagnostic plan

A. Schirmer tear test—Do not use topical anesthetic or any eye drops prior to this test. Normal values are greater than 15 mm in one minute.

B. Fluorescein stain—Dry eyes are prone to corneal ulceration. Do not confuse dye retention on a roughened surface with true ulceration.

C. Cytologic findings on conjunctival scraping—Routinely expect a purulent exudate. Bacteria (large and small cocci) are commonly present.

D. Culture is rarely indicated.

E. Palpebral reflex—Evaluate the animal for a facial nerve deficit or breed conformation indicating a predisposition to exophthalmos/lagophthalmos.

F. FA for distemper in puppies with severe KCS or in atypical breeds with acute KCS

G. FA for herpes in cats

H. Breeds known to be predisposed to KCS—cocker spaniel, English bulldog, West Highland white terrier, brachycephalic breeds

 4. Treatment

A. Topical 2% cyclosporine s.i.d. or b.i.d.

B. Artificial tears or lubricants

C. Oral pilocarpine as a lacrimomimetic

D. Topical mucolytics (Mucomyst)

E. Topical antibiotic/steroid preparations (unless corneal ulceration is present)

F. Parotid duct transposition in refractory cases

Retrobulbar Disease/Acute Exophthalmos

 1. Clinical findings

A. Exophthalmos is an abnormal protrusion of the globe.

B. The eye may appear red because of protrusion of the third eyelid or because of the conjunctivitis and keratitis that accompanies this condition.

C. The globe does not retropulse into the orbit.

 2. Associated disorders

A. Orbital abscess or cellulitis

B. Extension of tooth root abscess

C. Inflammation, infection, cyst, or neoplasia of the zygomatic or lacrimal glands

D. Extension of infection, neoplasia, inflammation, cyst from nasal sinuses

E. Metastatic orbital neoplasia

F. Traumatic proptosis

G. Myositis of extraocular or temporal muscles

 3. Diagnostic approach

A. History—As a generalization, retrobulbar abscesses tend to be acute and painful, whereas retrobulbar tumors are more chronic in nature and less painful.

B. Retrobulbar abscesses may cause fever and a left shift.

C. Skull radiographs are useful in determining bone lysis and evaluating tooth roots.

D. Oral examination may require sedation or anesthesia if the lesion is painful. Look for a mass or swelling behind the last molar.

E. Aspirate the mass for cytologic examination and culture.

1) General anesthesia is required.

2) In the mouth, aspirate from behind the last molar.

3) Obtain an aspirate from the orbit for cytologic examination and culture. Place the needle into the orbit on the opposite side from which the eye is deviated. Avoid perforation of the globe or optic nerve. Do not hesitate to aspirate from more than one area of the orbit.

F. Traumatic proptosis can be diagnosed on the basis of the animal's history and appearance.

G. If bilateral exophthalmos occurs in a clear, visual eye that retropulses into the orbit, consider myositis of the extraocular muscle. This can be confirmed by biopsy.

 4. Treatment

A. Drain the abscess from the mouth or orbit. Most abscesses that drain through the mouth are accompanied by swelling behind the last molar.

B. Systemic antibiotics

C. Systemic antiprostaglandins

D. Lubricants to protect the cornea

E. Orbital exenteration for retrobulbar neoplasia

F. Orbital exploratory surgery to remove a retrobulbar neoplasm, leaving the globe intact, is attempted only in select cases.

G. Systemic steroids for exophthalmos

secondary to myositis of the extraocular muscles

H. Temporary tarsorrhaphy for proptosis (See the section on ocular emergencies.)

Subconjunctival Hemorrhage

1. Clinical findings

A. Subconjunctival patterns may be petechial, ecchymotic, or diffuse.

B. In systemic disorders, hemorrhages may be found on other mucous membranes.

2. Etiology

A. Trauma

B. Disorders of hemostasis (see Chapter 4)

C. Rickettsial diseases

D. Excessive restraint around the head

E. Septicemia

3. Diagnostic approach

A. History

   1) Recent grooming, jugular venipuncture, excessive leash restraint, particularly in breeds with exophthalmic conformation

   2) Trauma

   3) Potential for exposure to rat poisons or ticks (vectors for rickettsia)

   4) Breeds associated with inherited bleeding disorders

B. CBC

C. Platelet count and estimation from blood smear

D. Rickettsial serologic tests

E. Coagulation profile

4. Treatment

A. Subconjunctival hemorrhage does not require treatment. Uncomplicated cases resolve within 10 to 14 days.

B. If the cause of the subconjunctival hemorrhage is associated with inflammation, administer topical steroids in the absence of corneal ulceration.

C. Treat any underlying systemic disorder.

Hyphema

1. Clinical findings

A. Hyphema is blood in the anterior chamber.

B. The source of the blood is the iris, ciliary body, choroid, or retinal vessels if detachment occurs.

2. Disorders

A. Trauma

   1) Proptosis

   2) Blunt trauma without rupture of the globe

   3) Penetrating ocular injury

B. Bleeding disorders

C. Anterior uveitis

D. Rickettsial diseases

E. FeLV

F. FIP

G. Retinal detachment

   1) Inherited retinopathies

   2) Secondary to buphthalmos

H. Intraocular neoplasia

I. Hypertension secondary to chronic renal disease, hyperthyroidism in cats, cardiomyopathy

J. FIV

3. Diagnostic approach

A. CBC, serum chemistry profile, and thyroxine (T_4) levels in cats

B. Coagulation profile (see Chapter 4)

C. Platelet count and estimation from smear

D. Examine mucous membranes for other signs of bleeding.

E. Serologic testing for rickettsial diseases

F. See the previous section on Anterior Uveitis (under Red Eyes) for an explanation of the appropriate systemic work-up.

G. Know the breeds that are predisposed to inherited retinopathies that can lead to detachment and hemorrhage. Because inherited retinopathies are bilateral and the fundus may not be visible in the eye with hyphema, examine the opposite (nonhemorrhagic) eye for fundic changes that are consistent with inherited retinopathies.

H. Physical examination for other abnormalities—fever, lymph node enlargement

I. Blood pressure measurement

J. Aqueous centesis is rarely beneficial.

K. Ultrasonography of the globe to detect detachments or intraocular masses

L. Examine the unaffected eye by penlight and ophthalmoscopy to detect any further evidence of systemic disease.

4. Treatment

   A. Treat specific systemic disorders.

   B. If hyphema is associated with trauma or uveitis, administer topical steroids and topical atropine, as for anterior uveitis.

   C. Limiting the animal's activity is helpful in preventing rebleeding, but is often impractical.

   D. Enucleation is necessary if an intraocular tumor is suspected.

Painful Eyes

1. Clinical signs of pain include epiphora, blepharospasm, redness, enophthalmos, and prolapse of the third eyelid.

2. Etiology

   A. Superficial corneal irritation (trigeminal nerve)

      1) Superficial corneal ulceration—It should be noted that, as a class of superficial ulcers, indolent ulcers are not always painful.

      2) KCS—Acute, severe KCS (Schirmer test values of less than 5 mm) is far more painful than chronic KCS.

      3) Entropion

      4) Trichiasis

      5) Distichiasis

      6) Ectopic cilia

      7) Nonpenetrating corneal foreign body

      8) Lid tumors or swelling

   B. Anterior uveitis

   C. Acute glaucoma

   D. Anterior lens luxation

   E. Acute exophthalmos

      1) Abscess or cellulitis

      2) Proptosis

   F. Acute conjunctivitis

   G. Iris prolapse

   H. Acute inflammatory eyelid conditions

      1) Blepharitis

      2) Hordeolum

      3) Blepharedema

3. Diagnostic plan

   A. Schirmer tear test (Do not use a topical anesthetic.)

      1) Normal values are greater than 15 mm in one minute.

      2) Omit this test if there is obvious epiphora.

      3) KCS is represented by values of less than 10 to 15 mm in one minute.

   B. Application of topical anesthetic

      1) Apply anesthetic following Schirmer tear test to facilitate the examination.

      2) If the ocular pain is diminished or alleviated by application of a topical anesthetic, this indicates trigeminal nerve irritation as the source of the pain. Look for causes of superficial corneal irritation.

      3) Topical anesthetics do not relieve the pain associated with intraocular or retrobulbar diseases.

      4) Never use topical anesthetics for treatment, even though they may provide transient alleviation of the pain.

   C. Fluorescein stain

      1) Superficial ulcers or abrasions are more painful than deep ulcers because the trigeminal nerve endings lie within the epithelial and anterior stromal layers.

      2) If an ulcer is present, examine the upper, lower, and third eyelids to determine if there is any source of mechanical irritation present (e.g., entropion, ectopic cilia, distichiasis, foreign body). Note that many breeds (of which the cocker spaniel is a classic example) routinely have distichiasis that causes no clinical problems. Do not attribute pain to distichiasis unless all other differential diagnoses have been ruled out.

   D. Tonometry

      1) Normal IOP is 15 to 30 mmHg.

      2) An increase in intraocular pressure is indicative of glaucoma.

      3) A decrease in intraocular pressure is seen with anterior uveitis or corneal perforation.

   E. Examine the pupil and its response to light.

      1) A miotic pupil is seen with anterior uveitis or severe ulcerative keratitis.

      2) A midrange to dilated pupil is seen with glaucoma or retrobulbar disease.

   F. Examine the anterior chamber. Cloudiness implies either severe external or intraocular disease.

   G. Localize any redness (see the previous section on Red Eyes). This may help to determine if the pain is attributable to intraocular disease (anterior uveitis, glaucoma) or extraocular disease (corneal ulcer, KCS).

H. Examine the relationship of the globe to the orbit.

1) Exophthalmos (See the section on exophthalmos under Red Eyes.)

a) Differentiate exophthalmos from buphthalmos. An exophthalmic globe (other than that related to breed conformation) resists retropulsion into the orbit. A buphthalmic globe can be pushed back into the orbit.

b) Acute exophthalmos (abscess, cellulitis, proptosis) is far more painful than chronic exophthalmos.

2) Enophthalmos—a clinical sign of pain. The third eyelid is often prominent. In the absence of pain, a prominent third eyelid evokes a different list of differential diagnoses. (See the section on Red Eyes [prominent third eyelid].)

4. Treatment—See specific disease entities.

Ocular Discharge

1. Serous ocular discharge may result from increased tear production (which implies pain or active inflammation) or normal tear production with an obstruction of the nasolacrimal system.

A. Diagnostic plan

1) If the eye is red and painful, refer to the previous section on Painful Eyes.

2) If the cornea and anterior chamber are clear, examine the eye for the presence of conjunctivitis. (If it is present, refer to the section on conjunctivitis under Red Eyes.)

3) If the eye is not inflamed, look for causes associated with abnormalities of the nasolacrimal drainage system.

a) Evaluate the patency of the nasolacrimal puncta. Irrigate the puncta with a nasolacrimal cannula. Flush through the upper punctum, and observe the flow from the lower punctum. Occlude the lower punctum; fluid will drain from the nose or the animal will swallow. This can easily be performed using topical anesthesia in tractable dogs and some cats. Sedation may be necessary for cats and excitable dogs.

b) Fluorescein dye test—Patency of the puncta is demonstrated if the dye is present at the nostril or in the mouth. A negative dye test does not confirm that the puncta are obstructed. This must be confirmed by failure to cannulate or irrigate each punctum.

B. Etiology

1) Imperforate (lower) puncta—This condition is relatively common. Because it is congenital, affected animals are presented at an early age. There is a breed predisposition in the cocker spaniel.

2) Stenosis

a) Congenital

b) Acquired—upper respiratory infection in cats, dacryocystitis, surgical trauma, foreign body, neoplasia

3) Patent but malpositioned or nonfunctional puncta—seen in breeds with facial conformation predisposed to medial entropion, exophthalmos, caruncular hair wicking, or idiopathic epiphora (seen in the poodle and Maltese)

4) Atresia of nasolacrimal drainage—uncommon

C. Treatment

1) Imperforate punctum—Using a 22- to 25-gauge nasolacrimal cannula, irrigate through the existing upper punctum. Watch for a bleb over the imperforate punctum. Incise the membrane with a No. 11 blade.

2) Stenosis—Some puncta closed by adhesions can be reopened surgically.

3) Tetracycline, 5 to 10 mg/kg/d for two weeks will decrease the staining of the hair. The staining usually returns if the tetracycline is discontinued. This therapy is used on an intermittent basis when there is excessive odor or moist dermatitis.

4) Never excise the gland of the third eyelid as a treatment for epiphora. This gland contributes significantly to the tear film; excision may cause a secondary dry eye.

5) Epiphora secondary to intraocular pain or extraocular irritation should be treated by removing the primary cause.

2. Thick ocular discharge

A. Characteristics

1) A purulent discharge which, on gross examination, appears yellow or green and is composed predominantly of polymor-phonuclear neutrophil leukocytes (PMNs)

2) The mucoid exudate is moist, greyish white, and found predominantly in the lower cul-de-sac or around the lids.

B. Disorders

1) Secondary to diseases of the eye-lids, cornea, conjunctiva, orbit, sinuses, or nasolacrimal system

2) Systemic infectious disease (e.g., canine distemper)

3) Concurrent dermatologic disease

4) Allergic disease

5) Enophthalmic breed conformation (Dobermans, setters, collies, weimaraners)

6) Ophthalmia neonatorum

a) Kittens two to six weeks of age (herpes, chlamydia)

b) Puppies 7 to 10 days of age, with eyelids still closed (Staphylococcus)

7) Microphthalmos

8) Phthisis

C. Diagnostic plan

1) Examine the animal for fever, na-sal discharge, respiratory involvement, otitis externa; check the vaccination history for distemper and upper respiratory infection (URI) in cats.

2) Schirmer tear test

a) Perform this test prior to instil-lation of topical anesthetic.

b) If the test value is less than 15 mm, refer to the section on KCS under Red Eyes.

3) Fluorescein stain

4) Conjunctival cytologic examina-tion—See the section on conjunctivitis under Red Eyes.

5) Conjunctival FA for feline herpes or canine distemper

6) Obtain a culture (prior to instilla-tion of topical anesthetic) if the discharge is nonresponsive to broad-spectrum antibiotics. A culture is not necessary if the diagnosis is KCS.

7) Irrigate the nasolacrimal system—Purulent exudate from the nasolacrimal sys-tem indicates dacryocystitis. Recurring ,dacry-ocystitis may indicate a foreign body or tumor within the nasolacriminal system.

a) Culture

b) Survey and contrast radio-graphs of the nasolacrimal system

c) Flushing of the nasolacrimal system with a viscous material (e.g., mineral oil) to dislodge foreign material followed by betadine flush

8) Eye position with respect to the orbit

a) Enophthalmos—If the eye is red, rule out causes of ocular pain (see the previous section on Painful Eyes). If the eye is uninflamed, consider passive accumulation of exudate secondary to breed conformation (deep-set eyes), microphthalmia, or phthisical eye.

b) Exophthalmos—Perform an evaluation for retrobulbar disease (see the previous section on Red Eyes).

9) Adnexal examination for signs of mechanical irritation—Examine both surfaces of upper, lower, and third eyelids for mechan-ical irritation.

D. Treatment—See specific disorders for treatment (e.g., KCS, bacterial conjunctivitis, ophthalmia neonatorum).

Acute Blindness

Acute blindness may occur with or without other systemic signs of illness. Certain types of acute blindness are reversible if treated promptly. The emphasis in this section is on diseases of the posterior segment (vitreous, choroid, retina, optic nerve).

1. Ocular penlight examination

A. Cloudy anterior segment (cornea, aqueous, iris, lens)

1) Bilateral anterior uveitis, glaucoma, and cataracts may cause acute blindness. Refer to the appropriate sections of this chap-ter for information on these diseases (sec-tions in Red Eyes and Gradual Vision Loss).

2) A complete listing of disorders that cause a cloudy anterior segment is provided in the section on Gradual Vision Loss.

3) Owners may interpret vision loss as acute when adapted animals are placed in unfamiliar surroundings.

B. Clear anterior segment—Refer to the following section on pupillary light reflexes.

2. Pupillary light reflexes (PLRs)

A. To draw meaningful conclusions from PLRs, the direct and consensual responses must be evaluated in each eye, and each eye must be assessed for vision.

B. Always use a bright light source to avoid erroneous conclusions at the outset of the examination.

C. The PLR distinguishes peripheral lesions (e.g., those involving the retina or optic nerve) from CNS lesions (e.g., those involving the optic tracts or visual cortex).

D. Blind animals with abnormal PLRs (dilated and poorly responsive to nonresponsive) have an interruption in the pathways for PLRs and vision. This implies a lesion cranial to the optic chiasm involving either both optic nerves or both retinas.

E. Blind animals with normal PLRs have a lesion caudal to the areas in the brain stem where pathways for PLRs diverge from those for vision. This implies a lesion in the visual cortex and is called cortical blindness. Refer to Chapter 17 for a discussion of diseases in this category.

F. Exceptions to the above generalizations may occur when retinal lesions cause blindness and yet the PLRs persist (e.g., disinsertion retinal detachments), or in early cases of sudden acquired retinal degeneration (SARD). A fundus examination and/or electroretinogram (ERG) maybe of value in these cases.

3. Ophthalmoscopic examination—dilated pupils

A. Normal fundus (no visible lesion)

  1) Sudden acquired retinal degeneration (SARD)

   a) In dogs, SARD accounts for the majority of cases of acute blindness with clear eyes.

    i. Affects middle-aged to older dogs

    ii. Frequently accompanied or preceded by a transient period of polyphagia, polyuria, and polydipsia

    iii. The cause is unknown.

    iv. Diagnostic approach

      A. CBC, serum chemistry profile, UA

      B. Evaluate for Cushing's disease.

      C. The laboratory work-up is usually normal.

      D. The ERG is absent. This confirms the diagnosis.

    v. Treatment

      A. None—The blindness is permanent.

      B. The signs of polyphagia and polydipsia eventually moderate. These animals do not progress to any other systemic disorder.

  2) Optic neuritis (retrobulbar)

   a) Optic neuritis refers to inflammation of the optic nerve. The fundus examination is normal when the visible portion of the optic nerve (optic disc/papilla) is not affected, and there is no concurrent chorioretinitis.

   b) Retrobulbar optic neuritis is differentiated from SARD by the ERG, which is normal in optic neuritis.

   c) Animals with optic neuritis respond to systemic steroids in some instances.

   d) For differential diagnosis, diagnostic plan, and treatment, refer to the section that follows on optic neuritis under Abnormal Fundus Examination.

B. Abnormal fundus

  1) Optic neuritis

   a) The optic disc is swollen with indistinct margins (papillitis). Hemorrhage on or around the disc may be evident. There may be accompanying chorioretinitis.

   b) Disorders—canine distemper, granulomatous meningoencephalomyelitis, reticulosis, systemic mycoses, FIP, FeLV, rickettsial diseases, toxoplasmosis, protothecosis, proptosis, blunt trauma, retrobulbar (orbital) mass (abscess, cellulitis, hematoma, cyst, neoplasia), lymphosarcoma or other neoplasms, lead poisoning, concurrent chorioretinitis and all its causes, and idiopathic optic neuritis

   c) Diagnostic approach

    i. CBC, serum chemistry profile, UA

    ii. Serologic examinations are

available for FIP, FeLV, Rocky Mountain spotted fever, *Ehrlichia canis* and *E. platys,* toxoplasmosis, and systemic mycoses. Note that ocular FIP is usually the dry form, and body cavity effusions are not present for analysis. Antemortem diagnosis is often presumptive, based on laboratory findings and exclusion of other diseases.

iii. FA for distemper on conjunctival scraping

iv. CSF analysis for neoplastic, inflammatory, infectious, and parasitic diseases if the blindness occurs with other neurological signs (seizures, ataxia, head tilt, neck pain)

v. Vitreous body centesis for cytologic examination and culture if there is exudate in the posterior segment

vi. The ERG is normal in diseases that cause optic neuritis.

d) Treatment

i. In the absence of active infection, treat optic neuritis with oral prednisolone, 1 mg/kg b.i.d. for 14 days, to prevent demyelination of the optic nerves. If there is a favorable response after one week (as evidenced by some restoration of vision and return of PLRs), then gradually taper the systemic steroids over a period of two to three weeks until an alternate-day maintenance regimen is achieved. If there is no response to systemic steroids at a dosage of 1 mg/kg b.i.d. after two weeks, then further steroid therapy is probably of no value for return of vision. (Refer to Chapter 17 for other neurological manifestations.)

ii. Avoid the use of systemic steroids in animals with systemic mycoses and protothecosis.

iii. Toxoplasmosis may be treated with clindamycin, 25–50 mg/kg divided BID–TID. Short term concurrent systemic steroid therapy may be used when blindness is present.

iv. Rickettsial diseases are treated with oral tetracycline, 20 mg/kg t.i.d.

v. Untreated optic neuritis leads to irreversible optic nerve atrophy.

vi. Some causes of optic neuritis tend to be progressive even in the face of steroid treatment. Inform the owner that there may be relapses of blindness as well as the onset of other neurological symptoms.

2) Retinitis or chorioretinitis

a) On fundus examination, dull, raised foci with indistinct margins, appearing grey in the tapetum and white or grey in the nontapetum, indicate active inflammation of the retina or choroid. Inactive areas tend to be flat, darkly pigmented, or hyperreflective and more sharply delineated. The causes overlap with those listed in the sections on optic neuritis, retinal detachment, and retinal hemorrhage.

b) Disorders—systemic mycoses, FeLV, FIP, toxoplasmosis, rickettsial diseases, canine distemper, protothecosis, lymphosarcoma, septicemia, and neoplasm

c) Diagnostic approach

i. The approach is the same as that used for optic neuritis with an abnormal fundic examination.

ii. Vitreous body centesis for cytologic examination and culture is particularly helpful for blastomycosis, bacterial infections, lymphosarcoma, and other neoplasms.

d) Treatment

  i. Treat the specific, underlying, systemic disease.

  ii. Avoid the use of systemic steroids in animals with infectious diseases.

3) Retinal detachment

a) Grey, elevated areas detected on fundic examination indicate retinal detachment. More extensive detachments can better be observed by penlight examination. The detached retina and its blood vessels are seen to be billowing directly behind the lens. Disinsertion (total) retinal detachment consists of the entire retina hanging ventrally and attached only around the optic disk.

  b) Etiology

   i. See the etiology section listed in the earlier discussion of retinitis or chorioretinitis.

   ii. Hypertension—renal failure, hyperthyroidism, cardiomyopathy

   iii. Any cause of hypoalbuminemia that can predispose an animal to serous effusion

   iv. Uveal effusion syndrome (immune-mediated)

   v. Chronic or severe anterior uveitis (particularly, lens-induced anterior uveitis)

   vi. Trauma

   vii. Intraocular surgery

   viii. Inherited retinopathies

   ix. Hyperviscosity syndromes

   x. Neoplasia

   xi. VKH

   xii. Ethylene glycol toxicity

  c) Diagnostic approach

   i. The approach is similar to that described earlier for optic neuritis and for retinitis or chorioretinitis.

   ii. Test for thyroid function in cats.

   iii. Measure blood pressure.

   iv. Consider the known breed predispositions for inherited retinopathies—springer spaniel, Labrador retriever, Sealyham terrier (retinal dysplasia), collie (collie eye anomaly), poodle, Lhasa apso, Shih Tzu (disinsertion [total] retinal detachment), and rottweiler (retinal detachment).

   v. In uveal effusion syndrome, the fluid beneath the retina is clear, signs of systemic disease are absent, and concurrent anterior uveitis may be present.

  d) Treatment

   i. For detachments associated with infectious diseases, treat the systemic disease. There is no specific treatment for the detachment, and the prognosis for vision is poor.

   ii. For detachments associated with hypertension, treat with propranolol or captopril and a spironolactone/thiazide diuretic. The prognosis for vision is guarded.

   iii. For uveal effusion syndrome, administer 1.1 mg/kg of prednisolone b.i.d. for 14 days; taper the dose over a period of weeks. The prognosis for vision is good if the condition is treated promptly.

   iv. Procedures for surgical reattachment are under investigation.

4) Retinal hemorrhage—Round, linear, globular, and keel-shaped areas of hemorrhage on fundic examination represent hemorrhage within and in front of the retina. Note that straight, parallel, regular red lines in the tapetum or nontapetum are normal choroidal blood vessels and do not represent hemorrhage. They are visualized because of the absence of tapetum or retinal pigment and should be expected in animals with lightly pigmented irises.

    a) Etiology
        i. See the etiology section under optic neuritis and retinitis or chorioretinitis listed earlier.
        ii. Rickettsial diseases
        iii. Disorders of hemostasis
        iv. Hypertension
        v. Anemia
        vi. Trauma
        vii. Thiamine deficiency
        viii. Hyperviscosity syndromes
        ix. Neoplasia
        x. Congenital vascular anomalies (tetralogy of Fallot)
    b) Diagnostic approach
        i. CBC, serum chemistry profile, UA
        ii. Platelet estimate on blood smear and platelet count
        iii. Serologic examination for rickettsia (Rocky Mountain spotted fever, *Ehrlichia canis* and *E. platys*), FeLV, FIP, toxoplasmosis
        iv. Blood pressure measurement
        v. Coagulation profile
    c) Treatment—Correct the underlying systemic disorder.

Gradual Vision Loss

Differentiate gradual from acute vision loss by the animal's history. (Acute blindness has already been addressed.) Gradual vision loss may seem acute to an owner if the animal decompensates when placed in an unfamiliar environment. Evaluate vision by menace response, by the animal's ability to negotiate an obstacle course or follow dropped cotton balls, or by an owner's interpretation of performance.

  1. Penlight examination
    A. Cloudy anterior segment (cornea, aqueous, lens)

    1) Corneal opacities
      a) Pigmentary keratitis
        i. Schirmer tear test to rule out KCS
        ii. Breed conformation for exophthalmos/lagophthalmos
        iii. Adnexal irritation—lower lid entropion, medial entropion, trichiasis, ectropion, distichiasis, ectopic cilia, prominent nasal folds
        iv. Degenerative pannus—Breed predisposition—German shepherd, dachshund, greyhound, Siberian husky
      b) Lipid keratopathy
        i. Diet
        ii. Hypothyroidism
        iii. Inherited dystrophy—Siberian husky, Airedale, Samoyed, beagle, sheltie, Afghan, collie, golden retriever
        iv. Sequela to corneal inflammation and neovascularization
        v. Fatty-base haircoat supplements
      c) Corneal edema
        i. Glaucoma (Perform tonometry to document.)
        ii. Anterior lens luxation
        iii. Endothelial dystrophy—inherited in Boston terrier, basset hound, Chihuahua
        iv. Anterior uveitis
        v. Interstitial keratitis—hepatitis vaccine reaction, infectious canine hepatitis, inflammatory
        vi. Ulcerative keratitis (positive fluorescein stain)
        vii. Persistent pupillary membranes
        viii. Healed ulcers
      d) Vascularized cornea
        i. KCS
        ii. Adnexal irritation

iii. Ulcerative and interstitial keratitis

iv. Blood stain secondary to hyphema

v. Eosinophilic keratitis

vi. Degenerative pannus

e) Mineral (calcium) keratopathy secondary to:

i. Ulcerative keratitis

ii. Uremia

iii. Lipid keratopathy

iv. Cushing's disease

2) Aqueous opacities

a) Flare—See the section on anterior uveitis under Red Eyes.

b) Keratic precipitates—See the section on anterior uveitis under Red Eyes.

c) Hyphema—See the section on hyphema under Red Eyes.

d) Hypopyon—See the section on ulcerative keratitis and anterior uveitis under Red Eyes.

e) Lipid flare

i. Diet

ii. Diabetes

iii. Pancreatitis

iv. Primary hyperlipemia syndrome of schnauzers

v. Cushing's disease

3) Lens opacities

a) Cataract

i. Inherited in toy, miniature, and standard poodles; cocker spaniels; miniature schnauzers; Boston terriers; Old English sheepdogs; golden and Labrador retrievers; Afghans; Irish setters; beagles; springer spaniels; Siberian huskies; Chesapeake Bay retrievers; Australian shepherds; pointers; German shepherds; Bedlington terriers; collies; bichon frises; cavalier King Charles spaniels; Himalayan cats

ii. Diabetes mellitus

iii. Traumatic rupture of lens capsule

iv. Esbilac feeding of puppies

v. Sequela to anterior uveitis

vi. Chédiak-Higashi syndrome in cats

vii. Dimethylsulfoxide (DMSO)

viii. Irradiation of the head

ix. Sequela to electrical shock

b) Nuclear sclerosis

i. Predictable benign cloudiness in animals older than six years of age

ii. Does not cause vision loss

B. Clear anterior segment

1) Test the animal for PLRs.

a) Normal PLRs

i. Cortical blindness—See Chapter 17.

ii. Early retinal disease—Confirm by ophthalmoscopic examination or ERG (see the discussion that follows).

iii. Metabolic disease—See Chapter 17.

b) Abnormal PLRs (both pupils dilated and poorly responsive)

i. Glaucoma

A. Tonometry—intraocular pressure greater than 30 mmHg

B. Breed predisposition—cocker spaniel, poodle, Norwegian elkhound, beagle, basset hound, Jack Russell terrier, wirehaired terrier, Manchester terrier, chow

ii. Retinal atrophy or degeneration (See the discussion that follows.)

iii. Optic nerve atrophy (See the discussion that follows.)

iv. Optic nerve hypoplasia (See the discussion that follows.)

c) Abnormal PLRs (anisocoria—See the separate section on anisocoria.)

2) Evaluate the posterior segment by ophthalmoscopic examination and ERG.

2. Ophthalmoscopic examination

A. Normal

1) SARD (See the earlier section on acute blindness.)

2) Early inherited retinal degeneration

B. Abnormal fundus

1) Retinal abnormalities

a) Focal to diffuse tapetal hyperreflectivity, generalized vascular attenuation, and optic disc pallor represent retinal atrophy.

i. Inherited progressive retinal atrophy (PRA)—poodle, cocker spaniel, Irish setter, collie, miniature schnauzer, Tibetan terrier, Norwegian elkhound, Gordon setter, Samoyed, Labrador retriever, springer spaniel, Abyssinian cats, Australian shepherd

ii. End-stage central progressive retinal atrophy (CPRA)—Labrador retriever, golden retriever, border collie, Shetland sheepdog (The abnormal fundus also has multiple pigment clumps in the tapetum.)

iii. Generalized retinal atrophy
A. Taurine deficiency
B. Idiopathic

iv. Sequela to chorioretinitis

v. Sequela to glaucoma (with concurrent optic nerve atrophy)

b) Linear or branching retinal folds with focal areas of tapetal hyperreflectivity represent retinal dysplasia.

i. Inherited in springer spaniels, Labrador retrievers, cocker spaniels, Sealyham terriers, Bedlington terriers, beagles, and Australian shepherds

ii. Canine herpesvirus

iii. Canine adenovirus

iv. Feline panleukopenia

2) Optic nerve abnormalities

a) A dull white or grey, circular or depressed optic disc with vessel attenuation characterizes optic nerve atrophy. There may or may not be concurrent retinal atrophy.

i. Optic neuritis

ii. Trauma

iii. Retinal degeneration

iv. Glaucoma

b) A small optic disc with normal retinal vessels characterizes optic nerve hypoplasia.

i. Inherited (poodles)

ii. Concurrent with microphthalmos and multiple ocular defects

c) A pit or focal depression in the optic disc represents an optic disc coloboma.

i. Inherited in collie eye anomaly

ii. Does not usually cause vision loss

3) Abnormal vitreous body

a) Most abnormalities are closely tied to retinal changes. See the section on abnormal retina under Acute Blindness.

b) Persistent hyperplastic primary vitreous (PHPV)

i. Congenital

ii. Focal to extensive retroleutal membrane

iii. Inherited in Dobermans

c) Inherited vitreoretinal dysplasia

d) In dogs, multiple small white opacities represent asteroid hyalosis. These deposits are benign and do not cause vision deficits.

3. ERG—The ERG measures the function of the photoreceptors.

A. Abnormal ERG (diminished to extinguished response)

1) SARD

2) Retinal degeneration—PRA, CPRA

3) Generalized retinal atrophy

4) Late glaucoma with concurrent retinal atrophy

B. Normal ERG

1) Focal retinal degeneration

2) Focal inherited retinopathy

3) Optic nerve hypoplasia

4) Optic nerve atrophy (unless there is concurrent retinal atrophy)

5) Cortical blindness

Anisocoria

Anisocoria is an asymmetry in the size of the pupils while they are under equal illumination. The afferent (sensory) arm of the PLR extends from the retina to the optic nerve to the brain stem. The efferent (motor) pathway extends from the parasympathetic nucleus of the third cranial nerve (midbrain) to the ciliary ganglion (within the orbit) to the iris sphincter. Because it is a brain stem reflex not involving the visual cortex, the PLR does not indicate whether an animal is visual.

Once this reflex is triggered, a freely mobile pupil is also dependent on a functional sphincter and dilator muscle within the iris, as well as intact parasympathetic and sympathetic innervation to these muscles.

1. Diagnostic approach
    A. Decide which pupil is abnormal.
    1) Assess both pupils for direct and consensual PLR.
        a) Use an adequately bright light.
        b) The temporal retina is the most sensitive area to light stimulation.
        c) If one pupil does not respond to light, the lesion is probably in the nonresponsive eye.
    2) Assess each eye for vision.
        a) Test the menace response or use a patch test to evaluate each eye.

b) Vision loss with anisocoria would localize the abnormal eye.
    B. Differentiate afferent from efferent lesions (see Table 18-1).
    1) If the lesion involves the efferent pathway, only the normal pupil will constrict, regardless of which eye is stimulated.
    2) With an afferent pupillary defect, neither pupil responds when the light is in the affected eye.
    3) Examine the pupils in dim light from a distance of three feet. The tapetal reflex will help outline their size. Both pupils should dilate equally. If the anisocoria persists, there is an efferent defect.
    4) Perform the swinging flashlight test.
        a) Direct the light into the normal eye for several seconds, and then direct it into the opposite eye. Repeat shining the light from one eye to the other several times.
        b) Each pupil is expected to be constricted in the presence or absence of the light because afferent stimulus to the iris sphincter either comes directly or consensually (decussation of optic nerve fibers at the optic chiasm).
        c) The following constitutes a positive swinging flashlight test.
            i. Both pupils constrict when the light is in the normal eye.

Table 18-1. **Differentiation between afferent and efferent lesions in a dilated pupil**

	Afferent Lesion (Retina, Optic Nerve)		Efferent Lesion (Pathways for Pupillary Constriction*)	
	Normal eye	*Affected eye*	*Normal eye*	*Affected eye*
Menace	Present	Absent	Present	Present
Pupillary light reflex				
Light in normal eye	Norma direct†	Normal consensual‡	Normal direct	No consensual
Light in abnormal eye	No consensual	No direct	Normal consensual	No direct

* For example, cranial nerve III and the iridal sphincter

† The direct pupillary light reflex is the reflex that is elicited in the eye being stimulated with the light.

‡ The consensual pupillary light reflex is the response in the eye that is not under light stimulation.

ii. On shifting the light to the affected eye, it is also constricted.

iii. With the light still shining in the affected eye, both pupils begin to dilate (because with an afferent pathway lesion the affected eye does not "see" the light).

iv. This response (a Marcus Gunn pupil) is pathognomonic for an afferent pupillary defect.

5) Assess each eye for vision.

a) Afferent lesions result in vision loss.

b) Efferent lesions do not result in vision loss unless associated with glaucoma or proptosis.

2. The abnormal pupil is dilated.

A. Etiology

1) Afferent lesions

a) Retinal atrophy

b) Retinal detachment

c) Severe chorioretinitis

d) Optic neuritis

e) Optic nerve atrophy

f) Optic nerve hypoplasia

g) Chronic gaucoma (optic nerve atrophy)

2) Efferent lesions

a) Oculomotor nerve from midbrain to orbit to iris sphincter

i. Proptosis

ii. FeLV

iii. Head trauma

iv. Key-Gaskell syndrome in cats

v. Orbital mass/Exophthalmos

vi. Idiopathic—This is not uncommon, particularly in older dogs.

b) Atrophy of the iris sphincter muscle (senile iris atrophy)

c) Topical parasympatholytic drugs

i. Atropine, tropicamide (Mydriacyl)

ii. Systemic atropine will not cause a dilated pupil (or anisocoria)

d) Posterior synechia

e) Glaucoma—hypoxia of the iris sphincter

B. Diagnostic plan

1) Question the owner about a history of previous use of eyedrops containing a mydriatic/cycloplegic.

2) Perform tonometry for glaucoma.

3) Perform focal illumination of the iris.

a) Atrophy

i. Holes or thinning of the iris stroma sufficient to prevent normal constriction

ii. Exclude all other causes before attributing anisocoria to iris atrophy.

b) Posterior synechia

4) Assess the animal's vision—Only glaucoma, proptosis, exophthalmos, or afferent pupillary lesions produce a vision deficit.

5) FeLV test

6) Key-Gaskell syndrome is an uncommon syndrome in cats accompanied by KCS, third eyelid prolapse, bradycardia, megaesophagus, constipation, and urinary incontinence.

7) Perform a fundus examination to rule out severe retinal or optic nerve disease.

8) Neurologic examination—Refer to Chapter 17 if other cranial nerve deficits or other neurologic symptoms are present.

3. The abnormal pupil is constricted.

A. Etiology

1) Anterior uveitis

2) Ulcerative keratitis may activate the oculopupillary reflex (C.N. V to C.N. III).

3) Posterior synechia

4) Horner's syndrome (loss of sympathetic innervation)

5) Increased parasympathetic input (head trauma)

6) Ophthalmic drops (miotics)

B. Diagnostic plan

1) Fluorescein stain for ulcerative keratitis

2) Penlight examination for changes in the anterior segment indicative of anterior uveitis (See the previous section on Red Eyes.)

3) Horner's syndrome

a) In addition to miosis, the other signs associated with Horner's syndrome are prolapse of the third eyelid, ptosis, and enophthalmos.

  b) Lesion of first-order neuron
   i. Hypothalamus to spinal cord at T1–T3
   ii. Additional symptoms are ataxia, paresis, seizures, and change in mentation
   iii. Trauma, neoplasia
  c) Lesion of second-order neuron
   i. Thoracic sympathetic trunk to cranial cervical ganglion located caudomedial to the tympanic bulla
   ii. May have concurrent forelimb paralysis
   iii. Brachial plexus avulsion, neoplasia, trauma, surgery
  d) Lesion of third-order neuron
   i. The third order neuron passes through the middle ear and joins a branch of the fifth cranial nerve behind the globe. The nerve terminates on the iris dilator muscle.
   ii. There may be concurrent peripheral vestibular symptoms (nystagmus).
   iii. Head or neck trauma or surgery, otitis, ear cleaning, idiopathic disorder
  e) Pharmacological testing (see Table 18-2)

   i. Horner's syndrome is often apparent on inspection.
   ii. Pharmacological testing is intended to localize the lesion. Unless the animal is systemically ill or has other neurologic deficits, it is reasonable to assume Horner's syndrome to be third order most frequently.
   iii. One drop of 10% phenylephrine is helpful in reassuring the owner that the eye itself is normal but has a loss of sympathetic tone.
  f) Thoracic and/or skull radiographs if other symptoms are present
  g) FeLV testing in cats
C. Treatment
  1) For anterior uveitis, administer topical atropine and steroids (unless contraindicated because of corneal ulceration).
  2) For severe ulcerative keratitis, treat with topical atropine and antibiotics and an anticollagenase agent (see the discussion of acetylcysteine under Descemetocele in the Ocular Emergencies section that follows).
  3) Synechiae—Topical mydriatic agents (atropine) may break down synechiae, depending on their extent and duration.
  4) In animals with Horner's syndrome, treat the underlying cause. No treatment is necessary for the miosis.
  5) Head trauma (see Chapter 17)

Table 18-2. **Pharmacologic testing for Horner's syndrome**

	Normal eye	First-order Horner's	Second-order Horner's	Third-order Horner's
First test: 1% hydroxyamphetamine hydrobromide (Paredrine)	Normal dilation	Normal dilation	Normal dilation	Incomplete or no dilation
Followed by 10% phenylephrine	Normal dilation	No dilation	No dilation	Normal dilation faster than in the unaffected eye owing to denervation hypersensitivity)

Ocular Emergencies

1. An ocular problem is considered an emergency if delayed treatment might result in blindness or if there is significant associated pain that requires attention.

2. The following are considered ocular emergencies:

    A. Proptosis

    B. Corneal laceration or perforation

    C. Ocular foreign body

    D. Anterior lens luxation

    E. Descemetocele

    F. Chemical keratitis

    G. Acute glaucoma

    H. Acute anterior uveitis

    I. Acute blindness

3. Although not emergencies, the following are also included in this section owing to their frequent association with ocular trauma:

    A. Lid lacerations

    B. Subconjunctival hemorrhage

    C. Hyphema

Proptosis

Proptosis is a protrusion of the eye from its normal position in the orbit.

Clinical Approach

1. Replace the eye as soon as possible.

2. Decide whether to replace the globe or enucleate the eye. Base the decision on the extent of muscle and optic nerve damage, not on the appearance of the eye, as most proptosed eyes look ghastly. If the globe is deviated but still well attached to the orbit, replace it. If the muscle damage is so severe that the globe hangs loosely, or if the optic nerve is obviously severed, then perform an enucleation.

3. Replacement and thorough examination require general anesthesia. Assess the animal as an anesthetic candidate if other traumatic injuries are present.

4. Prior to general anesthesia, perform a simple penlight inspection to assess the state of the pupil and the response of both pupils to light stimulation. A proptosed eye with a miotic pupil or a pupil that becomes miotic

upon replacement generally carries a better prognosis than one with a dilated pupil. Miosis is the normal response of the iridal sphincter to trauma. A dilated, nonresponsive pupil indicates severe damage to either the optic nerve, retina, or the parasympathetic innervation to the iris (ciliary ganglion). However, it is probably inadvisable to give any prognosis for vision when an animal with proptosis is initially presented. That assessment is best made after the temporary tarsorrhaphy is removed.

5. After administering general anesthesia:

    A. Stain the cornea with fluorescein.

    B. Assess the anterior chamber for the presence of hyphema to determine severity.

    C. Cleanse the cornea and adnexal area with eyewash or saline. Little to no clipping or preparation is preferred to avoid damage to an exposed globe or further trauma to already swollen and bruised tissues.

6. Globe replacement

    A. Use two strabismus hooks or sutures to pull the lids up and out as gentle pressure is applied to the globe.

    B. Perform a temporary tarsorrhaphy. Use stents to avoid excess pressure on the lids. The tarsorrhaphy prevents exposure and drying of the cornea while the retrobulbar swelling resolves (Fig. 18-1).

7. Precautions

    A. Do not administer IV mannitol. The pressure inside the eye is not elevated. In fact, it is apt to be lower than normal owing to the uveitis associated with the trauma. The protrusion of the eye is created and maintained by the constricting force of the lids.

    B. Do not perform a centesis on the eye. This can predispose the animal to intraocular bleeding and retinal detachment.

    C. Perform a lateral canthotomy only as a last resort in replacing the globe.

8. Postoperative care

    A. Topical atropine and steroid ointments for anterior uveitis associated with trauma (Use a topical antibiotic instead of a steroid if the cornea is ulcerated.)

    B. Systemic steroids—Administer oral prednisolone (1 mg/kg b.i.d.) for five days; then taper the dose over an equal number of days.

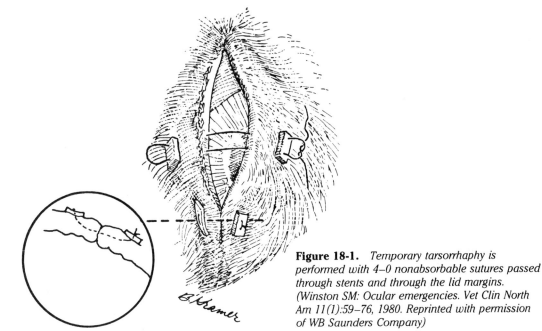

Figure 18-1. *Temporary tarsorrhaphy is performed with 4–0 nonabsorbable sutures passed through stents and through the lid margins. (Winston SM: Ocular emergencies. Vet Clin North Am 11(1):59–76, 1980. Reprinted with permission of WB Saunders Company)*

C. Systemic antiprostaglandins—Flunixin meglumine, 0.5 to 1 mg/kg IV

D. Systemic antibiotics for one week

E. Hot packs may be used for adnexal swelling.

F. Remove tarsorrhaphy in 7 to 14 days if the retrobulbar swelling appears to be resolved. If lagophthalmos (inability to close the lids) is still present, monitor the animal carefully for corneal ulceration. If the lagophthalmos persists and the corneal condition deteriorates, the tarsorrhaphy may have to be reapplied.

9. Potential unfavorable sequelae

A. Blindness

B. Frequently, an upward and lateral deviation of the globe occurs as a result of avulsion of the insertions of the medial rectus and inferior oblique muscles. The degree of deviation will lessen within six to eight weeks following the removal of the tarsorrhaphy. If the deviation causes a clinical problem, perform corrective surgery at a later date.

C. Phthisis bulbi—most common in eyes with severe hyphema

D. KCS

E. Lagophthalmos

Corneal Laceration

Clinical Approach

1. Treat a corneal laceration that is not full-thickness as you would a deep ulcer.

2. A full-thickness corneal laceration requires surgical correction.

Surgical Principles

1. Debridement, if necessary, should be undertaken judiciously.

2. Excise iridal tissue that has been prolapsed longer than two hours.

A. Because of the profound vascularity of this tissue in the animal eye, cautery* is recommended for removal of iridal tissue.

B. After cauterization, reposition the remaining viable iris within the anterior chamber.

3. Use suture material no larger than 6–0.

4. Suture through two thirds of the stroma. Sutures that penetrate the full thickness of the

---

* Accu-Temp Surgical Cautery Concept Inc, Clearwater, Florida

cornea create a nidus for the introduction of bacteria into the anterior chamber.

5. When the corneal closure is completed, if it is necessary to reform the anterior chamber, use a limbal injection of lactated Ringer's or Healon,† followed by an air bubble using a 25-gauge needle and syringe. This checks the integrity of the wound closure and prevents synechiae between the iris and the cornea.

6. Postoperative care

A. Treat the eye postoperatively with topical atropine, and topical and systemic antibiotics.

B. Administer systemic antiprostaglandins (flunixin meglumine, 0.5 to 1 mg/kg IV; or aspirin, 10 to 20 mg/kg b.i.d.).

Limbal Lacerations

1. Corneal lacerations adjacent to the limbus should be considered complicated wounds until proven otherwise. The defect may extend across the limbus and involve the sclera, even though the overlying conjunctiva is intact.

2. Incise the conjunctiva adjacent to the corneal wound so that the sclera can be visualized at the limbus. In the event of a scleral rent and uveal prolapse, reposition the uvea and suture the sclera with absorbable suture no larger than 6–0.

3. Handle the corneal section of the laceration as outlined earlier.

4. Postoperative care is the same as that for anterior uveitis, and involves administration of topical atropine, topical and systemic antibiotics, and systemic antiprostaglandins.

Ocular Foreign Bodies

1. Ocular foreign bodies may be described as nonpenetrating (cornea, conjunctiva) or penetrating.

2. The animal's pain may necessitate the administration of tranquilizers or general anesthesia for a thorough examination to be performed.

Therapeutic Approach

1. Superficial corneal or conjunctival foreign bodies

A. These can frequently be removed after administration of a tranquilizer and topical anesthestic.

B. Irrigation with eyewash may dislodge small, nonpenetrating particles.

C. Use a topical anesthetic and a 25-gauge needle to elevate any material that is superficially lodged in the cornea.

2. Penetrating foreign bodies

A. Gunshot wounds

1) The presence of corneal edema and hyphema may obscure examination of the eye, but a metallic foreign body can be confirmed by skull radiographs.

2) It is rarely feasible or beneficial to remove a gunshot pellet from within the eye or orbit.

3) The point of entry may reseal or need to be sutured.

4) Because the incidence of intraocular infection associated with gunshot injuries is low, most cases can be treated vigorously as a panuveitis using topical atropine, corticosteroids, and systemic steroids or antiprostaglandins (aspirin), and systemic antibiotics.

B. Other penetrating foreign bodies

1) The removal of an intraocular foreign body that penetrates the eye with less velocity than a gun-inflicted wound is influenced by the position and composition of the material involved.

2) A foreign body positioned within the anterior chamber may be removed through a limbal incision or at the point of entry.

3) The most irritating materials within the eye are metals that can oxidize (such as copper and iron), wood, and plant material. In addition to causing intraocular inflammation, wood and plant material may also introduce bacterial or fungal infection into the eye.

4) Precious metals, lead, glass, and rubber are chemically nonreactive, but the amount of ocular inflammation is influenced by what structures have been damaged.

† Healon is sodium hyaluronate, Pharmacia Medical Products Group, 800 Centennial Avenue, Piscataway, NJ 08855.

5) If the foreign body is a nonreactive material, if the ocular tissues penetrated are nonreactive to the insult, or if the surgical procedure would create more trauma than the foreign body itself, removal is contraindicated.

Anterior Lens Luxation

1. The lens may luxate or subluxate anteriorly or posteriorly for a variety of reasons.
   A. Breed predisposition—wirehaired, fox, Sealyham, Welsh, Manchester, Jack Russell, or Tibetan terriers; beagles; basset hounds; Brittany spaniels; Norwegian elkhounds
   B. Trauma
   C. Secondary to buphthalmos (enlarged globe caused by increased intraocular pressure)
   D. Secondary to chronic anterior uveitis (particularly in cats)
2. Anterior lens luxation
   A. An anterior lens luxation presents as a red, painful eye with variable amounts of corneal edema. With diffuse corneal edema, it may even be difficult to visualize the lens unless the anterior chamber is illuminated obliquely from the limbus.
   B. An anterior lens luxation may cause secondary glaucoma from blockage of the pupillary space or obstruction of aqueous outflow from the anterior chamber.
   C. This type of secondary glaucoma requires surgery to remove the lens.
   D. An anterior lens luxation is a more complicated surgical situation than an elective lens extraction and should be performed by a clinician who is familiar with intraocular surgical techniques.
3. Posterior lens luxation or subluxation—A posterior lens dislocation does not create the obstructive problem caused by an anterior lens luxation and is not necessarily either an emergency or a surgical problem if the IOP is not elevated.

Descemetocele

A *descemetocele* is the protrusion of Descemet's membrane through the floor of an ulcer by the pressure of the aqueous behind it. The term is also used to describe an ulcer that has extended to Descemet's membrane without the actual bulging of the membrane.

Clinical Approach

1. A descemetocele may be recognized as a clearing at the bottom of a deep ulcer. Descemet's membrane does not retain fluorescein stain, whereas any deep stromal ulcer does.
2. Medical therapy
   A. Treat a small ulcer that is down to Descemet's membrane with topical antibiotics and atropine.
   B. If the ulcer is "melting," add anticollagenase agents* (10% acetylcysteine or to, ical serum.)
   C. Topical medical adhesives
   D. Collagen lenses
   E. An animal with a descemetocele that is treated medically requires hospitalization and strict supervision, particularly in the case of brachycephalic breeds with a predisposition for axial ulcers that deepen precipitously.
3. Surgical approach
   A. Consider a conjunctival flap for large descemetoceles or for those that do not improve with medical therapy.
   B. A third eyelid flap serves more as a bandage than as a seal. Its greatest advantage is its technical simplicity.
   C. Postoperatively, treat the ulcer with an antibiotic and atropine. Anticollagenase agents are not generally necessary following surgery.

Chemical Keratitis

1. *Keratitis* is an inflammation of the cornea that may or may not be associated with concurrent corneal ulceration.
2. The inadvertent contact of soap with the cornea is a frequent cause of chemical keratitis. The soap may cause an ulcerative keratitis and anterior uveitis; this should be treated with a topical antibiotic and atropine.
3. Contact of acid or alkali with the eye is

---

* Mucomyst 20, Mead Johnson, Evansville, Indiana

the most common cause of severe chemical keratitis.

A. Alkaline agents

1) Alkaline agents are potentially far more destructive to the eye than acids.

2) Alkaline agents release hydroxyl ions into the tissue so that the initial ulceration continues to progress through the stroma.

3) In addition to the direct damage caused by contact with the alkali, the damaged corneal epithelial cells and PMNs that migrate into the area release a collagenase enzyme that itself digests the corneal stroma.

B. Acid agents

1) Acids are buffered by the ocular tissues and precipitate as they contact the corneal and conjunctival proteins.

2) Unlike alkali contact, the damage from acid contact is usually self-limiting.

Therapeutic Approach

1. If a known chemical (particularly an alkali) contacts an animal's eye, the initial treatment is immediate copious irrigation to dilute the chemical.

2. In most situations, tap water is available; this is useful for the extensive rinsing (up to 30 minutes in the case of alkali burns) that is necessary.

3. Use a topical antibiotic and atropine for the ulcerative keratitis and anterior uveitis that are associated with chemical keratitis.

4. Systemic antiprostaglandins are administered for pain.

5. Administer topical anticollagenase agents (acetylcysteine or serum) if keratomalacia ("melting") is present.

6. Corticosteroids are contraindicated until the ulcer epithelializes because they dramatically augment the potential of collagenase enzymes.

Prognosis

The prognosis for most soap burns is excellent. However, the prognosis for extensive alkali burns is guarded.

Acute Glaucoma

The reader should refer to the discussion of acute glaucoma presented in the previous section entitled Red Eyes (under Routine Ocular Complaints).

Acute Anterior Uveitis

Acute anterior uveitis is discussed in the earlier section on Red Eyes.

Acute Blindness

Refer to the section on Acute Blindness (under Routine Ocular Complaints) for a discussion of this entity.

Lid Lacerations

1. Suture a lid laceration as soon as possible for the best possible healing. This type of ocular injury does not carry the same degree of urgency as the previously discussed categories.

2. The vascular supply of the lids is so remarkable that a cosmetic primary repair can be achieved even several days after the injury.

Surgical Principles

1. As with all lid surgery, clipping and preparation should be done as carefully as possible to avoid subsequent lid swelling.

2. Irrigate contaminated lid lacerations with eyewash or saline.

3. If the laceration is not fresh, perform only minimal debridement of the edges.

4. Close lid lacerations in two layers.

5. Close the conjunctival layer using an absorbable suture no larger than 6–0.

6. A continuous mattress suture pattern is used, beginning at the apex of the laceration and working toward the free lid margin, with the suture in the fibroelastic layer of the conjunctiva.

7. Do not penetrate the palpebral side of the conjunctiva with the conjunctival sutures because this can create a nidus for corneal ulceration.

8. Close the skin with a nonabsorbable suture no larger than 4–0.

9. Carefully reappose the free lid margin and tarsal plate with a mattress suture.

10. Close the remainder of the skin with a simple interrupted suture pattern.

11. Postoperatively, treat the animal with systemic antibiotics and optional hot packs.

Subconjunctival Hemorrhage

The reader is referred to the discussion of subconjunctival hemorrhage that appears in the section on Red Eyes (under Routine Ocular Complaints).

Hyphema

Consult the section on Red Eyes (under Routine Ocular Complaints) for a discussion of hyphema.

Suggested Readings

Blogg RJ: The Eye in Veterinary Practice. North Melbourne, V. S. Supplies Limited, 1975.

Gelatt KN (ed): Textbook of Veterinary Ophthalmology. Philadelphia, Lea & Febiger, 1981.

Helper LC: Magrane's Canine Ophthalmology. 4th ed. Philadelphia, Lea & Febiger, 1989.

Ketring KL: In Seminars in Veterinary Medicine and Surgery. Arnoczky SP (ed). Vol. III. Philadelphia, Harcourt Brace Jovanovich, 1988.

Peiffer R: Small Animal Ophthalmology: A Problem-Oriented Approach. Philadelphia, W. B. Saunders, 1989.

Rubin L: Inherited Eye Diseases in Purebred Dogs. Philadelphia, Williams & Wilkins, 1989.

Rubin LF: Atlas of Veterinary Ophthalmoscopy. Philadelphia, Lea & Febiger, 1974.

Slatter DH: Fundamentals of Veterinary Ophthalmology. Philadelphia, W. B. Saunders, 1981.

Szymanski C: The Eye. In Holzworth J (ed): Diseases of the Cat Vol. 1. Philadelphia, W. B. Saunders, 1987.

Wyman M: Manual of Small Animal Ophthalmology. New York, Churchill Livingstone, 1986.

PART THREE

LABORATORY ABNORMALITIES AND PRINCIPLES OF FLUID MANAGEMENT

CHAPTER NINETEEN

Anemia

Justin H. Straus

•••••••••••••••••••••••

Basic Principles

1. Anemia results from RBC loss, excessive RBC destruction, or depressed RBC production.

2. Anemia is a manifestation of an underlying disease process.

 A. Anemia must be treated immediately when severe.

 B. The response to treatment is transient unless the cause is eliminated.

3. Classification

 A. Regenerative anemia (reticulocytosis, polychromasia)—RBC loss, excessive RBC destruction

 B. Nonregenerative anemia (lack of reticulocytosis)—depressed RBC production

 C. Acute versus chronic

 D. Microcytic versus normocytic versus macrocytic forms

 E. Hypochromic versus normochromic

4. RBC survival time

 A. Dog: 100–120 days

 B. Cat: 66–78 days

5. Neutrophil survival time: eight hours

6. Platelet survival time: eight days

7. Regenerative anemia

 A. RBC loss or excessive RBC destruction results in a regenerative anemia characterized by a reticulocytosis and increased polychromasia and anisocytosis.

 B. An increase in the number of reticulocytes is not seen until 72 hours after the onset of anemia, and it takes five to seven days

before peak reticulocytosis occurs. This may be longer in animals with multiple diseases.

 C. Hemolysis usually results in a greater degree of reticulocytosis than does hemorrhage, because the bone marrow has ready availability to iron derived from RBC destruction.

 D. Nucleated red blood cells (NRBC) in the absence of reticulocytosis are not an indication of regeneration.

Etiology

Nonregenerative Anemia

1. Nutritional disorders—iron deficiency, vitamin B_{12} deficiency, folic acid deficiency

2. Hypoplastic anemia, selective depression of erythrogenesis

 A. Chronic renal disease

 B. Chronic Addison's disease

 C. Hypothyroidism

 D. Chronic liver disease

 E. Chronic infection (bacterial, mycotic, viral)

3. Aplastic anemia (thrombocytopenia, granulocytopenia, anemia)

 A. Chemical agents (benzene derivatives, cyclic hydrocarbons, antimetabolites, alkylating agents, estrogens, chloramphenicol, phenylbutazone, trimethoprim-sulfa agents plus fenbendazole)

 B. Ionizing irradiation

C. Neoplasia
D. Ehrlichiosis
E. Myelophthisis (leukemia, leukemic lymphoma, multiple myeloma)
F. Idiopathic disease
G. Feline myeloproliferative disease
H. Parvovirus
I. Myelofibrosis
J. Myelodysplasia
4. Pure red cell aplasia
A. Feline leukemia virus (FeLV)
B. Immune mechanisms
C. Idiopathic disease
D. Drug-induced disorder (i.e., as a result of caparsolate use)
5. Congenital macrocytosis in the poodle

Regenerative Anemia

Secondary to Blood Loss

1. Trauma
A. Internal—contusion, fracture
B. External—laceration
2. Gastrointestinal parasites
3. Neoplasms bleeding into body cavities or externally (e.g., hemangiosarcoma)
4. Coagulation disorders (disseminated intravascular coagulation [DIC], factor deficiencies, vitamin K antagonists, thrombocytopenia)
5. Ruptured hematocysts
6. Gastrointestinal (GI) lesions (e.g., ulcerated neoplasms)
7. Urinary tract lesions (e.g., severe hemorrhagic cystitis, neoplasia)

Secondary to Hemolysis

1. Hemolytic anemia resulting from an intracorpuscular abnormality
A. Pyruvate kinase deficiency of the basenji and beagle
B. Lead poisoning (usually producing mild anemia)
2. Isoimmune hemolytic disease of the neonate
3. Hemolysis secondary to blood parasites
A. *Hemobartonella felis*
B. *Hemobartonella canis*
C. Babesiosis

4. Immune-mediated hemolytic anemia
A. Primary (idiopathic)—no other associated disease
B. Secondary—associated with another disease process (systemic lupus erythematosis [SLE], lymphosarcoma [LSA], lymphocytic leukemia, bacterial infections, granulomatous disease, viral disease, immune-mediated thrombocytopenia)
C. Secondary to drug administration (reported in humans following administration of cephalothin, penicillin, diphenylhydantoin, chlorpromazine, phenylbutazone, sulfonamide, and dipyrone; propylthiouracil administration in the cat)
5. Heinz-body anemias
A. Acetaminophen administration (feline)
B. Urinary antiseptics containing new methylene blue
C. Phenazopyridine administration (a urinary antiseptic)
D. Topical benzocaine
E. Onion intoxication
F. Unknown
6. Transfusion reactions

History

1. A thorough history is extremely important in the diagnosis of anemia because the primary problem must be determined.
2. The duration of signs may indicate whether the condition is acute or chronic.
3. The owner may note sudden weakness, acute collapse, tachypnea, dyspnea, or pallor of the mucous membranes in acute anemias. Usually in these cases, blood loss or accelerated RBC destruction is the cause.
4. Signs of chronicity are often vague (lethargy, depression, anorexia), but pale mucous membranes, weakness, and dyspnea may be noted. These signs may appear to be of sudden onset to the owner, however. Chronic anemias, characterized by a slower onset of signs are usually nonregenerative and attributable to decreased RBC production. Patients may be severely anemic but alert and ambulatory.
5. Rule out a traumatic cause in all cases.

6. Questions concerning drug administration (previous antibiotics) or toxin exposure (e.g., warfarin) are essential.

7. Signs referable to a specific body system may localize the primary problem to this area.

Physical Examination

1. The physical examination findings often are determined by the duration of illness, the severity of blood loss, and the underlying disease process.

A. Severe pallor in a relatively strong animal indicates a slowly progressive anemia and is almost always nonregenerative.

2. Physical examination may reveal:

A. Pale mucous membranes

B. Increased cardiac and respiratory rates

C. Heart murmur (secondary to decreased blood viscosity and increased turbulence; usually systolic in nature; I/VI to III/VI in intensity). In animals without valvular disease, the murmur is usually ejection in character (aortic/pulmonic); however, in the presence of mitral valvular disease, accentuation of the preexisting murmur may occur.

D. Weakness

E. Shock with acute hemorrhage

F. Petechial or ecchymotic hemorrhages of the oral mucous membranes, penis, vulva, or skin, suggesting thrombocytopenia

G. Icterus and pale mucous membranes suggesting a hemolytic process

H. Dark, tarry stool indicating significant intestinal blood loss

I. Retinal hemorrhages may be found on fundic examination in any anemic patient; they are not diagnostic of any specific disease process.

J. Splenomegaly may be found in immune-mediated hemolytic anemias or hypersplenism.

Diagnostic Approach

1. A CBC is indicated in every anemic patient.

A. A decrease in the packed cell volume (PCV) and total protein and the presence of reticulocytes suggest external blood loss.

B. The mean corpuscular volume (MCV) is an indication of overall RBC size.

1) The MCV is increased in regenerative anemias.

2) The MCV may be decreased in states of iron deficiency.

C. The mean corpuscular hemoglobin concentration (MCHC) indicates the concentration of hemoglobin per unit volume of RBCs.

1) A reduced MCHC accompanying microcytosis indicates iron deficiency.

2) A reduced MCHC accompanying macrocytosis and signs of regeneration is compatible with a regenerative anemia.

3) An elevated MCHC indicates hemolysis or laboratory error.

D. The reticulocyte count is an indication of the degree of regeneration present and must be interpreted in light of the PCV for a given patient. Polychromatic cells seen on peripheral blood smears are reticulocytes if the vital stain new methylene blue is used. Nonregenerative anemias lack significant reticulocytosis.

1) Reticulocytosis is first seen 72 hours after the onset of significant blood loss or hemolysis.

2) Peak reticulocytosis occurs within five to seven days.

3) Reticulocyte responses in dogs and cats are outlined in Table 19-1.

4) Cats produce aggregate and punctate reticulocytes. The aggregate type are seen to be polychromatic cells when stained with

*Table 19-1. **Reticulocyte responses in dogs and cats (%)***

	Dog	Cat
Normal	1.0	0–0.4
Slight	1–4	0–5.2
Moderate	5–20	3–4
Marked	21–50	5.0

Wright's stain; only these are counted when determining the reticulocyte count.

  5) The reticulocyte index is a crude determination of whether the reticulocyte response is appropriate for the degree of anemia.

$$\frac{\text{(patient's PCV)}}{\text{(normal PCV)}} \times \%\ \text{reticulocytes}$$

$$= \text{reticulocyte index}$$

A value greater than one indicates an appropriate response.

  E. Examination of the peripheral blood smear for RBC morphologic characteristics is essential for gaining information concerning regeneration and etiology.

  1) Basophilic stippling and nucleated RBCs—lead poisoning

  2) Spherocytes—immune-mediated hemolytic anemia

  3) Heinz bodies—Heinz-body anemia (Up to 10% of the RBCs in cats may normally contain Heinz bodies.)

  4) Schistocytes—DIC and other states of microangiopathic hemolytic anemia

  5) RBC agglutination—immune-mediated hemolytic anemia

  6) Nucleated RBCs with signs of regeneration indicate a regenerative anemia.

  7) Nucleated RBCs in the absence of reticulocytosis often indicate a bone marrow or splenic abnormality.

  8) Polychromatic cells are reticulocytes, and are seen in regenerative states.

  9) Blood parasites may be observed.

  10) In the cat, basophilic stippling is often associated with regeneration.

  F. Neutrophilia and thrombocytosis often are seen with regenerative anemias. These changes are believed to be the result of simultaneous stimulation of all the cell precursors in the bone marrow.

  2. The history, physical examination, CBC and reticulocyte count should enable the clinician to decide if the anemia is attributable to blood loss (regenerative anemia), increased RBC destruction (regenerative anemia), or decreased RBC production (nonregenerative anemia).

Diagnostic Tests for Blood Loss

  1. Fecal examination
  2. Urinalysis (UA)
  3. Chest roentgenography
  4. Abdominal roentgenography
  5. Blood chemistry profile
  6. Platelet count
  7. Clotting tests
  8. GI series
  9. Intravenous (IV) pyelography
  10. Cystography
  11. Ultrasonography

Diagnostic Tests for Increased RBC Destruction

  1. Blood smear examination for RBC defects and parasites
  2. UA
  3. Blood chemistry profile; direct and indirect bilirubin determination
  4. Coomb's test
  5. Chest roentgenography
  6. Abdominal roentgenography
  7. FeLV test
  8. ANA test and lupus erythematosus (LE) preparation
  9. Bone marrow biopsy
  10. Histoplasmosis or blastomycosis titers
  11. Blood culture
  12. Specific organ investigation
  13. Ultrasonography

Diagnostic Tests for Decreased RBC Production

  1. Blood chemistry profile
  2. Fecal examination
  3. UA
  4. Bone marrow biopsy
  5. Chest roentgenography
  6. Abdominal roentgenography
  7. Ultrasonography
  8. FeLV test, feline immunodeficiency virus (FIV) test
  9. Coombs' test, ANA, LE preparation
  10. Histoplasmosis or blastomycosis titer
  11. Blood culture

12. Specific organ investigation

   A. Triiodothyronine and thyroxine (T_3, T_4) determinations

   B. Adrenocorticotropic hormone (ACTH) stimulation test

   C. Bromsulphalein determination (BSP dye test), bile acid stimulation test

   D. Liver biopsy

   E. IV pyelography

Bone Marrow Biopsy

1. A bone marrow biopsy is indicated when more than one cell line is abnormal, when a selective red cell depression is present and extramarrow causes have been eliminated, and when no signs of regeneration are present.

2. A nonregenerative anemia usually reveals decreased erythroid precursors; rarely, normal bone marrow cellularity may be found.

3. A regenerative anemia discloses increased numbers of erythroid precursors.

4. Bone marrow infiltration by neoplastic cells (LSA, multiple myeloma) may occur.

5. Phagocytosis of RBC precursors may indicate an immune disorder directed at the RBC precursors.

6. Increased numbers of plasma cells may be seen in ehrlichiosis.

Selected Nonregenerative Anemias

Nutritional Anemias

1. Nutritional anemias are rare except for iron deficiency, which is the result of chronic blood loss.

2. Iron deficiency

   A. Seen most commonly in young animals whose iron stores are poor, in association with hookworm infestation or, sometimes, coccidiosis

   B. Neoplasia involving the intestines and resulting in ulceration and chronic blood loss may result in iron deficiency in older animals.

   C. A microcytic hypochromic anemia is

seen late in the disease state, but a regenerative response may be observed early because iron stores are not depleted and a response to the blood loss is initiated.

   D. Treatment of iron deficiency consists of transfusions, if necessary; treatment of hookworms in the young; adequate diet; and iron replacement therapy.

   E. Animals with intestinal neoplasia require supportive care and elimination of the tumor.

Bone Marrow Failure

1. Aplastic anemia is characterized by thrombocytopenia, granulocytopenia, and anemia, which indicate generalized bone marrow suppression.

2. Because of the much longer half-life of the RBC, an animal with acute aplastic anemia presents with signs referable to thrombocytopenia (blood loss) or leukopenia (infection). An animal with a more chronic disease process exhibits signs characteristic of anemia.

3. The numerous possible causes of this type of anemia are listed at the beginning of this chapter.

4. Pure red cell aplasia is the term used to describe those cases in which only the RBCs and their precursors are affected. The anemia is almost always severe (a PCV of 5 to 17), and the serum iron concentration is normal or elevated (150 to 400 μg/mL).

5. Pure red cell aplasia is usually idiopathic, but may be seen with FeLV. There are indications that immune disorders against the RBC precursor may lead to this condition in the dog and the cat.

6. In myelodysplastic syndromes, peripheral blood cytopenias are present, along with morphologically abnormal cells.

   A. Bone marrow biopsy usually discloses hyperplasia with an overabundance of immature blood precursors; however, normal numbers of cells may be found.

   B. This syndrome has been associated with FeLV infection in cats. In the dog, its cause is unknown.

   C. The need for transfusions is usually

dependent upon the rapidity of onset of the anemia, the actual PCV, and the etiology.

7. Treatment for aplastic anemia and pure red cell aplasia is supportive in nature, in the hope that remission may occur.

A. Recognition and removal of the cause may lead to remission. Obtain a thorough history of possible drug or toxin exposure and mismating injections.

B. When a specific etiology is found (e.g., Sertoli cell tumor or leukemic lymphoma), institute appropriate therapy.

C. Transfusions usually are not required until the PCV falls below 12% to 15% in the dog and 9% to 12% in the cat. Animals, especially cats, tolerate chronic anemias well. Use type A-negative (DEA 1.1, DEA 1.2) blood for dogs, if possible. Crossmatching after the first transfusion is highly recommended for both dogs and cats. To replace platelets, use fresh blood obtained in a plastic container; collection in glass bottles results in thrombocyte activation. Administer whole blood, 10 to 20 mL/kg of body weight, at a rate usually less than 10 mL/kg/h. Diarrhea or vomiting may occur if the blood is given too rapidly. If urticaria develops, discontinue administration. Transfused RBCs survive for approximately three weeks under ideal conditions.

D. Corticosteroids do not commonly induce remission in aplastic anemia in humans. However, if no etiology can be established, administer prednisolone in divided doses 1 mg/lb twice a day, for three to four weeks. Corticosteroids may help decrease bleeding when thrombocytopenia is present, and they may prolong survival of transfused RBCs.

E. Androgenic anabolic steroids (Anadrol-50, Winstrol V, Deca-Durabolin) are nonspecific stimulants of erythropoiesis. Thirty days are usually required before any improvement in RBC numbers is seen. Deca-Durabolin is currently believed to be the most effective of these agents. The dosage is 1 to 5 mg/kg, administered intramuscularly (IM) once weekly (not to exceed 200 mg).

F. Combined administration of corticosteroids and anabolic steroids may improve blood element production when each separately has failed.

G. Treat infection with appropriate bactericidal antibiotics. Administer prophylactic antibiotics to patients with neutrophil counts of less than 1000/mm³.

H. Hemorrhage, usually secondary to thrombocytopenia, may be a problem. Low-dose corticosteroids (e.g., prednisone, 0.25 mg/lb per day) often help prevent capillary bleeding. Platelet-rich plasma or fresh whole blood may be needed in cases of serious bleeding.

I. Immunosuppressive drugs may induce a remission in selected cases of pure red cell aplasia. Try oral cyclophosphamide (50 mg/m² for 4 days, then discontinue for 3 days) or oral azathioprine (2.0 mg/kg daily).

8. There have been reports of chloramphenicol causing a reversible nonregenerative anemia when administered to cats at therapeutic dosages. This is an uncommon condition that improves when drug administration is discontinued.

9. Estrogen-induced aplastic anemia of dogs may result from excessive exogenous estrogen administration (e.g., diethylstilbestrol [DES], estradiol) or from excessive endogenous production (e.g., Sertoli cell tumor, granulosa cell tumor). Reactions to exogenous estrogen administration may be idiosyncratic. The prognosis in all cases is extremely guarded.

A. Leukocytosis is seen one to two weeks after estrogen administration, followed abruptly by leukopenia or a normal WBC count at 20 to 25 days.

B. Thrombocytopenia also develops at this time; anemia appears later owing to the longer RBC life span.

C. If sublethal doses of estrogen are administered, the bone marrow may return to normal.

D. Treatment consists of platelet and RBC replacement therapy and antibiotics when leukopenia is severe. Oral lithium (25 mg/kg b.i.d.) was shown to be effective in one dog with estrogen toxicity.

E. This type of anemia can usually be avoided by administering DES at a dose of 1 mg/lb, not to exceed 20 mg per dog. Do not repeat doses as high as this for at least two months.

F. Estradiol is a much more potent estrogen; administer it at 1/10 the dose of DES. Complications with estradiol seem to exceed those with DES.

10. Ehrlichiosis is caused by infection with the rickettsial agent *Ehrlichia canis*.

A. Most affected animals experience only an acute phase of the disease characterized by pyrexia, lethargy, anorexia, and transient pancytopenia of two to four weeks' duration.

B. Some dogs, especially German shepherds, begin a chronic phase two to four months later. A severe pancytopenia is present and often results in either terminal hemorrhage or infection.

C. Diagnosis is made either by finding the characteristic intracytoplasmic morulae in mononuclear cells (which may be difficult in the chronic phase of the disease), or by determining the presence of antibody to *E. canis* with an indirect fluorescent antibody test.

D. Treatment consists of tetracycline, 22 mg/kg t.i.d. for 14 days. In severe chronic cases, supportive therapy, including transfusions and appropriate antibiotics, may be needed.

E. The prognosis is extremely guarded in severe chronic cases.

F. *E. equi* has been found to cause anemia and thrombocytopenia.

11. Infection with FeLV may result in a normocytic, normochromic, nonregenerative anemia, a panleukopenia-like syndrome, or a megaloblastic nonregenerative anemia.

A. The panleukopenia-like syndrome may occur during the viremic stage, and resembles closely true feline panleukopenia in which the neutropenia is very severe, thrombocytopenia is rarely found, and the anemia is mild. A percentage of these FeLV-positive cats rid themselves of the infection, become FeLV-negative, develop a normal blood picture, and show clinical improvement.

B. The panleukopenia-like syndrome that is seen with chronic FeLV infection is characterized by neutropenia, thrombocytopenia, and moderate to severe anemia.

C. In nonregenerative anemia only, bone marrow biopsy reveals an increased myeloid-to-erythroid ratio; in the panleukopenia-like

syndrome, all blood element precursors are reduced.

D. In the megaloblastic anemia the PCV is greater than expected for the degree of actual RBC counted. This is due to the larger size of the RBC. The MCV is increased in these cases.

E. Treatment, when deemed necessary, consists mainly of transfusions. Anabolic steroids may help in some cases.

F. It is believed by some that immune mechanisms are the cause of the nonregenerative anemia. These people advocate immunosuppressive dosages of prednisolone (0.5 mg/lb b.i.d.) or cyclophosphamide (500 mg/m^2 IV once every two weeks).

G. Administer antibiotics when neutropenia is severe.

12. The anemia of chronic disease (i.e., that associated with renal and hepatic disease, hypothyroidism, Addison's disease, chronic infection/inflammation, or neoplasia) is normocytic, normochromic, and nonregenerative. It can develop as early as two weeks after the onset of disease.

A. Serum iron concentration is reduced (30 to 80 μg/mL) and a mild to moderate degree of anemia is found (PCV of 18 to 35).

B. The anemia is probably attributable to the combination of:

1) Sequestration of iron in the reticuloendothelial macrophage system, resulting in a decreased iron supply delivered to the bone marrow

2) A decrease in erythropoietin production

3) A shortened RBC life span

C. Treatment is directed at the underlying disease condition.

1) Hypothyroidism and chronic Addison's disease—thyroid and glucocorticoid replacement, respectively

2) Chronic renal disease—anabolic steroid administration and blood transfusions, from which short-term benefits are derived

3) Recently human recombinant erythropoietin (r-HUEPO) has been used in cases of renal failure in dogs and cats and has effectively and safely corrected the anemia, though potential does exist for reactions to carrier proteins. In man it has also been shown to be effective in certain neoplastic conditions.

Regenerative Anemias

Blood Loss

1. Blood loss may be peracute, acute, or chronic, and the signs associated with the disease process depend on the rapidity of blood volume depletion.

2. Parasites, such as hookworms, coccidia, and fleas, are especially important in puppies and kittens as a possible cause of anemia and death.

A. Direct treatment is aimed at eliminating the parasites and restoring RBC mass.

B. Administer transfusions through the greater trochanter if a peripheral vein cannot be catheterized.

C. Intraperitoneal transfusions may destroy significant numbers of RBCs and result in a less rapid increase in the PCV.

D. Concomitant hypoglycemia is found frequently and must be treated.

E. Administer iron dextran, 10 mg/kg IM once, followed by ferrous sulfate, 100 to 300 mg orally per day for one to two months. Some clinicians prefer daily injectable iron, the dose of which should not exceed 25 mg in small dogs and 50 mg in large breeds.

F. Provide essential supportive care, including use of heating pads, adequate caloric intake, and fluid replacement.

3. Gastric or intestinal mucosal ulceration may initially result in a regenerative anemia, although late in the disease process, a nonregenerative anemia may be seen.

A. Tumor invasion and ulceration, peptic ulceration associated with liver disease, mast cell tumors, and idiopathic causes may result in significant blood loss.

B. Treatment is directed at eliminating the underlying disease process.

4. Neoplasms with bleeding into body cavities or external bleeding may cause a blood loss anemia that is often peracute in nature.

A. Vascular neoplasms, especially hemangiosarcoma, are prone to producing hemorrhage.

B. Typically, a middle-aged or older German shepherd presents with a peracute onset of weakness, anemia, and a fluid-filled abdomen. Surgical intervention reveals a ruptured splenic or hepatic hemangiosarcoma.

C. Periodic episodes of anemia may result from rupturing tumors and the resultant small amount of blood loss. In these cases, a reticulocytosis is present because adequate time for regeneration has elapsed.

D. It is very common to see nucleated RBCs with splenic hemangiosarcomas. This may be the result of a reduction in the "pitting" function of the spleen.

E. In peracute cases of bleeding, treatment consists of RBC and volume replacement, followed by surgical intervention to remove the bleeding tumor.

F. Always obtain chest roentgenograms in cases of abdominal bleeding to check for the presence of metastases.

5. An animal with a ruptured hematocyst may present exactly like one with a ruptured neoplasm. Diagnose and treat such animals by performing exploratory laparotomy, resection, and histopathologic examination.

6. Trauma may result in external or internal blood loss.

A. In the case of significant peracute blood loss, PCV and total protein values initially are normal. Body fluids redistribute within four to six hours; at that time, a decrease in these parameters occurs.

B. Hemorrhage into the abdomen or chest eventually is autotransfused by the body. Excessive bleeding into the pleural space, however, may compromise respiration, and the blood may need to be removed.

C. Tissue trauma with extravasation of blood and hemorrhage secondary to fractures may be substantial; little blood will be reabsorbed by the body.

D. Treatment depends on the extent and site of hemorrhage. Initially, obtain a PCV and total protein determination and begin volume replacement therapy with isotonic fluids. Whole blood transfusions may be needed. In specific cases, you may need to explore the chest, abdomen, or a fracture.

7. Bleeding disorders may result in peracute, acute, or chronic blood loss. They are discussed in Chapter 4.

8. In cases of severe hemorrhage into body cavities, the blood may be collected and autotransfused. Complications, such as hemolysis, microembolization, sepsis, tumor metastasis, and bleeding disorders, may occur.

Excessive RBC Destruction

1. Hemolytic anemias may be extravascular (RBC phagocytosis by the reticuloendothelial system, hyperbilirubinemia, bilirubinuria) or intravascular (hemoglobinemia, possible hemoglobinuria, and icterus).

2. Direct and indirect bilirubin determinations are not extremely useful in hemolytic disease.

A. Early in hemolytic disease, a greater percentage of indirect bilirubin will be detected.

B. A high direct bilirubin level in the presence of hemolytic disease and anemia points to either severe hemolysis or liver malfunction; this is because the liver normally can conjugate and excrete large amounts of bilirubin.

3. Hemolytic anemia may be seen in association with other disease processes (thrombocytopenia, glomerulonephritis); in these cases, it may be due to immune-mediated disorders.

Intracorpuscular Abnormalities

1. Pyruvate kinase deficiency of the basenji and beagle results in a chronic hemolytic anemia.

A. Pyruvate kinase is an essential enzyme in the Embden-Meyerhof glycolytic pathway, which supplies energy for RBC metabolism.

B. Membrane changes occur as a result of decreased cell energy, and the RBCs are prematurely removed by the spleen.

C. The disease is transmitted as an autosomal recessive trait. Documentation of the disorder is accomplished by assaying for pyruvate kinase activity. Carrier animals may be detected by assaying for the enzyme activity.

D. Reticulocytosis is marked, spherocytes are absent, and the anemia is macrocytic-hypochromic.

E. Late in the disease, bone marrow biopsy reveals myelofibrosis and osteosclerosis, which lead to decreased erythropoiesis, nonregenerative anemia, and death.

F. The average survival time is two to three years.

G. No definitive treatment is available. Splenectomy of affected children has resulted in some benefit, and may be of help in dogs if performed early. Late in the disease, the spleen may become a significant source of erythropoiesis.

2. Chronic lead poisoning may cause a mild to moderate, hypochromic, regenerative anemia.

A. Lead inhibits erythropoiesis by suppressing heme synthesis; it also leads to a decreased RBC half-life.

B. Increased numbers of nucleated RBCs, basophilic stippling, and polychromasia are present.

C. A history of GI and CNS signs, along with the laboratory findings just mentioned, is very suggestive of lead poisoning.

D. Definitive diagnosis is established by determination of blood lead levels.

E. Treatment consists of elimination of lead from the GI tract, corticosteroids for brain edema if seizures are excessive, and calcium EDTA to bind the blood lead and allow elimination by the kidneys.

F. Calcium EDTA, at a dose of 50 mg/lb/d diluted to 10 mg/mL in 5% dextrose, is administered subcutaneously (SQ) in divided doses q.i.d. for five days.

G. Signs may worsen initially after treatment is begun because more lead is entering the bloodstream from bones.

Extracorpuscular Abnormalities

1. Immune-mediated hemolytic anemia (IHA) occurs in both dogs and cats and is characterized by a regenerative anemia, spherocytosis (dog) and often the presence of autoantibodies against RBCs (positive direct Coombs' test).

A. Primary (idiopathic) IHA involves

only the RBCs themselves and accounts for 60% to 70% of the cases that occur in dogs. High concentrations of serum antibody to viral antigens in dogs with primary IHA suggest that idiopathic disease may follow viral infections.

B. Secondary IHA is associated with a wide variety of underlying conditions, including LSA; lymphocytic leukemia; reticulum cell sarcoma; SLE; immune-mediated thrombocytopenia; severe bacterial infections, such as subacute bacterial endocarditis; granulomatous disease, such as histoplasmosis; viral diseases; and drug administration. (Cephalothin, penicillin, phenytoin, chlorpromazine, phenylbutazone, sulfonamide, and dipyrone administration have been incriminated in humans.)

C. Two theories are currently accepted as to the cause of IHA:

1) A pathogenic change occurs in the RBC membrane and results in the formation of a new antigen and a subsequent immune response.

2) The immune system is unable to recognize "self" and, therefore, produces autoantibody.

D. The antibodies involved in canine IHA are immunoglobulin G (IgG) and IgM.

E. IgM and some subclasses of IgG can activate complement.

F. Attachment of antibody to the RBC membrane may result in phagocytic fragmentation of the membrane, leading to spherocyte formation. These cells have impaired deformability and are more susceptible to detention and accelerated destruction within the reticuloendothelial macrophage system.

G. Extravascular hemolysis occurs, with increased formation of unconjugated bilirubin. This compound is then transported to the liver where, in the absence of concurrent liver disease or severe hemolysis, it is conjugated and excreted into the biliary system. Hyperbilirubinemia and bilirubinuria may be seen.

H. Intravascular hemolysis may occur if complement is bound.

I. The clinical signs vary with the type of hemolysis and the onset of disease.

1) Complement-mediated intravascular hemolysis may result in peracute disease, sudden weakness and collapse, shock, severe anemia, hemoglobinemia, and hemoglobinuria.

2) Animals with acute disease involving extravascular hemolysis may present with weakness, fever, anemia, and possibly, jaundice.

J. Most dogs have splenomegaly, although hepatomegaly may be found when IgM antibody is present.

K. The owner may note darkly pigmented urine or feces.

L. Cold hemagglutinin disease involves antibodies that are most active at cold temperatures; it is often chronic, and is characterized by necrosis of the body extremities. Anemia is usually mild, if present. Clinical signs become evident when exposure to cold temperatures occurs.

M. Laboratory findings also vary with the severity and type of RBC destruction. In peracute cases, there is a lack of reticulocytosis. Later, however, a marked reticulocyte response occurs. Spherocytes are usually noted in the dog. Simultaneous bone marrow stimulation commonly results in a neutrophilic leukocytosis with a left shift. Hyperbilirubinemia and bilirubinuria are variable.

N. In some cases, blood agglutinates after being placed in a blood collection tube containing anticoagulant. Confirm agglutination by observing it microscopically on a slide after mixing a drop of blood with 0.9% NaCl solution. It must be differentiated from rouleau formation. Sometimes, autoagglutination occurs spontaneously in the absence of hemolytic disease.

O. In cats, spherocytosis is not seen because of the normally small size of their RBCs. Regenerative anemia will be found, and a positive Coombs' test can be determined using antifeline globulin.

P. Diagnosis of IHA is confirmed by the presence of a positive direct Coombs' reaction with an acute hemolytic anemia. Both false-positive and false-negative Coombs' reactions occur, however. For this reason, the diagnosis can also be established on the basis of an acute anemia accompanied by marked autoagglutination or a positive osmotic fragility test.

Q. Antiglobulin (Coombs') test

1) An antiglobulin (Coombs') test detects antibodies adhered to the RBC surface using antibodies against canine or feline antibodies.

2) The direct test is preferred. The indirect test is positive in less than 40% of the cases.

3) Possible causes of a false-negative test

a) The anti-C3 activity of commercial canine antisera is often poor.

b) Incorrect dilution of antiglobulin in cold agglutinin disease

c) Improper washing of RBCs

d) Non–species-specific antisera

e) Lack of anti-IgG or C3 antiglobulins

f) Rarely, IgA is the coating antibody.

g) Occasionally, the amount of antibody bound to the RBCs is too small to be detected by conventional tests.

h) Corticosteroid administration prior to testing

i) Use of other immunosuppressive drugs prior to testing

j) Drug-induced IHA (antibody is directed against the drug; not drug-induced chemical alteration of the RBC membrane)

4) Possible causes of a false-positive test

a) Reactivity to albumin or transferrin

b) Coincidental adherence of circulating immune complexes to RBCs

R. RBCs coated with antibody have increased RBC osmotic fragility.

1) At higher concentrations of an NaCl solution, they imbibe water and cannot maintain an intact cell membrane compared to normal RBCs.

2) Abnormal osmotic fragility is demonstrated in 85% of the cases of canine IHA.

3) Technique in canines

a) Normal canine RBCs maintain normal fragility at NaCl concentrations of greater than 0.54%.

b) Technique

i. A 0.54% concentration of NaCl may be obtained by combining three volumes of 0.9% NaCl with two volumes of water.

ii. Then add five drops of blood to 5 mL of the diluted solution.

iii. Incubate this solution for five minutes, centrifuge, and read.

A. Normal—intact RBCs present on the bottom of the tube, and a clear supernatant

B. Abnormal results—free hemoglobin will stain the supernatant somewhat

4) Technique in felines

a) Normal feline RBCs maintain fragility at NaCl concentrations of greater than 0.64%.

b) Technique

i. A 0.64% concentration of NaCl may be obtained by combining five volumes of 0.9% NaCl with two volumes of water. From this point on, the technique as well as the results are the same for dogs.

5) In both dogs and cats, a negative and positive control should be done (i.e., patient blood and 0.9% NaCl only, and patient blood with water).

S. Treatment of primary IHA is directed toward suppressing RBC destruction by the reticuloendothelial system.

1) Administer prednisolone or prednisone, 2.2 mg/kg, divided b.i.d. initially.

2) One author prefers dexamethasone administration (0.3 mg/kg/d)

3) Corticosteroids are more effective in IgG-mediated disease.

4) The majority of cases respond favorably, although in some cases, higher dosages may be needed. Spherocytosis persists, but fewer cells are destroyed.

5) Maintain the prednisolone dose of 2.2 mg/kg until the PCV rises to 30; then, taper the dose over a period of six to eight weeks.

6) Recurrence is uncommon, but is usually severe if it occurs.

7) Rarely, animals may require low-dose, every-other-day drug treatment the rest of their lives.

T. If corticosteroids fail to prevent the hemolysis, other immunosuppressive drugs may be used, such as cyclophosphamide (50 mg/m^2 s.i.d. for four days; then discontinue for three days) or azathioprine (2.0 mg/kg s.i.d. for seven days, and then every other day). The dose of corticosteroids can often be lowered when coupled with azathioprine or cyclophosphamide.

1) In addition to suppressing the reticuloendothelial system, these drugs rapidly destroy T and B lymphocytes, thereby decreasing antibody production.

2) These drugs are also indicated when marked autoagglutination is present, anemia is severe, a transfusion is to be given, moderate to severe icterus is detected, or adverse reactions to corticosteroids are noted.

U. Avoid blood transfusions if possible; if they are used, crossmatching is essential and the patient should be observed closely for reactions. The benefit derived may be transient if rapid destruction of transfused cells occurs.

V. Perform splenectomy when medical therapy is not successful and in cases of recurrent IHA.

1) IgG-coated RBCs are removed by the spleen, whereas IgM-coated RBCs are removed by the liver. Removal of antibody-coated RBCs by the liver also becomes significant when large numbers of antibody molecules are present.

2) The spleen is a major source of IgG antibody production.

3) Following splenectomy, the reticuloendothelial system in the liver may remove IgG-coated RBCs.

W. Plasmapheresis can be an effective emergency procedure before cytotoxic therapy has had time to bring about a beneficial response; however, it is available only at specific referral centers.

1) The technique removes anti-RBC antibody from plasma.

2) Other cells (RBCs, WBCs) are also removed, necessitating a transfusion.

3) Currently, the procedure can only be performed on dogs weighing more than 40 pounds.

X. Moderate to severe jaundice and IHA indicate rapid, severe hemolysis or concurrent hepatic disease. These clinical signs warrant a guarded prognosis and aggressive therapy.

Y. Some cases have been characterized by nonregenerative anemia, bone marrow erythroid hypoplasia, and a positive Coombs' test. Animals with these signs are corticosteroid-responsive, and such cases may represent immune-mediated destruction of erythrocyte precursors.

Z. Primary IHA must be distinguished from secondary IHA because this influences the management of the patient.

1) In secondary IHA, treatment of the underlying disease process is essential. Therapy may need to be initiated for primary IHA, as well.

2) Secondary IHA is often associated with SLE. In these cases, thrombocytopenia, polyarthropathy, and glomerulonephritis will be noted. Perform an ANA test or LE preparation to confirm the diagnosis.

2. Isoimmune hemolytic disease of newborn animals occurs when the fetus has a blood type that is incompatible with that of the mother, who has previously been sensitized with red cell products to produce isoantibodies. The newborn animal receives the antibodies when ingesting colostrum.

3. Drug-induced, immune-mediated hemolysis probably occurs in the dog and cat.

A. The RBCs themselves are normal. The drug alters the RBC antigen, or the RBC may be an "innocent bystander."

B. Treatment consists of halting the administration of all drugs currently being given.

C. Corticosteroids may be needed to prevent further RBC destruction.

D. A direct Coombs' test may yield a positive result.

4. *Hemobartonella felis* causes extravascular hemolysis in the cat.

A. The RBC with the *H. felis* organism on

its surface is recognized as abnormal by the reticuloendothelial system and is prematurely removed. Because large numbers of cats with *H. felis*-induced anemia have a positive Coombs' test, antibody against the organism RBC complex may be present.

B. Icterus and splenomegaly are common findings on physical examination.

C. *H. felis* infection rarely is a primary disease, and usually is associated with physical stress, concurrent disease, or immunosuppression (cat fight abscesses, FeLV or FIV infection, neoplasia).

D. The diagnosis is based on the presence of the organism and hemolytic anemia.

E. Repeat examination of the smear may be necessary because the organism is often transient or cyclic, and differentiation from stain artifact may be difficult. Use either Wright's or Giemsa stain. Air-dried blood samples are preferred for laboratory examination because the organism separates from RBCs preserved for several hours with EDTA.

F. Evaluate a patient with *H. felis* and nonregenerative anemia for causes of the latter. In these animals, the organism is present as a secondary cause of anemia and treatment is usually ineffective until the primary cause is eliminated.

G. Treatment involves removing the stress or treating the concurrent disease and administering drugs to eliminate the *H. felis.* Oral tetracycline, at a dosage of 22 mg/kg of body weight t.i.d. for two to three weeks, is effective. Drug-induced fever may occur in cats receiving tetracycline hydrochloride. Chloramphenicol may also be used.

H. Administration of thiacetarsamide sodium 1%, 5 mL/10 lb of body weight IV on two alternate days, is also effective.

I. Along with other therapy, some clinicians administer immunosuppressive doses of corticosteroids for one to two days to minimize further RBC destruction.

J. Blood transfusions may be needed in cases of life-threatening anemia.

5. *H. canis* rarely causes anemia in dogs that have not undergone splenectomy. These animals may test Coombs' positive. Treatment with tetracycline, 22 mg/kg t.i.d. for two to three weeks, is effective.

6. *Babesia canis* may cause intravascular hemolysis in the dog.

A. The organism is transmitted by the brown dog tick *Rhipicephalus sanguineus* and *Haemaphysalis leachi*; it invades and multiplies within canine RBCs.

B. Infection may present as an acute intravascular hemolytic episode or as a subacute disease with anemia, icterus, and bilirubinuria; alternatively, it may be so mild as to go unnoticed.

C. Stress, splenectomy, or concurrent disease may elevate the parasite load and result in clinical signs.

D. Diagnosis is based on finding the characteristic teardrop or pear-shaped organisms within infected RBCs. Oval, round, or ring-shaped bodies are also frequently found. It is common to see erythrophagocytosis of both normal and parasitized RBCs by mononuclear cells. In the acute stages, neutropenia and thrombocytopenia may be seen. A Coombs' test may be positive.

E. Concurrent infections with *E. canis* or *H. canis* may complicate infections with *B. canis*. Whenever Babesia species are found, thoroughly examine blood smears for *E. canis* morulae within the cytoplasm of mononuclear cells.

F. Diminazene aceturate (3.5 mg/kg of body weight IM) and Phenamidine (15 mg/kg of body weight SQ) are the drugs most commonly used for treatment. Other supportive therapy may be needed.

G. Dogs infected with Babesia species may become carriers.

7. Ehrlichiosis has been reported to result in a Coombs'-positive anemia. Immune-mediated phenomena appear to be involved in RBC destruction by this organism. However, the anemia is nonregenerative owing to the effect of the organism on erythroid precursor cells in the bone marrow.

8. Heinz-body anemias have been reported in the dog and cat.

A. Chemical oxidants that overload the cell's protective mechanisms result in methemoglobin formation. This is further oxidized to form precipitated globin (Heinz bodies).

B. A small number of Heinz bodies are normally found on peripheral blood smears from cats.

C. RBCs containing Heinz bodies may be removed prematurely by the spleen or they may be increasingly susceptible to intravascular hemolysis.

D. Cats receiving acetaminophen, urinary antiseptics containing methylene blue, and a urinary analgesic (phenazopyridine) have been reported to have developed hemolytic anemias with increased numbers of Heinz bodies. Icterus, hemoglobinuria, and methemoglobinemia were also seen.

E. Topical benzocaine has been implicated as a cause of Heinz-body anemia in the dog.

F. Onion toxicity could occur in the dog as it does in the cow.

G. Treatment involves discontinuing administration of the oxidizing agent, removing any remaining agent from the GI tract, and providing supportive care. In severe cases, blood transfusions may be necessary.

H. Acetaminophen intoxication in the cat is treated by administering N-acetylcystine (Mucomyst). The initial dose is 140 mg/kg orally, followed by 70 mg/kg orally every six to eight hours for four to five days.

1) In humans, ascorbic acid and new methylene blue are used to convert methemoglobin to functional oxyhemoglobin.

2) The efficacy of ascorbic acid in animals is not known; new methylene blue may compound the problem.

9. Zinc-induced hemolysis has been reported in dogs after ingestion of zinc-containing nuts and bolts used in pet carriers or pennies minted after 1983. Treatment consists of removing the source of zinc. Other supportive therapeutic measures may include blood transfusions and corticosteroids.

10. Hemolysis has been associated with DIC. (See Chapter 4.)

A. The mechanism for this is believed to be physical fragmentation of RBCs on intraluminal fibrin strands.

B. The anemia may be mild or severe, and has also been called a microangiopathic hemolytic anemia.

C. Some of the disease conditions in which a microangiopathic hemolytic anemia has been recognized include DIC in association with heat stroke, shock, transfusion reactions, the postcaval syndrome, and neoplastic disease.

D. Treatment is directed at the underlying disease process causing the DIC.

11. Severe hypophosphatemia (probably less than 1.0 mg/dL) may result in severe hemolysis with resultant hemoglobinemia and hemoglobinuria. This may be seen in animals with diabetes mellitus, although it is extremely rare. Correct the cause of the hypophosphatemia and provide phosphorus supplementation.

12. Incompatible blood transfusions may result in an IHA with hemoglobinemia and hemoglobinuria.

A. Early signs of transfusion reactions are restlessness, nausea, and vomiting. Later signs of hemolysis occur, and shock may develop.

B. Discontinue the transfusion if signs referable to hemolysis or cardiovascular collapse are noted.

C. Supportive therapy may be necessary.

13. Hemolysis may be associated with bacterial or viral infections.

A. Probable mechanisms involve adherence to RBCs and direct hemolysis, secretion of substances that directly lyse RBCs, antibody production against RBCs, and endotoxin release, resulting in secondary DIC.

B. Therapy involves treating the underlying infection and instituting other supportive measures. Administer corticosteroids to animals in which removal of RBCs by the reticuloendothelial system is so severe that anemia is life-threatening.

14. Hypersplenism is a syndrome in humans that consists of splenomegaly, accompanied by anemia, leukopenia and/or thrombocytopenia, and associated with a normal or hypercellular bone marrow and improvement in the blood picture after splenectomy.

A. Increased numbers of RBCs, platelets, or neutrophils are sequestered in the spleen.

B. Hypersplenism is a primary disease process when an underlying cause cannot be found. It can occur secondary to many disease states (myeloproliferative disorders, LSA, subacute bacterial endocarditis, connective tissue disorders).

C. The syndrome has not been documented in animals. However, some cases of chronic hemolytic anemia in the presence of splenomegaly have been reported to have responded to splenectomy.

Suggested Readings

Alsaker RD, Laber J, Stevens J, Perman V: A comparison of polychromasia and reticulocyte count in assessing erythrocyte regenerative response in the cat. J Am Vet Med Assoc 170(1): 39–41, 1977

Cowgill LD: Efficacy of recumbunant human erythropoietin (r-HUEPO) for anemia in dogs and cats with renal failure. Research Abstracts, Proceedings, Forum of the American College of Veterinary Internal Medicine, 1990.

Dodds WJ: Autoimmune hemolytic disease and other causes of immune-mediated anemia: An overview. J Am Anim Hosp Assoc 13: 427–442, July/Aug 1977

English RV, Breitschwerdt EB, Grindem CB, et al: Zollinger-Ellison syndrome and myelofibrosis in a dog. J Am Vet Med Assoc 192(10): 1430–1434, 1988

Ettinger SJ: Veterinary Internal Medicine. Philadelphia, WB Saunders, 1983

Finco DR, Barsanti JA, Adams DD: Effects of an anabolic steroid on acute uremia in the dog. Am J Vet Res 145: 2285, 1984

Fitchen J, Cline M: Recent developments in understanding the pathogenesis of aplastic anemia. Am J Hematol 5: 365–372, 1978

Greene CE, Kristensen F, Hoff EJ, Wiggins MD: Cold hemagglutinin disease in a dog. J Am Vet Med Assoc 170(5): 505–510, 1977

Hardy WJ, Jr: Feline leukemia virus non-neoplastic diseases. J Am Anim Hosp Assoc 17: 941, 1981

Harvey J, Sameck J, Burgard F: Benzocaine–induced methemoglobinemia in dogs. J Am Vet Med Assoc 175(11): 1171–1175, 1979

Harvey JW, Gaskin JM: Feline hemobartonellosis. 1978 Proceedings of the American Animal Hospital Association, pp. 117–124. South Bend, Indiana, American Animal Hospital Association, 1980

Jain NC, Finkl JG (eds): Symposium on clinical hematology. Vet Clin North Am 11: 2, 1981

Killingsworth CR: Use of blood and blood components for feline and canine patients. J Am Vet Med Assoc 185(11): 1452–1454, 1984

Kirk RW (ed): Current Veterinary Therapy VII. Philadelphia, WB Saunders, 1980

Kirk RW (ed): Current Veterinary Therapy VIII. Philadelphia, WB Saunders, 1983

Kirk RW (ed): Current Veterinary Therapy IX. Philadelphia, WB Saunders, 1986

Krantz S: Pure red-cell aplasia. N Engl J Med 291(7): 345–350, 1974

Lees GE, Polzin DJ, Perman V, Hammer R, Smith J: Idiopathic Heinz-body hemolytic anemia in three dogs. J Am Anim Hosp Assoc 15: 143–151, 1979

Maddux JM, Shaw EE: Possible beneficial effect of lithium therapy in a case of estrogen-induced bone marrow hypoplasia in a dog: A case report. J Am Anim Hosp Assoc 19: 242, 1983

Madewell BR, Feldman BF: Characterization of anemias associated with neoplasia in small animals. J Am Vet Med Assoc 176(5): 419–422, 1980

Maggio L: Anemia in the cat. Compend Contin Educ Vet Pract 1(2): 114–122, Feb 1979

Penny RHC, Carlisle CH, Prescott CW, Davidson HA: Effects of chloramphenicol on the haemopoietic system of the cat. Br Vet J 123: 145–152, 1967

Perman V: The anemic dog. Scientific Proceedings of the American Animal Hospital Association, pp. 13–20. South Bend, Indiana, American Animal Hospital Association, 1980

Prasse KW, Crouse D, Beutler E, Walker M,

Schall WD: Pyruvate kinase deficiency anemia with terminal myelofibrosis and osteosclerosis in a beagle. J Am Vet Med Assoc 166(12): 1170–1175, 1975

Schalm OW, Jain NC, Carroll EJ: Veterinary Hematology, 3rd ed. Philadelphia, Lea & Febiger, 1975

St. Omer VV, McKnight ED III: Acetylcysteine for treatment of acetaminophen toxicosis in the cat. J Am Vet Med Assoc 176: 911, 1980

Switzer JW, Jain NC: Autoimmune hemolytic anemia in dogs and cats. Vet Clin North Am [Small Anim Pract] 11: 405, 1981

Weiss DJ, Armstrong PJ: Non-regenerative anemias in the dog. Compend Contin Educ Vet Pract 6: 452, 1984

Weiss DJ, Miller ML, Crawford MA, et al: Primary acquired red cell aplasia: Response to glucocorticoid and cyclophosphamide therapy. J Am Anim Hosp Assoc 20: 951, 1984

Werner LL: Coomb's-positive anemias in the dog and cat. Compend Contin Educ Vet Pract 2: 96–101, Feb 1980

Zenoble RD, Stone EA: Autotransfusion in the dog. J Am Vet Med Assoc 172(12): 1411–1414, 1978

CHAPTER TWENTY

Disorders of Leukocytes

Marcia Carothers and C. Guillermo Couto

Evaluation of the leukogram is part of a CBC, and includes quantitation of the WBCs, as well as qualitative information via the differential cell count. Although a specific disease is rarely diagnosed by leukocyte evaluation, the information obtained from the CBC may be useful in narrowing the number of differential diagnoses, as well as in predicting the severity of disease and prognosis. Also, sequential CBCs may be helpful in monitoring an animal's response to therapy.

There are several methods of determining the WBC count. Manual diluting techniques involve the use of calibrated glass pipettes and disposable chambers (i.e., Unopette, Becton Dickinson, Rutherford, NJ). The WBC count is then determined using a hemacytometer. The inherent error in WBC counts using this technique is approximately 20%, even when technical skills are excellent. A variety of automated cell counters are available, and with proper standardization, inherent error using these techniques approximates 5%.

All nucleated cells are counted, including nucleated RBCs. In order to obtain a corrected leukocyte count, the following formula is used:

Corrected WBC count = initial WBC count

$$\times \frac{100}{100 + nRBC/100\ WBC}$$

Leukocytosis is the term used when the WBC count exceeds the upper limit of normal for the species in question. Leukopenia occurs when the WBC count is less than the lower limit of normal.

Depending on the laboratory, the differential WBC count may be reported in relative numbers (percentages) or absolute numbers (number per microliter). Interpretation should be based on *absolute* leukocyte numbers and not percentages, as the percentages may be misleading if the WBC count is very high or very low. See Table 20-1 for normal values in the dog and cat.

Neutrophils

Function

1. The primary functions of neutrophils are ingestion and killing of bacteria and fungi. Many processes, including margination, emigration, adhesion, chemotaxis, phagocytosis, degranulation, and bactericidal actions, have important roles in these functions.

2. Endogenous pyrogens (e.g., interleukin 2) may be secreted by neutrophils.

3. Leukocyte-derived mediators (i.e., proteases, elastases, collagenases, leukotrienes, etc.) also play an important role in inflammation and tissue injury.

Kinetics

1. Pluripotent hematopoietic stem cells give rise to neutrophils, as well as other blood

Table 20-1. **Normal laboratory values (per µL of blood)***

	Dog	*Cat*
Total WBC count	6,500–19,000	4,500–16,500
Neutrophils		
Band	0–300	0–300
Mature	3,000–11,500	3,000–13,000
Lymphocytes	1,200–5,200	1,200–9,000
Monocytes	200–1,300	0–700
Eosinophils	0–1,200	0–1,200
Basophils	Rare	Rare

* From The Ohio State University Veterinary Teaching Hospital, February 1988

cells, such as RBCs, megakaryocytes, lymphocytes, eosinophils, basophils, and monocytes. Differentiation into the blood cell lines is regulated by specific protein factors (colony stimulating factors). Granulocyte-colony stimulating factor (G-CSF) stimulates proliferation of neutrophils from the late progenitor stages. Macrophage-colony stimulating factor (M-CSF) stimulates the proliferation of monocytes. Other factors (granulocyte–macrophage colony stimulating factor [GM-CSF], interleukin 3 [IL 3], and interleukin 2 [IL 2]) stimulate proliferation at multiple stages of maturation (Fig. 20-1).

2. Neutrophils are produced in the bone marrow. Three theoretical neutrophil compartments exist. The *proliferation compartment* is composed of myeloblasts, progranulocytes, and myelocytes. The approximate maturation time from myeloblast to metamyelocyte is 48 to 60 hours. The *maturation compartment* consists of metamyelocytes and band neutrophils. The transit time through this compartment is 46 to 70 hours. The *storage compartment* is made up of mature neutrophils. Transit time in this compartment is approximately 50 hours. There is an estimated five-day supply of neutrophils in this compartment. Mature neutrophils leave the bone marrow by a random process that involves changes in cell deformability and adhesiveness.

3. Two neutrophil pools are present in the vascular compartment. The *marginal neutrophil pool* (MNP) consists of neutrophils that adhere to the vascular endothelium. The *circulating neutrophil pool* (CNP) consists of the neutrophils circulating in the blood. The *total blood neutrophil pool* (TBNP) comprises both the MNP and the CNP. The WBC count and differential are estimations of the neutrophil count in the CNP. In the dog, the size of the CNP is approximately equal to the size of the MNP. However, in the cat, the MNP is approximately two to three times the size of the CNP. The neutrophil has an average blood transit time of approximately 6 to 14 hours, with all the blood neutrophils being replaced every two to two and one-half days. Once the neutrophil has left the blood vessel, it normally does not return to circulation, and may be lost in the lungs, gut, urine, or saliva.

4. Neutrophils enter tissues by diapedesis through intracellular junctions between endothelial cells. The degree and duration of inflammation influences neutrophil migration to tissues.

Morphologic Characteristics

1. Normal neutrophils contain a clear cytoplasm with granules that stain neutral to pale pink and a polymorphic segmented nucleus with clumped chromatin when stained with Wright's or Romanowsky's stain.

2. Immature neutrophils have characteristic nuclear and cytoplasmic features that distinguish them from mature cells. Band neutrophils have mature cytoplasm with an indented nucleus and parallel nuclear membranes. Metamyelocytes contain a basophilic cytoplasm with an elongated, slightly indented (i.e., uniform) nucleus. Myelocytes possess a round nucleus with a fine chromatin pattern. Progranulocytes are slightly larger cells with fine azurophilic granules and an eccentric, round nucleus with a prominent nucleolus.

3. Toxic neutrophils contain cytoplasmic changes. Döhle bodies are small, bluish, cytoplasmic inclusions that consist of aggregates of endoplasmic reticulum; they are common in sick cats. Diffuse cytoplasmic changes include basophilia and vacuolation and indicate a more severe change. Toxic granulation consists of purplish cytoplasmic

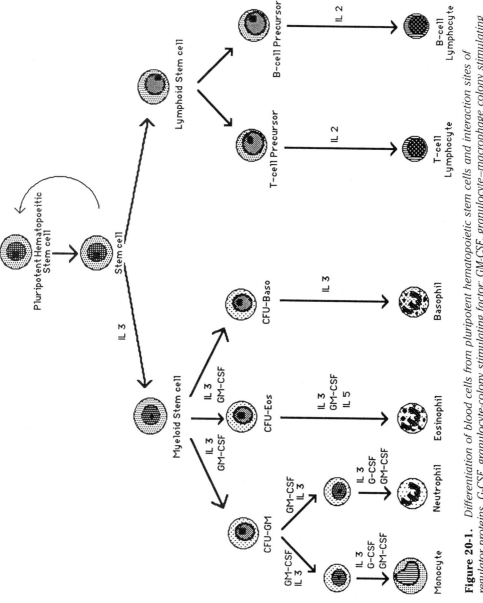

Figure 20-1. Differentiation of blood cells from pluripotent hematopoietic stem cells and interaction sites of regulator proteins. G-CSF, granulocyte-colony stimulating factor; GM-CSF, granulocyte–macrophage colony stimulating factor; M-CSF, macrophage colony stimulating factor; IL 2, interleukin 2; IL 3, interleukin 3; IL 5, interleukin 5; CFU-GM, colony forming units—granulocyte–macrophage; CFU-Eos, colony forming units—eosinophils; CFU-Baso, colony forming units—basophils.

granules and represents the most severe toxic change. Giant neutrophils, bands, and metamyelocytes are large and polyploidal cells that may result from skipped cell division. These cells are yet another manifestation of toxic changes, and are more common in the cat than in the dog.

4. Pelger-Hüet nuclear anomaly occurs when the nucleus fails to undergo division, but the nuclear chromatin and cytoplasm maturation is complete (i.e., the nucleus has a bandlike appearance with mature, clumped chromatin). These changes may also be apparent in the eosinophils and basophils. This anomaly may be acquired or inherited (autosomal dominant), but is usually considered to be benign.

5. Chédiak-Higashi syndrome is characterized by enlarged neutrophilic and eosinophilic granules. Other associated abnormalities include partial albinism, photophobia, increased susceptibility to infections, bleeding tendencies, and abnormal melanocytes. This lethal, autosomal recessive condition has been documented in Persian cats with smoke-colored haircoats and yellow eyes.

6. Nuclear hypersegmentation (i.e., four or more distinct nuclear lobes) may result from prolonged transit time. Hyperadrenocorticism, corticosteroid therapy, and the late stages of chronic disease may be associated with this change. This change may be also noted in poodles with macrocytosis.

Neutrophil Changes in Disease

Neutropenia

1. *Neutropenia* is an absolute decrease in circulating neutrophil numbers.
2. Etiology
   A. Decreased or ineffective production of cells in the proliferating pool
     1) Myelophthisis (neoplastic infiltration of the bone marrow)
      a) Myeloproliferative disorders
      b) Lymphoproliferative disorders
      c) Systemic mast cell disease
      d) Myelofibrosis
      e) Metastatic carcinoma (rare in small animals)

     2) Drug-induced
      a) Anticancer and immunosuppressive agents
      b) Chloramphenicol
      c) Griseofulvin
      d) Sulfa-trimethoprim combination
      e) Estrogen
      f) Phenylbutazone
      g) Phenothiazine derivatives
      h) Other
     3) Toxins
      a) Industrial chemical compounds (inorganic solvents, benzene)
      b) *Fusarium sporotrichioides* toxin
     4) Infectious diseases
      a) Parvovirus infection
      b) Retrovirus (feline leukemia virus [FeLV] and feline immunodeficiency virus [FIV]) infection
        i. Myelodysplastic or preleukemic syndromes
        ii. Cyclic neutropenia
        iii. Panleukopenia-like syndrome
      c) Histoplasmosis
      d) Ehrlichiosis
      e) Toxoplasmosis
      f) Early canine distemper virus infection
      g) Early canine hepatitis virus infection
     5) Idiopathic bone marrow hypoplasia/aplasia
     6) Cyclic neutropenia of grey collies
     7) Acquired cyclic neutropenia
   B. Sequestration of neutrophils in marginating pool
     1) Endotoxic shock
     2) Anaphylactic shock
     3) Anesthesia
   C. Sudden, excessive tissue demand or consumption
     1) Infectious diseases
      a) Peracute, overwhelming bacterial infection (e.g., peritonitis, aspiration pneumonia, salmonellosis, metritis)
      b) Viral (e.g., canine distemper or hepatitis, preclinical stage)
     2) Drug-induced
     3) Immune-mediated
     4) Paraneoplastic
     5) "Hypersplenism"

Neutrophilia

1. Neutrophilia is defined as an absolute increase in neutrophil numbers. It is the most common cause of leukocytosis.

    A. Mature neutrophilia—an increase in neutrophils without an increase in immature forms (i.e., bands)

    B. Neutrophilia with left shift—an increase in the number of both mature and immature neutrophils (bands > 300/μL)

    C. Regenerative left shift—a form of neutrophilia associated with increased numbers of immature neutrophils in which the number of immature forms does not exceed the number of mature neutrophils

    D. Degenerative left shift—occurs when the number of immature neutrophils exceeds the number of mature neutrophils. Neutrophilia may or may not be present. This usually implies a poor prognosis.

    E. Leukemoid response—a marked neutrophilia with a severe left shift (which includes metamyelocytes and myelocytes). Such a response indicates severe inflammatory disease and may be difficult to distinguish from chronic granulocytic leukemia.

    F. Granulocytic leukemia—a myeloproliferative disorder affecting mainly the neutrophils and causing marked leukocytosis with a large number of immature forms. There is asynchronous nucleocytoplasmic maturation characterized by giant forms, nucleoli in more mature-appearing neutrophils, and premature segmentation.

2. Etiology

    A. Physiologic or epinephrine-induced neutrophilia

        1) Associated with neutrophils released from the MNP. This transient response lasts 20 to 30 minutes following endogenous release of catecholamines. This neutrophilia occurs only in healthy animals and is most common in the cat

        2) Other CBC changes include erythrocytosis and lymphocytosis (primarily in cats)

        3) Causes

            a) Fear

            b) Excitement

            c) Exercise

            d) Seizures

            e) Parturition

            f) Hypertension

    B. Stress- or corticosteroid-induced neutrophilia

        1) Associated with a prolonged transit time in circulation and increased bone marrow release of neutrophils in the storage pool caused by endogenous or exogenous corticosteroids

        2) Other CBC changes include lymphopenia, eosinopenia, and monocytosis (the latter occurring only in dogs).

        3) Causes

            a) Pain

            b) Anesthesia

            c) Trauma

            d) Neoplasia

            e) Hyperadrenocorticism

            f) Metabolic disorders

            g) Debilitating disorders

    C. Inflammation or increased tissue demand

        1) The magnitude of the response is determined by the balance between the rate of bone marrow release and tissue emigration, and may vary with the species, location of inflammation, virulence of the etiologic agent, and inciting cause of the inflammation.

        2) Causes

            a) Infection (bacterial, viral, fungal, parasitic)

            b) Tissue trauma and/or necrosis

            c) Immune-mediated disorders

            d) Neoplasia

            e) Metabolic (uremia, diabetic ketoacidosis)

            f) Burns

            g) Abnormalities in neutrophil function

            h) Other (acute hemorrhage, hemolysis)

Lymphocytes

Function

1. There are two types of lymphocytes that are morphologically indistinguishable. T lymphocytes (thymic-derived) are involved in cell-mediated immunity, whereas B lymphocytes (bursa-derived) are associated with humoral immunity. Only about 10% of the total lymphocyte pool circulates in peripheral blood.

2. In healthy small animals, 70% of the blood lymphocytes are T lymphocytes.

Kinetics

1. Unlike other white cells, lymphocytes are long-lived and capable of transformation to more functional, active forms. Immature lymphoid precursors are present in the primary or central compartment (i.e., thymus, bone marrow, and bursa equivalent). These lymphocytes may differentiate or may provide precursors to the secondary or peripheral compartment (i.e., lymph nodes, spleen, and Peyer's patches). The lymphocytes of the peripheral compartment respond to antigenic stimulation and develop into T or B lymphocytes.

2. Lymphocytes recirculate via efferent lymphatics and the thoracic duct to the blood vasculature. This recirculation allows for generalized distribution of immunocompetent cells, exposure of lymphocytes to tissue antigens, relocation of antigenically exposed cells, and immune surveillance.

3. The number of circulating lymphocytes decreases with age.

Morphologic Characteristics

1. Normal lymphocytes contain a small amount of blue cytoplasm with a round nucleus and clumped chromatin. The nucleus may be slightly indented, but nucleoli are usually not present. Some lymphocytes contain prominent azurophilic cytoplasmic granules and are referred to as large granular lymphocytes (LGLs), or globoid leukocytes.

2. Reactive lymphocytes are slightly larger lymphocytes with nuclear folding, intense cytoplasmic basophilia with an occasionally pale zone (Golgi apparatus), and/or azurophilic granules. These lymphocytes occur in response to antigenic stimulation or, rarely, in cases of lymphoid neoplasm.

3. Lymphocytic leukemia may result in high circulating numbers (usually greater than 50,000/μL) of lymphocytes. Chronic lympho-

cytic leukemia is characterized by a predominance of normal-appearing lymphocytes. Acute lymphoid leukemia is characterized by circulating lymphoblasts. Involvement of the spleen, liver, bone marrow, and lymph nodes is common in these cases.

Lymphocytic Changes in Disease

Lymphopenia

1. *Lymphopenia* is defined as an absolute decrease in the lymphocyte count.

2. Etiology

A. Corticosteroid- or stress-induced (See the Neutrophilia section.)

B. Loss of lymph

1) Lymphangiectasia

2) Chylothorax (especially with repeated drainage)

C. Impaired lymphopoiesis

1) Chemotherapy

2) Irradiation

3) Prolonged corticosteroid usage

D. Viral disease (secondary to cell lysis, inhibition of cell production, and loss through denuded gastrointestinal [GI] mucosa)

1) Parvoviruses

2) Feline infectious peritonitis (FIP)

3) FeLV

4) FIV

5) Canine distemper

6) Canine infectious hepatitis

Lymphocytosis

1. *Lymphocytosis* is an absolute increase in lymphocyte number.

2. Etiology

A. Physiologic or epinephrine-induced (See Neutrophilia section.)

B. Prolonged antigenic stimulation (usually involving a mild increase in lymphocyte number)

1) Chronic infection

a) Ehrlichiosis (dogs)—Lymphocyte counts in dogs with ehrlichiosis may exceed 10,000/μL and may mimic chronic lymphocytic leukemia.

2) Allergic syndromes

3) Autoimmune disease
4) Postvaccination response
C. Leukemia
1) Lymphocytic (chronic)
2) Lymphoblastic (acute)
D. Hypoadrenocorticism

Eosinophils

Function

1. Although less effective when compared to neutrophils, eosinophils possess phagocytic and bactericidal capabilities against bacteria, mycoplasms, yeasts, and the like.
2. Parasiticidal activity, which is probably dependent on antibody or complement, or both, is an important function of eosinophils.
3. Eosinophils are involved in immediate hypersensitivity (type I) reactions. They possess substances that counteract the mediators released by mast cells, which may be important in modulating the immediate hypersensitivity response.
4. Eosinophilic granules may activate plasminogen, resulting in thrombosis.

Kinetics

1. Eosinophils are produced primarily in the bone marrow in response to GM-CSF, multi-CSF (IL 3), and IL 5. Storage of eosinophils also occurs within the marrow. Normally, only a small number of eosinophils are present in the peripheral circulation. Eosinophils migrate to tissues that have a close interaction with foreign material (i.e., gut, skin, and respiratory tract). Like neutrophils, eosinophils do not recirculate.
2. The transit time within the blood is approximately 24 to 35 hours.
3. The tissue eosinophil pool is significantly larger than the circulating pool. Eosinophils predominate in mucous membranes.

Morphologic Characteristics

1. Eosinophils have distinct pink to orange cytoplasmic granules and a segmented nucleus. Dogs have variably sized granules

when compared to those of cats, which are small and rod-shaped.
2. Eosinophilic leukemia may be characterized by large numbers of circulating eosinophils with immature forms, asynchronous maturation, and nuclear changes (i.e., prominent nucleoli, chromatin clumping, etc.).

Eosinophil Changes in Disease

Eosinopenia

1. *Eosinopenia* is defined as an absolute decrease in eosinophil numbers.
2. Etiology
A. Stress- or corticosteroid-induced (See Neutrophilia section.)
B. Acute inflammation and infection
1) Secondary to endogenous corticosteroid release
2) Tissue inflammation with production of eosinophilic chemotactic substances may lead to eosinopenia.

Eosinophilia

1. *Eosinophilia* is an absolute increase in eosinophil numbers.
2. Etiology
A. Parasitic disorders
1) Ancylostomiasis
2) Dirofilariasis
3) Ctenocephalidiasis
4) Filaroidiasis
5) Aelurostrongylosis
6) Ascariasis (larva migration)
7) Paragonimiasis
8) Demodicosis (in rare cases)
B. Hypersensitivity disorders
1) Atopy
2) Flea allergy dermatitis
C. Eosinophilic infiltrative disorders
1) Eosinophilic granuloma complex
2) Feline bronchial asthma
3) Canine PIE (pulmonary infiltrates with eosinophils)
4) Eosinophilic gastroenteritis/colitis
5) Feline hypereosinophilic syndrome
D. Infectious diseases
1) Upper respiratory viral disorders
2) Feline panleukopenia

3) FIP
4) Toxoplasmosis
5) Suppurative processes
  E. Neoplasia
    1) Mast cell tumors (systemic and cutaneous)
    2) Lymphomas
    3) Myeloproliferative disorders (e.g., eosinophilic leukemia)
    4) Solid tumors
  F. Miscellaneous
    1) Soft tissue trauma
    2) Feline urologic syndrome
    3) Cardiomyopathy
    4) Renal failure
    5) Feline hyperthyroidism
    6) Canine estrus

Basophils

Function

1. The function of the basophil is not completely known, but is thought to be similar to that of tissue mast cells. Both degranulate when antigen complexes with immunoglobulin E (IgE) on their surfaces, and both are involved in allergic and inflammatory reactions.
2. Basophils have a limited capability to phagocytize.
3. Basophils contain histamine and other vasoactive substances, as well as eosinophilic chemotactic factor.
4. Basophils may facilitate triglyceride metabolism.

Kinetics

1. Basophils originate in the bone marrow. The production of basophils appear to be antigen-specific and is similar to that of eosinophils and neutrophils.
2. Basophils migrate into tissues and survive for a short time (10 to 12 days).

Morphologic Characteristics

1. Normal basophils are characterized by reddish-violet cytoplasmic granules that may mask a lobulated nucleus. Canine basophils have larger and fewer granules compared to feline basophils, which have orange-gray colored granules against a grayish background.
2. Basophil granules are water soluble and may dissolve in some stained preparations.

Basophil Changes in Disease

Basopenia

Basopenia is an absolute decrease in basophil number. Because basophils are rare in circulation, basopenia is not significant.

Basophilia

1. *Basophilia* is defined as an absolute increase in basophil numbers that is usually associated with eosinophilia.
  A. Associated with IgE production
    1) Heartworm disease
    2) Allergic skin disease (type I hypersensitivity)
  B. Inflammatory diseases
    1) GI disease
    2) Respiratory disease
    3) Neoplasms
      a) Mast cell tumors
      b) Lymphomatoid granulomatosis
      c) Basophilic leukemia
  C. Associated with hyperlipoproteinemia
    1) Hyperadrenocorticism
    2) Hypothyroidism

Monocytes

Function

1. Monocytes transform into tissue macrophages, which may be fixed or migrate freely. These macrophages phagocytize microorganisms, senescent cells, and cellular debris.
2. Macrophages play an important part in regulating the immune response by presenting the antigen to the lymphocytes. Also, the macrophages secrete monokines that activate other immune cells (i.e., lymphocytes and neutrophils).

3. Macrophages may have cytotoxic effects (i.e., against tumor cells).

4. Secretory products of macrophages include monokines, endogenous pyrogens (IL 1), lysosomal hydrolases, prostaglandins, complement components, procoagulant factors, and so on. These products are important in phagocytosis, immune activation, and cytoactivity.

Kinetics

1. Monocytes originate in the bone marrow, where they probably spend a short time before randomly entering the peripheral circulation. The half-life of circulating monocytes in cattle is approximately 20 hours, but has not been well documented in the dog or cat.

2. Although many factors may stimulate production of monocytes, regulate the release of monocytes into circulation, influence monocytic migration into tissues, and affect the turnover time of the monocyte, these factors have not been identified fully.

Morphologic Characteristics

1. Monocytes are slightly larger than neutrophils. The cytoplasm stains blue-gray and may have a ground-glass or foamy appearance. Fine azurophilic granules may be present. The nucleus is pleomorphic with an indistinct membrane and fine, reticular chromatin.

2. Monocytic and myelomonocytic leukemias may be characterized by increased numbers of mature or immature monocytes in circulation. Promonocytes have a large nucleus with a fine chromatin pattern and nucleoli. Monoblasts may be similar to myeloblasts, with a moderate to deep blue cytoplasm and a round or oval nucleus with prominent nucleoli. However, unlike the myeloblasts, monoblasts may possess a clefted or undulating nuclear outline. These cells can be differentiated by using cytochemical stains (Table 20-2).

Monocytic Changes in Disease

Monocytopenia

1. *Monocytopenia* is an absolute decrease in monocyte numbers.

2. Monocytopenia is not important clinically.

Monocytosis

1. *Monocytosis* is defined as an absolute increase in monocyte numbers.

2. Etiology
  A. Chronic inflammation
    1) Infectious
      a) Bacterial (suppurative)
        i. Pyometra
        ii. Abscesses
        iii. Peritonitis
        iv. Pyothorax
        v. Osteomyelitis
        vi. Prostatitis
      b) Higher bacteria
        i. Nocardia
        ii. Actinomyces
        iii. Mycobacteria
      c) Intracellular parasites
        i. Ehrlichia
        ii. Hemobartonella

Table 20-2. **Typical cytochemical reactions in leukemic cells**

Cytochemical Markers	Lymphocytic Leukemia	Myelogenous Leukemia	Myelomonocytic Leukemia	Monocytic Leukemia
Peroxidase	Negative	Positive	Positive	Negative
Acid phosphatase	Negative	Positive	Positive	Negative
Sudan black B	Negative	Positive	Positive	Negative
Chloracetate esterase	Negative	Positive	Weak positive	Negative
Nonspecific esterase	Negative	Negative	Weak positive	Positive

d) Heartworms
2) Immune-mediated
   a) Hemolytic anemia
   b) Skin disorders (e.g., pemphigus, puppy strangles, systemic lupus erythematosus, etc.)
3) Granulomatous disease
   a) Systemic fungal disease
      i. Blastomycosis
      ii. Histoplasmosis
      iii. Cryptococcosis
      iv. Coccidioidomycosis
   b) Tuberculosis
B. Trauma with severe crushing injuries
C. Hemorrhage into tissues or body cavities
D. Stress- or corticosteroid-induced (in the dog)
E. Neoplasia
   1) Associated with tumor necrosis
   2) Myelodysplastic disorders
   3) Leukemia
      a) Myelomonocytic leukemia
      b) Monocytic leukemia
      c) Myelogenous leukemia (occasional)

White Blood Cell Neoplasias

Acute Leukemias

Acute leukemias are uncommon in small animals. These neoplasms are characterized by bone marrow infiltration by immature cells of myeloid, monocytoid, or lymphoid origin. Clinical signs are often vague and may include fever, lethargy, anorexia, lymphadenopathy, hepatosplenomegaly, respiratory distress, vomiting, and diarrhea. Hematologic changes may include leukocytosis, anemia, thrombocytopenia, and the presence of blasts. The accompanying biochemical changes may include azotemia, elevated liver enzyme activity, hypercalcemia, hyperphosphatemia, and hyperproteinemia. Diagnosis is based on morphologic and cytochemical characteristics of peirpheral blood and bone marrow. Various chemotherapeutic protocols have been used in treating acute leukemias, but the response has not been encouraging. Survival time is usually less than six months, with an average of one month.

Acute Lymphoblastic Leukemia

1. Acute lymphoblastic leukemia (ALL) is a progressive, malignant disease characterized by lymphoblasts in the bone marrow and other lymphoid tissues. The cytologic characteristics include round cells with a small rim of royal blue cytoplasm and a large, round nucleus with a fine to coarsely stippled chromatin pattern. A single nucleolus is usually present in the nucleus. Occasionally, large, azurophilic granules may be present in the cytoplasm. Most cytochemical stains usually yield negative results (see Table 20-2).
2. Signalment
   A. Canine: The age range reported has been 1 to 12 years, with a mean age of approximately 6 years. The male : female ratio has been reported to be 3 : 2. The disease has been commonly reported in large breeds (especially German shepherds).
   B. Feline: ALL is uncommon in cats.
3. Clinical signs—The clinical signs are usually nonspecific and include anorexia, lethargy, vomiting, diarrhea, dyspnea, lameness, polydipsia, polyuria, and weight loss. The physical examination may reveal pallor, hepatomegaly, splenomegaly, occasional mild lymphadenopathy, and fever. Neurologic abnormalities may be present.
4. Laboratory changes
   A. Usually a marked leukocytosis is present (WBC count > 100,000/μL), accompanied by circulating blasts, mild anemia (PCV > 25%), and thrombocytopenia (platelets < 100,000/μL).
   B. Increased liver enzyme activity, mild azotemia, and hypercalcemia may be noted on the biochemical profile.
   C. Bone marrow aspiration usually reveals a monomorphic population of lymphoblasts with decreased numbers of normal precursor cells.
5. Treatment
   A. Reported therapeutic approaches include chemotherapy (single and multiple

agents) and plasma/whole blood transfusions. Drugs utilized in the treatment of ALL include prednisone, vincristine, cyclophosphamide, cytosine arabinoside, L-asparaginase, and chlorambucil.

B. The major problems encountered in the treatment of this disease are persistent neutropenia and thrombocytopenia, which usually lead to sepsis and bleeding, respectively.

6. Prognosis—The response to therapy is poor, with average survival approximating four to six weeks. Death is usually attributable to sepsis, bleeding, or neurologic complications. Without therapy, survival time is one to two weeks.

Acute Myelogenous Leukemia

1. Acute myelogenous leukemia (AML) is a neoplastic disease of the granulocytic cell line. The peripheral blood picture usually reveals neutropenia with a disorderly left shift to myeloblasts. Neoplastic myeloid cells are susceptible to degenerative changes and may show cytoplasmic vacuolation and cell shrinkage. Myeloblasts are characterized by an irregularly shaped, slightly eccentric nucleus with fine, stippled chromatin and nucleoli, and abundant basophilic cytoplasm with occasional small, azurophilic granules. Granulocytic markers include peroxidase, acid phosphatase, chloracetate esterase, and Sudan black B (see Table 20-2).

2. Signalment

A. Canine—AML usually affects young dogs with an age range of 1.5 to 12 years and a mean of 4 years. No sex or breed disposition has been identified, but many of the reported cases occur in large breed dogs.

B. Feline—Most cats with AML are FeLV-positive. AML primarily affects young cats. No sex or breed predilection has been identified.

3. Clinical signs—The clinical signs and physical examination findings are similiar to those in ALL. Ocular changes (hyphema, glaucoma, and retinal detachment) have also been noted.

4. Laboratory changes

A. Leukocyte counts may be normal to moderately increased. Severe to moderate

anemia and thrombocytopenia may be present. An asynchronous left shift with myeloblasts is usually present.

B. Serum biochemical changes include increased liver enzyme activity and mild azotemia.

C. Bone marrow examination reveals displacement of marrow by neoplastic granulocytes with a disorderly maturation. Numbers of normal marrow precursors may be significantly depressed owing to this neoplastic infiltration.

5. Treatment—Chemotherapy using vincristine, cyclophosphamide, and 6-thioguanine has been tried with minimal response. A preliminary evaluation of drugs that induce cellular differentiation (i.e., cytosine arabinoside) has shown promising results.

6. Prognosis—The prognosis of AML is very poor. Survival rates, with or without therapy, are less than four months.

Acute Myelomonocytic Leukemia

1. Acute myelomonocytic leukemia (AMMoL) originates from the common granulocytic-monocytic precursor, and this form is the most common nonlymphoid leukemia occurring in dogs. The blasts are characterized by an oval to irregular nucleus with a fine, delicate chromatin pattern and occasional nucleoli. The cytoplasm may contain vacuoles or azurophilic granules, and may form pseudopods. Special cytochemical stains that yield positive results include both the granulocytic markers (chloracetate esterase, Sudan black B, peroxidase, and acid phosphatase) and monocytic marker (nonspecific esterase) (see Table 20-2).

2. Signalment

A. Canine—AMMoL is a disease of younger dogs (ranging in age from 1 to 12 years, with a mean of approximately 6 years). Female dogs appear to be at increased risk for development of AMMoL. No breed predilection has been reported.

B. Feline—AMMoL is a rare disease in cats.

3. Clinical signs—The clinical signs and physical examination findings are similar to those in AML.

4. Laboratory changes

A. The WBC count may be normal or moderately elevated (average of 50,000/μL). Monocytosis may be present. Mild to moderate anemia and thrombocytopenia are also usually present.

B. Elevated liver enzyme activity, azotemia, slightly decreased albumin concentration, and hypoglycemia have been reported.

C. Bone marrow aspirates usually reveal a large number of blasts with myeloid and monocytoid characteristics. Decreased numbers of normal marrow precursor cells are usually noted.

5. Treatment—Chemotherapy using prednisone, cytosine arabinoside, 6-thioguanine, vinblastine, and cyclophosphamide has been used, with and without plasmapheresis, with limited success.

6. Prognosis—Prognosis is poor, even with therapy. Survival times range from one day to six weeks (with a mean survival of approximately three weeks).

Acute Monocytic Leukemia

1. Acute monocytic leukemia (AMoL) is characterized by monocytoid blast cells that infiltrate the bone marrow. On cytologic examination, these cells are large, with an irregular, angular to oval nucleus with finely stippled chromatin and an occasional nucleolus. The cytoplasm is blue-gray with a ground-glass appearance, and may possess occasional vacuoles. Cytoplasmic pseudopods may also be present. Monocytic markers include alpha naphthyl butyrate esterase and alpha naphthyl acetate esterase.

2. Signalment

A. Canine—AMoL has been reported in dogs ranging in age from 2 to 12 years (mean of approximately 6 years). No sex or breed predilection has been noted, but large breed dogs are common in many reports.

B. Feline—The average age of the cats reported is four years. No sex or breed predilection has been noted.

3. Clinical signs—The clinical signs and physical findings are similar to those in AMMoL, with fever and weight loss being less common in AMoL.

4. Laboratory changes

A. The leukocyte count is usually markedly elevated (WBC count > 90,000/μL). Anemia and thrombocytopenia are usually mild, if present at all. Monocytosis may be present.

B. Serum biochemical changes include azotemia, elevated liver enzyme activity, and hyperphosphatemia.

C. Bone marrow evaluation may reveal a monomorphic population of monoblasts, with or without differentiation.

5. Treatment—Chemotherapy has included the use of prednisone, cytosine arabinoside, 6-thioguanine, and vincristine.

6. Prognosis—Despite the use of chemotherapy, average survival times have not exceeded those of untreated animals.

Other Acute Leukemias

Eosinophilic and mast cell leukemias are rarely reported in veterinary medicine. Mast cell leukemia is usually associated with systemic mastocytosis. Clinical signs, physical examination, and laboratory changes may be similar to those of the other acute leukemias, with neoplastic eosinophilic or mastocytic cells present in the peripheral circulation and the bone marrow. The prognosis is poor, even with chemotherapy.

Chronic Leukemia

Chronic leukemias are characterized by increased numbers of well-differentiated cells in blood and bone marrow, and generally have a longer and more slowly progressive course than do acute leukemias. Blast crises may occur in chronic myelogenous leukemia (CML), making the diagnosis more difficult. The response to therapy and the prognosis are usually better than for acute leukemias, except for patients with a blast crisis.

Chronic Lymphocytic Leukemia

1. Chronic lymphocytic leukemia (CLL) is characterized by a proliferation of small, nonfunctional lymphocytes (usually of B cell origin) in the peripheral blood and hematopoietic tissues. The lymphocytes are generally 7 to 9 μm in diameter with a large, round nucleus with clumped chromatin. Occasionally, large azurophilic cytoplasmic granules may be present. These cells (LGLs) are thought to be a subset of T lymphocytes (natural killer cells). All cytochemical stains generally yield negative results.

2. Signalment

A. Canine—CLL occurs in middle-aged to older animals. A 2 : 1 male to female ratio has been reported. No breed predilection has been identified, although a large number of reports have included English bulldogs.

B. Feline—CLL has rarely been recognized in older cats. The FeLV status of affected animals is variable.

3. Clinical signs—The clinical signs are usually vague and include lethargy, depression, anorexia, vomiting, diarrhea, fever, and intermittent lameness. The duration of these signs may range from a few weeks to months. The physical examination may be normal or may reveal mild to moderate peripheral lymphadenopathy, hepatosplenomegaly, or occasionally, pallor. A large number of dogs with CLL are asymptomatic, and are, therefore, diagnosed incidentally.

4. Laboratory changes

A. The leukocyte count is usually increased as a result of an absolute lymphocytosis; leukocyte counts may range from 5,000 to greater than 100,000/μL. A mild to moderate normocytic, normochromic anemia may also be present. The platelet count may be normal or slightly decreased.

B. Bone marrow examination usually reveals an excessive number of small lymphocytes which may increase in number as the disease progresses.

C. Serum chemistry values are generally normal except for an elevation in alkaline phosphatase activity and/or hypergammaglobulinemia.

D. Occasionally, a monoclonal spike is present in the beta-gamma region of the protein electrophoresis. The paraprotein is generally IgM. Bence Jones proteinuria is present in approximately half of those cases.

5. Treatment—The treatment of CLL is controversial, as many cases are asymptomatic

and discovered incidentally. Chemotherapeutic protocols that have been used successfully include an alkylating agent, such as chlorambucil; a corticosteroid, such as prednisone; and occasionally, a vinca alkaloid, such as vincristine. Continuous and intermittent therapeutic regimens have been used. Patients should be treated only when they are symptomatic or cytopenic (i.e., anemia, thrombocytopenia).

6. Prognosis—The prognosis for CLL is considerably better than for ALL. With or without chemotherapy, survival usually exceeds one to two years.

Chronic Myelogenous Leukemia

Chronic myelogenous leukemia (CML) is an uncommon disease in the dog and cat, and is characterized by an elevated granulocyte count with numerous mature and immature forms. White cell counts often are greater than 100,000/μL. A moderate anemia may also be present. Differentiation from other diseases, such as severe infections, immune diseases, and other neoplastic processes, may be difficult. Bone marrow examination reveals hyperplasia of the granulocytic cell line. Clinical signs are nonspecific and may include lethargy, anorexia, and weakness. Physical findings may reveal hepatosplenomegaly, ulcerative or nodular dermatitis, weight loss, and/or pallor. Progression of the disease to immature forms (a so-called blast crisis) may occur as a terminal event. The course of the disease is more prolonged compared to its acute counterpart. Therapy using hydroxyurea has been helpful in prolonging survival, but blast crises have developed in several dogs while receiving this type of therapy. The prognosis is guarded; however, survival times usually are in excess of one year.

Chemotherapy Protocols for Patients with Leukocytic Neoplasia

1. Lymphoma

A. Induction of remission

1) COAP protocol

a) Cyclophosphamide (Cytoxan)—

50 mg/m² of body surface area (BSA), orally, four days a week or every other day for eight weeks

    b) Vincristine (Oncovin)—0.5 mg/m² of BSA, intravenously (IV), once a week for eight weeks

    c) Cytosine arabinoside (Cytosar-U)—100 mg/m² of BSA, IV or subcutaneously (SQ), divided b.i.d., for four days

    d) Prednisone—40 to 50 mg/m² of BSA, orally, s.i.d. for one week; then, 20 to 25 mg/m² of BSA, orally, every other day for seven weeks

    e) *Note:* In cats, cytosine arabinoside is used for only two days, and the remaining three drugs (cyclophosphamide, vincristine, and prednisone) are administered for six weeks, rather than eight weeks.

  2) COP protocol

    a) Cyclophosphamide (Cytoxan)—50 mg/m² of BSA, orally, four days a week or every other day; or 300 mg/m² of BSA, orally, every three weeks*

    b) Vincristine (Oncovin)—0.5 mg/m² of BSA, IV, once a week

    c) Prednisone—40 to 50 mg/m² of BSA, orally, s.i.d. for a week; then, 20 to 25 mg/m² of BSA, orally, every other day

  3) CLOP protocol—the same as the COP protocol, but with the addition of L-asparaginase (Elspar) at a dose of 10,000 to 20,000 IU/m² of BSA, SQ, once every four to six weeks

  4) CHOP protocol (21-day cycle)

    a) Cyclophosphamide (Cytoxan)—100 to 150 mg/m² of BSA, IV, on day 1

    b) Doxorubicin (Adriamycin)—30 mg/m² of BSA, IV, on day 1

    c) Vincristine (Oncovin)—0.75 mg/m² of BSA, IV, on days 8 and 15

    d) Prednisone—40 to 50 mg/m² of BSA, orally, s.i.d. on days 1 through 7; then, 20 to 25 mg/m² of BSA, orally, q.o.d., on days 8 through 21

    e) Trimethoprim/Sulfadiazine—7 mg/lb, orally, b.i.d.

  5) AMC protocol

    a) Week 1—vincristine (0.025

mg/kg IV) and L-asparaginase (400 IU/kg intraperitoneally (IP)

    b) Week 2—cyclophosphamide (10 mg/kg IV)

    c) Week 3—vincristine (0.025 mg/kg IV) and L-asparaginase (400 IU/kg IP)

    d) Week 4—doxorubicin (30 mg/m² of BSA IV)

  B. Maintenance regimen

  1) Chlorambucil (Leukeran), 20 mg/m² of BSA, orally, every other week; and prednisone, 20 to 25 mg/m² of BSA, orally, every other day

  2) LMP protocol—chlorambucil (Leukeran) and prednisone, as above, plus methotrexate (2.5 to 5 mg/m² of BSA, orally, two or three times a week

  3) COP protocol—used every other week for six cycles, then every third week for six cycles, and then once a month thereafter

  4) AMC protocol—This protocol is used as induction and maintenance therapy.

  C. "Rescue" regimen

  1) The COAP protocol is instituted if the first relapse occurs while the animal is receiving Leukeran and prednisone, or Leukeran, prednisone, and methotrexate.

  2) ADIC protocol

    a) Doxorubicin (Adriamycin)—30 mg/m² of BSA IV, every three weeks

    b) DTIC (Dacarbazine)—1,000 mg/m² of BSA, IV drip, for six to eight hours once every three weeks

  3) L-asparaginase (Elspar)—10,000 to 30,000 IU/m² of BSA, SQ, every two or three weeks

  4) The CHOP protocol is used if the second relapse occurs during treatment with the COAP protocol, or if good response from Adriamycin was previously observed in the patient.

  5) Bleomycin (Blenoxane), 2 to 10 IU/m² of BSA/day, IV continuous drip, for three to five days; cytosine arabinoside (Cytosar-U), 100 mg/m² of BSA/day, IV continuous drip, for four days; and prednisone, 50 mg/m² of BSA, orally, s.i.d., or dexamethasone, 4 to 6 mg/m² of BSA, orally, s.i.d.

  6) Bleomycin, cytosine arabinoside, and prednisone, plus Adriamycin, 30 mg/m² of BSA, IV, every three weeks

---

* The duration of chemotherapy using this protocol is variable.

2. ALL

    A. COAP, CLOP, or COP regimens

    B. Vincristine, 0.5 mg/m^2 of BSA, IV, once a week; L-asparaginase (Elspar), 10,000 to 20,000 IU/m^2 of BSA, SQ, once every four weeks; and prednisone, 40 to 50 mg/m^2 of BSA, orally, s.i.d. on days 1 through 7; then 20 to 25 mg/m^2 of BSA, orally, q.o.d.

3. CLL

    A. Chlorambucil (Leukeran), 20 mg/m^2 of BSA, orally, every other week; prednisone, 20 mg/m^2 of BSA, orally, every other day

    B. Cyclophosphamide (Cytoxan), 50 mg/m^2 of BSA, orally, four days a week; prednisone, 20 mg/m^2 of BSA, orally, every other day

4. AML

    A. Cytosine arabinoside (Cytosar-U), 100 mg/m^2 of BSA/day, IV drip or SQ (divided b.i.d.), for four days; 6-thioguanine (6-TG), 40 to 50 mg/m^2 of BSA, orally, s.i.d. or q.o.d.

    B. Cytosar-U and 6-TG plus Adriamycin (10 mg/m^2 of BSA, IV, on days 2 and 4 of the cycle)

    C. Cytosar-U, 10 mg/m^2 of BSA, SQ, b.i.d. for two weeks, then on alternating weeks

5. CML

    A. Hydroxurea (Hydrea)—50 mg/kg, orally, divided b.i.d., daily or q.o.d. until the WBC returns to normal

6. Multiple myeloma

    A. Melphalan (Alkeran), 2 mg/m^2 of BSA, orally, s.i.d. for one week; then q.o.d.; prednisone, 40 to 50 mg/m^2 of BSA, orally, s.i.d. for one week, then 20 mg/m^2 BSA, orally, q.o.d.

    B. As in III.2

Approach to Diagnosis and Treatment

In order to identify the etiology of the disease process present in a given patient, a thorough history and physical examination should be performed. Once the problems are defined, then a logical diagnostic plan can be formulated. The serum chemical profile may be beneficial in identifying metabolic disease. A urinalysis may provide further information about the urinary tract. Radiographs may demonstrate mass lesions, organomegaly, lymphadenopathy, bony changes, or body fluid accumulations. A bone marrow aspirate may reveal abnormalities in a particular cell line or precursor cells. Fine-needle aspirates of masses or lymph nodes may identify neoplastic cells. Cultures, titers, and biopsies for histopathologic and immunofluorescence studies may also be useful.

Until the disease process has been identified, therapy is directed at supportive measures, such as administering IV fluids, blood products, and antibiotics. Once the diagnosis is established, specific treatment should be instituted.

Suggested Readings

Couto, GC: Oncology. In Sherding RG (ed): The Cat—Diseases and Clinical Management, pp 589–647. New York, Churchill Livingstone, 1989

Couto GC, Jacobs RM: Disorders of leukocytes and leukopoiesis. In Sherding RG (ed): The Cat—Diseases and Clinical Management, pp 557–572. New York, Churchill Livingstone, 1989

Duncan JR, Prasse KW: Veterinary Laboratory Medicine Clinical Pathology, pp 30–67. Ames, Iowa, Iowa State University Press, 1977

Hall RL: Leukocyte responses and abnormalities. In Fenner WR (ed): Quick Reference to Veterinary Medicine, 1st ed, pp 369–382. Philadelphia, JB Lippincott, 1982

Jain NC: Schalm's Veterinary Hematology, 4th ed, pp 103–139, 676–939. Philadelphia, Lea & Febiger, 1986

Prasse KW: White blood cell disorders. In Ettinger SJ (ed): Textbook of Veterinary Internal Medicine, pp 2001–2045. Philadelphia, WB Saunders, 1983

CHAPTER TWENTY-ONE

Interpretation of Biochemical Profiles

M. Judith Radin

···

General Approach

1. Because of the ease of obtaining samples, biochemical profiles, typically measuring 10 or more serum constituents, are a routine part of the patient's data base. As blood is circulated throughout the body, there is continuous exchange of ions, metabolites, and proteins between intracellular and extracellular fluids. Therefore, the composition of the serum, although not a direct measure of the intracellular environment, often reflects the integrity of cell and organ function. Various patterns of change can be expected in biochemical profiles as the result of cellular injury or organ dysfunction. These patterns reflect the leakage of cellular contents into the serum as well as loss of regulation of absorption, production, or excretion of serum components.

2. The biochemical profile will yield the most information when interpreted in conjunction with other parts of the patient's data base, including the history, physical examination, complete blood count, fecal examination, and urinalysis.

3. Often it is necessary to repeat chemistry screens and interpret serial changes.

A. Because the disease state is dynamic, the biochemical profile can be expected to change with the duration and severity of the disease process. Changes in some constitu-

ents will become more or less pronounced as the disease develops.

B. Serial profiles can be useful in monitoring the efficacy or, in some cases, the toxicity of therapy.

C. Sometimes it is necessary to repeat all or part of a profile to determine if a confusing alteration in a serum constituent is real and consistent or false, caused by laboratory or sample handling errors.

4. Normal values

A. A serum sample should be used for determination of a biochemical profile. Anticoagulants such as Na-K EDTA can inhibit enzyme assays as well as add ions such as sodium and potassium to the sample.

B. Because there may be variation in profile values due to the methods, equipment, or technique used, each laboratory must establish its own range of normal values for each species. It is especially important to know if this has been done when using a laboratory that deals primarily with human samples.

C. Some substances can interfere with the accurate measurement of a serum component depending on the methods used. Individual laboratories should furnish information concerning their specific methods. Problems commonly may be caused by hemolysis or lipemia.

1) Correct sample handling including

gentle venipuncture technique and timely removal of serum from the clot can minimize hemolysis.

    2) If possible, a 12-hour fasting sample should be drawn to eliminate postprandial lipemia; however, lipemia that is poorly responsive to fasting may occur in association with pregnancy and some disease states such as pancreatitis, the nephrotic syndrome, hypothyroidism, diabetes mellitus, hyperadrenocorticism, and liver disease. Idiopathic hyperlipemia also occurs in some miniature schnauzers.

    D. Age of the animal must be taken into account when determining if a value is normal. For example

    1) Alkaline phosphatase (ALP) may be increased two to three times the normal adult range in a young, growing animal because of bone growth and remodeling.

    2) Total protein values tend to be lower in young animals because of lower globulin concentrations compared to adults.

Components of a Biochemical Profile

Urea Nitrogen

1. Urea is produced from ammonia exclusively by the liver. Ammonia is generated from amino acid catabolism by cells of the body and by the intestinal flora.

2. Urea is excreted primarily by the kidneys.

3. Increases in urea nitrogen (SUN, also called BUN) (azotemia)

    A. Circulatory impairment can reduce glomerular filtration of urea (prerenal azotemia). This may occur with dehydration, heart disease, or shock.

    1) A urinalysis should reveal concentrated urine with a specific gravity greater than 1.030.

    2) Hematocrit and total protein values also may be increased.

    B. Renal disease in which greater than 75% of the nephrons are lost will result in impaired ability to excrete urea (renal azotemia). A low urine specific gravity (around

1.010) combined with evidence of dehydration (increased total protein and hematocrit) would indicate inability to concentrate the urine and impaired kidney function.

    C. Post-renal azotemia results from obstruction to urine flow at the level of the ureters, bladder, or urethra.

    1) If obstruction is of sufficient degree and duration, increased pressure in the urinary tract will damage renal parenchyma, resulting in secondary renal failure.

    2) Anuria, whether due to obstruction or primary anuric renal failure, may be accompanied by other changes in the biochemical profile including hyperkalemia, hyperphosphatemia, hypocalcemia, a variable degree of hyponatremia and hypochloremia, and hyperproteinemia.

    D. Mild increases are seen with increased protein catabolism (e.g., fever, exercise, starvation, burns, corticosteroids).

4. Decreases in SUN may occur with

    A. Anorexia

    B. Liver disease in which the capacity to convert ammonia to urea is decreased, for example

    1) Portosystemic venous anomolies

    2) End-stage liver disease or cirrhosis

Creatinine

1. Serum creatinine is derived from the breakdown of phosphocreatine, an energy storage molecule, found in skeletal muscle. Small amounts of creatinine also may be absorbed from meat in the diet.

2. The primary excretion route is through the kidneys; however, some may be lost through the gastrointestinal tract. This latter route becomes more important in renal disease with high serum creatinine concentrations. Consequently, serum creatinine levels may not increase proportionately to SUN in patients with renal disease.

3. Creatinine concentration will increase

    A. With renal disease in which greater than 75% of the nephrons are lost

    B. With dehydration and other causes of prerenal azotemia

    C. After a meal, especially one containing meat

D. Mildly with exercise

E. Mildly with muscle wasting due to increased catabolism

Glucose

1. Sources of serum glucose include dietary intake and gluconeogenesis or glycogenolysis by the liver. Blood level and cellular uptake are regulated by insulin and glucagon released from the pancreas. (See also Chapter 22.)

2. Hyperglycemia occurs with

A. Diabetes mellitus

B. Increased endogenous or exogenous glucocorticoids resulting in insulin resistance and augmented gluconeogenesis

   1) Hyperadrenocorticism

   2) Stress (e.g., after surgery)

   3) Exogenously administered corticosteroids

C. Excitement due to catecholamine release. This is especially seen in cats.

D. After a meal

E. Convulsions

F. Drugs such as xylazine, ACTH, morphine

G. Estrus or progestagen administration in some older female dogs

H. Megestrol acetate therapy in some cats

3. Hypoglycemia occurs with

A. Prolonged exposure of the serum to the clot in the sample tube resulting in use of glucose by blood cells. Sodium fluoride may be used as an anticoagulant to inhibit glucose oxidation. Because sodium fluoride will interfere with other tests, plasma from this tube cannot be used to run the rest of the biochemical profile.

B. Sepsis (variable)

C. Severe liver disease due to decreased insulin clearance and gluconeogenic capacity

D. Hypoadrenocorticism

E. Starvation

F. Intestinal malabsorption

G. Insulinoma (neoplasia of pancreatic beta cells)

H. Neoplasia in which glucose consumption by the tumor is high

I. Glycogen storage disease

Sodium

1. Sodium is the most abundant extracellular cation. It is excreted primarily by the kidney and blood levels are tightly regulated by the renin–angiotensin–aldosterone system. Aldosterone promotes sodium reabsorption by the kidney tubules in exchange for potassium.

2. Increases (hypernatremia) occur with

A. Dehydration

B. Hyperaldosteronism (rare)

3. Decreases (hyponatremia) occur with:

A. Anorexia or dietary deficiency

B. Diarrhea

C. Vomiting

D. Renal disease

E. Diabetes mellitus

F. Hypoadrenocorticism

G. Bladder rupture

Potassium

1. Potassium is primarily an intracellular cation, therefore its concentration in the serum is low and may not reflect body potassium status.

2. Excretion is through the kidney in exchange for sodium or hydrogen ions.

3. Serum concentrations are responsive to acid–base balance.

A. If the animal is acidotic, hydrogen ions will move into cells while potassium moves extracellularly.

   1) Serum potassium level will continue to be regulated by renal excretion, resulting in depletion of body stores. This potassium deficiency may be masked, however, because serum concentrations remain within the normal range.

   2) Consequently, care must be taken when correcting acidosis with fluid therapy because serious hypokalemia may result if potassium supplementation is not given concurrently.

B. Hypokalemia may occur during alkalosis as potassium moves into cells in exchange for hydrogen ions.

4. Increases (hyperkalemia) occur with

A. Renal failure

B. Urinary tract obstruction

C. Hypoadrenocorticism

D. Dehydration

E. Acidosis

5. Decreases (hypokalemia) occur with

A. Vomiting

B. Diarrhea

C. Hyperadrenocorticism

D. Alkalosis

E. Insulin therapy. Hypokalemia may occur in association with an influx of glucose into cells after insulin therapy. This is a potential complication seen when treating diabetic ketoacidosis.

F. Loop diuretic therapy (e.g., furosemide)

G. Fanconi syndrome

H. Anorexia

I. Primary hyperaldosteronism

J. Renal distal and sometimes proximal tubular acidosis

K. Developing renal disease in the cat

Chloride

1. Chloride is found in high concentrations in the extracellular fluid and its concentration is regulated by the kidney. During tubular reabsorption, bicarbonate ion initially is paired with sodium to maintain electrical neutrality. When bicarbonate is depleted from the filtrate, chloride is paired with sodium for further reabsorption.

2. Increases (hyperchloremia) occur with

A. Causes of metabolic acidosis, because more chloride is reabsorbed when filtered bicarbonate is low

B. Renal tubular acidosis

3. Decreases (hypochloremia) occur with

A. Vomiting, because chloride is paired with hydrogen ion during gastric acid secretion

B. Anorexia or malnutrition

C. Secretory diarrhea due to bacterial enterotoxins

D. Diabetes insipidus

E. Hypochloremia often is associated with hypokalemia.

Calcium

1. Serum calcium levels are regulated by the interaction of parathyroid hormone, calcitonin, and vitamin D.

2. The sources of serum calcium include absorption from the gastrointestinal tract in response to vitamin D and mobilization from bone in response to parathyroid hormone.

3. Excretion is mainly through the kidneys.

4. Calcium is deposited in the bone in response to calcitonin.

5. Calcium is found in two forms in the blood.

A. The ionized form, which is metabolically active and regulated hormonally

B. The inactive nonionized form, which is bound to albumin

C. Consequently, serum calcium levels vary with serum protein or albumin levels. In addition, hydrogen ions can displace bound calcium from albumin, resulting in a greater proportion of calcium in the ionized form and a lower total calcium concentration. This may be seen in conditions associated with acidosis.

6. Increases (hypercalcemia) occur with

A. Primary hyperparathyroidism

B. Pseudohyperparathyroidism

1) Lymphosarcoma

2) Apocrine gland carcinoma of the anal sac

C. Hypervitaminosis D

D. Osteolytic disease including primary and metastatic tumors and septic osteomyelitis

E. Multiple myeloma

F. Hypoadrenocorticism

G. Disuse osteoporosis

H. Renal failure (rare)

7. Decreases (hypocalcemia) occur with

A. Necrotizing pancreatitis—Calcium soaps are formed when fat surrounding the pancreas undergoes necrosis after enzyme release by damaged pancreatic acinar cells.

B. Hypoproteinemia

1) To determine if hypocalcemia is caused by hypoproteinemia, the following formula may be used

corrected calcium =
(actual serum calcium concentration
− actual serum albumin concentration)
+ 3.5

      a) If the corrected calcium falls within the normal range, then hypocalcemia is probably due to hypoproteinemia.

      b) If the corrected calcium is still low, look for other causes of hypocalcemia.

  C. Puerperal tetany (eclampsia)

  D. Hypoparathyroidism

  E. Hypercalcitoninism due to a thyroid C cell tumor

  F. Calcium may be normal to low with renal secondary hyperparathyroidism or nutritional secondary hyperparathyroidism.

  G. Fanconi syndrome

  H. Renal tubular acidosis

Phosphorus

1. Phosphorus, like potassium, is primarily located in cells and in bone. Consequently, its serum concentration does not necessarily reflect body stores.

2. Parathyroid hormone regulates serum phosphorus levels by decreasing tubular reabsorption in the kidney.

3. Phosphorus will move into cells in exchange for hydrogen ions and in conjunction with the influx of glucose in response to insulin therapy. Consequently, phosphorus concentrations often follow the patterns described for potassium.

4. Increases (hyperphosphotemia) occur with

  A. Nutritional secondary hyperparathyroidism

  B. Renal secondary hyperparathyroidism

  C. Anuria

  D. Hypoparathyroidism

  E. Fracture healing (mild increase)

  F. Ethylene glycol toxicity due to phosphate additives found in commercial antifreeze.

5. Decreases (hypophosphotemia) occur with

  A. Primary hyperparathyroidism

  B. Pseudohyperparathyroidism

  C. Hypercalcitoninism (thyroid C cell tumor)

  D. Insulin therapy in diabetic ketacidosis

  E. Fanconi syndrome

  F. Renal tubular acidosis

  G. Hyperadrenocorticism

Total Protein

1. Total protein consists of albumin and globulin fractions.

2. Total protein and albumin usually are measured in the serum. Globulin concentration is derived by subtracting albumin from the total protein determination.

3. Changes in total protein may reflect changes in albumin concentrations, globulin concentrations, or both, as outlined below.

Albumin

1. Albumin is synthesized by the liver. It is catabolized by peripheral tissues and has a half-life of seven to ten days.

2. Two major functions of albumin are

  A. Maintenance of osmotic pressure of the plasma

  B. As a carrier for transporting various hormones, ions, and drugs

3. Increases (hyperproteinemia) occur with dehydration. Concurrent elevations in total protein, globulin, and hematocrit (if the patient is not anemic) will occur.

4. Decreases (hypoproteinemia) occur with

  A. Protein-losing glomerulonephropathy (nephrotic syndrome)

  B. Protein-losing enteropathy

  C. Intestinal malabsorption

  D. Pancreatic exocrine insufficiency

  E. Parasites

  F. Starvation

  G. Liver disease with decreased production

  H. Increased catabolism with hyperadrenocorticism

  I. Hypergammaglobulinemic states— Synthesis of albumin by the liver is decreased.

  J. Fanconi syndrome

  K. Burns and other exudative skin lesions

Globulin

1. This portion of serum proteins includes the immunoglobulins and various transport proteins.

2. Increases may be seen with inflammation, infection, antigenic stimulation, neoplasia, or abnormal immunoglobulin production (multiple myeloma).

3. Mild decreases may be seen with immunodeficiency states and in young animals.

4. Fractionation into alpha, beta, and gamma portions can be done using electrophoretic techniques. This is not a routine part of the biochemical profile.

   A. Alpha globulins (acute phase reactive proteins) may increase with inflammation or liver disease.

   B. A polyclonal hypergammaglobulinemia may occur with chronic antigenic stimulation (e.g., canine erhlichiosis, feline infectious peritonitis).

   C. Monoclonal gammopathies usually are associated with abnormal immunoglobulin production in plasma cell dyscrasias.

   D. Rarely, a monoclonal gammopathy may occur with feline infectious peritonitis or canine erhlichiosis.

   E. Hypogammaglobulinemia may occur with immunodeficiency states where antibody production is impaired (e.g., combined immunodeficiency in basset hounds or weimaraners).

Bilirubin

1. Bilirubin results from the breakdown of heme by the mononuclear–phagocyte system. Hemoglobin from erythrocytes is the primary source of heme, but myoglobin and some heme-containing enzymes also contribute.

2. Prehepatic bilirubin (also called indirect, free, or unconjugated bilirubin) is released into circulation where it binds to albumin for transport to the liver.

3. The liver removes the unconjugated bilirubin from circulation, conjugates it with glucaronide (now called conjugated, direct, or posthepatic bilirubin), and excretes it into the bile.

4. Total bilirubin measurements include both forms of bilirubin. Hyperbilirubinemia will result from elevations in one or a combination of both forms, depending on the cause. Biochemical differentiation of conjugated and unconjugated bilirubin requires an additional procedure called the Van den Bergh test. The source of hyperbilirubinemia often may be ascertained using the history, physical examination, and other laboratory findings, however.

5. Unconjugated hyperbilirubinemia occurs with

   A. Moderate to severe hemolysis
      1) The hematocrit should be decreased.
      2) Blood film examination may help establish the cause.

   B. Mild hemolysis, if liver function is compromised

6. Conjugated hyperbilirubinemia occurs with

   A. Cholestasis
      1) Extrahepatic obstruction produces greater elevations in bilirubin than intrahepatic obstruction.
      2) Alkaline phosphatase should be elevated with cholestasis.

   B. Severe hepatocellular disease resulting in impaired secretion of bilirubin

7. Mixed conjugated and unconjugated hyperbilirubinemia occurs

   A. Most often

   B. With hemolysis associated with secondary hepatocellular injury from hypoxia

   C. With hepatocellular damage secondary to obstructive disease, resulting in a decrease in the liver's ability to uptake and conjugate bilirubin

   D. A rule of thumb suggests that if greater than 50% of total bilirubin is unconjugated bilirubin, hemolysis is indicated. If greater than 50% is conjugated, cholestasis or hepatocellular disease is indicated. Again, interpret this in conjunction with other clinical and laboratory findings.

Cholesterol

1. The main source of serum cholesterol is hepatic synthesis. Some also is absorbed from the diet by the small intestine.

2. Cholesterol is used for steroid hormone production. The major pathway for excretion is through the bile.

3. Increases occur with

A. Protein-losing nephropathies (nephrotic syndrome). The mechanism for this is not understood.

B. Hypothyroidism. Two thirds of the cases in one survey had hypercholesterolemia.

C. Cholestasis. Retention or reflux of biliary cholesterol as well as increased hepatic cholesterol production occurs.

D. Hyperadrenocorticism

E. Protein-losing enteropathy

F. Postprandial lipemia

G. Lipemia associated with diabetes mellitus, starvation, acute necrotizing pancreatitis, and steatitis (in the cat)

H. Idiopathic hyperlipoproteinemia in the miniature schnauzer

1) Cholesterol is moderately elevated.

2) Triglycerides are markedly increased.

4. Decreases occur with

A. Fat maldigestion

B. Portosystemic vascular anomalies in which there is increased conversion to bile acids.

Bile Acids

1. The use and availability of this test for liver function has become increasingly widespread in recent years.

2. Bile acids are formed by conjugation of cholesterol with an amino acid such as taurine or glycine in the hepatocytes. Bile acids are subsequently secreted into the bile and stored in the gall bladder between meals.

3. During a meal, bile acids are secreted into the intestinal tract to aid in fat absorption. Bile acids are reabsorbed in the ileum, filtered from the blood by the liver, and recycled.

4. In a normal fasted animal, bile acids are essentially absent from the blood. Levels may normally increase about four times by two hours after a meal.

5. Bile acid concentrations increase in all forms of liver disease due to a decrease in the ability of the liver to clear them from the

blood during enterohepatic circulation. In some cases of portosystemic vascular anomalies and cirrhosis, fasting bile acid concentrations may be only mildly elevated or within the normal range. Increases will be more pronounced if sampling is done two hours after a meal.

6. This may be the only abnormal parameter of liver disease seen in animals with portosystemic shunts.

Alanine Aminotransferase

1. This is a liver-specific enzyme in dogs and cats that increases with hepatocellular damage.

2. Increases may be seen with hepatic necrosis or with milder, reversible damage in which hepatocytes become "leaky" but do not die.

3. Examples in which alanine aminotransferase (ALT, formerly SGPT) may be increased include

A. Hepatitis

B. Neoplasia

C. Hepatic lipidosis secondary to metabolic disturbances

1) Diabetes mellitus

2) Megesterol acetate (Ovaban) therapy in cats

D. Steroid hepatopathy secondary to hyperadrenocorticism or glucocorticoid administration.

E. Hypoxia

F. Various toxins

G. Cholestasis if secondary hepatocyte injury occurs.

4. A single insult will result in elevations of ALT that decline over time. An ongoing insult results in sustained or increasing levels.

5. ALT may be within the normal range in patients with portosystemic shunts or in advanced cirrhosis.

6. Some drugs such as anticonvulsants can induce increased enzyme production in the dog. This does not seem to occur in the cat.

Asparate Aminotransferase

1. This enzyme is found in many tissues including liver, skeletal muscle, cardiac muscle, and erythrocytes.

2. In liver disease, asparate aminotransferase (AST, formerly SGOT) levels will follow those of ALT.

3. Increases also may be seen with muscle necrosis.

4. This enzyme should be interpreted in conjunction with ALT.

    A. Increased ALT with normal to mild increases in AST may indicate reversible, milder liver damage.

    B. Marked elevations in both AST and ALT may indicate hepatocellular necrosis.

    C. Increased AST with normal ALT may indicate that the source of the AST was not the liver.

Alkaline Phosphatase

1. Alkaline phosphatase (ALP) is present in many tissues including liver, bone, intestine, kidney, placenta, and some leukocytes. Only the isoenzymes produced by the liver, bone, or in response to corticosteroids have serum half-lives long enough to be clinically detectable.

2. It is possible to separate ALP isoenzymes using electrophoretic techniques, but this technology is not widely available. Recently, a simple assay for differentiating liver and steroid-induced ALP isoenzymes has been described for use with canine serum. The method is based on the greater inhibition of activity of the liver isoenzyme by levamisole, as compared to the steroid-induced isoenzyme. This method is readily adaptable to automated chemistry analyzers and is increasingly being adopted by clinical pathology laboratories. A drawback is that it will not allow differentiation between liver and bone isoenzymes. Whether or not a method for distinguishing ALP isoenzymes is available, interpretation of ALP concentrations in conjunction with the rest of the patient's data base will help clarify the clinical situation.

3. The liver isoenzyme of ALP will increase with

    A. Cholestasis, bile duct obstruction, or if there is sufficient hepatocellular swelling to cause intrahepatic cholestasis.

        1) Hyperbilirubinemia may be seen.

        2) Because of the shorter serum half-life and lower tissue concentrations of ALP, cats show variable response of ALP to cholestasis. Therefore, even small elevations in ALP (two to three times) are considered significant.

    B. Anticonvulsant drugs in dogs

4. The bone isoenzyme of ALP will increase with

    A. Bone growth and remodeling in young animals. A two- to three-fold higher concentration is expected compared with adults.

    B. Any disease in which bone remodeling or osteolysis occurs, such as

        1) Panosteitis

        2) Fractures

        3) Osteolytic neoplasms

        4) Secondary hyperparathyroidism

        5) Osteomyelitis

5. Liver production of a specific steroid-induced ALP isoenzyme occurs with increased endogenous (hyperadenocorticism) or exogenously administered glucocorticoids in the dog. Levels of this isoenzyme may become high and remain elevated for extended periods of time. This does not seem to occur in the cat.

Lactate Dehydrogenase

1. Lactate dehydrogenase (LDH) enzyme is found in most tissues, including liver, muscle, and erythrocytes.

2. Consequently, elevations are nonspecific.

Gamma Glutamyltransferase

1. Gamma glutamyltransferase (GGT) is found in liver, pancreas, and kidney; however, elevations in serum concentration usually are caused by the liver enzyme.

2. In small animals, increases in GGT reflect cholestasis and will parallel increases in ALP.

3. GGT may increase with glucocorticoid or anticonvulsant therapy.

4. Mild elevations occur in portosystemic vascular anomalies.

Amylase

1. Amylase is a pancreatic exocrine enzyme that is released into the circulation and peritoneal cavity after pancreatic necrosis. Other tissues that contain amylase include the liver and intestinal mucosa.

2. Causes of increased serum amylase concentrations include

A. Acute pancreatitis

1) Amylase concentrations will usually exceed two times the normal concentration.

2) In chronic pancreatitis with fibrosis, serum enzyme levels may be normal.

B. Renal failure—Amylase concentrations can increase 2.5 times the normal concentration due to decreased renal excretion and metabolism.

C. Hyperadrenocorticism

D. Liver disease

E. Upper gastrointestinal tract inflammation or obstruction

3. Be sure that the laboratory uses the amyloclastic or dye-starch procedures to measure amylase concentrations. The saccharogenic method may result in false elevations of amylase in dogs.

4. Amylase concentrations are not useful in cats.

Lipase

1. Lipase is a digestive enzyme produced by the pancreas and gastric mucosa. It has a short half-life of two hours. Levels tend to parallel serum amylase.

2. Hyperlipasemia occurs with

A. Acute pancreatitis, resulting in three-fold to four-fold elevations

1) Lipase determination is considered to be a better test than amylase assay for the dedication of pancreatitis. Lipase activities may remain elevated longer than amylase.

2) With chronic pancreatic fibrosis, levels may be normal.

3) Some cats with pancreatitis may not be identified using lipase.

B. Renal failure. Lipase concentrations may increase three to four times normal concentrations.

C. Hyperadrenocorticism

D. Dexamethasone treatment

E. Biliary tract disease, cirrhosis

Creatine Phosphokinase

1. Isoenzymes of creatine phosphokinase (CK, CPK) are found in skeletal muscle, cardiac muscle, and brain.

2. CK may be released from muscle as a result of leakage from reversible cellular damage or from necrosis.

A. Because of its short half-life, CK will begin to decrease within one to two days after cellular leakage ceases. CK concentration will decline more rapidly than AST.

B. If CK levels remain persistently high, muscle damage is ongoing.

3. Strenuous exercise may mildly increase CK concentrations.

4. Although brain CK isoenzyme concentrations increase in the cerebral spinal fluid in association with some forms of central nervous system disease, CK rarely crosses the blood–brain barrier in sufficient quantity to be detected in the serum.

Diagnostic Approach

1. Certain patterns of change in serum components are expected with disease in the various organ systems. Therefore, a helpful approach to interpreting the biochemical profile is to group constituents by organ system, rather than trying to interpret fluctuations in each value individually. For example

A. Renal disease (SUN, creatinine, electrolytes)

1) Look for elevations in SUN and creatinine caused by impaired glomerular filtration.

2) Potassium and phosphorus concentrations may be increased caused by decreased renal excretion.

3) Hyponatremia caused by sodium wasting may be present.

4) Hypocalcemia caused by impaired renal conservation, decreased vitamin D synthesis with subsequent decreased gastrointestinal absorption, and elevated phosphorus concentrations may be present.

B. Liver disease (ALT, AST, ALP, GGT, bilirubin, bile acids, glucose, cholesterol).

1) Hepatocellular injury or death may result in increased serum ALT, AST, and bile acids, and in decreased glucose (due to impaired gluconeogenesis).

2) Cholestasis is associated with increased ALP, GGT, bilirubin, bile acids, and cholesterol.

3) Combinations of hepatocellular injury and cholestasis can produce all of the changes mentioned above.

4) Portosystemic vascular anomalies or end-stage cirrhosis may be associated with little alteration in the serum biochemical profile.

C. Adrenal gland-related disease

1) The adrenal glands produce several important steroid hormones that regulate metabolism (glucocorticoids) and fluid and electrolyte balance (aldosterone and glucocorticoids). Insufficient or excess production of these hormones will result in alterations of those serum biochemical constituents that are regulated by the target organs for these hormones. This includes the liver (glucocorticoids) and kidney (aldosterone, glucocorticoids).

2) In hyperadrenocorticism, ALP concentration is increased because of increased liver production of the steroid-specific isoenzyme. Other liver enzymes such as ALT and AST may be elevated as disease progresses because of the development of "steroid hepatopathy." Other metabolic alterations include mild hyperglycemia and hypercholesterolemia. Alterations in serum electrolytes subsequent to mineralocorticoid and glucocorticoid effects on the kidney include a mild hypernatremia, hypokalemia, and hypophosphatemia in some patients.

3) In hypoadrenocorticism, prominent changes include hyponatremia and hyperkalemia (Na : K ratio < 20 : 1) caused by aldosterone deficiency. Mild hypercalcemia sometimes occurs. Prerenal azotemia (increased SUN and creatinine) may develop subsequent to hypovolemia, hypotension, and inadequate tissue perfusion. If the liver becomes hypoxic, elevations in ALT and AST may be seen. Occasionally, dogs with Addison's syndrome still produce sufficient quantities of mineralocorticoids so that the electrolyte alterations are not seen. In these cases, insufficient glucocorticoid production must be demonstrated using other tests, such as the ACTH stimulation test. Rarely, dogs with gastrointestinal disease and diarrhea may present with hyponatremia and hyperkalemia. They must be differentiated from those with true hypoadrenocorticism on the basis of ACTH stimulation testing.

2. Multiple problems in the patient can superimpose changes in serum constituents, resulting in biochemical profiles that are not "typical." For example

A. Anorexia

1) In anorexic patients with renal disease, the rises in serum potassium and phosphorus may be blunted as a result of decreased intake.

2) Anorexia will also exacerbate any tendency toward hypoglycemia or hypocalcemia.

B. Vomiting or diarrhea can cause marked alterations in acid–base status and electrolyte concentrations because of external losses of ions and failure of normal absorption.

3. By performing serial biochemical profiles, the progression of disease can be monitored by following patterns of change in serum constituents.

Suggested Readings

Center SA: Biochemical evaluation of hepatic function in the dog and cat. In Kirk RW (ed): Current Veterinary Therapy IX: Small Anim Pract, pp 924–936. Philadelphia, WB Saunders, 1986

Ettinger SJ: Textbook of Veterinary Internal Medicine: Diseases of the Dog and Cat, 2nd ed. Philadelphia, WB Saunders, 1983

Feldman EC, Peterson ME: Hypoadrenocorticism. Vet Clin North Am: Small Anim

Prac, pp 751–766. Philadelphia, WB Saunders, 1984

Kaneko JJ: Clinical Biochemistry of Domestic Animals, 4th ed. New York, Academic Press, 1989

Peterson ME: Hyperadrenocorticism. Vet Clin North Am: Small Anim Pract, pp 731–749. Philadelphia, WB Saunders, 1984

Strombeck DR, Farver T, Kaneko JJ: Serum amylase and lipase activities in the diagnosis of pancreatitis in dogs. Am J Vet Res 42: 1966–1970, 1981

CHAPTER TWENTY-TWO

Hypoglycemia and Hyperglycemia

Deborah J. Davenport and Dennis J. Chew

Glucose Abnormalities

1. A glucose plasma value of 70 to 120 mg/dL (with some variation dependent on laboratory method) is considered normal or euglycemic. In cases suspected of glucose abnormality, sample blood glucose values during a 24-hour fast, because postprandial increases in blood glucose are to be expected.

2. The existing blood glucose value is a function of intestinal absorption of glucose, hepatic production of glucose, and the amount of glucose consumed or taken up by peripheral tissues (Fig. 22-1).

3. The balance between hepatic production and peripheral uptake of glucose is greatly influenced by the hormones insulin, glucagon, cortisol, ACTH, growth hormone, and the sympathetic amines epinephrine and norepinephrine.

Gluconeogenesis

1. Glucose is synthesized from lactate, pyruvate, odd-chain fatty acids, and most amino acids.

2. Amino acids are quantitatively most important, with alanine as the major contributor.

3. Glucocorticoids, catecholamines, and glucagon all stimulate gluconeogenesis and raise the fasting blood glucose level.

4. Insulin inhibits gluconeogenesis and lowers the fasting blood glucose level.

5. During prolonged starvation the kidneys contribute half of the glucose synthesized.

6. Gluconeogenesis is the primary source of glucose after 24 hours of fasting.

7. Glucose-6-phosphate is manufactured from other nutrients and is converted to glucose by glucose-6-phosphatase.

Glycogenolysis

1. The breakdown of glycogen and the subsequent production of glucose occurs predominantly in the liver.

2. Other tissues (brain, muscle, heart) also contain glycogen.

3. Glucose-6-phosphatase is the enzyme necessary for free glucose formation.

4. Only the liver contains enough glucose-6-phosphatase to produce more glucose than it can use, resulting in subsequent release of excess glucose into the bloodstream.

5. Glucagon and epinephrine stimulate glycogenolysis. Glucagon acts in the liver only, whereas epinephrine acts in both muscle and liver.

6. Glycogenolysis and gluconeogenesis in the liver account for more than 90% of all endogenous production of glucose.

Normal Insulin Physiology

1. Proinsulin, a large single-chain polypeptide, is synthesized in beta cells of the pancreas.

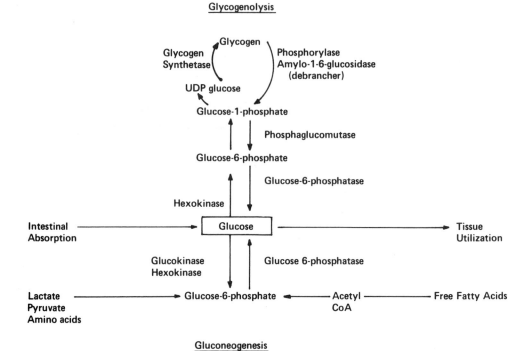

Figure 22-1.   *The existing blood glucose value depends on a balance between gluconeogenesis, glycogenolysis, intestinal absorption, and tissue use.*

2. Proinsulin cleaves into a connecting strand (C-peptide) and the smaller double-chain insulin molecule.

3. These are packaged within the cell in equimolar amounts and are released when stimulation of insulin secretion occurs.

4. The concentration of glucose in the blood perfusing the pancreas is the most important determinant of insulin secretion.

5. The route of glucose entry into the body and the blood glucose concentration determine the magnitude of insulin release. Glucose doses given orally result in a higher blood insulin concentration than an equivalent IV dose, because of release of GI hormones when glucose contacts the intestinal mucosa. (Gastric inhibitory polypeptide [GIP] may be of most importance.)

6. Amino acids, especially leucine and arginine, also stimulate insulin secretion.

7. Growth hormone and glucocorticoids cause a primary increase in circulating insulin. They also cause hyperglycemia, which could result in a secondary increase in insulin secretion.

8. There is also a constant secretion of insulin when no other stimulus is present (0.5 to 1.0 U/hr in humans), which should vary in direct proportion to the serum glucose concentration.

9. The precise mechanism of action of insulin is not known.

10. It is well established that tissues vary in sensitivity and responsiveness to insulin. With muscle and adipose tissue, insulin probably acts on cell membrane permeability, facilitating entry of glucose into these cells. The liver normally shows no permeability barrier to glucose. Insulin's effect in the liver appears to be on glycogen, inhibiting glycogenolysis and facilitating glycogen synthesis. The liver contains two enzymes for phosphorylation, a hexokinase that is insulin independent and a glucokinase that is insulin dependent (Table 22-1).

11. Insulin facilitates the uptake, use, and storage of glucose, fat, and amino acids. A deficiency of insulin leads to mobilization of body tissue stores for energy and reduces tissue uptake of ingested nutrients. Liver, muscle, and fat are the tissues predominantly affected (see Table 22-1).

Insulin Effects on Carbohydrate Metabolism

1. The liver is the most important site of insulin activity on carbohydrates.

2. The liver is more sensitive than adipose tissue or muscle to small increases in plasma insulin.

3. Insulin secretion after a carbohydrate meal promotes glucose uptake and storage in the liver.

4. Insulin also inhibits gluconeogenesis by inhibiting hepatic uptake of alanine, the key gluconeogenic precursor. This inhibition of gluconeogenesis requires greater concentrations of insulin than does inhibition of glycogenolysis.

5. The stimulatory effect of glucagon on glycogenolysis and gluconeogenesis is minimized by insulin.

6. The glucose retained within the liver is used for glycogen synthesis and triglyceride synthesis.

Insulin Effects on Protein Metabolism

1. Insulin facilitates transfer of amino acids from the intestine to muscle after protein ingestion. This effect is most marked for the branched-chain amino acids valine, isoleucine, and leucine. These amino acids are unique in their ability to escape liver uptake or metabolism after intestinal absorption, which accounts for more than 60% of the total amino acids entering the circulation after a protein meal.

2. Insulin increases the rate of protein synthesis in muscle and inhibits protein catabolism. This helps to maintain nitrogen balance in the interval between feeding and adds to its direct inhibitory effect on hepatic gluconeogenesis, because fewer amino acid precursors are available.

Insulin Effects on Fat

1. Insulin stimulates lipoprotein lipase, which increases uptake of endogenous triglycerides by adipose tissue.

2. Insulin inhibits a hormone-sensitive lipase in the fat cell, which otherwise catalyzes both the hydrolysis of stored triglycerides and the liberation of free fatty acids. A smaller concentration of insulin is needed to inhibit lipolysis than to affect glucose transport.

3. The major site of insulin-mediated fat synthesis is the liver.

4. Much of the insulin-mediated glucose uptake by the fat cells is used for alphaglycerophosphate formation, which is necessary

Table 22-1. **Action of insulin**

	Liver	*Adipose Tissue*	*Muscle*
Anticatabolic effects	Glycogenolysis	Lipolysis	Protein catabolism
	Gluconeogenesis		Amino acid output
	Ketogenesis		
Anabolic effects	Glycogen synthesis	Glycerol synthesis	Amino acid uptake
	Fatty acid	Fatty acid	Protein synthesis
			Glycogen synthesis

for esterification of fatty acids to form triglyc-erides. Some of this glucose is used for fatty acid synthesis.

Ketones

1. Ketone formation (beta-hydroxybutrate, acetoacetate, acetone) occurs when fatty acids are mobilized from adipose tissue and delivered to the liver, where they are oxidized to acetyl Co-A. Acetyl Co-A is further metabolized to ketones.

2. Low concentrations of ketones are normally present in blood and depend on the balance between production, use, and excretion.

3. Insulin has a suppressive effect on circulating blood ketones.

    A. Insulin reduces ketone formation by its antilipolytic effect and its stimulation of fatty acid synthesis.

    B. Insulin also decreases the liver's ability to oxidize free fatty acids. This is accomplished by lowering hepatic carnitine levels. Carnitine is important in the formation of acyl-carnitine transferase, an enzyme necessary in the transfer of fatty acids across the mitochondrial membrane to the site of beta-oxidative enzymes. Also, acyl-carnitine transferase is inhibited by malonyl Co-A, the first intermediate product in the synthesis of fatty acids from acetyl Co-A, which insulin enhances.

4. Uptake and oxidation of ketones by muscle are increased in the presence of insulin.

Normal Glucagon Physiology

1. Glucagon is secreted by the alpha cells of the islets of Langerhans. A glucagon similar to pancreatic glucagon also is believed to be excreted by the alpha cells of the gastric fundus and duodenum.

2. Glucagon is secreted in response to

    A. Insulin-induced hypoglycemia

    B. Starvation

    C. Ingestion of protein meals

    D. IV or oral administration of certain amino acids (arginine, alanine)

    E. Pancreozymin

    F. Gastroinhibitory polypeptide

    G. Exercise and stress

3. Glucagon stimulates hepatic glycogenolysis by increasing cyclic 3'5'-adenosine monophosphate (AMP), which leads to increased phosphorylase activity. Glucagon also inhibits hepatic glycogen synthetase through cyclic AMP. Both of these actions elevate plasma glucose concentration.

4. Glucagon stimulates gluconeogenesis by promoting hepatic uptake of amino acids.

5. Incorporation of amino acids into liver protein is inhibited by glucagon. This results in increased excretion of urinary nitrogen.

6. Lipolysis in liver and adipose tissue is stimulated in the presence of glucagon by activation of the adenyl-cyclase system. The resulting increased hepatic concentration of free fatty acids stimulates hepatic gluconeogenesis and ketogenesis.

7. Rapid increases of blood glucose inhibit secretion of glucagon.

8. Glucagon prevents hypoglycemia during nonglucose- (e.g., protein-) stimulated insulin secretion.

9. Glucagon antagonizes the inhibitory action of basal levels of insulin on hepatic glucose production in postabsorptive states.

Hypoglycemia

1. Hypoglycemia exists when measured blood glucose values are 50 mg/dL or less.

2. Hypoglycemia is not a disease but a secondary sign of an underlying disease that results in abnormal glucose homeostasis.

3. Hepatic glycogen stores begin to be exhausted within 24 hours of fasting. Adequate gluconeogenesis is needed to supply the necessary glucose.

4. The major detrimental effect of hypoglycemia is seen in the brain.

    A. The CNS depends almost exclusively on glucose as its energy substrate.

    B. Glucose entrance into the neuron occurs primarily by diffusion and is not insulin dependent.

    C. Cerebral cells have limited stores of glycogen and have a limited capacity to use protein and amino acid pools for energy.

D. Clinical features of hypoglycemia parallel those seen with cerebral hypoxia, although some histologic and physiologic differences exist.

1) Cerebral impairment probably reflects a decline in energy-rich phosphory-lated compounds, mainly adenosine triphos-phate (ATP), due to diminished glucose avail-ability for oxidation.

2) The acute changes in neurogluco-penia may result in cellular hypoxia with attendant increased vascular permeability, vasospasm, and vascular dilation. Neuron death from anoxia follows.

3) Acute histologic alterations include scattered petechiae, congestion, and nerve swelling; the lesions are identical to those of anoxia. In advanced cases, the brain shows spotty ischemic necrosis with shrunken neu-rons and pyknotic nuclei. The perineuronal spaces are enlarged from demyelination. These reactions are most marked in the cere-bral cortex, basal ganglia, hippocampus, and vasomotor centers. Most of the damage caused by hypoglycemia occurs in the brain, but peripheral nerve degeneration and demye-lination is sometimes encountered.

4) Prolonged, severe hypoglycemia may result in irreversible brain damage.

a) Hypoxic damage occurs be-cause of decreased metabolism and subse-quent lack of oxygenation of the neuron.

b) Cerebral edema is present.

c) Laminar necrosis is seen histo-logically.

Signs of Hypoglycemia

1. Clinical signs are related to the degree of hypoglycemia, the rate of decline of blood glucose, and the duration of hypoglycemia. Signs of hypoglycemia are similar regardless of the underlying cause.

2. Usually signs do not develop until the blood glucose level is less than 45 mg/dL. Cases have been reported of apparently clini-cally normal dogs with much lower blood glucose values.

3. Mild signs

A. Incoordination

B. Rear-leg weakness

C. Excessive appetite

D. Generalized weakness

4. Moderate signs

A. Amaurosis

B. Personality changes

C. Drowsiness

D. Confused mental states

E. Abnormal behavior (e.g., running, head pressing, barking, hysteria)

F. Muscle twitching

5. Severe signs

A. Seizures

B. Coma

6. Signs associated with a rapid decline in blood glucose levels are partly the result of activation of the autonomic nervous system and epinephrine release.

A. Shaking

B. Trembling

C. Tachycardia

D. Vomiting

E. Weakness

F. Hunger

G. Nervousness

7. Signs associated with a slower fall in blood glucose levels are mainly due to CNS depression (neuroglycopenia).

8. The signs of hypoglycemia are usually intermittent; consequently, consider hypogly-cemia in any case of episodic weakness (see Chapter 7). The signs may or may not be progressive depending on the underlying cause.

9. Whipple's triad

A. Signs of hypoglycemia are present, blood glucose is low, and the patient re-sponds to the administration of glucose.

B. The above criteria confirm that the signs are due to hypoglycemia.

C. No cause is indicated, however.

Causes of Hypoglycemia

Summary of Causes

Improper handling of blood sample*
Laboratory error

---

* Most important in small animals

Functional hypoglycemia
    Idiopathic neonatal disease*
    For working dogs, severe exercise
    Nutrient deficiency
        Starvation
        Competition from parasites
    Glucagon or epinephrine deficiency
Glycogen storagelike disease
    von Gierke's disease
    Cori's disease
Exogenous agents, iatrogenic
    Insulin excess*
    Sulfonylurea, salicylate, ethanol (humans)
Insulinoma (functional beta cell pancreatic tumor)*
Extrapancreatic tumor-induced disease
    Hepatoma*
    Pulmonary carcinoma
    Metastatic mammary carcinoma
    Melanoma
    Salivary adenocarcinoma
    Hemangiosarcoma
    Metastatic liver neoplasia
    Polycythemia vera
Severe hepatic disease or portovascular anomalies
Adrenocortical insufficiency*
Endotoxemia*
Hypopituitarism
Renal glycosuria
Pregnancy

1. Improper handling of blood samples may result in a faulty diagnosis of hypoglycemia in the patient.

  A. Whole blood kept at room temperature may undergo decrements in glucose values of 10 mg/h because of ongoing metabolism by the blood cells.

  B. Whole blood kept in a refrigerator at 4°C for 24 hours reveals a drop in glucose value of nearly 20 mg/dL.

  C. Whole blood may be acceptable for glucose determinations if collected into fluoride-anticoagulated (gray-stoppered) tubes. The fluoride poisons the cells' enzyme systems necessary for metabolic use of glucose.

* Most important in small animals

    1) Samples collected in fluoride tubes should not be used for dipstick glucose assays, however.

  D. Separated plasma stored at room temperature for 24 hours remains acceptable for glucose determinations, but longer holding results in much lower glucose values.

  E. Separated, refrigerated plasma yields reliable glucose determinations up to 48 hours; a drop in glucose value of 10 mg/dL may be anticipated in plasma samples refrigerated for 72 hours.

  F. Slight decrements in glucose value are seen in hemolyzed blood because of methodologic problems in the laboratory determination.

2. Laboratory error may occur. Evaluate an initial low glucose value for reproducibility.

3. Functional hypoglycemia

  A. Transient idiopathic neonatal hypoglycemia

    1) Occurs in toy and miniature breeds less than six months old

    2) Increased incidence in poodles, Yorkshire terriers, and Chihuahuas

    3) Cause unknown

      a) Related to stress (cold), starvation, GI disturbances

      b) Search extensively for parasites (including protozoa).

      c) An enzyme immaturity in the liver may be present.

      d) A deficiency in pyruvate or alanine (glucose precursors) may be present.

      e) The patient should outgrow the problem.

    4) Signs

      a) Weakness, collapse

      b) Severe depression

      c) Coma

      d) Hypothermia

      e) Seizures

      f) Loose stool or pasty perineum

    5) Diagnosis

      a) History of stress, anorexia, GI signs

      b) Typical signs in a puppy

      c) Lack of hepatomegaly

      d) Low blood glucose level or response to dextrose

      e) Response to IV glucagon

6) Treatment

a) Intravenous 50% dextrose, 1 mL/kg

    i. Administer to any puppy showing the above signs.

    ii. *Do not wait* for any blood glucose determinations.

b) Response is immediate (1 to 2 minutes)

c) If vein is too small

    i. Give glucose orally (Karo syrup) if animal is able to swallow.

    ii. Massage into gums—some is absorbed through oral mucosa.

    iii. Use the intramedullary canal of the femur.

d) Keep animal warm.

e) Examine feces for parasites; treat for roundworms whether you find eggs or not.

f) Advise owners to give frequent feedings; give corn syrup (Karo) if animal has another episode.

g) If problem recurs, no underlying cause is found, and owners are feeding frequently, try corticosteroids to increase the release of alanine from skeletal muscle.

B. Hunting dog hypoglycemia

1) Seen in working and hunting breeds (coonhounds, Labradors, setters)

2) Unknown cause

3) Historically, the animal is fed a regular meal the night before and nothing on the day of work.

4) Performs well for first one to three hours, then becomes weak, staggers and may have seizure. Rapid recovery.

5) Diagnosis

a) History, breed

b) Normal physical examination

c) Normal blood glucose in examination room

d) Blood glucose < 50 mg/dL during exercise

6) Treatment

a) Frequent feedings

b) Carbohydrate snacks throughout hunt

c) Protein-rich meal one hour before hunt

d) Main meal at end of day

e) Karo syrup (5 to 10 tablespoonfuls) in field

f) Some advocate adrenocorticosteroids and tranquilizers.

4. Glycogen storagelike disease is an inherited condition in which there is an absence or defective function of enzymes necessary for glycogenolysis. In some cases, the same enzyme also is necessary for gluconeogenesis (e.g., glucose-6-phosphatase)

A. von Gierke's disease

1) Type I glycogenosis

2) Breeds, miniature and toy

3) Simple autosomal recessive disease

4) Rare disease, not adequately documented in veterinary medicine

5) Glucose-6-phosphatase deficiency of liver, kidney, intestine

a) Hepatic glycogen degradation and gluconeogenesis are absent.

b) Marked hepatomegaly and renomegaly caused by glycogen accumulation; no functional impairment is present.

c) Diarrhea may exist.

d) In children, ketonemia, hypercholesterolemia, and hyperlipidemia are seen.

6) No response to exogenous glucagon or epinephrine administration

7) Clinical signs

a) Depression

b) Incoordination

c) Seizures

d) Coma

e) Hypothermia

8) Diagnosis based on age, history, signs

a) Recurrent episodes in young dog

b) Low blood glucose

c) Hepatomegaly helps distinguish it from idiopathic neonatal hypoglycemia.

d) Excess glycogen found on hepatic biopsy

e) Enzyme assay is possible.

9) Treatment

a) Poor prognosis for normalcy

b) If animal presents with seizures

or severe weakness, give 1 mL/kg 50% dextrose IV.

      c) May administer subcutaneous 2.5% dextrose in .45% saline after initial IV bolus.

      d) Good nursing care (e.g., increase body temperature)

      e) Frequent meals and frequent feedings are needed at home.

      f) Glucose added to meals helps.

      g) Nonbasic sugars and fats added to diet are of little help.

      h) Use steroids if all else fails.

  B. Cori's disease

    1) Type III glycogenosis

    2) Deficiency of amylo-1, 6-glucosidase

      a) This enzyme is needed for the production of a "smaller" glycogen molecule so that phosphorylase may act.

      b) Abnormal glycogen molecule accumulates in liver and kidneys.

    3) Signs similar to von Gierke's disease but less severe

    4) Diagnosis and treatment similar to von Gierke's disease

  5. Suspect insulin overdose in any diabetic patient presenting with hypoglycemia.

  6. Hyperinsulinism secondary to beta cell neoplasm

  A. Adenomas, carcinomas, hyperplasia, microadenomatosis

    1) Adenomas more common in humans (90%)

    2) Carcinomas more common in dogs (> 75%)

    3) Microscopic distinction of adenocarcinoma from adenoma is unreliable. Differentiation is best based on clinical staging (World Health Organization TNM, Table 22-2) and disease course.

    4) Clinical staging of beta cell neoplasms is important for prognosis. Endocrine pancreatic tumors are staged according to the World Health Organization TNM system (see Table 22-2).

    5) Right and left pancreatic lobes affected equally

  B. Age—older dogs affected (3.5 to 13 years)

Table 22-2. **Clinical staging system for pancreatic neoplasia**

T	Primary Tumor
	T0: no evidence of tumor
	T1: tumor present
N	Regional Lymph Nodes (RLN)
	N0: No RLN involved
	N1: RLN involved
	N2: distant LN involved
M	Distant Metastasis
	M0: no evidence of distant metastasis
	M1: distant metastasis present

  C. No breed predilection; increased incidence in large breed dogs

  D. No sex predisposition

  E. Described in cats and ferrets

  F. Duration of signs

    1) May be weeks or months

    2) Signs intermittent

  G. Hypoglycemia results from excessive, inappropriate insulin secretion. The negative insulin effects include

    1) Interference with mechanisms that enhance hepatic glucose output

      a) Decreased mobilization of amino acids from muscle and of glycerol from adipose tissue, resulting in decreased substrates reaching the liver for gluconeogenesis

      b) Decreased hepatic uptake of amino acids

      c) Decreased activity of hepatic enzymes that promote gluconeogenesis

      d) Decreased glycogenolysis

    2) Insulin increases glucose uptake and use in muscle, liver, and adipose tissue.

    3) Insulin increases amino acid uptake by muscle and therefore reduces the supply of amino acids for hepatic gluconeogenesis.

  H. Signs

    1) Episodic and intermittent

    2) Severity of signs increases with time.

3) No constant relation to eating, fasting, or exercise

4) Animals usually have signs other than seizure.

    a) Weakness, lethargy, collapse

    b) Caudal paresis

    c) Muscle twitching

    d) Amaurosis

    e) Personality changes

    f) Behavior changes

    g) Incoordination, disorientation, ataxia

    h) Seizures

    i) Coma

I. Physical examination is usually normal.

1) Obesity may exist.

2) Insulinomas are not palpable on physical examination.

J. Laboratory findings

1) Leukogram may disclose stress picture.

2) Chemistry profile

    a) Low blood glucose

    b) Hypokalemia may be present because of the hyperinsulin state.

    c) Liver metastases may result in mild elevation of liver enzymes.

3) Not observable radiographically

K. Diagnostic tests

1) Blood glucose

    a) May be normal on a random sample

    b) Below 60 mg/dL is questionable; below 50 mg/dL is significant.

    c) If highly suspect, enforce fast for 24 hours.

    d) If hypoglycemia is still not achieved, enforce fast for 48 to 72 hours.

    e) If 72-hour fast does not produce hypoglycemia, exercise and then evaluate serum glucose.

    f) All fasts should be supervised.

2) Immunoreactive insulin (IRI)

    a) Normal fasting value in canine is approximately 20 μU/mL (Johnson).

    b) Value greater than 54 μU/mL is clearly abnormal.

    c) Evaluate with concomitant blood glucose (see IRI-to-glucose ratio below).

    d) Usually elevated in insulinomas and below normal or normal in other causes of hypoglycemia

    e) The fasting IRI may be normal in insulinomas because of removal by the liver of secreted insulin before it appears in peripheral blood.

3) Glucose/immunoreactive insulin ratio (G : IRI)

    a) First testing technique described for the diagnosis of insulin-producing tumors

    b) Normal values 3.5 to 12.5 mg/μU

    c) Values < 2.5 mg/μU considered diagnostic

    d) False negative G : IRI values may occur.

4) Immunoreactive insulin/glucose ratio (IRI : G)

    a) Elevation provides the most reliable data to confirm diagnosis of insulinoma.

    b) Evaluate for inappropriate insulin secretion for the level of blood glucose.

    c) Insulin μU/mL: blood glucose mg/dL is normally less than or equal to .30.

    d) In patients with nonpancreatic-tumor hypoglycemia, the IRI : G is normal.

    e) Inappropriate elevation of plasma insulin in the presence of hypoglycemia remains the cornerstone for the diagnosis of pancreatic islet-cell disease.

    f) False negative IRI : G values may occur even in the face of profound hypoglycemia, however.

5) Amended insulin glucose ratio (AIGR)

    a) Use of this ratio is controversial

    b) Formula

$$\frac{\text{serum insulin } (\mu\text{U/mL}) \times 100}{\text{plasma glucose (mg/dL)} - 30}$$

    c) Values > 30 considered diagnostic for insulinoma

    d) False positive and false negative results have been reported.

L. Provocative tests

1) Rarely needed

2) Used in cases difficult to document (i.e., 72-hour fast, IRI, and IRI : G normal)

3) Rationale for tests

    a) Normally insulin is secreted in response to the blood glucose concentration.

    b) In insulinomas insulin is released intermittently or continuously at inappropriate times and inappropriate levels for the concomitant blood glucose.

    c) Glucose, tolbutamide, glucagon, and leucine stimulate the release of insulin.

    d) The provocative tests are designed to accentuate the release of insulin from the abnormal beta tissue.

    e) In decreasing order, the normal beta cell responds to glucose, tolbutamide, glucagon, and leucine; the neoplastic beta cell responds to glucagon, tolbutamide, leucine, and glucose.

    f) Always have patient fast before testing.

    g) Have IV catheter in place.

    h) Have glucose available in case hypoglycemia develops during test.

    i) *Note:* never leave patient unattended.

4) Intravenous glucose-tolerance test

    a) Give .5 g dextrose/lb IV

    b) Samples at 0, 15, 30, 45, 60, 90, 120 minutes

    c) Normal

        i. Peak blood glucose > 300 at 15 minutes with gradual return to normal by 60 minutes

        ii. Plasma IRI levels rise concomitantly but return to resting values by 60 minutes.

    d) Diagnostic test

        i. Lower and flatter curve

        ii. Return to resting glucose sooner than expected

        iii. Inappropriate insulin secretion

    e) Advantage—easy test

    f) Disadvantage—not diagnostic in some cases

5) Glucagon-tolerance test

    a) Procedure

        i. Give .03 mg/kg glucagon IV not to exceed total of 1 mg

        ii. Samples of glucose at 0, 1, 3, 5, 10, 30, 45, 60, 90, 120 minutes

        iii. Measure insulin levels simultaneously.

    b) Action of glucagon

        i. Normally produced by alpha cells of the islets of Langerhans

        ii. Stimulates insulin production by direct action on beta cells (one to two minutes) and indirectly by its gluconeogenic and glycogenolytic properties (15 to 30 minutes)

        iii. Insulinogenic effects exaggerated in the presence of an insulinoma

    c) Normal

        i. Blood glucose values greater than 150 mg/dL

        ii. Insulin levels rarely above 50 μU/mL

    d) Abnormal

        i. Decrease in blood glucose one to two minutes after injection (rapid release of insulin)

        ii. Blood glucose concentrations < 135 mg/dL

        iii. Hypoglycemia by 60 to 90 minutes (highly diagnostic)

        iv. One minute after injection, plasma IRI values > 50 μU/mL or an average increase of > 18 μU/ml from fasting to 1 minute.

        v. Plasma IRI/G ratio > .7 μU/mL at one minute

    e) Advantage—easy test

    f) Disadvantage—time-consuming, expensive

6) Tolbutamide test

    a) Procedure

        i. Give 20 mg/kg up to 1 g

tolbutamide IV in 20 ml of saline

    ii. Samples at 0, 10, 20, 30, 60, 90, 120, 150 minutes

  b) Action of tolbutamide

    i. Augments insulin release from beta cells

    ii. Potentiates insulin action at cellular level

  c) Normal—Percentage decrease of blood glucose from fasting is equal to 40%.

  d) Abnormal—diagnostic

    i. Percentage decrease > 70%

    ii. Hypoglycemia sustained longer in dogs with insulinomas (three hours)

  e) *Note:* test is dangerous.

    i. Effects last 18 hours.

    ii. If initial concentration of blood glucose is less than 50 mg/dL, do not perform.

    iii. If signs of hypoglycemia develop, discontinue test and administer glucose IV.

7) L-leucine test

  a) Procedure

    i. Give 150 mg/kg suspended in water PO.

    ii. Samples at 0, 5, 10, 15, 30, 45, 60 minutes

  b) Action

    i. May potentiate peripheral action of insulin

    ii. Especially stimulates neoplastic beta cells to release insulin

  c) Normal—no reduction in glucose

  d) Abnormal

    i. Forty percent reduction in blood glucose from fasting within 30 minutes

    ii. Excessive insulin secretion

  e) Advantage—highly diagnostic

  f) Disadvantage—hypoglycemia

8) Epinephrine

  a) Procedure

    i. Give 1 ml epinephrine IM

    ii. Blood samples at 0, 30, 60, 90, 120 minutes

  b) Action—Expect hyperglycemia by glycogenolysis.

  c) Decreased hyperglycemia seen with

    i. Depletion of hepatic glycogen

    ii. Unresponsiveness to glycogenolytic stimulation, as in hyperinsulinism

    iii. In insulinomas, the increase in fasting glucose is < 35 mg/dL after one hour.

  d) Advantage—?

  e) Disadvantage—nonspecific

M. Treatment

  1) Surgery is the treatment of choice.

  a) NPO for two to three days postoperatively (Pancreatitis is not an uncommon postoperative complication.)

  b) Glucocorticoids for two days presurgically

  c) Five percent dextrose drip during and after surgery. Discontinue if hyperglycemia develops.

  d) Very gentle handling

  e) Local excision if possible

  f) Partial pancreatectomy if tumor is not palpable

  g) Careful search for metastases to lymph nodes, liver, omentum, spleen, bowel, and mesentery

  h) Intravenous infusion of methylene blue dye (3 mg/kg) may be useful in identification of pancreatic islet-cell tumors. (Heinz body anemia may develop.)

  i) Always biopsy regional lymph nodes.

  j) If complete pancreatectomy is done, treat patient for pancreatic insufficiency and diabetes mellitus.

  k) In some cases, treatment for diabetes mellitus is needed even if entire pancreas is not removed. It is thought that the normal beta cells atrophy in the face of the hyperinsulinism; this may be transient or permanent.

  l) Most carcinomas already have micrometastasis or macrometastasis by the time surgery is performed.

m) If primary tumor is difficult to remove, be sure to perform a biopsy.

n) If metastasis is seen, remove primary tumor and excise solitary metastasis, if possible. Use medical therapy as an adjuvant.

o) Monitor electrolytes (especially K), glucose, amylase, and BUN postoperatively.

p) Supplement fluids with potassium chloride postoperatively because patient is NPO.

q) Dogs with metastatic disease usually continue to be hypoglycemic after surgery.

2) Medical

a) The goal of medical management is to reduce the severity and frequency of clinical signs.

b) Recommended when extensive metastasis is present

c) Indicated when patient is an extreme surgical risk

d) Frequent feedings (three to six small meals daily) are necessary. Avoid the use of diets containing large quantities of simple sugars (i.e., semimoist foods), which are rapidly absorbed from the gastrointestinal tract.

e) Acute hypoglycemia should be treated with sugar-water or syrup.

f) Limit exercise to minimize glucose consumption.

g) Glucocorticoids (prednisone at 0.25 to 0.5 mg/kg PO q12h)

h) Diazoxide

i. Inhibits insulin release

ii. 5 mg/kg PO q12h up to 40 mg/kg PO q12h

iii. May cause arrhythmias, sodium retention and vomiting

iv. Hyperglycemia effects of diazoxide are potentiated by hydrochlorothiazide (2 to 4 mg/kg q24h).

i) Propanolol, phenytoin, and L-asparaginase may decrease insulin production, release, or both. These agents have not been well-investigated in the dog or cat.

j) Alloxan is a chemotherapeutic agent that destroys normal beta cells but usually has little effect on neoplastic beta cells.

k) Streptozotocin

i. Destroys beta cells

ii. Complete remissions in humans have been accomplished.

iii. Antibiotic derived from the bacterium *Streptomyces achromogenes*

iv. Severely nephrotoxic and heptatotoxic

N. Prognosis

1) Clinical stage 1 cases have significantly longer disease-free intervals and survivals after tumor excision than stage 2 and stage 3 patients (see Table 22-2).

2) Clinical stage 2 and 3 patients may survive as long as two years with medical treatment and frequent feedings.

7. Extrapancreatic, tumor-induced hypoglycemia

A. Tumor types

1) Hepatoma

2) Pulmonary carcinoma

3) Metastatic mammary carcinoma

4) Melanoma

5) Salivary adenocarcinoma

6) Hemangiosarcoma

7) Metastatic liver neoplasia

8) Polycythemia vera

B. Theories concerning production of hypoglycemia

1) Block of hepatic glucose output

2) Excessive glucose consumption by tumor tissue, with a high rate of anaerobic glycolysis

3) Inhibition of lipolysis

4) May be related to high plasma insulinlike activity (ILA)

a) In the majority of cases, immunoreactive insulin (IRI) levels have been low.

b) In humans, tumors have been found with high ILA measured by a radioreceptor assay.

5) Somatostatin-secreting tumor

a) Inhibits glucagon release or synthesis

b) Inhibits insulin release

C. Diagnosis
    1) Physical examination and radiographic evidence of neoplasia
    2) Normal IRI level in the majority of cases
D. Therapy
    1) Removal of tumor
    2) Streptozotocin is being tried experimentally.
    3) Diazoxide has not been helpful.
  8. Diffuse hepatic disease
    A. Hypoglycemia is relatively rare in hepatic disease.
    B. The liver is essential in maintaining glucose homeostasis by way of gluconeogenesis and glycogenolysis.
    C. Experimentally, 80% of hepatic tissues must be destroyed before hypoglycemia develops.
    D. The development of hypoglycemia indicates nothing about the reversibility of the hepatic disease.
    E. Associated with
      1) Diffuse, acute hepatitis
      2) Diffuse, hepatic necrosis
      3) Terminal cirrhosis
      4) Hepatic lipidosis
      5) Portovascular anomalies
      6) Severe liver metastases
    F. Diagnosis is made by other clinical and laboratory signs of hepatic disease.
    G. Therapy
      1) Glucose bolus may be needed in crisis situation.
      2) Persistent hypoglycemia necessitates IV drip.
      3) Dextrose is said to be "liver sparing."
      4) Give frequent feedings in chronic disease.
  9. Adrenocortical insufficiency (Addison's disease)—see Chapter 14.
    A. Hypoglycemia is not a frequent finding in canine hypoadrenocorticism.
    B. Hypoglycemia is due to reduction in gluconeogenesis resulting from deficiency of glucocorticoids.
    C. Glucocorticoid deficiency alone may be seen (i.e., Na : K ratio > 23 : 1), or may be in combination with mineralocorticoid deficiency (i.e., Na : K ratio < 23 : 1).

D. Corrected by exogenous administration of glucocorticoids
  10. Endotoxic hypoglycemia
    A. Increased hepatic glycogenolysis occurs, as well as decreased hepatic gluconeogenesis.
    B. Glucose uptake and glucose oxidation are enhanced.
    C. Mechanism unknown, but insulin or compounds with insulinlike activity are suspected.
    D. Seen with parvovirus infection, hemorrhagic gastroenteritis (HGE), gram-negative septicemia
    E. Treatment
      1) IV glucose bolus if symptomatic
      2) Dextrose in IV drip to maintain normal blood glucose
      3) Treat the underlying condition.
  11. Hypopituitarism
    A. Deficiency of ACTH and growth hormone may result in hypoglycemia.
    B. Rare cause of hypoglycemia in dogs
    C. Seen in German shepherds as a congenital defect
    D. May be acquired because of traumatic, inflammatory, or neoplastic pituitary lesions
    E. Confirm diagnosis by growth hormone and ACTH stimulation studies
  12. Renal glycosuria
    A. Loss of glucose from renal tubular disorders is seen in canine Fanconi's syndrome and in some cases of chronic and acute renal injury.
    B. The loss of glucose into the urine has not yet been reported to cause hypoglycemia in dogs, although it has been observed in two instances by one of the authors, when anorexia also was present.
  13. Hypoglycemia of pregnancy is extremely rare in dogs.

• •

Hyperglycemia

  1. Hyperglycemia exists when plasma or serum glucose values are in excess of 130 mg/dL.

2. Determine plasma or serum glucose values on samples from animals that have fasted 12 to 24 hours.

3. Clinical signs referable to hyperglycemia are uncommon until the plasma or serum glucose value remains consistently in excess of 180 mg/dL.

Causes of Hyperglycemia

Summary of Causes

Laboratory error
Postprandial hyperglycemia*
Diabetes mellitus*
Stress-induced hyperglycemia*
Endocrine
    Hyperadrenocorticism*
    Pheochromocytoma*
    Hyperthyroidism
    Iatrogenic or spontaneous growth hormone excess
    Glucagon-secreting tumor
Uremia*
Iatrogenic hyperglycemia
    Glucose infusions
    Peritoneal dialysis
    Partial or total parenteral nutrition
    Diazoxide
    Thiazide diuretics
    Glucocorticoids (high or prolonged dose)
Intracranial injury
Pancreatitis*
Pancreatectomy
Hyperosmolality, severe

1. Because laboratory error of a random nature may occur, determine the reproducibility of hyperglycemia.

2. Postprandial hyperglycemia normally occurs immediately after a carbohydrate-rich meal (i.e., semimoist diets).

3. Diabetes mellitus (DM) is the most important cause of hyperglycemia in small animals and is considered to be the result of the absolute or relative lack of insulin. Overt diabetics have glucosuria and serum glucose values consistently in excess of 200 mg/dL.

* Most important in small animals

4. Stress-induced hyperglycemia may occur as a result of the outpouring of catecholamines from anxiety, fright, strenuous exercise, or seizures.

A. The magnitude of this elevation is variable but may occasionally result in serum glucose greater than 300 mg/dL, especially in cats.

B. This elevation is transient and the blood glucose returns to normal if a blood sample is obtained when the animal is in a quietly resting state.

5. Mild hyperglycemia (130 to 170 mg/dL) may be seen in dogs with hyperadrenocorticism because of the effects of increased levels of circulating cortisol. Chronic hyperadrenocorticism may result in islet cell exhaustion with resultant DM and more severe elevation in serum glucose (> 200 mg/dL).

A. Pheochromocytoma also may cause mild hyperglycemia through increased levels of circulating and epinephrine. The level of hyperglycemia varies according to the functional status of the neoplastic adrenal medulla.

B. Hyperthyroidism in humans may be associated with hyperglycemia. This association has not been noted in feline or canine hyperthyroidism except in those animals with concurrent DM.

C. Iatrogenic or spontaneous growth hormone excess may be associated with hyperglycemia or frank DM as well as acromegaly in small animals.

1) Spontaneous growth hormone excess may occur as a consequence of pituitary neoplasia (most common in cats) or as a complication of progesterone production during diestrus in intact female dogs.

2) Administration of progestational compounds may result in iatrogenic growth hormone overproduction.

6. Uremia is often associated with mild (130 to 170 mg/dL) hyperglycemia caused by poorly defined factors in the uremic environment that cause insulin antagonism.

7. Parenteral infusion of glucose-containing fluids routinely causes hyperglycemia when the rate of glucose infusion exceeds glucose removal from the vascular space by translocation into cells, metabolism, and renal excretion.

A. Peritoneal dialysis with hypertonic solutions containing glucose may result in hyperglycemia. This is particularly troublesome when glucose used in the dialysate has a 3.0% or greater concentration; it may result in severe hyperglycemia and hyperosmolality.

B. Partial or total parenteral nutrition often uses high concentrations of glucose as a caloric source. During infusion mild hyperglycemia is usually present, and severe hyperglycemia results if these fluids are administered too rapidly.

C. Various drugs may cause hyperglycemia, including diazoxide, thiazide diuretics, and glucocorticoids.

8. Intracranial injury may be associated with hyperglycemia.

9. Pancreatitis may be associated with hyperglycemia and the development of DM either secondary to islet cell destruction or possibly due to other neuroendocrine responses.

10. Partial (> 90%) or complete pancreatectomy results in hyperglycemia.

11. Severe hyperosmolality may be associated with hyperglycemia because of a decreased ability to release insulin.

Signs of Hyperglycemia

The signs of moderate to severe hyperglycemia (> 180 to 200 mg/dL) are referable to the osmotic load presented for glomerular filtration. These signs are polyuria with compensatory polydipsia. Hyperglycemia also contributes significantly to increasing serum osmolality, resulting in cellular dehydration (see Chapter 25 on osmolality). Other signs are referable to the underlying cause of hyperglycemia, such as hypertension in pheochromocytoma and hepatomegaly in hyperadrenocorticism or DM.

Uncomplicated Diabetes Mellitus—Background and Treatment

1. Diabetes mellitus is the only disease resulting in persistently high serum glucose values and requiring treatment directed toward correction of the serum glucose concentration. Hyperglycemia seen in other disorders abates as the underlying condition is successfully treated (e.g., adrenolectomy or o′-p′-DDD therapy in hyperadrenocorticism, adjusting the fluid rate of solutions used in parenteral nutritional support).

2. The metabolic dysfunctions seen in diabetes primarily reflect the degree to which there is an absolute or relative deficiency of insulin.

A. Minimal deficiency results in inability to store foodstuffs properly and leads to glucose intolerance.

B. A major deficiency allows accumulation of metabolic fuels when fed but also results in excessive mobilization of endogenous fuels during fasting (fasting hyperglycemia, elevated fatty acids, and amino acids).

C. In the most severe form of deficiency, overproduction of glucose and a marked increase in catabolic processes (lipolysis, proteolysis) occurs.

3. Pathophysiology in uncomplicated DM

A. Insulin deficiency and resulting hyperglycemia are present.

B. Inability to use glucose signals the hypothalamic eating center to increase appetite.

C. Osmotic diuresis develops when hyperglycemia exceeds the renal threshold for glucose and results in glycosuria accompanied by compensatory polydipsia.

D. Weight loss may occur even in the face of increased caloric intake because of the body's inability to use foodstuffs properly, the existing catabolic state, and the calories lost in the urine.

4. History (uncomplicated)

A. Polydipsia

B. Polyuria

C. Polyphagia (possible previous obesity)

D. Most common in middle-aged or older female dogs; older cats of either sex

E. Rapid onset of cataracts may occur (dogs only, not reported in cats).

1) As excess glucose enters the lens, sorbitol is produced by alternate metabolic pathways for glucose metabolism and is confined to the lens.

    2) Sorbitol then acts as an osmotic agent and fluid enters the lens, irreversibly disrupting lens fibers.

  5. Physical examination

    A. Cataracts ±

    B. Hepatomegaly, fatty infiltration

    1) Improper glucose use leads to excessive fat mobilization.

    2) The liver is unable to use all the glycerol and fatty acids for energy and much of it is converted to hepatic lipid.

    3) Decreased protein synthesis in the liver results in decreased lipoprotein triglycerides that are unable to leave the liver. Hepatic lipid formation occurs.

    4) Triglycerides are unable to enter other body tissues because of the lack of lipoprotein lipase activity, an enzyme normally activated by insulin.

    C. Obesity, normal, or low body weight

    D. Physical examination is often otherwise normal.

  6. Laboratory examination

    A. Thorough laboratory evaluation (complete blood count [CBC], biochemical profile, urinalysis) of all diabetic patients is recommended.

    B. CBC usually normal

    C. The blood-chemistry profile is usually normal except for a serum glucose > 150 mg/dL.

    1) In most cases serum glucose is > 200 mg/dL.

    2) Glucose-tolerance tests are rarely necessary (serum glucose 150 to 200 mg/dL).

    3) Beware of stress hyperglycemia, especially in the cat (may be > 300 mg/dL).

    4) Increased liver enzymes may be seen secondary to fatty infiltration of the liver.

    5) Lipemia may be present due to decreased activity of lipoprotein lipase, an enzyme activated by insulin, which is necessary for the metabolism of lipoproteins and chylomicrons.

    D. Urinalysis

    1) Glycosuria is present.

      a) Renal threshold for glucose in dogs is approximately 180 mg/dL.

      b) Renal threshold for glucose in cats is approximately 300 mg/dL.

    2) A mild ketonuria may be present.

    3) The presence of pyuria dictates the need for a urine culture and sensitivity, because asymptomatic urinary infections may exist.

    E. Do not make a diagnosis of DM based on an elevated blood glucose determination unless concomitant glycosuria is present.

  7. Therapy

    A. The objective of therapy should be to lower blood glucose to the point where the clinical manifestations of diabetes such as polydipsia, polyuria, polyphagia, and weight loss are eliminated while hypoglycemia is avoided.

    B. It is not necessary to lower the serum glucose rapidly because the animal has had an elevated serum glucose for several weeks to months.

    C. Remember that hypoglycemia is life threatening, consequently hyperglycemia is preferable.

    D. Diabetics are best managed and regulated at home. Whenever possible, keep them there.

    E. Although used widely in humans, oral hypoglycemic agents are used infrequently in veterinary medicine because most canine and feline diabetics are insulin deficient and prone to ketosis.

    1) Sulfonylureas stimulate insulin secretion from beta cells and decrease hepatic gluconeogenesis.

    2) Biguanides delay absorption of food and promote glucose uptake by peripheral tissues.

    F. Insulin

    1) Adequate control of diabetic dogs and cats is usually achieved by administering insulin once daily and following a strict feeding regimen throughout the day.

    2) Most insulins are of beef or pork origin.

    3) Insulins are classified as short-acting, intermediate-acting, or long-acting based on their onset and duration of action (Table 22-3).

    4) NPH and protamine zinc insulins

Table 22-3. **Commonly used insulin preparations**

Type of Insulin	Onset*	Maximal Effect*		Duration of Action*	
		Dog	Cat	Dog	Cat
Regular	.25	2–4	2–4	6–8	6–8
NPH	3	8–12	2–8	18–24	6–12
Lente	3	10–12	?	18–28	?
Protamine zinc	3–4	14–20	3–12	24–36	12–24

* Hours after subcutaneous administration

are most often selected for use in dogs and cats, respectively.

    5) Dosage—.5 to 1.0 U/kg, subcutaneously

    a) Administer insulin approximately 30 minutes before the morning meal. The evening meal should be fed six to eight hours later (approximately two hours before the expected peak of insulin activity). Each meal should meet approximately half of the caloric requirements.

    b) Usually requires two to four days for the dog's or cat's response to insulin administration to equilibrate. During this time period, blood glucose is monitored at the expected time of peak of insulin activity only.

    c) After a two-to-four day equilibration period, close monitoring of blood glucose is instituted. Blood glucose concentration is monitored before insulin administration and every two hours afterward. Morning and evening meals are fed as before. Ideally this monitoring should continue for a 24-hour period. This allows determination of the time of peak insulin effect.

    d) Glucose can be monitored using standard laboratory methods or by reagent sticks with or without a corresponding automated test strip analyzer. Whole blood samples may be obtained using 26-gauge needles when using reagent sticks. When initiating insulin therapy in cats, the use of an indwelling jugular catheter facilitates frequent blood sampling and minimizes stress-induced alterations in blood glucose.

    e) Ideally glucose concentrations will reach their nadir (approximately 80 mg/dL) 10 to 12 hours after insulin administration and peak (approximately 200 mg/dL) 24 hours after insulin administration.

    f) The time of the afternoon meal may need to be altered after determination of the time of peak insulin effect using the values determined by serial monitoring of blood glucose. The afternoon meal should be fed approximately two hours before the peak insulin effect.

    g) Insulin dose may need to be increased if blood glucose values exceed 200 mg/dL or decreased if blood glucose falls below 80 mg/dL. Changes in insulin dose are usually made in .5 to 1.0 unit increments.

    h) If the duration of effect of the insulin selected for use in diabetic patients is less than 20 hours, a change in insulin type or administration schedule may be necessary. Often a change to protamine zinc insulin or to twice-daily administration of isophane (NPH) insulin is effective.

    6) Always use corresponding insulin syringes and insulin (e.g., NPH U-40 insulin and U-40 insulin syringes).

8. Home management and monitoring

    A. After the diabetic animal's glucose curve has been completed and the veterinarian is confident that the majority of the day's blood glucose determinations will be < 200 mg/dL, the animal can be discharged to the owner. The insulin type, dose, administration schedule, injection technique, and feeding schedule should be discussed thoroughly with the owner.

B. Insulin needs may change from day to day because of alterations in exercise, food intake, and environmental stress. Therefore, do not attempt to fine tune the patient's therapy in the hospital.

C. Initially, the diabetic patient should be reevaluated every one to two weeks until glucose control is obtained. The owner should administer insulin and feed their pet as usual before admitting the dog to the veterinary hospital for serial blood glucose determinations throughout the day. Any necessary adjustments in insulin dose, type, administration schedule, and feeding times can be made based on these blood glucose concentration determinations.

D. It is essential that the same amount of food be fed every day.

1) Ideally, a high-protein, low-carbohydrate, low-fat diet should be provided.

2) Avoid semimoist commercial products because they contain large quantities of simple sugars.

3) Feed obese animals amounts that will result in weight loss.

4) Tell owners to monitor these patients closely at home because their insulin needs will change with variations in weight.

E. Keep exercise constant daily; exercise increases glucose receptors on muscle and increases their avidity for insulin, thereby decreasing insulin needs.

F. Once stabilization has been achieved, the patient should be reevaluated every two to four months with a complete history, physical examination, review of the client's diary (see below), and blood glucose determinations made throughout the day.

G. If recrudescence of clinical signs of diabetes recur, i.e., polydipsia/polyuria/polyphagia (PD/PU/PP), the animal should be reevaluated immediately.

H. Home monitoring should consist of determination of appetite, attitude, water intake, and urine output. In addition, some owners are willing to determine urine glucose one or more times daily. These determinations can be made with the use of commercial reagent sticks. Ideally, urine glucose

should be negative at the time of the evening meal. If persistent glycosuria, ketonuria, or both develop, the owner is instructed to return the patient to the hospital for further evaluation. Owner observations and urine values can be recorded in a daily diary.

I. Because of difficulties in interpretation of urine glucose values, particularly persistent morning glycosuria or persistent negative urine glucoses, insulin therapy should not be adjusted based on urine glucose monitoring alone.

9. Hypoglycemic reaction

A. If only weakness occurs, oral supplementation with Karo syrup or honey is adequate.

B. If seizures, collapse, or coma occur

1) Have owner massage Karyo syrup or honey onto gums while on the way to the veterinary hospital.

2) Give 50% dextrose 1 mL/kg IV bolus.

3) Maintain on IV dextrose drip because duration of action of insulin has not been completed.

4) Decrease the insulin dosage the next day.

5) Severe hypoglycemia and seizures may result in cerebral anoxia and cerebral edema; steroids are then indicated and mannitol may be needed.

C. If hypoglycemia is seen every day an hour before feeding, then give the second meal earlier.

D. If hypoglycemia is consistently noted earlier in the day, the peak of insulin activity may be earlier than expected. A change in insulin type or administration schedule may be indicated.

E. Investigate collapse or weakness at times other than peak action (i.e., draw blood glucose). Other disease processes, such as severe hyperglycemia, may be involved.

F. Somogyi effect

1) Hypoglycemia occurs and the body responds with an outpouring of glucagon, cortisol, and epinephrine.

2) This raises the blood glucose and the next morning 2^+ to 4^+ glycosuria occurs.

3) If the owner is altering insulin dose daily based on morning urine glucose determinations, he increases the insulin dose and further precipitates a hypoglycemic attack.

      4) This effect usually indicates an earlier peak action of insulin.

10. Estrus and pregnancy

      A. Estrus increases insulin needs.

      B. During pregnancy, insulin needs are increased; diabetic patients may develop ketosis.

      C. Spay all females as soon as they are regulated so that wide fluctuations in insulin requirements and ketosis may be prevented more easily.

11. Surgery of the diabetic patient

      A. Do not change insulin dosage and feeding the day before.

      B. On the day of surgery give half the necessary insulin dosage and do not feed the animal.

      C. Perform the surgery early in the morning.

      D. Administer 5% dextrose during surgery.

      E. Give half of the total daily food intake 8 to 10 hours after giving the insulin.

      F. If possible, send the animal home in the afternoon when it is fully recovered from anesthesia.

      G. The next day, administer twice the amount of insulin given the day of surgery.

12. Glycosylated hemoglobin

      A. Determination of the quantity of glucose that becomes irreversibly bound to hemoglobin during the lifespan of a red blood cell

      B. Useful in humans for assessment of blood glucose control over a prolonged period of time

      C. Rarely used in veterinary medicine

      D. Not accurate in cats

13. Prognosis and client education

      A. Be positive with clients.

      B. Explain that diligence will be needed to maintain a near-normal life for the pet. Most uncomplicated diabetics do well if they have a conscientious owner.

      C. Well-controlled diabetics have lived as long as six years after diagnosis.

      D. Be sure everything is clearly understood before the client undertakes the control

of a diabetic patient. Euthanasia is the most common cause of death in diabetic dogs and cats.

14. Inability to regulate glucose adequately suggests that

      A. Insulin was not stored properly (i.e., refrigerated) or is outdated.

      B. Insulin was not properly agitated before injecting.

      C. Improper method of injection was used.

      D. Concurrent infection exists. (Respiratory tract, urinary tract, and skin are most common places.)

      E. Changes in food intake or diet schedule occurred.

      F. There were changes in exercise.

      G. Estrus is occurring.

      H. Underlying disease such as hyperadrenocorticism and hypothyroidism are elevating plasma glucose concentration.

      1) A diabetic, Cushingoid dog cannot be regulated properly unless the Cushing's disease is controlled.

      2) Regulation is difficult and may be dangerous while o′-p′-DDD is being given.

      3) In these cases, it is better to give too little insulin.

      I. Production of antibodies against insulin is occurring.

      J. There is production of antibodies against the insulin receptor.

      K. The duration of action of insulin is shorter (the "transient insulin response").

      1) Some animals metabolize insulin more rapidly than others.

      2) Try ultralente or protamine zinc insulin because they have a longer duration of action (see Table 22-3).

      3) Split-dose insulin therapy using NPH may be needed.

      a) Administer insulin in the morning and then 12 hours later (.5 hours before evening meal).

      b) Although this regimen is difficult to maintain, some clients will follow it.

Complicated Diabetes Mellitus

Complicated DM occurs in any patient presenting with DM, and with systemic signs of disease not seen in the uncomplicated cases. The patient may or may not be ketoacidotic.

1. Historical signs

  A. Anorexia

  B. Vomiting

  C. Diarrhea

  D. Heavy, labored breathing (Kussmaul's respiration)

  E. Weakness, depression

  F. Weight loss

  G. Coma

2. Physical examination (not all signs are expected in each patient)

  A. Dehydration

  B. Kussmaul's respiration (seen with ketoacidosis)

  C. Acetone odor on breath

  D. Depression

  E. Abdominal pain on palpation

  F. Icterus

  G. Coma

  H. Hepatomegaly

  I. Fever

  J. Shock

3. Laboratory examination

  A. The CBC may show a stress picture. Neutrophilia with a left shift may be present if infection or pancreatitis is present.

  B. The serum glucose is > 150 mg/dL and usually > 300 mg/dL, in some cases approaching 1000 mg/dL.

  C. BUN, creatinine

    1) Usually elevated from prerenal causes (dehydration, vomiting, diarrhea)

    2) Primary renal disease with DM may be seen as the cause of azotemia.

      a) Specific gravity should be > 1.030 if prerenal azotemia exists.

      b) Urinary sediment may be "active" if pyelonephritis or tubular damage is present (pyuria, casts, bacteria, dilute urine).

  D. Serum sodium is generally normal or low. Eliminate fictitious hyponatremia (pseudohyponatremia, see Chapter 25) due to severe hypertriglyceridemia as the cause for low sodium concentration. This often can be done visually by observing the plasma.

    1) Total body sodium is usually decreased regardless of the measured sodium concentration.

    2) Sodium is lost in urine from the increased osmotic diuresis induced by glycosuria and by renal excretion of the sodium-ketone and potassium-ketone salts.

    3) The presence of hyponatremia may indicate patients who are predisposed to cerebral edema when therapy is instituted, as follows: insulin therapy leads to decreased plasma glucose, which leads to decreased serum osmolality; brain hyperosmolality persists longer, causing fluid to enter the intracellular space, leading to intracellular edema.

  E. Serum potassium

    1) A deficit in total-body potassium is always present with ketoacidosis; the deficit may be as large as 10 mEq/kg of body weight (BW).

    2) In some cases plasma potassium concentration is normal or elevated despite the large decrease in total body stores because acidosis results in translocation of intracellular K^+ to the extracellular fluid. Volume contraction results in decreased renal loss of K^+ when severe oliguria or anuria is present.

    3) Initial hypokalemia is particularly ominous because treatment causes potassium to drop even further and life-threatening hypokalemia may develop. Potassium falls during treatment for various reasons.

      a) Dilution from rehydration

      b) Continued urinary potassium loss due to volume expansion and increased delivery to the kidney. As much as half of supplemented potassium may be lost in the urine.

      c) Correction of acidosis results in translocation of some K^+ into cells.

      d) Increased cellular uptake of potassium occurs because of the action of insulin.

  F. Phosphorus

    1) Total phosphorus stores are deficient in most diabetics, especially in those that are ketoacidotic.

      a) Depletion is due to increased tissue catabolism accompanied by increased renal excretion, impaired glucose use, and cellular phosphorus uptake.

      b) Serum phosphorus may be low, normal, or elevated.

c) Prerenal azotemia or oliguria may result in an elevation of the serum phosphorus even though total stores are depleted.

2) Phosphorus is important in the formation of 2,3-diphosphoglycerate, a substance that binds with hemoglobin and decreases its affinity for oxygen.

3) Treatment with potassium phosphate supplementation along with, or as a substitute for, potassium chloride supplementation may be helpful.

G. Serum amylase may be elevated mildly from prerenal causes or more markedly from concomitant pancreatitis.

H. Liver enzymes may be elevated from fatty infiltration. Pancreatitis also may cause localized hepatic inflammation and enzyme elevations. With severe hepatic involvement or bile duct inflammation secondary to pancreatitis, elevation of the serum bilirubin may be seen

I. Urinalysis (UA)

1) Glycosuria present

2) Ketonuria may or may not be present.

3) Sediment may disclose inflammatory elements.

4) Specific gravity variable

J. Ketonemia and ketonuria result mainly from increased hepatic ketone body formation.

1) Increased levels of free fatty acids from adipose tissue result from insulin deficiency.

2) Ketogenic pathways within the liver are activated by lack of insulin; specifically, increased activity of acylcarnitine transferase occurs.

3) Decreased use of ketones for energy by muscle and brain results in increased substrate delivery to the liver. Diabetic dogs use ketones less rapidly than normal dogs because of lack of insulin.

K. Blood gases disclose varying metabolic acidosis.

1) Acetoacetate and beta-hydroxybutyrate accumulate and add H^+ to the body because they are strong acids.

2) Decreases in pH stimulate ventilation; this results in increased rate and depth of respiration (Kussmaul's) with subsequent decrease in P_{CO_2}.

3) Poor perfusion of tissues from dehydration and shock also contributes to metabolic acidosis.

4) Lactic acidosis may occur as an uncommon cause of acidosis and coma in a diabetic patient. The onset of acidosis in this condition is usually within hours, in contrast to the development of ketoacidosis, which develops over several days. A large anion gap is present in both lactic acidosis and ketoacidosis.

L. Roentgenograms (radiographs)

1) Abdominal films may disclose signs compatible with pancreatitis.

2) Pyometra with DM is not uncommon.

3) Pneumonia may be evident on thoracic films.

4. Possible coexisting disorders

   A. Pancreatic disorders

      1) Acute pancreatitis

      2) Chronic relapsing pancreatitis

      3) Pancreatic exocrine insufficiency

   B. Renal disease

      1) Pyelonephritis

      2) Chronic interstitial nephritis

   C. Other bacterial infections

      1) Cystitis

      2) Pneumonia

      3) Pyometra

   D. Severe fatty infiltration of the liver

   E. Congestive heart failure

5. Prognosis

   A. Guarded for complicated DM

   B. If an animal can be stabilized, it usually does well with a diligent owner.

Goals of Treatment in Complicated Diabetes Mellitus

Rehydration
Lower blood glucose
End to ketone production
Correct electrolyte imbalances (K^+ most
   important)
Treatment of acidosis only if severe (pH <
   7.1)
Treatment of coexisting disorders

1. Therapy

A. Fluid therapy

1) Aseptic technique in placing intravenous catheters is crucial because diabetics are known to be more susceptible to infections in this setting. The routine use of antibiotics to cover the possibility of sepsis is controversial. Use an appropriate antibiotic in patients with known concurrent infection.

2) Therapy for shock consists of adequate volume replacement and glucocorticoids (even though they are antagonistic to the action of insulin).

3) .9% sodium chloride is the fluid of choice.

a) It corrects sodium depletion rapidly.

b) Use lactated ringers alternatively.

4) Estimate percent of dehydration and calculate needs (see Chapter 24).

5) Half of the calculated fluid needs for dehydration and maintenance fluids may be given in the first six hours to expedite correction of the dehydration.

6) In case of severe oliguria or anuria, take care not to overhydrate the animal.

a) Insert a urinary catheter to monitor urine output.

b) A jugular catheter allows central venous pressure (CVP) monitoring.

7) After the rapid period of dehydration correction, start potassium supplementation.

8) After the first 18 to 24 hours, lactated Ringers may be substituted for the .9% NaCl unless a normal serum sodium level has not been attained.

B. Lowered serum glucose and decreased ketoacidosis are accomplished simultaneously.

C. Potassium supplementation

1) Because all diabetics are potassium-depleted, start supplementation early in the treatment regimen.

2) The rate of IV potassium administration must not exceed .5 mEq/kg/h.

3) Add potassium to the fluids only after the rapid rehydration period (approximately six hours) to avoid exceeding the maximum rate of IV potassium infusion.

4) Adjust supplementation according to the serum potassium concentration by using the sliding scale of Scott (see Chapter 25).

5) Daily serum potassium determination is needed at least as long as the animal is being supplemented intravenously. More frequent determinations may be needed during the initial stages of insulin administration.

6) Once the animal begins eating, taper and then stop potassium supplementation.

7) In the face of anuria or oliguria, potassium supplementation is dangerous.

a) Other factors may further reduce serum potassium levels (insulin, acidosis correction, rehydration), however, and life-threatening hypokalemia may occur.

b) Supplement potassium at a lower level and use either an ECG or serum potassium levels to monitor for toxicity.

D. Therapy for metabolic acidosis

1) Use no alkali therapy unless the *p*H is less than 7.1.

2) Rapid correction of acidosis could decrease the oxygen-carrying ability of blood or result in paradoxical CSF acidosis; fatal hypokalemia also may occur.

3) Rehydration, electrolyte correction, and insulin administration slowly correct the acid–base imbalance and minimize complications.

4) In the face of severe metabolic acidosis, supplement $NaHCO_3$ in the IV fluids and do not give it as a bolus.

a) Calculate the mEq $NAHCO_3$ needed

$$= .4 \times \text{body weight in kg} \times \text{base deficit in mEq/L}$$

b) Give one fourth of calculated dose in two hours and administer the rest over 24 hours (see Chapter 26).

Insulin Treatments

1. Insulin treatment, *low-dose intramuscular method*

A. Earlier theories about insulin resistance in ketoacidosis and the necessity for large doses of insulin are being abandoned.

B. Advantages of this method

1) Accurate measurement of administered insulin

2) Minimal equipment and supervision

3) Gradual decline of serum glucose

4) Unlikely development of hypoglycemia or severe hypokalemia

   a) A steady decline in the blood glucose is desirable. Too rapid a decrease may result in cerebral edema because the blood glucose concentration decreases more rapidly than the CSF concentration, possibly widening the CSF–plasma osmotic gradient.

  C. Method

1) Use regular (crystalline) insulin.

2) Dose—.25 U/kg initially, followed by hourly injections of .1 U/kg until the blood glucose is less than 250 mg/dL

3) When treating small animals (< 10 kg), accuracy in insulin dosage will be improved by diluting the insulin 1 : 10 with commercial insulin diluent or sterile saline.

4) Measure blood glucose hourly before each intramuscular injection. Use reagent sticks with or without a corresponding automated test strip analyzer.

5) Expect a mean of about four hours to lower blood glucose to < 250 mg/dL (range two to seven hours). Expect an average decline in blood glucose of about 88 mg/dL/h (range 42 to 176 mg/dL/h) using this technique.

   a) When the blood glucose reaches 250 to 300 mg/dL, add 50% dextrose to the animal's fluids to make a 5% dextrose solution.

   b) Also monitor electrolytes and supplement potassium, sodium, and phosphorus as necessary (see above).

6) Change to subcutaneous regular insulin injections every six hours when the blood glucose is below 250 mg/dL.

   a) Monitor blood glucose every one to two hours and adjust insulin dosage accordingly before each insulin injection.

   b) Continue regular insulin injections every six hours, even after the plasma glucose is reduced to below 200 mg/dL.

    i. Insulin is needed for the use of ketone bodies already present.

    ii. Discontinuation of insulin results in further tissue breakdown.

   c) As a source of carbohydrates, and to prevent hypoglycemia, maintain fluid therapy with a 2.5 or 5% dextrose drip until the animal is eating. Oral supplementation is contraindicated in the presence of pancreatitis, however.

7) Change to daily longer-acting insulin injections (NPH, protamine zinc insulin) only when the patient has stabilized.

   a) Usually make this change when the animal is clinically much improved, eating, not vomiting, and maintaining fluid and electrolyte balance.

   b) Start NPH in the morning for management convenience.

   c) If anorexia or vomiting from any cause should recur during this period, discontinue NPH insulin and reinstitute regular insulin and a 2.5 or 5% dextrose infusion.

  2. Insulin treatment, *continuous IV method*

  A. Advantages over intermittent bolus therapy

1) Constant physiologic levels of insulin are more easily attained.

2) Timing and dosage of subsequently administered insulin is not a problem.

3) There is less chance for hypokalemia to develop.

4) There is less chance for hypoglycemia to develop.

5) There is a rapid decline in serum insulin concentration once the infusion is stopped because insulin has a short half-life. This allows a quicker response if hypoglycemia or hypokalemia were to develop.

  B. Method

1) Add 5 U of regular (crystalline) insulin to 500 mL of isotonic solution to get a concentration of 1 U insulin in each 100 mL of fluid.

2) Infuse insulin at a rate of .5 to 1.0 U per hour; this is equivalent to 50 to 100 mL per hour of the above solution. Administer by means of an infusion pump, buretrol, or pediatric infusion set to ensure delivery of accurate volume.

3) Achieve hydration with another solution setup and possibly another IV line.

4) Measure serum glucose values every .5 to 1.0 hours and slow or stop the infusion when a glucose concentration of 200 mg/dL or less is achieved.

5) At that time, initiate subcutaneous regular insulin injections at six-hour intervals as described above.

3. Insulin treatment, *intermittent method*

A. Use only regular (crystalline) insulin.

B. Dose

1) Administer .5 to 1.0 U/kg; use the lower dose in large dogs and cats, the higher dose in small dogs.

2) If the animal is dehydrated, do not give insulin subcutaneously because, when a rehydrated state is reached, excessive absorption could occur.

3) Use the IM route until a rehydrated state is attained.

4) If the animal has high blood glucose, is comatose, or is severely ketotic, some authors recommend the administration of half of the insulin dose by an intravenous route and the remainder intramuscularly.

5) Perform blood glucose determinations every one to two hours.

a) Blood glucose values should be available because low doses of insulin might reduce the blood sugar markedly and unpredictably in any given patient.

b) A steady decline in the blood glucose is desirable.

6) When the blood glucose reaches 250 to 300 mg/dL, add 50% dextrose to the patient's fluids to make a 5% solution.

7) Adjust the patient's insulin dose every six hours according to results of previous blood glucose determinations.

8) Continue regular insulin injections every six hours, even after the plasma glucose is reduced to below 200 mg/dL.

Cerebral Edema

1. A complication seen in small animal medicine

2. Veterinarians have not had much experience in the treatment of cerebral edema associated with DM.

3. Consider furosemide (Lasix) and mannitol for treatment of the condition.

4. Treat coexisting disease or disorders.

Hyperosmolar, Nonketotic Diabetic Coma

Hyperosmolar, nonketotic diabetic coma is a syndrome characterized by severe hyperglycemia, hyperosmolality, depressed level of consciousness, and dehydration in the absence of ketoacidosis. In humans, hyperosmolar coma may be the first sign of DM. This condition is rarely encountered in dogs and cats.

1. Severe signs may occur when serum osmolality is in excess of 375 mOsm/kg.

2. The osmolality can be calculated or measured (see Chapter 25).

3. The lack of a low level of ketosis may be related to the much smaller amount of insulin needed to prevent lipolysis compared with that needed to prevent gluconeogenesis and glycogenolysis.

A. Extreme hyperosmolality could have an effect on intermediary metabolism. It could result in an inhibitory effect on adipose tissue lipolysis and reduce the amount of free fatty acids presented to the liver; thus, it could prevent increased ketogenesis.

B. Growth hormone and cortisol are lipolytic agents. There have been studies in humans showing decreased levels of these hormones in hyperosmolar diabetic patients.

4. Profound osmotic diuresis from persistent hyperglycemia results in a loss of water in excess of electrolytes.

5. Intracellular dehydration of the brain leads to neurologic abnormalities.

6. Serum sodium may be high, normal, or low.

A. Hyponatremia occurs when the hyperglycemia draws water from the cells into the plasma to maintain a normal serum osmolality.

B. Serum sodium also is affected by urinary loss.

C. When fluid loss and dehydration become severe, hypernatremia may develop.

7. Patients with high blood glucose concentrations are most likely to develop cerebral edema.

A. The presence of idiogenic osmoles helps to maintain intracellular hydration of neurons.

B. A rapid decrease in blood glucose because of therapy could result in the development of an unfavorable osmotic gradient.

8. In dogs, studies have shown that a sudden decrease of sustained hyperglycemia may lead to increased CSF pressure and cerebral edema.

A. Studies in rabbits show that

1) Acute hyperglycemia (at two hours) results in loss of water from the brain and intracellular volume contraction.

2) By four hours, brain volume and hydration are returned to normal.

3) Apparently, osmotically active particles that prevent water loss, even in the presence of hyperosmolality, are present within the brain.

4) These particles originally were thought to be sorbitol but are now referred to as *idiogenic osmoles*.

B. Idiogenic osmoles seem to disappear slowly.

C. With insulin, brain osmolality falls slower than plasma osmolality, and a gradient develops.

D. Clinically, when the blood glucose concentration is rapidly reduced below 300 mg/dL, cerebral edema develops.

E. Plasma glucose concentrations decrease more rapidly than CSF glucose concentrations; this widens the CSF–plasma osmotic gradient.

F. The above factors could all lead to larger CSF–plasma osmotic gradients and result in intracellular edema of neural tissue.

9. Treatment objectives and procedure

A. To correct dehydration and hypotension

B. To correct electrolyte imbalances

C. To lower the blood glucose concentrations slowly and steadily by judicious use of regular insulin

D. Do not administer alkali if there is no significant acidosis.

E. Use .45% NaCl if normonatremia or hypernatremia is present, so that minimal additions to the hyperosmolar state occur. Use 0.9% NaCl if hyponatremia is present.

F. Administer regular insulin (.25 U/lb); give half of the dose IV and the other half IM.

1) Take a blood glucose determination in two hours.

2) If no significant decrease has occurred (decrease < 100 mg/dL), repeat the insulin dose.

3) Administer regular insulin every six hours after serum glucose determination and urine glucose and ketone determinations have been made.

4) When the blood glucose falls below 300 mg/dL, add dextrose to the IV fluids.

5) To prevent cerebral edema, avoid a precipitous decline in blood glucose.

10. Potassium supplementation

A. Start after the initial rehydration period (six hours).

B. Guidelines are the same as for other complicated diabetics.

Miscellaneous

1. Cases of transient DM do exist; this is especially true for cats.

2. After acute pancreatitis, dogs may develop transient DM. Warn the owner of this and instruct the owner to contact the veterinarian if a steady decline in insulin requirements is seen.

Suggested Readings

Hypoglycemia

Caywood DD, Klausner JS, O'Leary TP, et al: Pancreatic insulin-secreting neoplasms: Clinical, diagnostic, and prognostic features in 73 dogs. J Am Anim Hosp Assoc 24: 577–584, 1988

Nelson RW, Foodman MS: Medical management of canine hyperinsulinism. J Am Vet Med Assoc 187: 78–82, 1985

Rogers KS, Luttgen PJ: Hyperinsulinism. Comp Cont Ed Pract Vet 10: 829–841, 1985

Hyperglycemia

Chastain CB, Nichols CE: Current concepts on the control of diabetes mellitus. Vet Clin North Am [Small Anim Pract] 14: 859–872, 1984

Chastain CB, Nichols CE: Low-dose intramuscular insulin therapy for diabetic ketoacidosis in dogs. J Am Vet Med Assoc 178: 561–564, 1981

Feldman EC, Nelson RW: Canine and Feline Endocrinology and Reproduction. Philadelphia, WB Saunders, 1987

CHAPTER TWENTY-THREE

Urinalysis

Dennis J. Chew

A properly collected and performed urinalysis (UA) may yield valuable information about the urinary system or may reflect some systemic disorder.

Collection of Urine

1. Urine may be collected after voiding, manual expression, catheterization, or cystocentesis.

2. Generally, try to collect urine specimens in the A.M., because this is usually the most concentrated specimen of the day.

3. Transfer the urine to the laboratory in a vessel that is clean and free of chemical contamination.

4. Perform the UA as soon as possible, and refrigerate the specimen if it cannot be performed within 30 minutes.

Methods of Urine Collection

Voided

1. Midstream-voided specimens are most desired, because the initial void stream mechanically flushes out contamination from the distal urethra and vagina or prepuce.

2. Voided specimens taken from the cage or floor are less desirable but still may be of some benefit if the contamination factor is considered.

3. Voided specimens may be sufficient for interpretation; however, when contamination with cells, protein, or bacteria is a concern, collection by another method is recommended to confirm the abnormality.

4. This is the method of choice in the initial evaluation of hematuria, since the remaining methods can all add RBC from trauma during collection.

Expressed

1. This method is particularly suitable for obtaining a urine specimen from cats and small dogs.

2. It is more difficult to express urine from the bladder in the male dog or cat.

3. Trauma during attempts to expel urine from the bladder may add RBC and protein to the urine specimen. The degree of difficulty in expressing the urine specimen should be noted.

4. Do not attempt to express urine specimens for collection if the animal has urethral obstruction, major bladder-tissue devitalization, or recent major bladder trauma, or if a recent cystotomy has been performed.

5. Rupture of a normal bladder can occur if too much digital pressure is applied; rupture of a diseased bladder may occur more readily.

6. Contamination from the distal urethra, vagina, or prepuce also must be considered when evaluating urine obtained by this technique.

7. If attempts to express urine are unsuccessful, be prepared to collect a voided specimen. Animals frequently urinate when returned to the cage after bladder palpation.

Catheterized

1. This technique should be performed in as sterile a manner as possible.

2. Direct visualization of the urethral orifice in females is preferred over "blind" sterile-glove techniques. This may be accomplished with vaginal speculums, otoscopic speculums, or the use of human anuscope equipment.

3. Much of the contamination of the vagina, prepuce, and perineum is bypassed with this technique, but remember that the distal urethra is not bypassed. The distal urethra may not be sterile.

4. Introduction of bacteria into the bladder during catheterization may result in urinary tract infection.

5. Rupture of the diseased urethra or bladder may occur when too much force is applied to the catheter. Faulty technique also may result in rupture of the normal urethra or bladder.

6. Trauma during catheterization may add RBC, protein, and epithelial cells to the specimen.

Cystocentesis

1. This technique bypasses contamination from the distal urethra, vagina, prepuce, and perineum.

2. Reflux of urine from the proximal urethra and prostate into bladder urine may occur, and abnormal elements may be discovered on samples taken by cystocentesis.

3. Do not use this technique for collection of urine if the urethra is obstructed, bladder atony exists, severe bladder trauma or devitalization exists, or a recent cystotomy has been performed.

4. The technique results in the least non-urinary contamination of the urine sample

and the fewest number of WBC in normal urine.

5. Trauma from the needle tip during aspiration may result in iatrogenic hematuria.

6. Cystocentesis is the technique of choice for urine collection when a urine culture is desired, and to confirm proteinuria and microscopic bacteriuria reported by other collection techniques.

Performing the Urinalysis

1. Examine fresh urine.

2. Warm refrigerated urine to room temperature before examination.

3. Perform a complete UA.

    A. Specific gravity

    B. Reagent strip testing

    C. Sediment examination after centrifugation

4. Perform the UA under identical conditions in your laboratory so that comparison and serial evaluation of results may be made.

5. Read reagent strip color reaction at time intervals suggested by manufacturer. Compare intensity of color reaction that occurs with standards provided by the manufacturer. Read color reactions in good lighting and record the results.

6. Urinary sediment (microscopic examination)

    A. Initially, scan under low power to identify the location of abnormal elements; then switch to high dry magnification to characterize further and identify the abnormal elements.

    B. Count at least 10 microscopic fields and average the number of elements per field.

    C. Record casts as the number per low-powered field. Record RBC, WBC, and epithelial cells as the number per high-powered field.

Interpretation of the Urinalysis

1. Proper interpretation requires that a complete UA be performed (specific gravity, re-

---

Sample Urinalysis Form

Patient identification _____
Source of specimen: Void   Express   Cath.   Cysto.
Volume submitted _____ mL
Color _____   Casts:
Appearance _____   Hyaline _____/Lpf
Specific gravity _____   Granular _____/Lpf
pH _____   Other _____/Lpf
Protein _____   WBC _____/hpf
Occult blood _____   RBC _____/hpf
Glucose _____   Epithelial cells _____/hpf
Ketone _____   Crystals _____
Bilirubin _____   Bacteria _____
Urobilinogen _____   Miscellaneous _____

---

agent strip testing, and microscopic evaluation of urinary sediment).

2. Always note how the sample was obtained, because the method used may influence certain results greatly.

Physical Properties

Color

1. Normal color is yellow to amber, due mostly to the pigment urochrome.
2. Abnormal color
  A. Deep amber
    1) Highly concentrated urine
    2) Increased amounts of bile pigments in the urine
  B. Red to reddish-brown
    1) Intact RBC (hematuria), most common
    2) Hemoglobinuria
    3) Myoglobinuria, uncommon
    4) Porphyrins, rare
  C. Dark brown to black—Conversion of hemoglobin in acid urine to methemoglobins is most likely.
  D. Green
    1) Increased biliverdin in urine as bilirubin in urine is oxidized
    2) *Pseudomonas spp.* urinary infection

    3) Methylene-blue administration (greenish-blue urine)
  E. Remember that many drugs may alter urine color as the parent compound or metabolites are excreted into urine.

Appearance (Turbidity, Transparency, Clarity)

1. Normal urine is usually clear when evaluated in a clear tube or in good lighting.
2. Cloudy urine may be normal in some dogs and cats that are found to have no other abnormality on further analysis.
3. Abnormal appearance, cloudy or hazy
  A. Excessive RBC
  B. Excessive WBC
  C. Epithelial cells
  D. Bacteria or fungi
  E. Spermatozoa
  F. Prostatic fluid
  G. Mucous
  H. Crystals
4. Abnormal appearance, flocculent
  A. Aggregates of WBC
  B. Clumps of epithelial cells
  C. Very small calculi

Specific Gravity

1. Measure specific gravity (SG) using a refractometer. Older methods using hydrometers (urinometer) are not as accurate. New dipstrip methods to determine human SG may not be accurate in dogs and cats.

2. Most refractometers measure up to an SG of 1.035 in humans. To determine the SG accurately beyond this, add equal portions of distilled water and urine, then redetermine the SG. Multiply the numbers to the right of the decimal point by a factor of 2 to determine the actual SG.

3. Use veterinary refractometers designed specifically for use in dogs, cats, and horses to avoid the need to dilute with distilled water, because the scale is much larger to accommodate these species.

4. SG is influenced by the number of particles, molecular weight, and molecular size of the substances in solution in urine.

    A. 1000 mg/dL glucose elevates the SG approximately .004.

    B. 1000 mg/dL protein elevates the SG approximately .003.

5. Some degree of urine concentration is usually seen from normally hydrated dogs and cats.

    A. Random SG from these healthy animals often has a value in excess of 1.020 in dogs or 1.030 in cats.

    B. Some normal dogs and cats routinely exhibit in excess of a 1.040 SG.

    C. One random dilute urine SG does not always imply disease. Repeated dilute SG justifies a search for possible urinary and extraurinary causes of dilute urine.

    1) Primary renal disease

    2) Pituitary insufficiency (diabetes insipidis)

    3) Liver disease

    4) Cushing's disease (hyperadrenocorticisim)

    5) Diabetes mellitus

    6) Psychogenic polydipsia

    7) Pyometra

    8) Hypercalcemia or hypokalemia

6. Dehydrated dogs and cats should be elaborating very concentrated urine (>1.030) if their kidneys are healthy.

7. If at all possible, SG should be measured before the administration of any drug or fluid therapy, because these may alter the SG.

8. SG is the only parameter on the UA that may reflect renal function accurately.

9. Use the SG as a guide to note the relative concentration of abnormal elements in the sample (e.g., 6 RBC/hpf on a 1.065 SG specimen may have less significance than 6 RBC/hpf on a 1.010 SG specimen).

Chemical Properties (Reagent Strip Evaluation)

pH

1. *p*H in urine from normal dogs and cats is usually acidic but may range from 5.5 to 7.5.

2. Abnormal *p*H

    A. Persistently alkaline urine most often reflects urinary tract infection with urease-producing bacteria. (Urinary tract infection need not alter the urine *p*H.)

    B. Alkaline urine may be elaborated transiently after meals (postprandial alkaline tide).

    C. Bacterial contamination of the urine sample may result in alkaline urine by liberation of ammonium from urea, if the sample sits before examination.

    D. Urinary *p*H may or may not correlate with acidemia or alkalemia seen in systemic disorders and is not considered a reliable predictor of acid–base balance in the body.

    E. Urinary acidifiers and alkalinizers alter urinary *p*H.

Protein

1. Reagent strips allow a qualitative and semiquantitative measurement of proteinuria. These strips are much more sensitive to albumin than to other urinary proteins.

2. Normal urine from dogs and cats may have positive determinations for protein.

3. Trace to +1 readings (20 to 30 mg/dL) are considered normal if the urine is concentrated. Extremely concentrated urine (>1.060 SG) may result in a +2 reading (100 mg/dL) that does not signify pathologic proteinuria.

4. The protein reading, when positive, should be integrated immediately with sediment findings.

A. If associated with inflammatory cells, the protein probably entered the urine along with the cells.

B. If associated with no inflammatory cells or if associated with excessive numbers of casts, the protein probably entered the urine from the kidney.

5. Localization of proteinuria

A. Prerenal proteinuria occurs when low-molecular-weight proteins pass excessively through normal glomeruli.

1) Bence–Jones proteins

2) Hemoglobinuria

3) Myoglobinuria

B. Renal proteinuria

1) Abnormal glomerular filter permeability

a) Glomerulonephritis

b) Amyloidosis

c) Glomerular atrophy

2) Abnormal tubular reabsorption of filtered proteins

3) Addition of protein to urine from intrarenal inflammation

4) Combinations

C. Postrenal proteinuria usually occurs in association with increased numbers of RBC and WBC in urinary sediment. Lesions resulting in proteinuria may be hemorrhagic or inflammatory and may arise from the

1) Ureter

2) Bladder

3) Urethra

4) Genital secretions

Glucose

1. Glucose is not present in detectable quantity in urine from normal dogs and cats.

2. Refrigerated urine specimens may result in false-negative results; they should be warmed to room temperature before testing.

3. Causes of glucosuria

A. Diabetes mellitus is the most common clinical disorder resulting in hyperglycemia and glucosuria. Pancreatitis, hyperadrenocorticism, pheochromocytoma, and hypothalamic lesions may on occasion be associated with hyperglycemia and glucosuria.

B. IV fluids containing gluc... result in hyperglycemia and gluc...

C. Cats may have transient hyp... mia and glucosuria after severe stress... excitement. Some cats with severe uret... obstruction have glucosuria, although the mechanism is unknown.

D. Glucosuria associated with a normal blood glucose may be encountered with decreased renal tubular function.

1) Primary renal glucosuria

2) Fanconi syndrome

3) Norwegian elkhound renal disease and other familial nephropathies

4) Acute intrinsic renal failure

a) Nephrotoxic tubular injury (drugs)

b) Ischemic tubular injury

Ketones

1. Ketones are not present in normal urine.

2. Ketonuria indicates abnormal fat and energy metabolism.

A. Diabetic ketoacidosis is the most common clinical condition resulting in ketonuria and is associated with glucosuria.

B. Long-standing starvation also may result in ketonuria; however; glucosuria is absent.

C. Chronic catabolic diseases

D. Persistent fever

E. Persistent hypoglycemia (non–insulin-mediated)

Occult blood

1. Reagent strips react in the presence of heme pigments.

A. Intact erythrocytes

B. Free hemoglobin

C. Myoglobin

2. The reaction is more sensitive to the presence of free pigment than to that found inside intact RBC.

3. Reagent strips detect the presence of hematuria long before it becomes macroscopically visible.

4. Normal dog or cat urine does not have a positive reaction for occult blood.

occult blood should
.re-sediment findings for

...tes seen in urinary
..n that hematuria is the cause
.e occult blood reaction.
ence of erythrocytes in urinary
.means that the occult blood reac-
.due to either liberated hemoglobin or
,lobin.

C. Hemoglobinuria may occur after severe intravascular hemolysis or lysis of RBC that were once within urine.

D. Myoglobinuria follows severe muscle-cell damage.

6. Positive occult blood reactions are most commonly due to erythrocytes, sometimes due to freed hemoglobin, and uncommonly due to myoglobin.

7. Contamination of the sample with flea feces may uncommonly result in a positive reaction for occult blood.

White Blood Cells

1. Designed to detect esterase of human WBC

2. Not sensitive in dogs; unknown in cats

3. Not recommended for routine use

Bilirubin

1. Urinalysis samples must be fresh, or bilirubin may be oxidized to biliverdin or hydrolyzed to unconjugated bilirubin and will not be detected.

2. Bilirubin is not detectable in urine from normal cats.

3. As many as 60% of normal dogs may have detectable bilirubinuria. Trace to +1 reactions may be measured, particularly if the urine specimen is highly concentrated.

4. Any bilirubin detected in feline urine is considered abnormal.

5. In dogs a +2 to +3 reaction is considered significantly abnormal. Lesser reactions on dilute urine specimens also may be significant.

6. Only conjugated bilirubin can be filtered into the urine.

7. The dog has a low renal threshold for conjugated bilirubin, allowing bilirubinuria to be detected before elevations in serum bilirubin occur.

8. Causes of pathologic bilirubinuria

  A. Prehepatic

    1) Hemolysis may result in liver dysfunction because of anemia and hemosiderosis leading to subsequent regurgitation of conjugated bilirubin from within the liver into the plasma.

    2) In dogs hemoglobinuria may result in bilirubinuria after tubular transformation of the filtered hemoglobin.

  B. Hepatic diseases

  C. Posthepatic—Obstruction of the common bile duct results in the highest magnitude of bilirubinuria.

  D. Febrile disorders and starvation may result in small quantities of bilirubinuria.

9. Significant hepatic and posthepatic pathology may exist without the detection of bilirubinuria.

Microscopic Examination of Urinary Sediment

1. Evaluation of the urinary sediment requires proper identification of cells (RBC, WBC, epithelial cells), casts, organisms, and crystals.

2. It is not always possible to identify accurately all elements within urinary sediment owing to altered morphology encountered from the hostile environment of urine.

3. Normal urine sediment contains very few cells or casts and should not have visible organisms.

4. Normal values for urinary sediment cannot be established between laboratories because of methodologic differences in performing the analysis and in setting up the sediment for microscopy.

5. Sediment identification is aided greatly if fresh urine is analyzed immediately and if supravital staining (Sedi-stain) is used.

6. Microscopy is greatly facilitated by using reduced-contrast illumination.

7. Remember to consider how the urine was collected when interpreting sediment findings.

8. Remember to consider urine concentration (SG) in an attempt to determine the effect on relative concentration of all elements within the sediment.

9. Urine sediment findings must be integrated with other aspects of the UA, patient history, physical examination, and other pertinent laboratory findings.

10. Cells

  A. RBC

    1) Some RBC in low numbers may be found in normal urine from dogs and cats.

    2) Approximately normal ranges

      a) 0 to 8/high power field if by void

      b) 0 to 5/high power field if by catheter

      c) 0 to 3/high power field if by cystocentesis; traumatic values easily exceed 50/high power field, however.

    3) Always consider the degree of trauma encountered during the collection process when evaluating excess numbers of RBC.

    4) *Hematuria* refers to excessive numbers of RBC in urine.

    5) Origin of RBC—The finding of RBC in urine does not localize where the excessive entry of RBC into urine is occurring, unless the RBC are included in casts (thereby incriminating the kidney). RBC entry must be considered possible from the

      a) Kidney

      b) Ureter

      c) Bladder

      d) Urethra

      e) Vagina or prepuce

    6) Urinary causes for hematuria

      a) Trauma

      b) Urinary calculi

      c) Urinary tract infection

      d) Urinary neoplasia

      e) Renal infarction

      f) Any necrotic urinary lesion

      g) Nephritis

      h) Nephrosis

      i) Prostatic disease

      j) Cystitis (nonbacterial) or urethritis

      k) Urinary parasites

      l) Coagulopathy (warfarin, disseminated intravenous coagulation or DIC, thrombocytopenia)

    7) Nonurinary causes for hematuria

      a) Estrus

      b) Draining pyometra

      c) Endometritis

      d) Vaginal disease

      e) Preputial or penile lesions

  B. WBC

    1) As with RBC, small numbers of WBC may be found in urine from normal dogs and cats.

    2) Approximately normal ranges

      a) 0 to 8/high power field if by void

      b) 0 to 5/high power field if by catheter

      c) 0 to 3/high power field if by cystocentesis

    3) *Pyuria* refers to excessive numbers of WBC in urine.

    4) The anatomic origin of WBC in urine is not defined unless WBC are found within casts, thereby incriminating the kidney. WBC entry must be considered possible from the

      a) Kidney

      b) Ureter

      c) Bladder

      d) Urethra

      e) Vagina or prepuce

    5) Causes of pyuria

      a) Urinary tract inflammation

      b) Contamination from an inflammatory process within the vagina or prepuce

    6) Urinary tract infection is the most common cause of pyuria.

      a) Clumps of WBC may occur with urinary infections.

      b) Search carefully for organisms that might account for the pyuria.

      c) Bacteria may be visible (free floating; between clumps of WBC; or, when phagocytized, within WBC).

      d) Fungal organisms or yeasts are rarely the cause of pyuria.

7) It may be difficult to identify WBC accurately once significant morphologic degeneration has occurred.

C. Epithelial cells

1) Squamous epithelial cells

a) Usually of no diagnostic importance

b) Small numbers per high power field seen normally in urine collected by void or catheterization

c) Estrus may greatly increase the numbers of squamous epithelia in urine.

2) Renal epithelial cells

a) There is no reliable way to differentiate the small epithelium of renal tubular origin from small transitional epithelial cells unless epithelial cells are included within casts (thereby incriminating renal origin for the epithelium).

b) Nephritis

c) Nephrosis

3) Transitional epithelial cells

a) Occasional transitional epithelial cells are seen per high power field in urine from normal dogs and cats.

b) Excessive numbers of transitional epithelial cells may be associated with

i. Urinary infection

ii. Mechanical abrasion (urolithiasis or catheter technique)

iii. Neoplasia

iv. Chemical irritation (cyclophosphamide therapy)

c) Clumps of epithelial cells may be seen with neoplasia but also may be seen as a hyperplastic response to infection.

d) Cytologic study of clumps of epithelial cells is often needed to differentiate neoplasia from hyperplasia.

11. Casts

A. Casts are cylindrically shaped molds of aggregated proteins or cells formed within tubular lumina.

B. Very few casts are found in normal urine.

1) 0 to 2 hyaline casts/low power field

2) 0 to 1 granular cast/low power field

3) 0 other types of casts

C. *Cylindruria* refers to excretion of abnormal casts or increased numbers of casts.

D. Cylindruria helps to document the presence of renal disease but does not refer to level of renal function.

E. Hyaline casts

1) Often associated with conditions having proteinuria

2) May occur even though kidneys are normal, as in fever, severe exercise, and diuretic therapy (humans). In these instances hyaline casts are a transient finding.

3) Persistent finding of hyaline casts suggest renal pathology.

a) Glomerular

b) Tubular

F. Cellular casts

1) RBC casts

a) Not frequently observed in urine specimens from dogs and cats

b) Renal trauma; bleeding into tubular lumina is the most common cause.

c) Glomerulonephritis, uncommonly associated

d) Acute interstitial nephritis, rarely find a pure RBC cast, but may be mixed with other cells

2) WBC casts (pus casts)

a) Pyelonephritis, most common cause

b) Any active interstitial nephritis

c) Acute tubular necrosis

d) Exudative glomerulonephritis (humans)

e) May exist as a mixed cast with other cells

3) Epithelial-cell casts

a) Severe tubular-cell injury is implied.

b) Often associated with nephrotoxic or ischemic renal disease

c) Pyelonephritis

d) May exist as a mixed cast with other cells

G. Granular casts

1) Granules in these casts may represent aggregates of serum proteins from a glomerulopathy or cellular breakdown products from tubular degeneration.

2) Excessive numbers of granular casts suggest accelerated tubular degeneration in many instances but also may indicate glomerular damage.

H. Waxy casts

1) Waxy casts are thought to be the final stage of granular-cast degeneration

2) Because this degree of degeneration requires the greatest amount of intrarenal time, substantial intrarenal stasis or local oliguria is implied when waxy casts are found.

3) Most commonly associated with chronic renal diseases; can be seen in any disorder resulting in increased formation of intrarenal cellular or granular cast formation.

12. Organisms

A. Bacteria should not be visible in urine sediment from normal dogs and cats if the sample was collected properly.

B. Visible bacteriuria usually means that bacterial urinary tract infection exists.

C. Amorphous debris may be confused with bacteria, particularly during Brownian motion, resulting in a false-positive recording for bacteria.

D. Urinary infection may exist even though bacterial organisms are not visible in the wet mount of sediment (false-negative).

E. Suspected urinary infection should be confirmed by additional testing.

1) Quantitative urine culture

2) Gram stain of urine sediment

F. Fungal organisms or yeasts are most often contaminants encountered during collection, during transportation to the laboratory, or from bottles of stain. True fungal infection may exist rarely, often in a clinical setting of urinary obstruction and prolonged use of antimicrobials. Immunosuppressive therapy (including corticosteroids) also may contribute to true fungal urinary infection.

13. Crystals

A. Crystals often are in normal urine.

B. Expect greater numbers of crystals when the sample is highly concentrated (high urinary specific gravity), refrigerated, or if the urinary *p*H favors precipitation.

C. Crystals may occur after the excretion into urine of endogenous substances or those from outside the body.

D. Crystal formation is enhanced when excretion of a substance increases or its urinary concentration increases as a consequence of dietary intake, abnormal metabolism, or defective renal tubular reabsorption.

E. Reference to urinary *p*H can be helpful when trying to identify crystals.

F. Most likely to form in alkaline urine

1) Struvite

a) May be normal or associated with urolithiasis

2) Amorphous phosphate

a) May be normal or associated with urolithiasis

3) Calcium phosphate

a) Urolithiasis

4) Calcium carbonate

a) Urolithiasis

5) Ammonium biurate

a) Liver disease

b) Portosystemic shunt

G. Most likely to form in acid urine

1) Uric acid

a) Urolithiasis

b) Metabolic defect

2) Cystine

a) Urolithiasis

b) Metabolic defect

3) Calcium oxalate

a) Normal

b) Ethylene glycol poisoning

c) Urolithiasis

4) "Hippurate-like"

a) Are not really hippurates

b) Another hydrated form of calcium oxalate

c) Ethylene glycol poisoning

H. Bilirubin crystals can be normal in dogs, especially males, but also can indicate liver disease or hemolysis.

I. Bilirubin crystals are never normal in cats.

J. Many therapeutic agents that form crystals that are difficult to identify are excreted into urine.

1) Sulfas frequently form crystals.

Suggested Readings

Chew DJ: Urinalysis. In Bovee KC (ed): Canine Nephrology. Media, PA, Harwal Publishing Co., pp. 235–274, 1984

Finco DR: Kidney Function. In Kaneko JJ (ed): Clinical Biochemistry of Domestic Animals, 4th ed. pp. 496–542, 1989

Osborne CA, Stevens JB: Handbook of Canine and Feline Urinalysis. St. Louis, Missouri, Ralston Purina Co., 1981

PART FOUR

PRINCIPLES OF FLUID AND ELECTROLYTE BALANCE

CHAPTER TWENTY-FOUR

Disorders of Fluid Balance and Fluid Therapy

Dennis J. Chew, Catherine W. Kohn, and
Stephen P. DiBartola

Normal Distribution of Body Water

1. Total body water (TBW) ranges from 50% to 70% of body weight for adults.

A. Sixty percent of body weight (BW) is used as an approximation of TBW (Figures 24-1 and 24-2).

1) A number of factors affect the percent of body weight that is water.

a) Age—In young puppies 70% to 80% of body weight is water.

b) Pregnancy and lactation—An increased percentage of body weight is water.

c) Obesity—Percent of body weight that is water is decreased since fat contains little water.

d) Fluid accumulation in body cavities (e.g., ascites, pleural effusion)—An increased percentage of body weight is water.

B. TBW consists of approximate division into two thirds intracellular water (40% BW) and one third extracellular water (20% BW)

1) The volume of distribution for administered water may have fast and slow phases for equilibration.

a) Fast phase equilibration approximates about one half (30% BW) intracellular and one half (30% BW) extracellular water.

2. Extracellular fluid (ECF) is further divided

A. Plasma volume—about 5% BW

B. Blood volume—about 8% BW (includes plasma volume)

C. Interstitial—about 15% BW (includes transcellular fluid)

D. Transcellular fluid—about 3% BW (subgroup of interstitial fluid)

1) CSF, bile, GI fluids

2) Slow equilibration with ECF

3. Fluid flux between compartments is a dynamic process and may occur rapidly.

4. The volume of water retained within a compartment of body water is related to the number of osmotically active particles present in the space.

5. All body fluid compartments are isosmotic. Water and solutes shift across semipermeable membranes to maintain isotonicity of body fluid space.

6. Starling's forces are important determinants of plasma volume. Plasma oncotic pressure and tissue hydrostatic pressure are forces that favor maintaining plasma volume. Plasma hydrostatic pressure and tissue oncotic pressure are forces favoring egress of fluid from the plasma volume.

Figure 24-1. *The diagram illustrates compartmentalization of total body water in an average, normal mammal. TBW = Total Body Water; ICF = Intracellular Fluid; ECF = Extracellular Fluid; IF = Interstitial Fluid; BW = Body Weight*

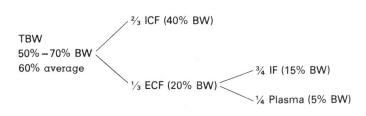

Water Balance in Health

1. Normal sources of fluid input to maintain TBW

A. Consumed water

B. Water in food

C. Metabolic water generated by nutrient or tissue oxidation

2. Normal sources of fluid loss from TBW

A. Urine, 12 to 24 mL/lb/day (sensible losses)

B. Feces, respiration, sweating, 10 mL/lb/day (insensible losses)

3. The volume of water added to TBW equals the volume of water lost from TBW in a healthy patient (input volume − output volume = 0). This is known as zero water balance.

4. Physiologic control mechanisms exist that are important in maintaining zero water balance. Failure of these normal mechanisms results in rapid development of dehydration in the patient.

A. Thirst

B. Renal mechanism

1) ADH

2) Aldosterone

C. Gastrointestinal mechanism, altered absorption

D. Metabolic water from oxidation of body tissues

5. Daily maintenance water needs of healthy animals

A. 20 to 30 mL/lb/day, adults. Values near 20 mL/lb/day are chosen for large dogs; values near 30 mL/lb/day are chosen for smaller animals. (Figure 24-3)

B. 30 to 50 mL/lb/day, young puppies

6. Maintenance water replacement of 20 to 30 mL/lb/day meets the requirements of both sensible and insensible loss.

$$\text{Insensible} + \text{Sensible needs}$$
$$10 \text{ mL/lb/day} + \tfrac{1}{2} \text{ to } 1 \text{ mL/lb/hr}$$
$$(12 \text{ to } 24 \text{ mL/lb/day})$$

7. Alternatively refer to standard charts (see Figure 24-3) or tables (Table 24-1) to select maintenance fluid volumes.

8. Maintenance needs for water are those that replace normal daily obligate fluid loss from the body that would otherwise result in dehydration.

9. Remember that maintenance water needs are a function of metabolic rate, ambient temperature and humidity, body temperature, respiratory rate, and dietary intake. As such, it may not be possible to predict or calculate maintenance fluids accurately on occasion.

Figure 24-2. *The following illustrates an approximate volumetric compartmentalization of water in a 10-kg beagle.*

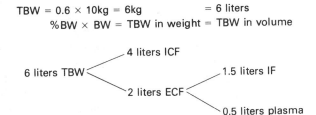

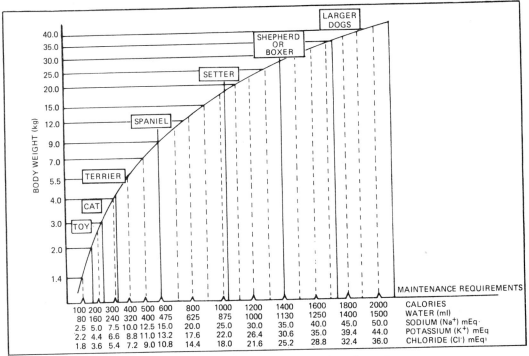

Figure 24-3. *Maintenance requirements of calories, water, and electrolytes of caged dogs and cats. (Finco after Harrison JB, from J Am Anim Hosp Assoc 8:179, 1972)*

Water Balance in Disease—Dehydration

1. A negative water balance (dehydration) exists when loss of water from is greater than gain of water into TBW. In this chapter, the term dehydration includes both pure water loss (uncommon) and loss of fluids with varying quantity of electrolytes.

2. Losses of water and electrolytes are assumed to come from the ECF initially, followed by compensatory movement of water and electrolytes from other compartments, if any.

3. The form of dehydration may be named according to

    A. The character of the fluid lost from or added to the body (whether isotonic, hypertonic, or hypotonic)

    B. The character of the body fluids after loss or gain of fluid has occurred, thus, hy-

pertonic fluid loss leaves hypotonic fluid in the body, and hypotonic fluid loss leaves hypertonic fluid in the body. Hypertonic fluid retention results in hypertonicity of body fluids. Hypotonic fluid retention results in hypotonicity of body fluids.

4. NaCl and water may be lost (dehydration) or retained (hydration) in varying proportions (isotonic, hypotonic, hypertonic). Serum (Na) is a relative quantity that may change.

5. In disease states, water and salt losses may occur in any ratio along the continuum between primary water loss with little or no salt loss (water deprivation) and primary salt loss with little accompanying water loss.

6. Because Na is the most abundant cation in ECF, it has become customary to characterize dehydration in relation to the serum concentration of this electrolyte (Table 24-2).

    A. Hypertonic dehydration—The plasma is hyperosmolar and hypernatremic, causing cells to give up intracellular water to the ECF

Table 24-1. **Daily water requirements for dogs**

Body Weight (kg)	Total mL Water per Day	Milliliters per Kilogram
1	140	140
2	232	116
3	312	104
4	385	96
5	453	91
6	518	86
7	580	83
8	639	80
9	696	77
10	752	75
11	806	73
12	859	71
13	911	70
14	961	68
15	1011	67
16	1060	66
17	1108	65
18	1155	64
19	1201	63
20	1247	62
25	1468	59
30	1677	56
35	1876	54
40	2068	52
45	2254	50
50	2434	49
60	2781	46
70	3112	44
80	3431	43
90	3739	41
100	4038	40

From Ross L: Fluid Therapy for Acute and Chronic Renal Failure. Vet Clin North Am 19: 343–359, 1989

Table 24-2. **Types of dehydration**

	Serum Na$^+$	ECF		ICF	
		Volume	Tonicity	Volume	Tonicity
Hypertonic dehydration*					
Pure water loss	↑ ↑	↓	↑ ↑	↓ ↓	↑ ↑
Loss of hypotonic fluid†	↑	↓ ↓	↑	↓	↑
Isotonic dehydration†	N	↓ ↓ ↓ ↓	N	N	N
Hypotonic dehydration					
Loss of hypertonic fluid	↓	↓ ↓ ↓ ↓ ↓	↓	↑	↓
Loss of isotonic fluid, replaced by an equal volume of water†	↓ ↓	↓ ↓ ↓	↓ ↓	↑ ↑	↓ ↓

*In the following classification scheme the adjective preceding the word "dehydration" describes the tonicity of the fluid that remains in the body.
†Most common clinical disorders; N = No change; number of arrows = magnitude of change in parameter

in an attempt to reestablish iso-osmolality. This brings about intracellular dehydration, which tends to minimize decreases in volume of ECF. Because ECF volume changes are blunted, minimal changes in packed cell volume (PCV) and total protein (TP) are observed.

B. Isotonic dehydration—Proportional losses of water and salt are iso-osmotic with body fluids, resulting in no change in plasma osmolality or sodium concentration. Consequently, no shifts of water between ECF and cells take place. PCV and TP are normal.

C. Hypotonic dehydration—Losses of relatively more salt than water result in hyponatremia and hypoosmolality. In an attempt to equilibrate the ECF and intracellular fluid (ICF) osmolality, water from the ECF is taken up by the cells, resulting in intracellular overhydration and ECF dehydration. This results in increases in PCV and TP, decreased effective blood volume, and a tendency toward shock.

Examples of Physiologic Principles

1. Given, 10-kg beagle

	Volume (Liter)	Tonicity (mosm/kg)	Total mosm
ECF	2	300	600
ICF	4	300	1200

A. ECF osmolality = ICF osmolality after equilibration

B. Assume NaCl is impermeant.

2. Hypertonic dehydration

A. Pure water loss of 1 L from the ECF occurs and the animal has no access to water. Water transfers from the ICF to the ECF to equalize osmotic pressure. Calculate the new osmolality of body fluids.

New ECF osmolality = New ICF osmolality

$$\text{Osmolality} = \frac{\text{mosm}}{\text{volume in liters}}$$

ECF osmolality = ICF osmolality

$$\frac{600 \text{ mosm}}{(1 + X) \text{ liter}} = \frac{1200 \text{ mosm}}{(4 - X) \text{ liter}}$$

$$600(4 - X) = 1200(1 + X)$$

$$X = .67 \text{ liter}$$

x = volume of solute-free water moving between compartments

$$\text{ECF}_{osm} = \frac{600 \text{ mosm}}{1.67 \text{ liter}} = \frac{360 \text{ mosm}}{\text{liter}}$$

$$\text{ICF}_{osm} = \frac{1200 \text{ mosm}}{3.33 \text{ liter}} = \frac{360 \text{ mosm}}{\text{liter}}$$

B. Hypotonic fluid loss results in loss of 1 L of ECF. The fluid lost contained $\frac{200 \text{ mosm}}{\text{liter}}$. As in above example, water now moves out of the ICF to the ECF to equalize osmotic pressure between the compartments. Calculate the new osmolality of the body compartments.

Present osmoles of ECF
= previous value − 200 mosm
= 600 − 200
= 400 mosm

New ECF$_{osm}$ = New ICF$_{osm}$

$$\frac{400 \text{ mosm}}{(1 + X) \text{ liter}} = \frac{1200 \text{ mosm}}{(4 - X) \text{ liter}}$$

X = .25 liter
= volume of solute-free water moving between compartments

$$\text{ECF} = \frac{400 \text{ mosm}}{1.25 \text{ liter}} = \frac{320 \text{ mosm}}{\text{liter}}$$

$$\text{ICF} = \frac{1200 \text{ mosm}}{3.75 \text{ liter}} = \frac{320 \text{ mosm}}{\text{liter}}$$

Notice that more intracellular water moved into the extracellular space in the first example (i.e., more cellular dehydration occurs with loss of pure water). Notice also that the ECF volume is maintained during pure water loss to a greater degree than when electrolytes are lost also.

3. Isotonic dehydration—Loss of 1 L of isotonic fluid from the ECF occurs. Calculate the new osmolality of body fluids rapidly, before any shifts can occur from Starling's forces.

New ECF$_{osm}$ = New ICF$_{osm}$
Present osmoles of ECF
= previous total − 300 mosm
600 − 300 mosm = 300 mosm

$$\frac{300 \text{ mosm}}{(1 + X) \text{ liter}} = \frac{1200 \text{ mosm}}{(4 - X) \text{ liter}}$$

X = 0 = no movement of
solute-free water occurs
between compartments

$$ECF_{osm} = \frac{300 \text{ mosm}}{1 \text{ liter}} = \frac{300 \text{ mosm}}{\text{liter}}$$

$$ICF_{osm} = \frac{1200 \text{ mosm}}{4 \text{ liter}} = \frac{300 \text{ mosm}}{\text{liter}}$$

4. Hypotonic dehydration—Loss of 1 L of hypertonic fluid from the ECF occurs. The osmolality of the lost fluid is 400 $\frac{\text{mosm}}{\text{liter}}$. Solute-free water moves from the ECF to the ICF to equalize osmotic pressure. Calculate the new osmolality of body fluids.

New ECF$_{osm}$ = 600 − 400 = 200 mosm

$$\frac{200 \text{ mosm}}{(1 - X) \text{ liter}} = \frac{1200 \text{ mosm}}{(4 + X) \text{ liter}}$$

X = .286 liter = volume of
solute-free water movement
out of ECF into cells

$$ECF_{osm} = \frac{200}{.714} = \frac{280 \text{ mosm}}{\text{liter}}$$

$$ICF_{osm} = \frac{1200}{4.286} = \frac{280 \text{ mosm}}{\text{liter}}$$

Underlying Causes of Dehydration

1. Decreased intake of water (hypodipsia, adipsia)
   A. Lack of food intake also decreases available water (water from oxidation and that which is present mechanically).
   B. Appetite and thirst centers may be depressed in systemically ill animals.
   C. Accidental or deliberate deprivation of adequate water and food.
2. Increased loss
   A. Urinary (polyuria)
   B. Gastrointestinal (vomiting, diarrhea)
   C. Respiratory (fever, panting)
   D. Skin (burns, large wounds)
   E. Excessive salivation

Detection of Dehydration

1. History often leads the clinician to suspect dehydration and to assess its magnitude

more accurately. Question the owner about volume of intake (adipsia, hypodipsia, polydipsia, or normal intake of water). Because volume of water intake may, in part, be a function stimulated by food intake, note also the presence or absence of anorexia. Abnormal losses of body fluid may be detected by positive client responses to questions about vomiting, diarrhea, polyuria, panting, excessive salivation, or other bodily discharge. The duration of these historical signs affects the magnitude of clinically detectable dehydration.
   2. Acute loss in the animal's body weight is substantially due to loss of water. A very recent weight from the animal before the present illness must exist to make a valid comparison. An acute loss in body weight of 1 lb suggests a decrease of 500 mL in TBW.
   3. Physical examination provides general guidelines for detecting dehydration, but the magnitude of dehydration assessed will vary from clinician to clinician. Signs of listlessness and depression may exist but may be partially attributable to the underlying disease process or to concomitant electrolyte and acid–base abnormalities. As dehydration becomes more severe, sunken globes, dryness of mucous membranes, tachycardia, diminished capillary refill, and signs of shock may occur.
      A. Normal skin pliability (skin turgor) depends on hydration of the tissues in the area tested. Choose skin from the trunk as a test area. Avoid dependent areas and skin from the neck. Normal skin returns immediately to its initial position when lifted a short distance and released. Dehydrated skin shows varying degrees of slow return to the original position. The clinician assigns increasing percentages of dehydration to abnormal skin turgor of increasing severity (Table 24-3).
      B. Clinical detection of dehydration is not possible if less than 4% to 5% of body weight in water has been lost. Skin turgor of obese animals may appear normal despite dehydration, owing to the large amounts of subcutaneous fat. The skin of an emaciated animal with normal hydration may fail to return to its normal position owing to a lack of subcutaneous fat and elastic tissue. Conse-

Table 24-3. *Physical assessment of dehydration*

Percent of Dehydration	Signs
<4	Not detectable
4–5	Subtle loss of skin elasticity
6–8	Definite delay in return of skin to normal position; eyes may be sunken in orbits; slightly prolonged capillary refill time; possibly dry mucous membrane
10–12	Tented skin stands in place; prolonged capillary; refill time; eyes sunken in orbits; dry mucous membranes; possible signs of shock (increased heart rate, weak pulses)
12–15	Signs of shock present, death imminent

quently, the possibility of underestimating dehydration in obese individuals and overestimating dehydration in emaciated animals exists. Avoid cervical skin as a test area because extra skin in this area confuses the result. Skin turgor changes in long-haired animals are more difficult to detect than those in short-haired animals. In addition, dry mucous membranes may occur in animals that pant continually and in those given anticholinergics (atropine like). Sunken globes also may be seen in catabolic diseases in which tissue behind the globe is reduced or atropy of the muscles of mastication has occurred.

4. Laboratory evaluation of hydration

A. PCV and plasma-protein (PP) or total-protein (TP) determinations may support the clinician's physical detection of dehydration or may suggest that intravascular dehydration exists when physical examination did not disclose dehydration. The magnitude of intra-vascular volume depletion (dehydration) may be estimated after evaluating the degree of abnormality in the simultaneous determination of PCV and TP. PCV and TP values may be within limits of normal even though dehydration exists, if the dehydration is a result of

acute hemorrhage or if compensatory shifts of body water into the vascular compartment have occurred. PCV and TP determinations may be simply, rapidly, and inexpensively made using microchematocrit techniques and a Goldberg refractometer with only a few drops of blood. Evaluate the PCV and TP routinely as a pair to avoid misleading information that could be obtained from evaluation of either parameter alone (Table 24-4.)

B. Urinalysis (UA) is important in all cases of suspected dehydration. An animal that is clinically dehydrated has already undergone its own endogenous water-deprivation test, which should result in the elaboration of concentrated urine (urine specific gravity [SG] > 1.030) if the kidneys are healthy. An elevated SG represents the healthy kidney's response to decreased perfusion. The finding of dilute urine (< 1.030 SG) from a dehydrated animal immediately incriminates the kidneys as a major cause of, or contributor to, the dehydration. Further evaluation of renal function is then indicated.

1) Urine for analysis of specific gravity must be obtained before administration of any fluid or diuretic therapy, because this therapy may alter the specific gravity and make accurate interpretation difficult or impossible.

2) Other components of the UA may provide useful information about the condition underlying dehydration. Changes in urinary pH may reflect systemic acid–base alterations (see Chapter 23 for further discussion). Glucosuria is most commonly encountered in diabetes mellitus and is nearly pathognomonic for this condition if ketones are detected simultaneously. Urinary sediment evaluation may show casts. The presence of casts may be derived from some preexisting renal pathology, independent of dehydration, or it may represent a degenerative process secondary to renal ischemia resulting from the dehydration.

C. Serum osmolality, see above under type of dehydration (see Chapter 25)

D. Serum electrolytes Na, K, Cl—Abnormalities in the serum concentration of these electrolytes may occur in dehydrated animals. Assessment of these changes helps to charac-

Table 24-4. **Simultaneous assessment of PCV and TP**

PCV(%)	TP (g/dL)	Possible Interpretation
↑	↑	Dehydration
↑	N or ↓	Splenic contraction Erythrocytosis Hypoproteinemia with dehydration
N	↑	Hyperproteinemia disorder Anemia with dehydration
↓	↑	Anemia with dehydration Anemia with preexisting hyperproteinemia
↓	N	Non–blood-loss anemia, normal hydration
N	N	Normal hydration Dehydration after secondary compartment shift Dehydration with preexisting anemia and hypoproteinemia Acute hemorrhage

terize the nature of fluid lost from the body (see Types of Dehydration and Chapter 25 on Sodium, Potassium, Chloride).

E. Blood gases—Abnormalities in blood-gas values may appear in dehydrated animals owing to loss or gain of certain body fluids, activity of the underlying disease process itself, or decreased perfusion of major organ systems (see Chapter 26 for specific discussion).

Replacement Volume

1. Using previously known body weight
   A. Example

$$\begin{array}{r} 40 \text{ lb on day 1} \\ - \underline{38 \text{ lb on day 2}} \\ 2 \text{ lb difference (reflects weight of} \\ \text{water lost acutely)} \end{array}$$

1 lb H_2O = 500 mL H_2O

$$2 \text{ lb} \times 500 \frac{mL}{lb} = 1000 \text{ mL}$$

   B. Consequently, 1000 mL of volume replacement should correct this dehydration. This technique emphasizes the importance of accurate measurement and recording of body weights at frequent intervals.

2. Using clinical estimates of dehydration
   A. Example, 40-lb dog estimated at 10%

dehydration. How any mL of fluid infusion should correct this dehydration?

% dehydration × body weight (lb)
$$= \text{lb fluid deficit}$$
$$10\% \times 40 \text{ lb} = 4\text{-lb deficit}$$

$$4 \text{ lb deficit} \times \frac{500 \text{ mL}}{lb} = 2000 \text{ mL deficit}$$

   B. Example, 18-kg dog estimated at 10% dehydration

% dehydration × body wt (kg) = liter deficit
10% dehydration × 18 kg = 1.8 kg = 1.8 L
$$= 1800 \text{ mL deficit}$$

Planning Daily Fluid Therapy

Questions in Cases Requiring Fluid Therapy

1. Is dehydration or overhydration present? If so, to what magnitude?

2. Is the ECF hypertonic, isotonic, or hypotonic?

3. Is there a serious acid–base abnormality?

4. Is there an abnormality in the concentration of any specific important electrolyte?

The answers to these questions will aid you in making the following decisions

1. The optimal route for fluid administration
2. The optimal volume of fluid to be given
3. The best type of fluid to meet the animal's needs
4. The optimal rate of fluid administration

Volume of Fluid Administration

1. Calculation of fluid volume requirements may dictate the route that fluids will need to be given.
2. Fluid volume needs usually take precedence over the type (quality) of fluid that is best for the patient.
3. Add together maintenance volume needs with those calculated from assessment of dehydration.
4. Note contemporary fluid losses that occur while fluid therapy is being given.
    A. Diarrhea
    B. Vomiting
    C. Oozing of serum from burns or extensive wounds
    D. Blood or other fluid lost during surgical procedures
    E. Rapid accumulation of fluid into body cavity effusions.
5. Approach the calculation of total fluid-volume requirement in a step-by-step manner and then total these separate volumes (Figures 24-3 and 24-4).
6. Alternatively, prescribe fluid volume as a multiple of maintenance volume to include correction for dehydration.
7. As can be seen from Table 24-5, most animals will require 2 to 3 times maintenance volume both to correct dehydration and to supply maintenance needs.

Routes of Fluid Administration

1. The route of fluid therapy depends on the nature of the clinical disorder, its severity, and its onset (acute vs chronic), and the composition of fluids to be given.
2. The oral route is useful in supplying high-caloric-density preparations (that are necessarily hypertonic) to maintain nutrition and hydration. This route cannot be used if vomiting or diarrhea is present and should not be used in animals whose fluid losses have been sudden or extensive. Forced fluid and food may be given orally, by nasogastric intubation (#8 French feeding tube for most dogs and #5 French feeding tube for cats; the tube is first coated with lidocaine cream), or by pharyngostomy tube. Gruels of blended canned dog foods and a polyelectrolyte solution such as Pediolyte may be given by pharyngastomy intubation.
3. Subcutaneous administration of fluids is common in dogs and cats; choose isotonic or mildly hypotonic fluids to enhance absorption. Do not give 5% dextrose in water as an isotonic solution by this route in cases of severe dehydration; it allows the possibility of delayed absorption, with consequent equilibration of ECF electrolytes into the pocket of pooled, nonabsorbed subcutaneous fluid.
    A. Absorption of subcutaneous fluid is unreliable in conditions of shock, severe dehydration, or hypothermia due to peripheral vasoconstriction. Never rely on this route for the emergency replacement of fluid. Mini-

Replacement volume (correction of dehydration)
(% dehydration × wt (lb.) × 500 = ml)
          +
Insensible needs = 19 ml/lb/day
          +   } Maintenance
Sensible needs = 10–20 ml/lb/day   requirement
                    or measured urine output
          +
Ongoing (contemporary) losses = (usually estimated)
_____
Total quantitative needs

Figure 24-4. *Calculation of fluid volume requirements as shown leads to more accurate fluid volume management of the patient.*

Table 24-5. **Maintenance and dehydration fluid volume requirements***

Maintenance (M) +Dehydration (%)†	mL/lb/day	Factor × Maintenance
M + 1	35	1.16
M + 2	40	1.33
M + 3	45	1.50
M + 4	50	1.67
M + 5	55	1.80
M + 6	60	2.00
M + 7	65	2.17
M + 8	70	2.33
M + 9	75	2.50
M + 10	80	2.70

*Maintenance defined as 30 mL/lb/day.

†Maintenance + dehydration needs are listed as mL/lb/day.

From Chew DJ: Parenteral fluid therapy. In Sherding RG (ed): The Cat: Diseases and Clinical Management. New York, Churchill Livingstone, 1989, pp 35–80. Reprinted with permission.

mally dehydrated animals may be corrected by this route, or dehydration in the anorexic animal may be prevented. In general, treat the critically ill or massively dehydrated animal initially with intravenous fluids and then switch to subcutaneous fluids as the problems resolve.

B. The volume of fluid that can be administered subcutaneously is limited by the individual's skin elasticity. Animals differ in their abilities to tolerate the infused load comfortably. Choose the site of the subcutaneous infusions somewhere on the trunk so that the fluid does not gravitate into the limbs. Avoid areas with surgical wounds because fluid may dissect the healing tissues. Subcutaneous infusions may be given under gravitational forces through an IV administration tubing or by direct injection from a large-volume hypodermic syringe.

4. Use intravenous fluid administration whenever accurate delivery of fluid volume and potent pharmacotherapeutic agents are required. Give hypotonic, isotonic, and hypertonic fluids by this route as the need arises. Rapid infusions of fluid volume may be readily accomplished by this route. The cost of

using this route is more expensive owing to the IV catheter equipment and the increased personnel time required for catheter care (bandaging, adjusting drip, etc.)

IV Catheter Care

1. Always perform aseptic catheter placement. This includes wide clipping of hair surrounding the vein and a surgical scrub. After securing the catheter in the vein, place a gauze sponge with an antimicrobial cream over the puncture site.

2. Catheter complications include thrombophlebitis, thromboembolism, bacteremia, bacterial endocarditis, and catheter-fragment foreign body.

3. To minimize problems

A. Place catheter aseptically.

B. Do not allow catheter to remain in a given vein longer than 48 to 72 hours.

C. Monitor patient for fever, leukocytosis, and heart murmurs.

D. Keep catheter site clean.

E. When the catheter is not in use, heparinize it to avoid clotting. Use heparinized saline (.9% saline with 5 U heparin/mL).

Vein Selection

1. The jugular vein and cephalic vein are most commonly chosen for indwelling IV catheterization. The lateral saphenous and femoral veins also may be used. I prefer use of the jugular vein in cats and small dogs. Advantages of using the jugular vein include the ability to measure central venous pressure (CVP), use of large-bore catheters for more rapid infusions, ready administration of hypertonic solutions and other irritating drugs due to greater dilutional effects from greater blood flow, and ease of obtaining serial blood samples from the IV line, if care is exercised to avoid clotting within the line. The prime disadvantage of peripheral-limb veins is that limb position often changes the rate of fluid infusion owing to partial or complete occlusion of the indwelling catheter. Nineteen-gauge catheters are often used in cats and small dogs; 17-gauge catheters are generally used in larger animals. Larger-bore catheters may be of value in emergency situations.

2. Intraperitoneal fluid administration is not used widely.

A. Severely anemic puppies and kittens may be transfused by this route when a vein cannot be catheterized.

B. May be considered for rewarming very hypothermic animals

C. Use isotonic to mildly hypotonic fluids when used for rehydration.

3. Intraosseous route

A. Rarely used until recently; should be considered more often

B. Blood and crystalloid solutions can be infused safely.

C. Bone marrow of femur, tibia, or humerus is catheterized with a bone-marrow needle and secured in place.

D. Rapid access to circulation when venous catheterization is not successful or possible.

Rate of Fluid Administration

1. The rate of fluid administration depends on the extent and rapidity of the fluid loss, as well as on the composition of the fluid to be infused. Rapid or extensive fluid losses demand rapid replacement. In chronic disorders, it is not always necessary to replace the dehydration deficit rapidly. Some clinicians prefer to calculate the dehydration deficit, add it to the daily maintenance requirements, and distribute this fluid load over 24 hours. Others prefer to replace the dehydration deficit over the first few hours (referred to as "front-end loading"). The decision depends on the status of the individual animal. The literature recommends deficit replacement of 75% to 80% on the first day and the remaining 25% deficit the second day. It is my opinion that this is unnecessary and that dehydration can be corrected safely within 24 hours in most cases.

2. Maximal infusion rates may be necessary in the treatment of shock or severe dehydration. One blood volume per hour of isotonic fluid (40 mL/lb/h for a dog; 30 mL/lb/h for a cat) is recommended as the maximal rate of IV fluid infusion without the use of CVP monitoring.

3. Measure urine output during rapid fluid infusion as a guide to organ perfusion. With persistent oliguria, be careful about maximal fluid infusion and monitor CVP to avoid overhydration.

4. In less critical conditions, distribute fluids equally throughout the day. Physiologically this may be advantageous because it allows more time for adequate equilibration of water and electrolytes between the body compartments. Ideally, a constant or continuous infusion of IV fluids over a 24-hour period would accomplish this. This ideal situation may not be possible if very small volumes of fluid are being infused or if monitoring of the IV lines is available for part of the day only. Employ intermittent infusion over the maximal practical number of hours for your practice as an alternative. With this technique, infuse the total calculated daily volume over the number of hours that the IV drip can be observed, then flush the catheter with heparinized saline and cap it until the infusion can be resumed the next day. Consider a dose of subcutaneous fluids to tide over the animal's fluid needs until IV fluids can be resumed.

5. A rate of IV fluid infusion of 10 mL/lb/h is recommended in uncomplicated anesthesia and surgery cases. Nearly all potent inhalent anesthetics cause vasodilatation with subsequent reduction in effective circulating volume.

Calculation and Monitoring
Volume of IV Drip Rate

1. Intravenous administration sets are available in standard "macrodrip" volumes of 10, 15, or 20 drops/mL. Pediatric administration sets also are available in the "minidrip" volume of 60 drops/mL. Patient size and volume of fluid to be infused allows the clinician to choose between the minidrip and macrodrip systems.

2. Example—10-lb dog, 10% dehydrated

$0.1 \times 10 \text{ lb} \times 500 \text{ mL/lb}$
$$= 500 \text{ mL fluids}$$
(= dehydration deficit)

$30 \text{ mL/lb/day} \times 10 \text{ lb}$
$$= 300 \text{ mL fluids/day}$$
(= maintenance requirements)

Hence: 300 + 500
= 800 mL given over 24 hours

Macrodrip: $\dfrac{800 \text{ ml}}{24 \text{ h}} = 33 \text{ mL/h}$

$\dfrac{33 \text{ mL}}{h} \times \dfrac{1 \text{ h}}{60 \text{ min}} \times \dfrac{10 \text{ drops}}{mL}$

= 5.5 drops/min = 1 drop/10 to 12 sec

A. This case would probably be easier to manage using a pediatric drop set (minidrip)

$\dfrac{33 \text{ mL}}{h} \times \dfrac{1 \text{ h}}{60 \text{ min}} \times \dfrac{60 \text{ drops}}{mL}$

= 33 drops/min = 1 drop/2 sec

1) Note that when using a minidriop of 60 drops/mL that the calculated mL/h is equal to minidrips/min.

B. This same case could be handled differently. Assume that dehydration is corrected rapidly within 4 hours because of the clinician's assessment of the animal's critical

condition. In this instance, 300 mL of maintenance fluids remain to be infused over a 20-hour period after dehydration has been corrected.

$$\frac{300 \text{ mL}}{20 \text{ h}} = \frac{15 \text{ mL}}{h}$$

1) Macrodrip

$\dfrac{15 \text{ mL}}{h} \times \dfrac{1 \text{ h}}{60 \text{ min}} \times \dfrac{10 \text{ drops}}{mL}$

= 2.5 drops/min
= 1 drop/24 sec

2) Minidrip

$\dfrac{15 \text{ mL}}{h} \times \dfrac{1 \text{ h}}{60 \text{ min}} \times \dfrac{60 \text{ drops}}{mL}$

= 15 drops/min
= 1 drop/4 sec

3. Once the drip set has been adjusted to the desired rate, mark the IV bottle with adhesive tape as indicated below to monitor the hourly volume of fluids received. This allows adjustment for individual variations (e.g., animal changing position of limb that contains the catheter). This bottle has been marked for an animal that is supposed to be getting 100 mL/h (approximately 17 drops/min with a 10 drop/mL drip set).

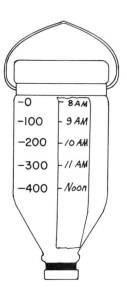

–0	8 AM
–100	9 AM
–200	10 AM
–300	11 AM
–400	Noon

	First 4 Hours	*Second 4 Hours*	*Third 4 Hours*
IV fluid volume infused	$\dfrac{10\ mL/lb}{6}$	$\dfrac{10\ mL/lb + x\ mL}{6}$	$\dfrac{10\ mL/lb + y\ mL}{6}$
Volume urine produced	x mL	y mL	z mL

4. In dehydrated animals with either severe oliguria or diuresis, actual measurement of urine output may be helpful in accurate matching of the needs of the animal to the fluid therapy. Without this system, there is a tendency to overestimate the actual fluid needs in an oliguric animal (resulting in over-hydration) and to underestimate the fluid needs in an animal undergoing extensive diuresis (resulting in failure to correct dehydration). In this technique, divide the day into six 4-hour intervals. The hour interval is chosen based on the severity of the condition. It could be chosen every hour, or every 6 or 8 hours, as the need dictates. Determine fluid needs for this fractional period using both

calculated insensible $\left(\dfrac{10\ mL/lb}{6} \right)$ and mea-

sured sensible (urine-volume) losses. The measured volume of sensible losses from the previous 4-hour period is given back to the patient in the next 4-hour period. An example follows of how this technique works after initial dehydration deficits have been replaced. Replace previously calculated dehydration needs first, then proceed as shown in the table above.

A. Carry this out in identical fashion for an additional three time periods. This type of attention to fluid volume is of benefit in the initial management of critically ill animals, particularly when CVP and renal status are uncertain.

B. Rate of IV fluid infusion is important when considering potassium-rich fluids and those containing a large quantity of alkali. Infuse potassium-rich fluids at a maximal rate of 0.5 mEq K^+/kg/h to avoid toxicity (see Chapter 25 on Disorders of Potassium). Too-rapid infusion of alkali in the form of $NaHCO_3$ may cause hyperosmolality, seizures or tet-

any, and paradoxical CSF acidosis (see Chapter 26 on Disorders in Acid–Base Balance).

5. For small dogs and cats consider the use of a Buretrol or similar device to accurately premeasure the fluids to be administered over the next few hours.

A. Fluids from the reservior bag are then periodically used to reload the administration set.

B. This method minimizes the chances of overhydration because it allows more accurate delivery of small volumes.

6. Infusion pumps

A. Enter mL/h or drops/min depending on the type of machine.

B. Electronic drip counter ensures accuracy of delivery.

C. Most are equipped with alarm system if fluids are not running.

D. Expensive if new

1) Refurbished used machines may be surprisingly affordable.

Quality (Type) of Infusion Fluid

1. Fluids are classified by
   A. Intended function
      1) Maintenance
      2) Replacement
   B. Crystalloid vs colloid
   C. Osmolality/tonicity
      1) Hypotonic
      2) Isotonic
      3) Hypertonic
   D. Similarity to normal plasma
   E. See Table 24-6 for a summary of available fluids and supplements.

2. Maintenance solutions are designed to replace the normal daily losses of hypotonic fluids and electrolytes. They also are designed to meet potassium requirements of healthy animals. Consequently, the electrolyte

Table 24-6. Composition of solutions used in fluid therapy

	Glucose* (g/L)	Na+ (mEq/L)	Cl− (mEq/L)	K+ (mEq/L)	Ca2+ (mEq/L)	Mg2+ (mEq/L)	Buffer† (mEq/L)	Osmolarity (mosm/L)	Cal/L	pH
Dextrose and Electrolyte Solution Composition										
5% dextrose	50	0	0	0	0	0	0	252	170	4.0
10% dextrose	100	0	0	0	0	0	0	505	340	4.0
2.5% dextrose in .45% NaCl	25	77	77	0	0	0	0	280	85	4.5
5% dextrose in .45% NaCl	50	77	77	0	0	0	0	406	170	4.0
5% dextrose and .9% NaCl	50	154	154	0	0	0	0	560	170	4.0
.45% NaCl	0	77	77	0	0	0	0	154	0	5.0
.85% NaCl (normal saline)	0	145	145	0	0	0	0	290	0	5.0
.9% NaCl	0	154	154	0	0	0	0	308	0	5.0
3% NaCl	0	513	513	0	0	0	0	1026	0	5.0
7% NaCl	0	1197	1197	0	0	0	0	2394	0	—
Ringer's solution	0	147.5	156	4	4.5	0	0	310	0	5.5
Ringer's lactated solution	0	130	109	4	3	0	23(L)	272	9	6.5
2.5% dextrose in Ringer's lactated solution	25	130	109	4	3	0	28(L)	398	94	5.0
5% dextrose in Ringer's lactated solution	50	130	109	4	3	0	28(L)	524	179	5.0

2.5% dextrose in half-strength Ringer's lactated solution	25	65.5	55	2	1.5	0	14(L)	263	89	5.0
Normosol-M in 5% dextrose‡	50	40	40	13	0	3	16(A)	364	175	5.5
Normosol-R‡	0	140	98	5	0	3	27(A) 23(G)	296	18	6.4
Plasma-Lyte§	0	140	103	10	5	3	47(A) 8(L)	312	17	5.5
Plasma-Lyte M in 5% dextrose‡	50	40	40	16	5	3	12(A) 12(L)	376	178	5.5
Plasma	1	145	105	5	5	3	24(B)	300	—	7.4
Additives and Special Solutions										
20% mannitol	200(M)	0	0	0	0	0	0	1099		
7.5% NaHCO₃	0	893(B)	0	0	0	0	893(B)	1786	0	
8.4% NaHCO₃	0	1000(B)	0	0	0	0	1000(B)	2000	0	
10% CaCl₂	0	0	2720	0	1360	0	0	4080	0	
14.9% KCl	0	0	2000	2000	0	0	0	4000	0	
50% dextrose	500	0	0	0	0	0	0	2780	1700	4.2

*All glucose, with one exception: M, mannitol.

†Buffers used: A, acetate; B, bicarbonate; G, gluconate; L, lactate.

‡CEVA Laboratories.

§Baxter Healthcare.

From Chew DJ, DiBartola SP: Manual of Small Animal Nephrology and Urology, pp. 308–309. New York, Churchill Livingstone, 1986.

composition (concentration) of these solutions differs markedly from that of plasma; it contains a much lower sodium content than plasma and much higher concentrations of potassium. Maintenance solutions are not designed for rapid infusion.

A. Normosol-M or Normosol-M in D_5W are examples of commercially available maintenance fluids (Table 24-6). One part lactated Ringer's combined with two parts 5% dextrose in water approaches a maintenance solution if additional K^+ is added.

B. Maintenance solutions for use in veterinary practice have not been specifically chosen for use until recently. Once dehydration has been corrected and ongoing contemporary loss of fluid minimized, hypotonic fluids for maintaining hydration may be used selectively. Most clinicians continue to use a polyionic isotonic solution (e.g., lactated Ringer's) to maintain hydration. This practice is not harmful if renal function is adequate to excrete the unneeded electrolytes and if additional K^+ is added to the infusion.

C. Estimates of maintenance electrolyte needs can be taken from Table 24-3 when individually formulating fluids for infusion.

3. Replacement fluids are designed to correct specific deficits in plasma concentration or total body quantity of electrolytes and alkali (sodium, potassium, chloride, bicarbonate, calcium, phosphorus).

A. Commercially available fluids may provide replacement needs as formulated by the manufacturer.

1) Frequently specific additives to stock commercial solutions will be required to provide replacement needs for a specific substance, however.

B. Lactated Ringer's solution or 0.9% NaCl may be a replacement fluid for sodium, but not for potassium (see Table 24-6).

4. The selection of replacement or correcting fluids to be infused into the body is based on knowledge of the type of fluid lost from or gained to the body.

5. As a general rule, give back to the patient fluid that matches the volume and electrolyte content lost from the body.

A. Avoid supplying substances that have been retained by the body or are present in too high a plasma concentration.

B. Volume and electrolyte composition of fluid lost from the body is not often documented in veterinary medicine. In some instances, fluid is lost to the use of the body, but not actually lost from the body, as in cases of sequestered fluid (e.g., intestinal obstruction). In these cases it is not possible to document the quantity and quality of fluid loss.

6. Integration of the history and physical examination provides clues to the nature (quality) of fluid lost from the body. A history of water deprivation or severe hypodipsia alone with no other routes of fluid loss should raise the clinician's suspicion that hypertonic dehydration exists (mostly obligate hypotonic fluid loss has occurred). This patient requires a solute-poor (mostly water) solution. A history of severe diarrhea suggests that major loss of electrolytes, including HCO_3, probably has occurred; give this patient a polyionic isotonic solution with alkali supplementation. A history of severe vomiting and a pyloric obstruction suggest the existence of metabolic alkalosis and severe chloride depletion. The fluid of choice for this patient is .9% saline or Ringer's solution, with K^+ supplementation added to either fluid. Knowledge of the underlying disease process allows you to make an educated guess about the nature of the fluid-balance disorder, however, shortcomings in planning fluid therapy without laboratory testing do exist, as listed on page 577.

7. Biochemical evaluation of serum plasma samples may give insight into the type of fluid lost from the body. Returned serum values for electrolytes and osmolality indicate what is left in the ECF after the losses have occurred. These values represent relative concentrations rather than absolute values.

A. As a general rule, after return of serum laboratory data, choose an IV solution for infusion that is devoid or poor of the electrolyte that is present in relatively excessive quantity and that is rich in quantity of the relatively deficient electrolyte.

B. The electrolytes that are most valuable in this type of evaluation include Na, K, Cl, and HCO₃. Specific treatment of the extremes in excess or deficiency of these parameters is important and is discussed in Chapter 25, Disorders of Electrolytes and Osmolality, and Chapter 26, Disorders in Acid–Base Balance.

8. Most fluids available for infusion are called *crystalloids.* Crystalloid solutions contain substances capable of passing a semipermeable membrane only. In contrast, others, called *colloid* solutions, contain particles such as protein that are not capable of crossing a semipermeable membrane. Whole blood and plasma are the most commonly used colloidal solutions in veterinary medicine. Low-molecular-weight dextrans may be used as an alternative commercial colloidal solution, but expense and adverse reactions such as pyrexia have limited their use. Table 24-6 provides quantitative information on the composition of the more commonly used solutions.

9. Fluids also are categorized on the basis of osmolality or tonicity.

A. Tonicity of selected fluid is compared with that of normal plasma.

B. Tonicity of selected fluid also is compared with that of patient's plasma (relative tonicity).

C. .45% NaCl in H_2O is an example of a hypotonic fluid.

D. .9% NaCl is an example of an isotonic fluid when compared with normal plasma, but could be effectively hypotonic when given to a patient with an elevated serum sodium and osmolality (e.g., 170 mEq/L Na and 350 mosm/L).

E. In general, select hypotonic fluids when increased serum osmolality exists.

F. Select isotonic or mildly hypertonic fluids when decreased serum osmolality exists.

G. Select isotonic fluids to correct dehydration in patients with normal serum osmolality.

H. Select isotonic fluids for rapid infusion.

I. Select hypotonic fluids for maintenance needs.

J. The dextrose portion of fluids contributes only transiently to tonicity of fluids when metabolized to water.

K. .45% NaCl in 2.5% dextrose is isotonic to normal plasma, but is hypotonic when dextrose is gone.

Shortcomings of Patient Evaluation and Selection of Appropriate Fluids Without Laboratory Tests

1. There are no objective facts.
2. The guesses could be wrong.
3. The patient may be unusual.
4. There is no objective means of monitoring response to treatment.

Water Balance in Disease—Overhydration

1. Clinical overhydration (hydremia, positive water balance) occurs much less commonly than dehydration in animals and is more likely to be seen in patients with compromised cardiovascular or renal status. Forces from Starling's hypothesis of the capillary are again operative, as in dehydration. When intravascular overhydration occurs, increased intravascular hydrostatic pressure and decreased plasma oncotic pressure favor egress of fluid from the intravascular space to the interstitial space (edema).

2. Positive water balance exists when input of water into TBW is greater than loss of water volume from the TBW. As with dehydration, overhydration may occur to varying degrees within the body water compartments.

Causes of Overhydration

1. Increased input of water into TBW
A. Spontaneous oral intake, unlikely
B. Acutely catabolic diseases resulting in increased metabolic water
C. Iatrogenic, from IV fluid administration
2. Decreased output of water from TBW—oliguric primary renal failure

3. Combinations of increased input and decreased output
4. Fluid-compartment shifts
   A. Pleural effusion
   B. Abdominal effusion
   C. Sequestered GI fluid

Detecting Overhydration

1. Physical examination
   A. Gelatinous feeling of skin and subcutaneous tissue
   B. Serous nasal or ocular discharge
   C. Chemosis
   D. Subcutaneous edema
   E. Pulmonary edema, tachypnea or rales
   F. Vomiting or diarrhea
2. Body weight increased suddenly and inappropriately
3. Increased CVP when measured
4. Decreased PCV and decreased PP due to dilution of intravascular volume

Treatment of Overhydration

1. Stop all IV infusions. This may be all that is needed, because normal compensatory physiologic mechanisms may then rid the body of excess fluid.
2. Give diuretics, furosemide (Lasix) 1 to 2 mg/lb IV; if no effect within 15 minutes, double the dose and give again.
3. Peritoneal dialysis may be necessary. Use very hypertonic dialysate to remove water from body in life-threatening circumstances in which excess water cannot be removed by other means.
4. Give morphine to increase compliance of pulmonary vessels.
5. Phlebotomy may be used to decrease blood volume when other methods have been unsuccessful.

Monitoring Efficacy of Fluid Therapy

1. Physical examination is an important monitor during fluid therapy. Evaluate the patient several times daily during the initial fluid management to document rehydration, prevent overhydration, and detect contemporary fluid loss. Normalizing skin turgor, moist-

ening mucous membranes, strengthening pulses, increasing perfusion (decreasing refill time), and increasing alertness are goals of successful fluid therapy. Continued surveillance of the patient prevents overhydration. (See previous section, Water Balance in Disease—Overhydration.)
2. CVP helps to prevent overloading the heart and resultant pulmonary edema when administering fluids rapidly. Monitor CVP with a jugular catheter, the tip of which is level with the right atrium. Normal CVP is 0 to 10 cm H_2O. A sudden increase in CVP during fluid therapy indicates the inability of the cardiovascular system to accommodate the rate of fluid administration. Reduce the rate of administration accordingly.
3. Body weight changes are very useful in monitoring hydration. An acute gain or loss of 1 lb suggests an increase of 500 mL body water. An anorexic animal, however, loses 0.1 to 0.3 kg body weight per day per 1000 calories of daily caloric requirement, owing to tissue catabolism. Determine and record body weight accurately at least once daily.
4. Follow PCV and TP serially during fluid therapy. Relative change in these two parameters suggests adequacy or inadequacy of fluid therapy (Table 24-7).
5. Urinalysis has value in monitoring fluid therapy because larger volumes of urine output imply improved organ perfusion. This

Table 24-7. **Interpretation of changes in PCV and PP during fluid therapy**

PCV	PP	Possible Interpretation
↓*	↓	Repletion of intravascular volume (rehydration) overhydration
—	—	Rehydration keeping pace with current fluid loss; i.e., balance exists
↑	↑	Ongoing fluid loss occurring faster than fluid replacement
↑	↓	Continuing fluid loss with possible loss of capillary integrity and loss of PP from intravascular space

*Arrows refer to direction of change compared to PCV and PP values before instituting fluid therapy (Modified from Kohn CW: "Preparative Management of the Equine Patient with an Abdominal Crisis." *Veterinary Clinics of North America: Large Animal Practice* 1(2): 289–311, 1979.

increased urine output may be detected indirectly as urine of high SG becomes less concentrated. The presence of more dilute urine does not guarantee that successful rehydration is occurring; too-rapid IV infusion may result in transient intravascular volume expansion and diuresis, even though the nonvascular compartments still need fluid volume. The appearance of more dilute urine also may denote the onset of primary renal failure.

6. Determine serial serum electrolyte values in severely dehydrated animals receiving fluid therapy. Ideally, animals that had serum electrolyte deficiency or excess will show improvement toward normal values after appropriate therapy. Also follow electrolyte determinations in those cases that had initially normal values to detect the possible consequences of volume expansion and changes in the underlying disease process.

7. Blood gases are valuable in characterizing the nature of fluid losses and assessing the effectiveness of therapy to return blood-gas parameters to normal.

Possible Causes of Failure to Correct Dehydration Adequately

1. Calculation errors, mathematical

2. Error in assessment of initial degree of dehydration

3. Larger contemporary losses than expected

4. Too-rapid infusion resulting in diuresis and loss of fluid from body

5. Mechanical catheter problems, calculated volume not infused

6. Increased insensible loss not appreciated (fever, panting)

7. Increased sensible loss not appreciated (polyuria)

Transfusions

1. Fresh whole blood, stored whole blood, stored packed red blood cells or fresh-frozen plasma, and platelet-rich plasma may be used according to specific need.

2. In private practice fresh whole blood will be used most often, although stored whole blood may be used occasionally.

3. Fresh whole blood indications
  A. RBC and plasma needed
  B. Coagulation factors needed
  C. Platelets needed
4. Stored whole blood indications
  A. RBC and plasma needed
5. Stored packed RBC
  A. RBC needed in absence of need for protein or albumin (normovolemia)
6. Fresh-frozen plasma
  A. Coagulation factors
7. Platelet-rich plasma
  A. Platelets needed
8. Use of whole blood or packed RBC
  A. Anemia with normal blood volume— Dogs and cats with a PCV of 10% to 15% or less may need whole blood or packed RBC infused as an emergency procedure, depending on how rapidly the anemia developed and on other stresses. In animals with immune-mediated hemolysis, avoid blood transfusions if possible until the hemolytic process is controlled by corticosteroids or other immunosuppressive drugs.
  B. It is generally desirable that animals undergoing anesthesia have a PCV of 20% or more.
  C. Hemorrhagic shock—Hypovolemia from blood volume loss that is significant enough to cause shock requires replacement of volume and RBC. Blood loss may be obvious (external) or concealed. Concealed blood loss may occur in the thoracic or abdominal cavities, the lung, the retroperitoneal space, or tissue surrounding fractured bones. Less severe conditions of blood loss may be stabilized with crystalloid-solution infusion and the gradual production of new RBC by the patient.
    1) <15 mL/lb blood loss is readily treated with crystalloids.
    2) 15 to 20 mL/lb blood loss benefits from plasma.
    3) ≥25 mL/lb blood loss requires whole blood.

Blood Donors

1. Exsanguination and euthanasia of a healthy donor
  A. Blood type will be unknown, but

crossmatching may be used if multiple transfusions of same blood is given to the canine recipient.

B. Criteria for use of these donors should be identical to those listed below in the discussion of permanent donors.

2. Permanent donor—in-hospital resident or donor on call nearby (client or staff owned)

A. These animals should be in good physical health, tractable, and large enough to provide adequate blood volume at each bleeding. Dogs and cats can be bled every 2 weeks if necessary at 10 mL/lb; however, bleeding at 3-week intervals is recommended for routine collection.

B. Dogs should be negative on testing for heartworm, *Brucella canis, E. cani,* and *Babesia.* Cats should be FeLV, FIV, and Hemobartonella negative. Routine hematology should be normal for both. Endoparasites and ectoparasites should be absent as extra sources of blood loss.

C. Dogs have eight blood groups but only three are important RBC antigens; canine-erythrocyte antigens (CEA) 1, 2, and 7. Dogs negative for these RBC antigens are desirable as donors because these RBC are not readily destroyed in recipient's body even after multiple transfusions.

1) CEA-1 (DEA 1.1) is the most important because it stimulates isoantibodies the most.

a) 40% incidence

2) CEA-2 (DEA 1.2) also is important.

a) 20% incidence

3) CEA-7 has a 40% incidence.

4) The universal donor should be CEA-1 and CEA-2 negative; the ideal donor also is CEA-7 negative.

5) Naturally occurring isoantibodies to CEA-1 or CEA-2 do not exist.

6) Low titer isoantibodies occur in 15% of dogs, mostly against CEA-7.

D. Greyhounds are excellent blood donors because of the low frequency of significant RBC antigens, high PCV, and ease of venous access.

E. Blood typing for dogs can be done at Tufts University and Michigan State University.

F. Typing for cat blood groups is not routinely available commercially.

1) Cats have three blood groups; A, B, or AB (unrelated to human or dog typing).

a) Most cats in the U.S. are blood type A. Less than 1% cats in U.S. are type B.

b) In Australia nearly 25% of cats are type B.

c) 25% of type A cats have weak naturally occurring anti-B isoantibodies.

d) 95% of type B cats have strong anti-A isoantibodies.

3. Autotransfusion

A. In this instance, the donor and recipient of the blood transfusion are the same. When massive blood loss suddenly occurs in the patient's thoracic or abdominal cavity, this blood may be retrieved preoperatively, stored, and infused; or collected at the time of surgery, anticoagulated, and reinfused.

B. Autotransfusion is contraindicated if the bleeding occurred because of direct effects of cancer or infection because it may induce metastases or sepsis. Other complications include damage to RBC during collection and resulting hemolysis; coagulation abnormalities such as thrombocytopenia and disseminated intravascular coagulation (DIC); microemboli of platelet aggregates, cellular aggregates, fat, and air. The use of in-line micropore filters (40 μm) is recommended.

C. Do not collect blood for autotransfusion if it has been in contact with serosal surfaces of the thorax or abdomen for more than 24 hours.

D. Autotransfusion has merit when demand for blood severely exceeds either banked donor blood volume or available fresh donor blood volumes. This source of blood is already warm and does not require crossmatching.

4. Collection and storage of whole blood

A. Euthanasia donors are anesthetized with a barbiturate, intravenous fluids infused to prevent hypotension, and then exsanguinated from cardiac puncture or from femoral-artery catheterization. Expect to collect about 30 mL/lb from dogs. Blood is collected most often from permanent canine donors using jugular venapuncture and a vacuum glass bottle or plastic bags with acid citrate dextrose (ACD) solution or citrate phosphorus dextrose (CPD) solution as the anticoagulant.

Plastic blood bags may be used for collection by gravity flow or by use of a vacuum pump. Plastic bags result in less damage to RBC, less inactivation of certain clotting factors, and less aggregation of platelets.

   B. Refrigerated dog blood anticoagulated with ACD or CPD maintains reasonable viability of RBC when stored at 4°C, for at least 3 weeks, and possibly as long as 6 weeks. Trauma during collection of blood, storage conditions, and infusion all effect RBC survival once blood is in the patient. Adequate levels of 2,3-DPG are maintained in stored dog blood for at least 3 to 4 weeks. Diminished 2,3-DPG content in RBC decreases their ability to release O_2 to the tissues. Even when 2,3-DPG levels are low in stored blood, they may be restored to normal value within hours of transfusion. The degree of 2,3-DPG depletion in stored dog blood does not parallel the amount of decrease observed in stored human blood.

   1) Gentle agitation of blood periodically during storage may help prolong post-transfusion viability of RBC.

   C. Cat blood often is not stored for long periods, but collected at the time of need.

   1) 1 mL CPDA per 5 to 7 mL blood in a 50 to 60 mL syringe

   2) Sedation with ketamine–valium is recommended to facilitate collection.

   a) Avoid acepromazine because of hypotensive effects.

   3) Heparin as anticoagulant is not recommended.

   a) Activation of platelets

   b) No nutrient support for RBC, therefore must be infused shortly after collection (24 to 36 hours).

   i. 625 U/50 mL blood

   4) Refrigerated cat blood stored in ACD solution maintains high RBC viability for at least 30 days.

   a) 1 mL ACD per 4 mL blood

   D. With prolonged storage of whole blood, hemolysis occurs. If you observe a dark discoloration of the plasma, discard this blood. Hemolysis results in increased K^+ content of the plasma, but intracellular K^+ content in canine RBC is much less than that seen in human RBC. Consequently, hyperkale-

mia from infusion of aged, stored canine blood is much less likely to occur.

   5. Administration of blood

   A. Most often blood is given intravenously. On occasion you may use the intraperitoneal (IP) or intramedullary (IM) route (also referred to as the intraosseous route).

   1) 50% of IP RBC absorbed by 24 hours, 65% by 48 hours.

   2) 95% RBC in circulation minutes after intraosseous injection.

   B. Gently agitate stored blood and warm to body temperature before infusion, if a crisis situation does not exist. Warming of blood prevents loss of body heat from the patient. It also reduces the viscosity encountered in cold blood, making it easier to ensure adequate infusion rate. Drip blood through a commercially available administration set with a nylon-mesh filter (170 μm) to trap microemboli and platelet aggregates. Use coiled polyethylene tubing as part of the infusion line; submerge it in warm water to maintain warmth of the infused blood.

   C. If large volumes of blood are to be infused rapidly, use blood that is freshly collected or that has been stored less than 10 days to ensure that the 2,3-DPG concentration and oxygen dissociation curve will be adequate for immediate delivery of O_2 to the tissues. Less critical cases do not require this because 2,3-DPG and a normal oxygen dissociation curve soon regenerate from blood stored longer.

   D. Do not infuse crystalloid solutions containing calcium (e.g., lactated Ringer's) through the same IV lines as blood. These CA^{2+}-containing solutions may negate the effect of the anticoagulant in the blood resulting in microthrombi. Do not infuse hypotonic solutions, or hemolysis might occur. .9% NaCL is usually the fluid of choice to infuse with RBC.

Volume of Blood Administered

   1. Hemorrhagic shock—Required volume is extremely variable, but in combination with crystalloid solutions, aim to keep the PCV higher than 20%. Whole blood is not usually indicated in initial phases of shock from blood loss, but may be needed when severe blood loss has occurred. PCV and TP have been shown, in some cases of hemorrhagic shock, to remain normal for four hours, which limits their usefulness in making a decision about whether or not to give blood.

2. Anemia, normovolemic

A. General rule 1—1 mL whole blood/lb to raise PCV by 1% (assume anticoagulated donor PCV = 40% for dog and 30% for cat); .5 mL packed RBC/lb to raise recipient PCV 1% (assume donor packed RBC = 80% for dogs).

B. General rule 2—

mL of anticoagulated = recipient blood
blood required   volume (mL)
for transfusion   40 mL/lb—dog
(from donor)   30 mL/lb—cat

$$\times \frac{\text{desired PCV} - \text{actual PCV of recipient}}{\text{PCV of anticoagulated donor blood}}$$

3. Assumptions when using this formula include

A. Loss or destruction of RBC is not occurring rapidly at this time.

B. RBC stay within intravascular space.

C. Expanded plasma volume is not reduced immediately by compensating physiologic mechanisms.

D. If "extra" plasma volume perceived by the body is rapidly corrected (e.g., by diuresis), then this formula closely estimates requirements of donor blood needed to raise PCV to expected values (see below).

E. Actual calculation in this example only raises PCV to 25%, as is expected if plasma volume is not rapidly decreased.

1) Example 1 (using rule 1)—20-lb dog; 10% PCV, recipient; assume PCV 40% donor.

a) How many mL of whole blood should be infused to raise the recipient's PCV from 10% to 30%?

b) Because it will take approximately 1 mL/lb of whole blood to raise the PCV 1%, it will take about 20 mL/lb to raise the PCV 20% (from 10% to 30%)

20 mL/lb × 20 lb
          = 400 mL whole blood needed

2) Example 2 (using rule 2)—20-lb dog; actual patient (recipient) Hct = 10%; Hct of anticoagulated donor blood = 40%

a) How many mL of anticoagulated donor blood is needed in transfusion to raise the patient's PCV from 10% to 30%?

Volume required (mL)

$$= 40 \text{ mL/lb} \times 20 \text{ lb} \times \frac{30\% - 10\%}{40\%}$$

$$= 800 \text{ mL} \times \frac{20\%}{40\%}$$

$$= 400 \text{ mL of donor anticoagulated} \\ \text{blood needed}$$

Initial Whole Blood Volume Administration

1. Cats—50 to 60 mL

2. Dogs—50, 100, 250, 500, or 1,000 mL based on size

3. Hemorrhagic shock, replace with estimated volume of loss

4. Serially recheck PCV to determine adequacy of replacement

Rate of Whole Blood Administration

1. Normovolemic = 10 mL/lb/24 h

2. Hypovolemic = 10 mL/lb/h

3. Heart failure = 2 mL/lb/h

4. Warm blood to near body temperature not to exceed 37°C

A. Immerse blood bags in warm water bath or infuse blood through coils travelling through warm water.

B. Do not overheat; this can result in agglutination of RBC, hemolysis, and precipitation of plasma proteins.

5. Finish RBC infusion within four hours to prevent potential complications of infection in stored blood.

A. Slowly infuse blood for first 15 to 20 minutes to monitor for any severe adverse reactions.

6. Do not rerefrigerate unused blood that has warmed to 10°C (about 30 minutes at room temperature).

7. Use or discard all blood products that

have been entered (needle puncture) within 24 hours regardless of refrigeration.

Selection and Administration of Donor Blood

1. Choose blood from the same species.
2. Administer blood from known CEA-1– negative donor if possible, even for first-time transfusion so as to not sensitize recipient to subsequent RBC infusions.
3. If blood type of donor is not known, perform a major cross-match.
  A. Donor RBC and recipient sera, then evaluate for microagglutination or hemolysis
    1) Subtle reactions in dogs and cats compared with people
  B. This helps to rule out possibility of immediate hemolytic reaction on this transfusion, but does not guarantee that sensitization will not occur (i.e., with exposure, the same blood may not be acceptable to infuse in the future).
4. Perform a cross-match if multiple transfusions are anticipated.
5. Perform a minor cross-match if multiple plasma transfusions are anticipated.
  A. Donor plasma and recipient RBC are evaluated.
6. If immediate oxygen carrying capacity is required in a crisis situation, choose fresh blood or that which has been stored for 10 days or less.
7. Antihistamines are routinely administered 10 to 15 minutes before starting a transfusion at some institutions to reduce or eliminate transfusion reactions.
8. Avoid the use of transfusions to animals with immune-mediated hemolytic anemia unless absolutely necessary. Make sure such patients are pretreated with corticosteroids in immunosuppressive doses.
9. When a transfusion reaction occurs
  A. Stop or severely slow the rate of further blood infusion
  B. Increase rate of crystalloid fluid infusion
  C. Antihistamines, corticosteroids
  D. Epinephrine for anaphylaxis/collapse not responsive to the above

Complications of Blood Transfusion

1. Shortened RBC lifespan due to RBC antigen sensitization (particularly during repeated transfusions) is the most common problem. This is more likely to occur when nontyped donors are used.
  A. Associated with postive Coombs' test
2. Hemolysis is uncommon.
  A. Dogs lack appreciable levels of naturally-occurring isoantibodies, so immediate intravascular hemolysis due to immune mechanisms will not occur with the first transfusion. Once patient's sensitized and reexposed to the same antigenic type of RBC, hemolysis can be rapid.
  B. Type B cats that receive type A blood may experience a severe and immediate reaction, including death after the first transfusion.
  C. Aged blood or blood damaged during collection, storage, or infusion may undergo hemolysis without influence of immune mechanisms.
3. Plasma/WBC reactions may include fever, chills, tremors, emesis, urination, weakness, or urticaria.
4. Blood contaminated during collection and storage may result in fever and septicemia. Bacterial growth may impart a dark brown color from breakdown of hemoglobin.
5. Fever may be septic or nonseptic.
6. Transmission of infectious agents from improperly screened donor blood
7. Vomiting may occur when blood is infused too rapidly or from the development of hypervolemia.
8. Hypervolemia, particularly when whole blood rather than packed RBC is infused to an initially normovolemic animal
9. Hypothermia can occur when chilled blood is administered quickly in large quantity, particularly to smaller animals.
10. Cardiac arrhythmias can result from hypothermia, hypocalcemia, and possibly from emboli.
11. Embolization can occur from microaggregates that localized most commonly in the lung.

12. Disseminated Intravascular Coagulation (DIC)

13. Abnormal coagulation due to dilution of clotting factors with large volumes of packed RBC, or with infusion of aged or nonfresh plasma lacking viable coagulation factors. Poor platelet function of stored blood also can contribute.

14. Nephrosis due to hemoglobinuria from hemolysis is uncommon.

15. Hypocalcemia can result if too much citrate is added as the anticoagulant and then blood is infused rapidly.

    A. Ionized hypocalcemia wil occur but total calcium measurements will be normal.

    B. Citrate is normally metabolized quickly by the liver. Animals with liver disease may be at increased risk to suffer signs of low ionized calcium.

Plasma

1. Either fresh-frozen plasma or fresh plasma are used to supply clotting factors in a coagulopathy (hemophilia, von Willebrand's disease, warfarin toxicity, and DIC).

    A. Fresh-frozen plasma has been frozen within six hours of collection and has been stored frozen for less than one year.

    B. Fresh plasma has been removed from RBC within four hours of collection and used within 24 hours.

    C. Fresh whole blood may be used alternatively; it also will supply platelets.

    D. Give 5 mL/lb plasma twice daily until bleeding stops, or give a dose before anesthesia and surgery.

2. It is not necessary to use plasma for routine volume expansion. Crystalloids or dextrans suffice in most instances.

    A. Hemorrhagic shock may benefit from the infusion of plasma to help maintain effective circulating blood volume if whole blood is not available.

3. It is nearly impossible to treat severe hypoproteinemia or hypoalbuminemia with units of plasma (each unit of plasma contains little protein compared with the body deficit) if ongoing protein losses are large.

    A. This particularly true with protein-losing enteropathies or nephropathies.

    B. Some patients with severe edema do respond to plasma infusion temporarily (increased oncotic pressure), even when they failed to respond to diuretics.

Suggested Readings

Auer L, Bell K, Coates S: Blood transfusion reactions in the cat. J Am Vet Med Assoc 180: 729–730, 1982

Authement JM, Wolfsheimer KJ, Catchings S: Canine blood component therapy: product preparation, storage, and administration. J Am Anim Hosp Assoc 23: 483–493, 1987

Bell FW, Osborne CA: Maintenance fluid therapy. In Kirk RW (ed): Current Veterinary Therapy X: Small Anim. Prac., pp 37–43. Philadelphia, WB Saunders, 1989

Carlson GP: Fluid, electrolyte, and acid–base balance. In Kaneko JJ (ed): Clinical Biochemistry of Domestic Animals, pp 543–575. San Diego, Academic Press, 1989

Clark CH, Woodley CH: The absorption of red blood cells after parenteral injection at various sites. Am J Vet Res: 1062–1066, 1959

Cornelius LM: Fluid therapy in small animal practice. J Am Vet Med Assoc 176(2): 110–114, 1980

Finco DR: Fluid therapy. In Kirk RW (ed): Current Veterinary Therapy VI. Philadelphia, WB Saunders, 1977

Greene CE: Practical considerations of blood transfusion therapy. AAHA Proceedings 47th Meeting: pp 187–191, 1980

Hayes A, Mastrota F, Mooney S, Hurvitz A: Safety of transfusing blood in cats (Letter). J Am Vet Med Assoc 181: 4–6, 1982

Muir WW, DiBartola SP: Fluid therapy. In Kirk RW (ed): Current Veterinary Therapy VIII: Small Anim Prac, pp 28–40. Philadelphia, WB Saunders, 1983

O'Rourke LG: Practical blood transfusions. In Kirk RW (ed): Current Veterinary Therapy VIII, 408–411. Philadelphia, WB Saunders, 1983

Schaer M: General Principles of fluid therapy

in small animal medicine. Vet Clin North Am Small Anim Pract 19: 203–213, 1989

Schall WD: General principles of fluid therapy. Vet Clin North Am Small Anim Prac 12: 453–462, 1982

Tanger CH: Transfusion therapy for the dog and cat. Compend Contin Educ Pract Vet 4: 521–527, 1982

Tasker JB: Fluids, electrolytes, and acid-base. In Kaneko JJ (ed): Clinical Biochemistry of Domestic Animals. New York, Academic Press, 1980

CHAPTER TWENTY-FIVE

Disorders of Electrolytes and Osmolality

Dennis J. Chew and Stephen P. DiBartola

Disturbances in Electrolytes

Like body water, electrolytes have a compartmental distribution between the fluid spaces. Dramatic differences of distribution exist between intracellular and extracellular electrolytes, but the osmolality is identical for both compartments. Sodium, chloride, and biocarbonate are located predominantly in the extracellular fluid (ECF); potassium, magnesium, organic phosphates, and proteinates predominate in the intracellular fluid (ICF). Concentration of electrolytes in the ECF is closely approximated by analyzing readily obtained plasma or serum. These values for electrolytes represent relative rather than absolute quantity of the electrolyte in the plasma. No accurate method is available currently to measure the concentration of intracellular electrolytes. Remember that plasma electrolyte concentration may not reflect intracellular electrolyte concentration.

Clinical Approach

If a significant electrolyte abnormality is returned from the laboratory, repeat the determination to ensure the accuracy of the abnormality. Serial electrolyte evaluation provides far more valuable clinical information than a single sample, particularly while monitoring therapy.

Physiology and Regulation of Normal Serum Sodium

1. Nearly all ingested sodium is absorbed by the gut. In the steady-state, the amount of ingested sodium will nearly equal the amount excreted in the urine.

2. Changes in dietary sodium intake are accompanied by parallel changes in urinary sodium excretion after a short period of adaptation.

3. Renal handling of sodium involves glomerular filtration followed by extensive tubular reabsorption ($> 99\%$ reabsorbed in health).

4. Most sodium is located in the extracellular water. Low intracellular sodium content and concentration is maintained by the activity of cell membrane sodium–potassium ATPase pumps rather than selective membrane permeability.

A. Intracellular sodium for muscle is about 12 mEq/L, or less than 10% of its extracellular concentration.

5. Normal serum sodium determined in most laboratories is 140 to 155 mEq/L in dogs and 145 to 160 mEq/L in cats, and is maintained within a narrow range for an individual animal.

6. Sodium and its attendant anions account for about 95% of the osmotically active substances in the extracellular water.

7. Adjustments in water balance (thirst and vasopressin [ADH]) work to maintain normal serum osmolality and serum sodium concentration.
8. Adjustments in sodium balance maintain normal extracellular fluid volume. These include the effects of glomerulotubular balance, aldosterone, atrial natriuretic peptide, and renal hemodynamic factors.
   A. Extracellular fluid volume expansion increases sodium excretion.
   B. Extracellular fluid volume contraction decreases sodium excretion.

Disorders of Sodium and Osmolality*

Hyponatremia

1. Hyponatremia exists when the measured sodium value returns less than 140 mEq/L in dogs and less than 145 mEq/L in cats.
2. Mechanisms causing hyponatremia
   A. Inadequate salt intake—Lack of salt intake alone does not result in hyponatremia.
   B. Loss of salt
   C. Gain of water
   D. Gain of salt with more gain of water
   E. Combinations of the above

Etiology of Hyponatremia

Salt Depletion
Inadequate intake
Renal loss
   Diuretics†
   Salt-losing nephropathy
   Hypoadrenocorticism†
Extrarenal loss
   Gastrointestinal (GI)†
   Uroperitoneum (ruptured urinary tract)
   Burns
   Large wounds
   Body-cavity lavage
   Peritoneal dialysis
   Chylothorax

* See also characterization of dehydration, Chapter 24.
† Most common conditions in veterinary medicine. See text for further discussion.

Salt Dilution
Isotonic loss with water replacement*
Iatrogenic water load (hypotonic IV fluids)*
Secondary hyperaldosteronism
Congestive heart failure
Nephrotic syndrome
Severe liver disease
Psychogenic polydipsia (marginal)
Syndrome of inappropriate secretion of antidiuretic hormone (ADH)
Hyperglycemia
Mannitol administration

Pseudohyponatremia
Hyperlipemia*
Hyperproteinemia—severe

Laboratory Error

3. Renal loss of sodium due to diuretic abuse may be seen, particularly with concurrent anorexia. Dogs with hypoadrenocorticism classically have hyponatremia due to failure of renal-salt conservation. Primary nephropathy occasionally may be characterized by major salt loss into the urine.
4. Extrarenal losses of sodium occur commonly through the GI tract. Opportunity for salt loss is high with diarrhea or vomiting.
5. Lack of intake of salt from food magnifies the intensity of hyponatremia in patients with excessive salt losses from the body. If water intake is maintained, hyponatremia becomes more obvious because water is added as a dilutional component.
6. Occasionally, hypertonic fluid loss such as that encountered in burns, large oozing wounds, body-cavity lavage, or peritoneal dialysis may result in hyponatremia.
7. Dilution of body sodium with excessive water may be seen in patients with secondary hyperaldosteronism. This may occur in congestive heart failure, severe liver disease (cirrhosis), or nephrotic syndrome; these patients are unable to dilute their urine maximally.
8. Dilution of plasma also may occur after IV administration of salt-free solutions, particularly in patients that are unable to initiate a brisk diuresis.

* Most common conditions in veterinary medicine. See text for further discussion.

9. Physiologic hyponatremia may occur when severe hyperglycemia exists. This hyperglycemia results in increased osmolality of the ECF and a compensatory shift of water into the ECF that expands the ECF volume. Infusion of mannitol or other impermeant solute also may create dilutional hyponatremia.

10. The syndrome of inappropriate secretion of ADH may result in hyponatremia.

    A. ADH released despite absence of normal osmotic or nonosmotic stimuli (hypovolemia)

    B. Rare in animals

    C. It has been seen in humans secondary to CNS disease, pulmonary disease, neoplasia, and certain drugs.

    D. Documented in dogs with dirofilariasis, undifferentiated carcinoma, and possibly dogs with glucocorticoid deficiency.

    E. ADH may be abundantly released after major traumatic injury and as a result of anesthesia.

      1) Excess fluid therapy during this period may predispose the patient to hyponatremia.

11. Drugs may stimulate the release of ADH or potentiate its renal effects.

    A. Barbiturates

    B. Beta-adrenergic drugs

    C. Cholinergic drugs

    D. Chlorpropramide

    E. Clofibrate

    F. Narcotics

    G. Nitrous oxide

    H. Vincristine

12. Severe hypothyroidism with myxedema coma is a rare condition associated with hyponatremia reported in dogs.

    A. Mechanism may involve nonosmotic ADH release and decreased distal tubule fluid delivery.

13. When the plasma is severely lipemic or hyperproteinemic, pseudohyponatremia may result as an artifact.

    A. The standard laboratory determination of sodium measures the sodium content in plasma water relative to the total plasma volume.

      1) Flame photometer is the most common method.

    B. Normally, plasma volume is about 93% water and 7% protein.

    C. When components such as lipid or additional protein contribute to the plasma volume, the relative amount of plasma water is decreased; consequently, the reported value of sodium per volume of plasma also is lowered. The abnormal component of plasma creates a displacing volume that sodium does not occupy.

    D. The concentration of sodium in plasma water may actually be normal.

      1) Plasma or serum osmolality in these cases is normal because, owing to their size and insolubility in water, these displacing macromolecules do not add significant numbers of particles to serum water.

    E. Ion-specific electrode methods measure the concentration of electrolyte in the aqueous phase of plasma by potentiometry.

      1) Concentration of sodium is unaffected by amount of nonaqueous substances if direct potentiometry

      2) Indirect potentiometry involves an initial dilution of sample that will allow pseudohyponatremia to occur, however.

    F. The laboratory method used to determine sodium concentration must be known to determine if pseudohyponatremia is a possibility.

14. Chylothorax occasionally results in hyponatremia in experimental and clinical animals. The mechanism is unknown.

15. The differential diagnosis of hyponatremia may be grouped by serum osmolality into those with decreased, normal, or increased osmolality.

    A. Those patients with hyponatremia and decreased serum osmolality may be divided further into those with volume depletion, volume excess, or those with normal volume. (See Figure 25-1.)

Clinical Signs of Hyponatremia

Signs are mainly weakness and contraction of effective extracellular fluid volume, possibly resulting in shock. Severe hyponatremia of sudden onset results in intracellular overhydration (edema), including cerebral edema and resultant depression.

    Severity of signs is a function both of the

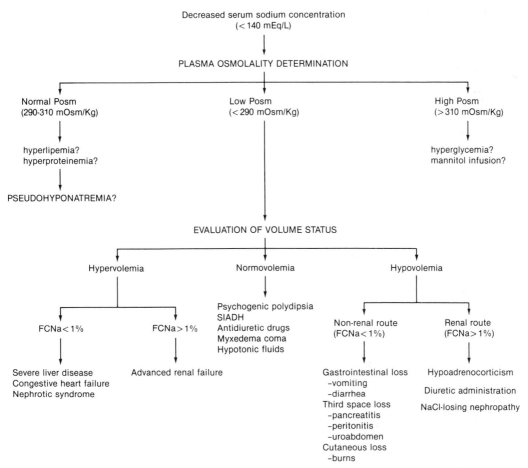

Figure 25-1. *Diagnostic approach to the patient with hyponatremia. FC$_{Na}$ = fractional clearance of sodium. Normal values in dogs <1%. From DiBartola SP. Hyponatremia, Vet Clin North Am. 19: 215–230, 1989.*

serum sodium level and of how rapidly the fall in sodium concentration developed. Much more severe signs are seen if the decreased serum sodium developed rapidly than if it developed slowly.

Anorexia and vomiting may be caused by hyponatremia. Abdominal cramps, paralytic intestinal ileus, and muscular twitching also may be seen. Neurologic signs include both focal and diffuse deficits, with occasional seizures. Permanent brain damage may be caused by protracted hyponatremia. There are no consistent ECG changes in hyponatremia.

Treatment of Hyponatremia

1. Stop IV infusion of salt-free solution if the cause is iatrogenic.

2. Treat the underlying cause of water retention or salt loss.

3. In hyponatremia with severe clinical signs, consider infusing hypertonic saline solution initially.

A. Loop diuretics may be given at same time if patient is overhydrated.

4. In patients with moderately symptomatic hyponatremia and normal cardiovascular and renal status, administer .9% saline. In most cases this is sufficient for sodium repletion because renal conservation of sodium and excretion of excess water corrects the deficit.

5. Water restriction should be started if the cause is psychogenic polydipsia or if it is caused by the rare finding of syndrome of inappropriate ADH (SIADH).

   A. Lithium or demeclocycline can be considered for treatment of SIADH.

6. Pseudohyponatremia does not require treatment since sodium concentration in plasma water is normal.

7. Do not attempt total immediate correction of the Na deficit because of the dangers of overcorrection.

   A. Particularly true when hyponatremia is chronic

      1) Acute severe symptomatic hyponatremia in dogs or cats is rare.

   B. Rapid correction of chronic hyponatremia may result in central nervous system demyelination, but this is controversial.

   C. Persistent hyponatremia can result in brain damage, particularly if acute.

   D. We suggest an initial acute sodium correction of 10 mEq/L.

   E. Thereafter, repeat the sodium determination and give further emergency Na repletion if clinically necessary.

Sample Calculation

An owner brings in a 10-kg dog with Na of 110 mEq/L; the dog is depressed. How many milliliters of 3% saline is needed to raise the serum sodium to 120 mEq/L?

10 kg dog × 0.3
   = Volume of distribution for sodium*
   = 3 kg = 3 L

$$\frac{110 \text{ mEq}}{L} \times 3 \text{ L} = 330 \text{ mEq sodium}$$

   initially in ECF of dog

At $\frac{120 \text{ mEq}}{L} \times 3 \text{ L} = 360 \text{ mEq sodium}$

   existing after addition of sodium
   to same volume.

---

* 30% volume of distribution for sodium = volume of ECF.

360 mEq desired
− 330 mEq already present

   30 mEq additional sodium required

3% NaCl contains $\dfrac{513 \text{ mEq}}{L}$ Na

$$\frac{\dfrac{30 \text{ mEq needed}}{513 \text{ mEq available}}}{L}$$

   = 0.058 L = 58 mL of 3% saline

58 mL of hypertonic 3% saline could be infused rapidly. Perform repeat determination of Na⁺ to evaluate effects of this therapy. Assumptions for this evaluation are that substantial volume expansion does not occur and that all the sodium given stays in the ECF.

Hypernatremia*

1. Hypernatremia exists when the measured sodium value is greater than 155 mEq/L in dogs and greater than 160 mEq/L in cats (Table 25-1).

2. Mechanisms causing hypernatremia

   A. Loss of water

   B. Gain of sodium

   C. Combinations of the above

3. Associated ECF volume

   A. Pure water loss results in relative preservation of ECF volume.

   B. Hypotonic fluid loss results in decreased ECF volume.

   C. Gain of salt results in expansion of ECF volume.

4. Underlying conditions resulting in hypernatremia

   A. Lack of adequate water intake while obligate hypotonic losses continue results in hypernatremia and hypertonic dehydration.

   B. Excessive intake of sodium may be the cause. Spontaneous oral intake of sodium causing hypernatremia is very uncommon in small animals. Iatrogenic overadministration of sodium-containing fluids is more common and may result in hypernatremia, particularly in cases with oliguria or marginal renal function.

---

* See also characterization of dehydration, Chapter 24.

Table 25-1. **Etiologies for hypernatremia in pets**

Hypernatremia Association with Water Loss	Hypernatremia Associated with Salt Gain
Pure Water Loss	
Increased Na$^+$ and normal ECF volume	Increased Na$^+$ and increased ECF volume
Pituitary diabetes insipidus	Increased salt intake
Nephrogenic diabetes insipidus	Dietary
Heat stroke	Sea water
High environmental temperature	Saline emetics
Fever	IV hypertonic fluids
Inadequate access to water (CNS disease, infirmity)	IV sodium bicarbonate
	Hyperaldosteronism
Burns	Hyperadrenocorticism
Hypotonic Water Loss	
Increased Na$^+$ and decreased ECF volume	
Diarrhea	
Vomiting	
Oral hyperalimentation	
Osmotic diuresis	
Acute renal failure	
Chronic renal failure	
Diabetes mellitus	
Diuretic use	
IV solute administration	
Hypoadrenocorticism	

Abbreviations: ECF = extracellular fluid; IV = intravenous.
From Hardy RM: Hyponatremia. Vet Clin North Am [Small Anim Pract] 19:231–240, 1987.

C. Cases with near-terminal chronic renal disease may have such marked impairment of glomerular filtration rate (GFR) that sodium retention occurs. A case with less advanced chronic renal pathology tends to have normal or slightly low serum sodium values.

D. Primary hyperaldosterism has been reported once in a dog.

E. Loss of water and sodium from the body may result in hypernatremia if relatively more water is lost than sodium (hypertonic dehydration due to hypotonic loss).

F. Essential hypernatremia (primary adipsia or hypodipsia)

1) Defect in central thirst and osmoreception of hypothalamus; may have partial ADH deficiency too.

2) Very uncommon in dogs, rare in cats

Signs of Hypernatremia
Most of the signs of hypernatremia arise from the CNS. The more rapid the development of hypernatremia, the more severe the neurologic signs are likely to be. Acute hypernatremia results in acute hyperosmolality of ECF favoring shrinkage of brain cells; these changes are minimized in chronic hypernatremia. Depression progressing to coma, sei-

zures, and possibly permanent brain injury may result from severe hypernatremia. Acute severe hypernatremia in experimental cats may result in cerebral hemorrhage and subdural hematomas. Weakness is often seen, sometimes arising from neuronal changes and sometime attributed to direct effect on muscle cells. The ECG is usually normal. If derangement of the hypothalamic thirst center is not the cause of the hypernatremia, intense thirst may be seen.

Treatment of Hypernatremia

1. Stop infusions of sodium-rich IV fluids (.9% saline, Ringer's).
2. Reduce supplementation with sodium salts (e.g., $NaHCO_3$).
3. Consider use of natriuretic diuretics (Lasix) to enhance removal of excess sodium if cause was iatrogenic.
4. Correct ECF hypovolemia with isotonic fluids first (.9% NaCl; lactated Ringer's solution).
  A. Although istonic to normal plasma, these fluids are effectively hypotonic.
5. Infuse sodium-poor solutions (5% dextrose in water, 2.5% dextrose in .45% saline) to replenish water and thereby dilute the present concentration of plasma sodium after volume depletion has been corrected.
6. Do not correct chronic hypernatremia too rapidly because brain cells may have undergone a protective adaptation resulting in osmotically active intracellular particles called *idiogenic osmoles* (osmolytes).
  A. The production of idiogenic osmoles serves to maintain cellular hydration in the face of chronic ECF hyperosmolality.
  B. Sudden correction of chronically hyperosmolar ECF could result in cellular overhydration if a parallel reduction in number of idiogenic intracellular osmoles does not occur also.
  C. Clinically, the animal initially responds to infusion of hypotonic fluid but then deteriorates mentally as further hypotonic fluid infusion is continued.
  D. Seizures can occur during therapy for hypernatremia, usually indicating too rapid correction.
    1) Cerebral edema

E. Some authors recommend correction of severe hypernatremia over 2 to 3 days, or a decrease of .5 to 1.0 mEq/L/h during rehydration.
  F. Less severe hypernatremia can be corrected more quickly without apparent harm.
7. Add water to food is diagnosis is essential hypernatremia.

Disorders of Serum Osmolality

1. Serum osmolality is maintained within a narrow range in healthy animals. Normal serum osmolality of dogs and cats is 285 to 310 mosm/kg. Osmolality may be measured (freezing-point depression or vaporization osmometry), or it may be estimated by various indirect formulas. Diseases may result in hyperosmolality or hypo-osmolality, or they may not affect osmolality. Changes in osmolality due to impermanent substances in the ECF result in body water shifts until all compartments are isosmotic.
2. Changes in serum osmolality usually parallel changes in serum sodium concentration because sodium and its attendant anions represent most of the osmotically active particles normally present in ECF. Na^+ shifts are always accompanied by an equal number of anions to maintain electroneutrality.
3. Indirect formulas for the estimation of serum osmolality vary in their accuracy and should be species-correlated. Studies in the dog have confirmed inaccuracy in several of the frequently published formulas. Two formulas found to be accurate at one veterinary institution are

$$2 \ (Na + K) \ \text{closely estimates}$$
$$\text{measured osmolality if azotemia}$$
$$\text{or severe hyperglycemia}$$
$$\text{do not exist.}$$

$$1.86 \ (Na + K^*) + \frac{\text{glucose}}{18} + \frac{BUN†}{2.8} + 9$$

closely estimates measured osmolality (when azotemia or hyperglycemia do exist).

---

* Na and K measured in mEq/L.
† Glucose and BUN measured in mg/dL.

Table 25-2. **Use of osmole gaps in evaluation of body fluids**

Serum Osmolality	Osmole Gap	Probable Interpretation
↓ Calculated Normal measured	↑	Pseudohyponatremia (↑ abnormal plasma macromolecules)
↓ Calculated ↓ Measured	N	True hypoosmolality (hyponatremia)
Calculated > measured	↓ or negative value	Laboratory or mathematical error
↑ Calculated ↑ Measured	N	Hyperosmolality due to loss of water, measured osmotic solute (glucose, BUN)
N or ↑ calculated ↑ ↑ measured	↑	Hyperosmolality due to addition of unmeasured osmotically active solute

4. The second formula closely estimates patient serum osmolality; use it in dogs with substantial azotemia or hyperglycemia. The 9 mosm/kg added to the end of the second equation is an estimate of normal osmotic particles that are not normally measured.

5. The second formula shows that each additional elevation in blood glucose of 100 mg/dL contributes an increased osmolality of 5.5. A rise in BUN of 100 mg/dL raises the osmolality by 35.

6. The difference between the calculated and measured serum osmolality should be small. In normal dogs, it is presently valued at 0–10 mosm/kg. This difference is called the *osmole gap.*

(Measured − calculated)
$$\text{osmolality} = \text{osmole GAP}$$

Principle of the Osmole Gap

1. Although calculated osmolality and measured osmolality alone are helpful in evaluating disorders in osmolality, these and the calculated osmole gap yield more useful information.

2. The greater the magnitude in the osmole gap, the greater the quantity of unmeasured solute in the patient's serum.

3. Certain disease states may significantly increase the osmole gap (unmeasured solute present; Table 25-2 and list below).

4. Evaluation of the osmole gap may be useful in initial diagnoses and serially in prognosis after initiation of therapy.

5. Hyperosmolar states caused by a loss of water have a normal gap; hyperosmolar states caused by diseases adding unmeasured solute have an increased gap.

Increased Osmolar Gap; Hyperosmolality Due to Addition of Unmeasured, Osmotically Active Solute

Ethylene glycol*
Other poisoning
    Ethanol
    Salicylate
    Drugs
Lactic acidosis
Shock (partly due to lactic acid)
Septicemia
Lymphosarcoma (LSA)
Cirrhosis

6. The greatest veterinary value in using the osmolar gap may lie in the initial evaluation and diagnosis of possible ethylene-glycol intoxication. Large increases in osmotically active ethylene-glycol solute in the serum may be detected shortly after ingestion and for 24 hours thereafter. Most other veterinary diseases do not cause the level of hyperosmolality and osmolal gap encountered during the initial phases of ethylene-glycol poisoning.

7. General guidelines for "tolerable" abnormal increases in osmolality usually offer an upper limit of 345 to 350 mosm/kg for the dog and cat.

---

* Most important consideration in veterinary medicine.

8. Increases in osmolality due to freely permeable particles between water compartments do not result in shifts of water.

    A. Serum hyperosmolality due to urea or ethanol does not result in net movement of water because they are freely permeable to cells.

    B. Rapid IV infusion of urea results in movement of water out of cells. An osmolality gradient exists until urea has time to equilibrate within the cells, then water shifts cease. Consequently, it is better to consider the "effective" osmolality gradient that is generated.

9. Osmolality, corrected for the quantity due to urea, allows more accurate assessment of osmotic forces capable of causing fluid shifts (see above).

Corrected osmolality

$$= \text{measured osmolality} - \frac{\text{BUN*}}{2.8}$$

$$= \text{"effective" osmolality}$$

10. In dehydration mostly due to water loss (hypertonic or hypernatremic dehydration), the serum osmolality may be used to estimate fluid deficit. This formula may be applied *only* to hypertonic dehydration.

Sample Calculations

1. How much solute-free solution is needed to acutely return the serum osmolality of a 10-kg dog from 320 to 300 with normal BUN and glucose?

$$\text{Fluid deficit (L)} = \frac{320 - 300}{300} \times 0.6 \times 10 \text{ kg}$$

$$= \frac{20}{300} \times 6 \text{ kg} = .4 \text{ L} = 400 \text{ mL}$$

2. How much solute-free solution is needed to return the serum osmolality of a 10-kg dog from 350 to 300 with BUN at 112 mg/dL? In this case the measured serum osmolality (Sosm) must first be corrected to account for the ineffective osmotic activity contributed by the freely permeable urea.

---

* BUN is reported in $\frac{\text{mg}}{\text{dL}}$.

$$\text{BUN} = 112 \frac{\text{mg}}{\text{dL}} \div 2.8$$

$$= \frac{40 \text{ mosm}}{\text{kg}} \text{ contributed by urea}$$

$$\text{Corrected osmolality} = 350 - 40 = 310$$

$$\text{Fluid deficit (L)} = \frac{310 - 300}{300} \times 0.6 \times 10 \text{ kg}$$

$$= \frac{10}{300} \times 6 \text{ kg} = .2 \text{ L} = 200 \text{ mL}$$

Disorders in Potassium Balance

Normal Physiology and Regulation of Potassium

1. Potassium (K^+) is the major intracellular cation and is thereby largely responsible for maintenance of intracellular volume.

2. Over 95% of body potassium is stored within cells, with only 2% to 5% of body K^+ in the extracellular fluids.

    A. Approximately 40 mEq/kg is considered normal body potassium capacity.

3. The ratio of intracellular to extracellular K^+ concentration is important in determining cellular membrane potential. Rapid alterations in extracellular K^+ concentration alter this ratio and predispose an animal to arrhythmias and conduction disturbances in excitable tissues (heart, nerve, muscle).

4. Approximately 90% of ingested K^+ is excreted by the kidney and 10% in the feces. Under special circumstances (as in chronic renal failure) the colon may adapt to increase K^+ excretion into feces.

5. Daily potassium intake equals daily loss in healthy dogs and cats. Daily requirements are 2.2 to 44 mEq (see Figure 24.3).

6. The healthy kidney is well evolved as an organ of K^+ excretion. Its ability to conserve K^+ is less well developed. Obligatory losses of K^+ in urine occur even during severe dietary K^+ restriction.

7. Plasma or serum concentration of K^+ stays within a narrow range (4.0 to 5.5 mEq/L) despite wide variation in dietary K^+ intake. This control is maintained by secretion of insulin, the sympathetic nervous system, and renal or adrenal mechanisms.

8. Renal handling of potassium

A. Potassium is filtered freely by glomerular filtration and is either passively or actively reabsorbed along the entire nephron.

B. In the distal nephron, aldosterone facilitates potassium secretion. Aldosterone stimulates active transport of K^+ from peritubular fluid into the tubular cell. Through passive diffusion, potassium moves out from the cell into the tubular fluid as the concentration of intracellular K^+ increases. This effect may occur without simultaneous changes in Na^+ excretion.

C. Plasma aldosterone concentration is regulated both by the renin–angiotensin system and by direct stimulation of the adrenal cortex from hyperkalemia.

D. Tubular flow rate past the secreting site of the distal nephron is also important. Potassium excretion here depends on the maintenance of a favorable gradient between K^+ concentration in tubular fluid and K^+ concentration within the tubular cell. A gradient favorable to continuing secretion of K^+ into tubular fluid is maintained at high rates of tubular flow because maximal secretion of K^+ into the tubular fluid occurs rapidly. Diminution of this gradient occurs at low rates of tubular flow.

E. The healthy kidney adapts to a chronically high intake of K^+ (potassium load) by intrinsic renal mechanisms that are not understood. An acute potassium load results in a more limited renal excretory response for K^+.

9. Plasma or serum K^+ concentration may not reflect total-body potassium because the extracellular concentration of a predominantly intracellular electrolyte is being measured.

A. During chronic wasting of body muscle mass, approximately 3 mEq K^+ is lost per gram of protein nitrogen lost. In chronic disease associated with loss of muscle mass, serum K^+ is likely to be normal, although total-body K^+ stores are diminished.

B. As K^+ is lost from extracellular fluid, K^+ from intracellular stores tends to move into the ECF, thereby masking the ECF K^+ loss.

C. Interpret serum or plasma potassium concentration values in light of the animal's acid–base balance. Acute acidosis or alkalosis results in translocation of K^+ between cellular and extracellular compartments. As a general rule for every change in blood pH of .1 U, there is a simultaneous inverse change in serum K^+ of .6 mEq/L. For example, consider a patient with a pH of 7.1 and a serum K^+ of 4.5 mEq/L. When the acidosis is corrected (pH now 7.4), serum K^+ will be 2.7 mEq/L; hypokalemia will exist if K^+ supplementation has not been provided.

1) This is true if metabolic acidosis is due to inorganic causes (i.e., these changes are not seen if it is due to lactic acidosis).

Hypokalemia

1. Hypokalemia exists when measured values of serum K^+ are less than 4.0 mEq/L.

A. Hypokalemia usually becomes clinically important at concentrations less than 3.5 mEq/L.

B. Hypokalemia from all causes may be more common in cats than in dogs.

2. Hypokalemia may indicate

A. A total-body deficit of potassium

B. Translocation of K^+ into cells with no real total-body deficit (also referred to as redistributive hypokalemia)

3. Negative K^+ balance (K^+ intake $- K^+$ loss = negative value)

A. Inadequate K^+ intake

B. Increased K^+ losses

1) GI

2) Urinary

C. Often decreased K^+ intake in combination with increased K^+ loss

4. Signs of hypokalemia are divided into metabolic, neuromuscular, cardiovascular, and renal.

A. Metabolic—Impaired tolerance to carbohydrates may exist as an elevated fasting blood glucose determination. Pancreatic insulin secretion is decreased because it is dependent on K^+.

B. Neuromuscular—These signs are common, particularly if the K^+ is less than 2.5 mEq/L.

1) Muscle weakness, cramps, and paresthesias may be seen.

    a) Weakness in dogs may involve the rear limbs preferentially.

    b) Trunkal weakness in cats may be the most obvious sign, sometimes resulting in ventroflexion of the head and neck.

    2) Myopathy may result from chronic hypokalemia.

        a) Recently documented in cats

    3) Mental depression, lethargy, and confusion may exist; coma and delirium occur rarely.

    4) Weakness of the smooth muscles in the GI tract may result in decreased bowel motility and ileus. Similarly, the bladder may sometimes be paralyzed, resulting in urine retention.

    5) Anorexia, vomiting, constipation, delayed gastric emptying, and abdominal cramps also may result from hypokalemia.

    6) With extreme hypokalemia, death from respiratory-muscle paralysis may occur.

    C. Cardiovascular—ECG changes may be detected when the serum K^+ is less than 3.0 mEq/L; however, the presence of these abnormalities in dogs with hypokalemia is questionable. When present, these findings may include ST-segment depression, flattening or T-wave inversion, presence of a U wave, increase in P amplitude, PR-interval prolongation, and prolonged QRS duration (in severe hypokalemia). Sinus bradycardia, first-degree and second-degree heart block, atrial flutter, paroxysmal atrial tachycardia, atrioventricular dissociation, and ventricular fibrillation have been seen. Myocardial necrosis may be seen in severe potassium depletion, but the previously listed abnormalities probably arise from the hypokalemia and not from this necrosis.

    D. Renal—Hyposthenuria may be an important renal abnormality created by the hypokalemia. Concentrating ability is progressively lost as the K^+ deficit becomes more severe. Psychogenic stimulation of the hypothalamic centers for thirst from the hypokalemia may be contributory. A fall in GFR may occur if K^+ depletion is chronic, and intrarenal lesions also may result.

    1) A syndrome of K^+ depletion, hypokalemia, and primary renal failure recently

has been described in cats (feline kaliopenic polymyopathy/nephropathy syndrome).

Causes of Hypokalemia (or Potassium Depletion)

    1. Translocation of K^+ from ECF to ICF

        A. Increased pH (decreased H^+), alkalosis

        B. Increased plasma HCO_3^-

        C. Increased plasma insulin

        D. Increased plasma glucose (non-diabetic)

        E. Diuretic administration

        F. Catecholamines

            1) Beta-2 agonist effect

        G. Severe hypothermia

            1) Catecholamine-induced?

    2. Decreased K^+ intake

        A. Anorexia*

        B. Fluid administration deficient in K^+

        C. K^+-deficient diet

            1) Recently described in cats, particularly so if diet is highly acidifying.

    3. Gastrointestinal loss

        A. Vomiting*

        B. Diarrhea*

        C. Overuse of enemas, laxatives, or exchange resins

    4. Urinary loss

        A. Parenchymal renal disease

            1) Renal tubular acidosis

            2) Fanconi's syndrome

            3) Chronic renal disease (occasionally)

                a) May be more common in cats than in dogs.

            4) Amphotericin-B chronic administration, gentamicin administration

            5) Postobstructive diuresis*

                a) Urethral obstruction in feline urologic syndrome (FUS)

                b) Urinary calculi

            6) Diuretic phase of primary acute renal failure*

        B. Diuretic therapy

        C. Hypomagnesemia

---

* Most common and important causes of hypokalemia in dogs and cats.

D. Increased mineralocorticoid effect (hyperaldosteronism)

E. Impermeant anion effect (penicillin, carbenicillin)

F. Chronic metabolic acidosis

5. Spurious

A. Dilutional from failure to adequately clear IV line from heparinized saline flush

6. Parenteral fluid therapy with inadequate K+ supplementation

A. Volume expansion contributes dilutional component.

B. Increased renal tubular flow rate increases K+ loss into urine.

7. Paradoxic hypokalemia during K+ supplemented fluid administration.

A. Described in K+ depleted cats with renal disease.

Treatment of Hypokalemia

The patient's clinical signs and the degree of hypokalemia determine how aggressively and by what route correction is attempted. Patients with serum K+ values less than 2.5 mEq/L generally are treated, even if no specific signs referable to hypokalemia are present. Patients with serum K+ values near 2.0 mEq/L may require emergency replacement of potassium. Potassium values of 2.5 to 3.0 mEq/L usually require supplemental potassium if anorexia is present. Cases with K+ values of 3.0 to 3.5 mEq/L may require supplemental K+ if the disease process predicts either continuing anorexia or losses of potassium.

Oral K+ Replacement

During the recovery phase of many diseases, as appetite returns, correction of hypokalemia occurs with the intake of regular foodstuff. If anorexia persists or adequate intake of food is not sufficient for K+ replacement, commercially available K+ supplementation is available (Kay Ciel, 20 mEq/15 mL; Kaon, 20 mEq/15 mL). It is advisable to mix these preparations with an equal volume of water, or emesis frequently results from intake of the irritating liquid. Enteric tablets of K+ are available but not recommended, owing to problems with absorption and gastrointestinal

ulceration. Oral supplementation may be of no value in animals that are vomiting. The dosage of oral K+ is based on serial evaluation of serum K+ determinations.

Subcutaneous K+ Replacement

Solutions containing up to 30 mEq K+/L may be used safely by the subcutaneous route without local irritation. The likelihood of systemic toxicity due to hyperkalemia is low because of the prolonged time required for subcutaneous fluid absorption. This route is inadequate when serious deficits of potassium and water exist.

Intravenous K+ Replacement

1. As a general rule, the rate of K+ administration (mEq/h) is more important to toxicity levels than the total mEq K+ administration.

A. To avoid hyperkalemia, do not exceed 0.5 mEq K+/kg/h replacement.

B. 0.1 to .2 mEq/kg/h is usually adequate during repletion (Willard).

2. 3 to 5 mEq/kg/day of K+ may be required to treat moderate to severe hypokalemia (Schaer).

3. Sliding scale of Cornelius bases the total daily dose of potassium on the prevailing K+ concentration.

A. Mild K+ depletion

  1) K+ = 3.0 to 3.7 mEq/L

  2) Give 1 to 3 mEq/kg/day K+.

B. Moderate K+ depletion

  1) K+ = 2.5 to 3.0 mEq/L

  2) Give 4 to 6 mEq/kg/day K+.

C. Severe K+ depletion

  1) K+ < 25 mEq/L

  2) Give 7 to 9 mEq/kg/day K+.

4. If serum K+ values are available for evaluation on at least a daily basis, use the following sliding scale of Scott for guidelines to the level of K+ supplementation (Table 25-3). Accuracy of K+ repletion using this technique assumes an accurate estimation of fluid needs. Do not infuse potassium-rich fluids rapidly for correction of dehydration or shock. For rapid correction of both hypokalemia and dehydration, use two separate infusion lines with different rates for the potassium-rich (slow) and the potassium-poor (fast) fluids.

Table 25-3. **Modified sliding scale of Scott for treatment of hypokalemia or those with potassium depletion and normal serum potassium**

Serum K⁺ (mEq/L)	mEq K⁺ to Add to 250 mL Fluids	mEq K⁺ to Add to 1L Fluids	Maximum Infusion Rate* (mL/kg/h)
<2.0	20	80	6
2.1–2.5	15	60	8
2.6–3.0	10	40	12
3.1–3.5	7	28	18
>3.5<5.0	5	20	25

*At 0.5 mg/kg/h.

From Chew DJ: Parenteral fluid therapy. In Sherding RG (ed): *The Cat: Diseases and Clinical Management.* New York. Churchill Livingstone, pp 35–80, 1989. Reprinted with permission.

Fluid volume chosen is usually that for maintenance, but can include dehydration needs also if fluid infusion is evenly distributed over 24 hours and renal function is good.

5. Reevaluate serum to determine the efficacy of therapy and to adjust the level of administered potassium. If losses of K⁺ continue from the disease process, give the same level of K⁺ supplementation the next day even though the serum K⁺ value may have returned to normal. In this instance, on-going supplementation is necessary to keep the serum K⁺ within the normal range. If the previous level of K⁺ supplementation proved inadequate to raise the serum K⁺ value, choose the next higher level of K⁺ supplementation.

6. Risk for development of hyperkalemia while on K⁺ supplementation

    A. Oliguria/anuria

    B. Acidosis

    C. Rapid correction of alkalosis

    D. Emaciated patient with limited cellular uptake reservoir

        1) Total body K⁺ capacity may be reduced to 20 to 30 mEq/kg in severe to moderate wasting respectively (normal is about 40 mEq/kg).

    E. Rapid infusion of K⁺-containing fluids

7. Temper K⁺ administration guidelines when conditions listed in 6A to 6E are present.

    A. Give less K⁺.

    B. Monitor more closely

8. Taper the amount of K⁺ supplementation rapidly as the animal starts to eat; further IV supplementation usually is unnecessary.

9. Another technique of K⁺ repletion involves a standard concentration of 30 mEq K⁺ added to 1 L of fluid. This is a mild supplementation of K⁺ (equal to 7 to 8 mEq/K⁺/250 mL fluid) and may safely be given intravenously to animals presumed to be potassium deficient on the basis of history and physical examination (e.g., diabetes mellitus) when ready access to serum K⁺ is not available.

10. Parenteral potassium supplementation is available in the form of potassium chloride or potassium phosphate.

    A. Potassium chloride is more commonly used, often at 2 mEq K⁺/mL.

11. Calculated K⁺ deficits also may be estimated by the following formula:

Potassium deficit equals
(Normal K⁺ − present K⁺)
$$\times \text{ volume of K⁺ distribution}$$
$$= \frac{mEq}{L} \times L$$

    A. Because K⁺ is primarily an intracellular ion, its volume of distribution is greater than ECF. Forty percent of body weight is used empirically to compensate for anticipated intracellular deficit and uptake.

    B. Calculated needs using this method

provide far less K⁺ than that when using the sliding scale of Scott.

12. Potassium may be supplemented to fluids before development of hypokalemia (prophylactic use).

    A. Use when fluids are expected to be given for more than 24 hours.

    B. Use lowest end of modified sliding scale of Scott.

        1) 5 mEq K⁺/250 mL or 20 mEq K⁺/1000 mL

    C. Depends on gradual transfer of K⁺ into cells plus excretion of additional unneeded K⁺

    D. Alternatively, 0.5 mEq K⁺/kg/day has been recommended as a starting point to deter development of hyperkalemia while on fluids (Willard).

Sample Calculations

1. You evaluate a 10-kg (22-lb) dog with 8% dehydration

$$\frac{2.6 \text{ mEq}}{\text{L}} = \text{serum K}^+$$

$$4.0 = \text{normal K}^+$$

    A. Method 1

3 to 5 mEq/kg
= 30 to 50 mEq K⁺ potentially needed
                        per day

    B. Method 2

$$\text{Deficit of K}^+ = 4.0 - 2.6 = \frac{1.4 \text{ mEq}}{\text{L}}$$

Subacute volume of distribution (Vd) for K⁺ =40% of body weight

$$\text{Vd} = .4 \times 10 \text{ kg} = 4 \text{ kg} = 4 \text{ L}$$

$$\text{K}^+ \text{ deficit} \times \text{Vd} = \text{mEq K}^+ \text{ needed}$$

$$\frac{1.4 \text{ mEq}}{\text{L}} \times 4 \text{ L}$$

= 5.6 mEq K⁺ needed for initial replacement.

Additional K⁺ will be needed for maintenance and ongoing loss of K⁺ (See Figure 24-3, which indicates about 14 mEq K⁺ needed for daily maintenance. Total K⁺ administration by this method = 5.6 + 14 = about 20 mEq. Compared with the sliding scale of Scott, this calculation is conservative for replacement K⁺ values.

    C. Method 3, using the technique of Scott and the same dog

$$\frac{2.6 \text{ mEq}}{\text{L}} = \text{serum K}^+$$

Use 10 mEq K⁺ supplementation to each fluid volume of 250 mL.

Dehydration needs
$$= \% \text{ dehydration} \times \text{wt (lb)}$$
$$\times 500 = \text{mL}$$
$$= .08 \times 22 \times 500$$
$$= 880 \text{ mL}$$

Maintenance

$$= \frac{30 \text{ mL}}{\text{lb}} \times \text{weight (lb)} = \text{mL}$$

$$= \frac{30 \text{ mL}}{\text{lb}} \times 22 \text{ lb} = 660 \text{ mL}$$

Total fluid needs
$$= \text{maintenance} + \text{dehydration}$$
$$= 660 \text{ mL} + 880 \text{ mL} = 1540 \text{ mL}$$

    1) K⁺ supplementation from this sliding scale is at 10 mEq K⁺ for each 250 mL of fluid volume to be infused. (This is equivalent to 40 mEq K⁺ supplementation/L.) This dog will receive approximately 60 mEq K⁺ over a 24-hour period as fluid needs are infused. The K⁺ supplementation includes both replacement and maintenance considerations for K⁺.

    2) Day 2—Hydration is normal.

$$\frac{2.9 \text{ mEq}}{\text{L}} = \text{serum K}^+$$

$$\text{Wt} = 24 \text{ lb (wt. gained by rehydration)}$$

    3) How much K⁺ and fluids should be infused on day 2?

$$\text{Dehydration needs} = 0$$

Maintenance = 30 mL/lb
$$= 30 \text{ mL} \times 24 \text{ lb} = 720 \text{ mL}$$

Total fluid volume to be infused
$$= \text{about 720 mL (three 250 mL}$$
$$\text{bottles approximately)}$$

    4) K⁺ supplementation from the sliding scale is still at 10 mEq K⁺/250 mL volume

Figure 25-2. *Typical ECG in hyperkalemia. Note the absence of a P wave (atrial standstill) and the peaked T wave typical of moderate hyperkalemia.*

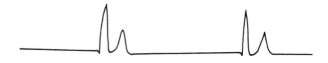

infused fluid. Since the fluid volume for day 2 is much lower than for day 1, the total amount of K⁺ infused must be proportionately lower. Approximately 30 mEq of K⁺ is supplemented over a 24-hour period while the calculated volume of fluid is infused.

Hyperkalemia

1. Hyperkalemia exists when serum K⁺ values are 6.0 mEq/L or greater.
2. Hyperkalemia may indicate either a positive potassium balance (K⁺ intake − K⁺ loss = positive value) or a translocation of K⁺ from the ICF to the ECF with no real change in total-body potassium.

Signs of Hyperkalemia

1. Some animals display surprisingly little physical examination abnormality even though the serum K⁺ may be in excess of 7.0 mEq/L.
2. Neuromuscular—Weakness or paralysis may be seen. Paralysis of the respiratory muscles may occur, resulting in death. Paresthesias may be present.
3. Cardiovascular*—The effect of hyperkalemia on the heart is the single most important concern because the patient may die from serious arrhythmia or cardiac asrystole. Effects on the heart are unlikely if the serum K⁺ is less than 7.0 mEq/L and more likely if serum K⁺ is greater than 8.0 mEq/L. ECG changes due to hyperkalemia are magnified by hyponatremia, hypocalcemia, acidosis, and hypermagnesemia. Dogs tend to maintain

*Most important in dogs and cats.

cardiac contractility even in the face of severe hyperkalemia and arrhythmia.

Progressive ECG Abnormalities

1. Increased amplitude, peaked T waves
2. ST-segment depression
3. Decreased amplitude R wave
4. Increased P–R interval
5. Decreased-amplitude P wave; atrial standstill
6. Increased Q–T interval
7. Increased QRS duration
8. Sinoventricular rhythm (sine-wave appearance)
9. Ventricular fibrillation or standstill
10. Bradycardia is a hallmark of hyperkalemia, but its absence does not exclude significant hyperkalemia. ECG detection and following of hyperkalemia is generally considered reliable in dogs and cats (Figures 25-2 and 25-3).

Causes of Hyperkalemia

1. Pseudohyperkalemia
   A. *In vitro* generation and release of K⁺ from cells may occur with clot formation in serum samples, if marked increases in platelets or white blood cells are present.
      1) Leukocytosis (>100,000)
      2) Thrombocytosis (>1,000,000/mm³)
   B. Hemolysis—If blood stands for a long time before the serum is harvested, some intracellular K⁺ may leak into the serum. Hemolyzed RBC that have been damaged during venapuncture or old stored blood may have plasma with increased K⁺ values, but

Figure 25-3. *This ECG tracing is representative of sinoventricular rhythm seen in advanced hyperkalemia.*

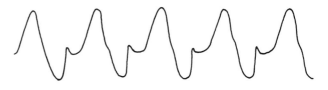

the amount of added K^+ in the plasma is small in dogs.

    1) Akita dogs may have enough K^+ in their RBC to make this artifact pronounced.

  C. Repeated K^+ determination on plasma is normal or if cells are quickly separated from serum

  D. Tight tourniquets or vigorous limb exercise (as in struggling) may create local generation of K^+ and acidosis. This is reflected in the venous blood drawn from that limb.

  2. Decreased renal excretion of K^+

  A. Oliguric primary renal failure (see Chapter 12)*

    1) Acute

    2) Chronic, near terminus

  B. Hypoadrenocorticism (canine Addison's disease; see Chapter 14)*

    1) Lack of mineralocorticoid

    2) Volume depletion

    3) Acidosis

  C. Pharmacologic blockade of K^+ secretion (K^+-sparing diuretics)

    1) Spironolactone

    2) Triamterene

    3) Amiloride

  D. Hypoaldosteronism

    1) Hyporeninism

    2) Addison's disease

  E. Oliguric postrenal failure*

    1) Urinary-tract obstruction

      a) FUS with urethral obstruction (see Chapter 13)

      b) Urolithiasis

    2) Tear in excretory pathway

      a) Ruptured bladder*

      b) Ruptured urethra

      c) Ureteral avulsions

  F. Isolated renal K^+ secretory defect (rare)

  3. Translocation or leak of K^+ from ICF to ECF

  A. Acidosis, metabolic or respiratory*

  B. Rapid cellular release from injured and catabolic tissue resulting in autoinfusion of K^+

    1) Crushing injury

    2) Surgery

    3) Overwhelming infections

    4) Chemotherapy with massive necrosis of neoplastic tissue

    5) Succinylcholine depolarization

    6) Acute digitalis intoxication

    7) After arginine infusion

    8) Tumor lysis syndrome after cancer therapy

    9) Rhabdomyolysis

  C. Lack of insulin

  D. Hyperthermia

  4. Increased intake of K^+

  A. Excessive oral supplementation

  B. Over-rapid IV infusion of K^+-containing fluid*

  C. Inadequate mixing of K^+ supplement into flexible plastic IV fluid bags

  D. High-dose K^+ penicillin IV (1.7 mEq K^+ administered with 1,000,000 U penicillin)

  E. Use of KCL as a salt substitute, with concurrent Na restriction in heart-failure patients

  F. Rapid transfusion of old blood, minimal effect in the dog

  5. Acute increases in ECF osmolality

  A. Glucose

  B. Mannitol

  C. Saline

    1) More commonly results in hypokalemia after hypertonic saline

  D. Sudden increases in ECF osmolality promote transfer of intracellular water to the extracellular water. This sudden movement of water may draw intracellular K^+ by the solvent-drag effect.

  6. Chylothorax

  A. Mechanism unknown

  7. Failure to flush K^+ supplemented fluids from IV lines before withdrawing sample from the same line.

Treatment of Hyperkalemia

  1. Stop all oral and IV K^+ supplementation.

  2. Remove the underlying cause of hyperkalemia if possible (e.g., relieve urethral obstruction immediately, supply volume and adrenocorticoids in hypoadrenocorticism).

  3. Aim acute treatment at restoring the intracellular-to-extracellular K^+ ratio, thus tempo-

*Most important in dogs and cats.

*Most important in dogs and cats.

rarily stabilizing cell-membrane potential. Use bicarbonate, or glucose and insulin as listed below to encourage translocation of ECF K^+ to an intracellular location.

A. Use 1 to 2 mEq/kg $NaHCO_3$ IV as a slow bolus. Translocation of K^+ into cells is favored by an increased pH and by some direct effect of the bicarbonate ion. This measure alone is usually effective in correcting the hyperkalemia transiently and may be seen within minutes as a return toward normal of the ECG.

B. $\frac{1}{4}$ to $\frac{1}{2}$ U/lb regular insulin IV with 2 g glucose/U insulin. Insulin administration promotes the transfer of glucose and K^+ into cells. Provide additional glucose simultaneously to prevent hypoglycemia from the exogenously administered insulin. This technique has been used safely and successfully but offers no advantage over the administration of sodium bicarbonate.

C. Direct antagonism of the toxic effects of hyperkalemia at the myocardial level may be obtained with calcium. Slowly infuse 2 to 10 mL of a 10% calcium-gluconate solution IV to effect under direct ECG visualization. This measure is not widely used in veterinary medicine.

1) As much as .5 to 1.0 mL/kg of 10% calcium gluconate IV over 10 to 15 minutes has been recommended.

D. If the underlying cause of the hyperkalemia cannot be corrected, chronic treatment measures are necessary to sustain life.

1) Dietary restriction to foods containing only carbohydrates and fats is ideal.

2) Ion-exchange resins may be helpful in removing K^+ from the body in exchange for sodium. Give sodium polystyrene sulfonate (Kayexalate) at 20 to 30 g PO tid to qid. Simultaneously, give 20 mL of 70% sorbitol to promote liquid stools that enhance K^+ excretion. Vomiting animals may require this treatment through an inflated Foley catheter as a retention enema.

3) If these procedures fail to lower the serum K^+ adequately, and if renal function does not respond to IV fluid treatments (see Chapter 12, Renal Failure), consider dialysis.

4. Not all cases of hyperkalemia require specific treatment for the hyperkalemia. This depends on the magnitude of hyperkalemia, the animal's clinical status, and the likelihood that normal physiologic mechanisms will restore serum K^+ if underlying abnormalities are corrected entirely or at least improved.

Disorders in Calcium Balance

1. The extracellular fluid concentration of ionized Ca^{++} is maintained within a narrow range.

2. Parathyroid hormone (PTH), vitamin D, and calcitonin work in an integrated manner as the primary regulators of calcium homostasis. Calcium is absorbed from the intestine, stored in bone, and excreted by the kidney.

A. PTH actions promoting Ca^{++} in plasma

1) Mobilization of Ca^{++} from bone

2) Increased renal tubular reabsorption of Ca^{++}

3) Increased urinary excretion of phosphorus

4) Enhancement of intestinal calcium absorption

5) Increased activity of 1-hydroxylase in renal tissue promotes conversion to active vitamin D.

B. Vitamin D actions—Predominant effect is to increase intestinal absorption of calcium and phosphorus.

C. Calcitonin promotes lowering of plasma calcium.

3. Normal serum total calcium values for mature dogs are near 10.0 mg/dL, with some variations caused by diet and analytic method.

A. Young dogs that are growing rapidly may have calcium values in excess of 12.0 mg/dL that are considered normal.

B. Older dogs (> 8 yr) may have calcium values close to 9.0 mg/dL that are considered normal.

C. Standard laboratory measurements determine total calcium in plasma or serum.

D. Total plasma calcium consists approximately of ionized (50%), complex (10%), and protein-bound (40%) fractions.

E. Ionized calcium is the fraction that is considered biologically active, although ionized calcium measurements are not available routinely for evaluation.

    1) Ion-specific methods for potentiometric determination of ionized calcium may be helpful in the evaluation of selected cases with suspected calcium disorders.

    2) Calculated ionized calcium values derived from automated serum biochemical panels are sometimes reported, but the validity of this calculation has yet to be proven.

  4. Ionized calcium is important in maintaining the normal excitability of nervous and muscular tissues. Extreme alterations in calcium concentration (hypercalcemia or hypocalcemia) often result in clinical signs of a neuromuscular disorder.

  5. Disorders of serum or plasma calcium concentration are being recognized with increasing frequency. Abnormal calcium concentrations may be detected before signs are directly attributable to severe calcium disturbance.

  6. The ideal evaluation of patients with suspected calcium disorders includes

    A. Total calcium

    B. Ionized calcium (not calculated)

    C. Phosphorus

    D. N-terminal or intact PTH assay validated for dogs and cats

      1) Becoming more widely available

      2) Affordable at some laboratories

    E. Calcitriol

      1) Limited availability

      2) Expensive

  7. The practical evaluation of patients with calcium disorders includes serum total calcium, phosphorus, and occasional measurement of PTH.

  8. Formulas may be used to estimate the contribution of protein binding of calcium to the total calcium reported from the laboratory.

    A. Corrected total calcium = calcium (mg/dL) − albumin (G/dL) + 3.5

    B. Corrected total calcium = calcium (mg/dL) − .4 (total protein G/dL) + 3.3

    C. Validated for use in dogs only

      1) Recently reported invalid for use in cats

D. Most cases with hypoproteinemia/ hypoalbuminemia and low total calcium will "correct" to normal or near normal values.

  E. Occasional cases with normal calcium and low proteins will "correct" to hypercalcemia range.

  F. The fact that "corrected" total serum calcium values are normal does not guarantee that ionized calcium is normal, however.

Hypocalcemia

Etiology of Hypocalcemia

  1. Hypoalbuminemia
  2. Chronic renal failure
  3. Acute renal failure
  4. Puerperal tetany (eclampsia)
  5. Hypoparathyroidism
  6. Acute pancreatitis
  7. Intestinal malabsorption
  8. Ethylene-glycol intoxication
  9. Hypovitaminosis-D
  10. Hypomagnesemia
  11. Chelation by edetate (EDTA)
  12. Blood transfusion (too much citrate anticoagulant/volume blood)
  13. Massive soft-tissue mineralization
  14. Treatment with drugs/fluids

Signs of Hypocalcemia

  1. Hypocalcemia exists when serum Ca^{++} is less than 9.0 mg/dL in dogs and less than 8.0 mg/dL in cats.

  2. Signs of hypocalcemia are similar regardless of the underlying cause.

    A. Muscular evidence

      1) Tremors

      2) Twitching

      3) Cramps or spasms

    B. Nervous signs

      1) Generalized seizures

      2) Gait change (stiff-legged gait)

      3) Ataxia or paresis

    C. Behavioral changes

      1) Restlessness

      2) Panting

      3) Dementia

      4) Over-excitability

5) Aggressive behavior

6) Howling

D. Tachycardia, possibly with prolongation of the Q–T interval of the ECG

E. Hyperthermia

F. Polydipsia or polyuria (possibly psychogenic)

3. The magnitude of hypocalcemia is not always a reliable indicator of the signs that the patient will demonstrate.

4. Even though hypocalcemia persists, clinical signs may be intermittent (episodic).

Causes and Treatment of Hypocalcemia

1. Hypoalbuminemia is the most common cause of hypocalcemia, because low serum albumin decreases the protein-bound fraction of calcium that is measured. Hypocalcemia tends to be mild (7.5 to 9.0 mg/dL); there are no attendant clinical signs because ionized calcium remains normal.

A. Look for causes of protein-losing nephropathy, protein-losing enteropathy, failure of hepatic protein synthesis, and blood loss.

2. Chronic renal failure is a common cause of hypocalcemia.

A. Decreased kidney transformation of 25-OH vitamin D_2 to $1,25(OH_2)D_3$ (Calcitriol) occurs as a consequence of diminishing functional renal mass.

B. Elevated serum phosphorus occurs eventually as severe reductions in glomerular filtration take place.

1) The elevated plasma phosphorus tends to depress levels of ionized calcium through a reciprocal effect favoring movement of calcium from extracellular fluid to bone fluid.

2) Increased serum phosphorus also can depress the activity of 1-alpha hydroxylase, the renal enzyme necessary to facilitate activation to calcitriol.

C. Even though hypocalcemia of less than 7.0 mg/dL may occur, it is uncommon to develop seizures or signs attributable to serum calcium deficiency. The protective effects of the metabolic acidosis that usually accompanies renal failure minimize the clinical

signs of hypocalcemia. Acidosis increases the fraction of biologically active ionized calcium.

D. If possible, direct treatment at correcting the underlying renal functional abnormalities. Initiate vitamin-D and calcium-salt supplementation after hyperphosphatemia has been controlled. Avoid over-zealous alkali therapy to prevent symptomatic episodes of hypocalcemia (see Chapter 12, Renal Failure).

3. Acute renal failure may result in significant phosphorus retention in plasma. It may thereby depress plasma calcium concentration by the reciprocal effects of mass action between phosphorus and calcium. As with chronic renal failure, these animals are not usually directly symptomatic of hypocalcemia. Supplementation with vitamin D and calcium salts usually is not necessary, because these animals usually either die or recover adequate renal function (see Chapter 12).

4. Puerperal tetany (eclampsia) often occurs 1 to 3 weeks postparturition in small-breed bitches. Queens and large-breed bitches may occasionally be affected.

A. Neuromuscular signs with tetany are typical.

B. Serum calcium often less than 7.0 mg/dL; phosphorus values also are reduced.

C. Imbalance of flow in and out of the bone pool is responsible for the hypocalcemia and hypophosphatemia.

D. Acute treatment

1) Control tetany or seizures as described below

2) Remove puppies from the bitch for at least 24 hours, or permanently, if possible.

E. Chronic treatment

1) Give supplemental vitamin D and calcium during lactation.

2) Corticosteroids are advocated by some as helpful, but their value is questionable.

3) Feed a balanced calcium–phosphorus diet (1 : 1 or less) during gestation to keep the parathyroid glands "primed" for lactation, when they will be greatly needed.

5. Hypoparathyroidism may cause hypocalcemia because of a deficiency in plasma PTH concentration.

A. Iatrogenic surgical removal of the parathyroid glands deliberately or inadvertently during other neck surgery may occur. Compromised blood supply to the parathyroids also may result in hypoparathyroidism.

   1) This is most common after bilateral thyroidectomy in cats with hyperthyroidism.

      a) Hypoparathyroidism can be permanent.

   2) Unilateral thyroidectomy occasionally may result in hypocalcemia.

      a) Usually within one to three days of surgery

      b) Often transient, but may take weeks to months before remaining parathyroid gland is capable of resuming normal function

   B. Lymphoplasmacytic parathyroiditis of unknown cause may result in hypoparathyroidism. An immunologic or autoimmune process is suspected in the etiopathogenesis.

   C. Idiopathic atrophy

   D. The diagnosis may be confirmed by measurement of low concentrations of PTH by radioimmunoassay at the time of low serum calcium. Mild hyperphosphatemia may be detected because of the lack of PTH-induced phosphaturia. Parathyroid histopathology helps to confirm the nature of the underlying disease in the parathyroid glands.

6. Hypocalcemia of varying degree, often attributed to saponification (calcium-soap formation) of the peripancreatic fat, is sometimes associated with acute pancreatitis. The degree of hypocalcemia cannot be accounted for entirely by saponification, however; other unknown mechanisms are contributory.

7. Intestinal malabsorption may be associated with hypocalcemia when severe steatorrhea occurs. Loss of fat-soluble vitamin D and loss of calcium exist with the steatorrhea.

8. Ethylene-glycol intoxication (radiator fluid) sometimes results in symptomatic hypocalcemia due to chelation of calcium from the plasma by metabolites of ethylene glycol.

9. Hypovitaminosis D is a possible but unlikely cause of hypocalcemia.

10. Hypomagnesemia is an as yet unreported cause of hypocalcemia in small animals. Hypomagnesemia may result in deficiency of a cofactor needed in the production of cyclic AMP and release of parathyroid hormone.

11. Submission of plasma samples collected in EDTA-anticoagulated tubes for analysis results in fictitious hypocalcemia.

12. Anticoagulated blood that contains too much citrate for the volume of blood administered can result in binding of patient plasma calcium to the extra citrate if the volume of transfused blood is large.

13. Soft-tissue calcium uptake can occur after massive trauma or rhabdomyolysis.

14. Treatment with drugs/fluid

   A. Dilutional hypocalcemia can occur after the rapid infusion of calcium-free fluids.

   B. The rapid intravenous infusion of phosphate-supplemented fluids may depress serum calcium.

   C. The rectal administration of phosphate-containing enemas may allow systemic phosphate absorption and subsequent hypocalcemia.

      1) Especially in cats

   D. $NaHCO_3$ administration may decrease both ionized and total calcium.

Treatment of Hypocalcemia

1. None required if due to decreased albumin or total protein

2. Acute management of symptomatic hypocalcemia (tetany, seizures, hyperthermia)

   A. Treatment must be individualized in each case.

      1) The clinical signs of hypocalcemia often abate, even though normocalcemia has not yet been achieved.

      2) It is not necessary to achieve a 10.0 mg/dL serum calcium value during therapy. Adequate treatment results in serum calcium determination of 7.0 to 9.0 mg/dL.

   B. Give slow infusion of calcium salt IV

      1) 10 to 15 mg/kg elemental calcium over 10 to 20 minutes (Peterson)

      2) Too-rapid infusion of calcium may result in cardiac arrest.

         a) Stop infusion temporarily if bradycardia develops.

         b) Suggest ECG monitoring.

      3) Calcium gluconate is most commonly used salt (see types of calcium salt below).

   C. Consider alcohol bath or fan-cooling

if body temperature is greater than 105°F from seizures or muscle tremors.

D. Do not expect animal to immediately become normal in spite of fact that serum calcium has been normalized.

1) Lag of 30 to 60 minutes can occur (Russo).

3. Subacute management—maintenance of serum calcium

A. Continue calcium salt in fluids.

1) Give 60 to 90 mg/kg/day elemental calcium (Peterson).

2) As much as 5 to 10 mg/kg/h may be necessary to maintain normocalcemia in some instances (120 to 240 mg/kg/day equivalent).

4. Types of calcium salts for injection

A. Calcium gluconate 10% (93 mg calcium in 10 mL)

1) 0.465 mEq/mL calcium

2) 9.2 mg/mL elemental calcium

3) 1.0 to 1.5 mL/kg for initial control

4) 2.5 mL/kg every six to eight hours for maintenance

5) IV route

B. Calcium chloride 10% (272 mg in 10 mL)

1) 1.36 mEq/mL calcium

2) 27.2 mg/mL elemental calcium

3) .4 to .6 mL/kg for initial control

4) IV route

C. Calcium gluceptate 22% in 5 mL

1) 18.0 mg/mL elemental calcium

2) .5 to .8 mL/kg for initial control

3) IV or IM

D. Calcium glycerophosphate and lactate (Calphosan) 1%

1) .08 mEq/mL

2) 1.9 mg/mL elemental calcium

3) 30 to 45 mL/kg SQ to provide maintenance control

E. Calcium glycerophosphate + lactate calphosan 10%

1) 18.7 mg/mL elemental calcium

2) 3 to 5 mL/kg to provide maintenance control

3) IM only

F. Both calcium glycerophosphate preparations (see 4D and 4E) contain phosphate, which may not be advisable depending on the cause of hypocalcemia.

5. Do not mix calcium salts in fluids that contain lactate, acetate, or bicarbonate.

6. Do not inject calcium salts through IV lines containing anticoagulated blood.

7. Avoid aggressive calcium salt administration if serum phosphorus remains high.

A. Risk of soft tissue mineralization

8. Start vitamin D and calcium salt supplementation orally as soon as possible.

9. Taper off parenteral calcium salts two to three days after oral medication is started.

10. Oral medication—loading doses (Peterson)

A. Dihydrotachysterol (DHT)—drug of choice most often

1) .03 to .06 mg/kg/day for two to three days

2) .02 to .03 mg/kg/day for next two to three days

3) .01 mg/kg/day until changed after evaluation of serum calcium

4) Quicker onset and less duration of action than vitamin D_2; also renal hydroxylation of compound is not necessary.

5) 1 mg DHT = 120,000 U vitamin D_2 (3 mg)

B. Vitamin D_2

1) 4000 to 6000 U/kg/day for one to two weeks

2) 1000 to 2000 U/kg/day maintenance

3) Maximal effect may take weeks to see (significant stores in fat).

C. 1,25 dihydroxy vitamin D_3 (Rocaltrol .25 μg)

1) Not often used because of expense and inconvenient liquid capsule formulation

2) Very rapid onset; short half-life; little storage

D. Oral calcium supplementation at 50 to 100 mg/kg/day elemental calcium during initial treatments to ensure adequate intestinal calcium for absorption

1) Calcium gluconate

2) Calcium lactate

3) Calcium chloride

4) Calcium carbonate

E. Reduce the calcium-salt dosage gradually as the full action of vitamin D takes place. In cases with persistent hyperphosphatemia continue calcium-salt supplementation, because this calcium in the intestinal lumen binds with phosphorus and reduces its entry into the body.

11. The risk of developing hypercalcemia during treatment is significant and may be heralded by the development of polyuria and polydipsia (see following discussion of hypercalcemia).

Hypercalcemia

1. Hypercalcemia exists when serum or plasma calcium measurement exceeds 12.0 mg/dL in mature dogs, or is greater than 11.0 mg/dL in cats. Hypercalcemia occurs in cats much less commonly.

2. Hypercalcemia may result from increased resorption of bone calcium, increased GI absorption of calcium, increased protein binding of calcium, and decreased removal of calcium by the kidney.

3. Signs of hypercalcemia are similar regardless of the underlying cause.

   A. Urinary
      1) Polyuria and polydipsia
      2) Dehydration, prerenal azotemia
      3) Primary renal failure
   B. Gastrointestinal
      1) Anorexia
      2) Vomiting
      3) Constipation
   C. Musculoskeletal
      1) Generalized muscle weakness
      2) Lameness from bone pain if demineralization is present
   D. Neurologic
      1) Depression
      2) Stupor or coma
      3) Seizures or muscle twitching
   E. Cardiovascular
      1) Arrhythmia, including ventricular fibrillation with severe hypercalcemia
      2) Decreased Q–T interval
      3) Increased P–R interval

4. The severity of clinical signs is related both to the amount of elevation of serum calcium and to the speed at which elevation occurred. The severity of clinical signs in hypercalcemic patients is greatly influenced by concomitant electrolyte and acid–base disturbances.

5. Patients with serum calcium values in excess of 16.0 mg/dL generally have the most severe signs.

6. Malignancies account for most cases of hypercalcemia in small animals. Hypercalcemia in a patient without obvious cause calls for a search to rule out cancer as a possibility.

Conditions Associated with Hypercalcemia

Nonpathologic
Nonfasting
Laboratory error
Spurious
   Lipemia
   Detergent contamination of sample/tube
Physiologic growth of young

Transient and Inconsequential
Hemoconcentration
   Hyperproteinemia
Hypoadrenocorticism(?)
Severe environmental hypothermia

Pathologic and Consequential
Malignancy associated
   Humoral hypercalcemia of malignancy
      Lymphosarcoma
      Adenocarcinoma, anal sac apocrine gland
      Others
   Local osteolytic
      Multiple myeloma
      Hematopoietic neoplasia (myeloproliferative)
      Lymphosarcoma
      Metastatic/primary bone neoplasia (focal and multifocal)
Hypoadrenocorticism (Addison's-like disease)
Chronic renal failure
Hypervitaminosis D
   Iatrogenic
   Plants
      Cestrum diurnum
      Solanum malacoxylon
      Triestum flavescens
   Rodenticide
   Granulomatous disease
      Blastomycosis

Primary hyperparathyroidism
    Adenoma/adenocarcinoma
    Hyperplasia (diffuse and nodular)
Acute renal failure
Skeletal lesions (nonmalignant)
    Osteomyelitis (bacterial and mycotic)
    Hypertrophic osteodystrophy (HOD)
    Disuse osteoporosis (immobilization)
Excessive intestinal phosphate binders
Excessive calcium supplementation (calcium
    carbonate)
Human
    Thiazide diuretics
    Hypervitaminosis A
    Milk-alkali syndrome
    Thyrotoxicosis
    Pheochromocytoma
    Postrenal transplantation
    Aluminum exposure

Causes of Hypercalcemia

1. Make sure that hypercalcemia is not an artifact from lipemia.

    A. Lipemia can cause markedly elevated calcium values to be reported.

    B. Evaluate serum calcium on fasting sample.

2. Recognize that young growing dogs may have serum calcium values greater than normal.

3. Hypercalcemia is recognized uncommonly in cats.

4. Make sure that hypercalcemia is a repeatable finding.

    A. Mild transient (nonrepeatable) hypercalcemia is common.

5. Hemoconcentration can result in mild transient hypercalcemia.

    A. Hyperproteinemia from volume contraction and increased calcium binding

    B. Volume contraction signals kidneys to increase tubular reabsorption of calcium.

    C. Most dehydrated animals do not develop hypercalcemia, however.

6. Malignancy-associated hypercalcemia is the most common cause of persistent hypercalcemia.

    A. Always rule out cancer first.

    B. Lymphosarcoma is the most common tumor associated with hypercalcemia in dogs.

From 10% to 40% of LSA dogs may have hypercalcemia. Anterior mediastinal or visceral involvement in hypercalcemic dogs with LSA usually is present with or without peripheral lymphadenopathy.

    C. Perirectal apocrine-gland carcinomas are another group of tumors associated with pseudohyperparathyroidism. The tumor may not be obvious unless a rectal exam discloses a mass lesion associated with the anal sac. This syndrome occurs mainly in older female dogs, although rare cases of affected male dogs have been seen. Metastasis to the internal iliac lymph node occurs most frequently, with some metastasis to lung.

    D. Primary or metastatic tumors of bone occasionally cause hypercalcemia (myeloma, LSA).

7. Hypoadrenocorticism sometimes presents with hypercalcemia in addition to other classic electrolyte abnormalities. This hypercalcemia is transient and disappears rapidly when standard treatment for hypoadrenocorticism is initiated.

8. Primary renal failure may occasionally result in hypercalcemia, although hypocalcemia or normocalcemia occur in most cases.

    A. Chronic renal failure

    B. Acute renal failure, diuretic phase

    C. Mechanisms may include increased ionized calcium, or increased calcium complexes without increased ionized calcium.

    D. Hypercalcemia may cause renal disease. In some cases it is difficult to tell whether hypercalcemia is causing the renal failure or whether renal failure is causing the hypercalcemia.

9. Hypervitaminosis-D results in hypercalcemia. Hyperphosphatemia of variable degree is often also present. Serum alkaline phosphatase may be mildly elevated.

    A. The most important cause has emerged after ingestion of rodenticides containing cholecalciferol.

    B. Dietary oversupplementation by breeders or veterinarians

    C. Over-zealous treatment of hypoparathyroidism

    D. Cestrum diurnum (day-blooming jasmine) is a house plant containing high concentrations of vitamin D_3 that could result in hypervitaminosis-D. This plant appeals to cats that enjoy eating house plants.

10. Primary hyperparathyroidism occasionally occurs in older dogs. A functional lesion in the parathyroid glands leads to excessive production of PTH.

    A. Adenoma most common in the neck

    B. Adenoma uncommon at heart base, embryologic remnant

    C. Carcinoma rarely

    D. Tumors not palpable

    E. Increased serum calcium, decreased serum phosphorus, and increased serum alkaline phosphatase may be seen.

    F. Bone demineralization and soft-tissue mineralization possibly seen on roentgenograms

11. Nonmalignant skeletal lesions occasionally are the cause of hypercalcemia.

    A. Osteolytic lesions may result in hypercalcemia if an extensive degree and high rate of bone destruction occur.

    B. Disuse osteoporosis occurs uncommonly in recumbent animals that are unable to move around owing to severe musculoskeletal or neurologic injury.

12. Rarely, contamination of the serum sample with detergent (as with reused and cleaned syringes or tubes) can cause increased serum calcium to be reported.

Treatment

1. Remove the underlying cause, which will most commonly be neoplasia.

    A. Excision

    B. Chemotherapy

    C. Radiation therapy

    D. Immunotherapy

    E. Hypercalcemia resolves if tumor mass is sufficiently reduced; it returns as regrowth of the tumor occurs.

2. Stop all vitamin D supplementation if this is the cause.

3. Treat infections that may be causing osteolysis.

4. Provide supportive care.

    A. Fluid therapy is the most important initial step.

        1) Correct dehydration to dilute the existing concentration of plasma calcium.

        2) Volume expansion with .9% NaCl promotes a diuresis rich in sodium and calcium.

    B. Furosemide diuresis promotes calciuresis.

        1) 1 mg/kg tid minimal amount

        2) As much as 1 mg/kg/h may be necessary.

        3) Ensure adequate IV fluid replacement to avoid dehydration and worsening of hypercalcemia.

    C. Glucocorticoids may be of value in diminishing GI absorption of calcium, decreasing bone resorption, and increasing renal excretion of calcium.

        1) 2 to 4 mg/kg prednisone divided twice daily

        2) Obtain biopsies before start of this treatment, otherwise lymphosarcoma may be difficult or impossible to definitively diagnose.

    D. Sodium bicarbonate IV may lower serum ionized and total calcium.

        1) The effect is rapid and may be helpful during a hypercalcemic crisis.

        2) 2 to 4 mEq/kg as a slow IV bolus

    E. The use of diphosphonates, calcitonin, mithramycin, EDTA, and peritoneal dialysis for treatment of hypercalcemia that does not respond to the more conventional therapies listed above can be considered.

    F. The combination of fluid therapy and furosemide can result in a fall of serum calcium of about 3 mg/dL.

        1) Do not expect this to return serum calcium to normal if initial hypercalcemia is severe.

    G. Glucocorticosteroids result in rapid decrease in serum calcium if the cause is lymphosarcoma.

        1) Expect minor reduction in serum calcium when due to other causes.

    H. Dietary calcium restriction is helpful in the control of hypercalcemia when caused by hypervitaminosis D.

        1) Lean ground beef and rice

        2) Non–calcium-containing intestinal phosphate binders helpful when accompanied by increased serum phosphorus

5. Treatment of renal failure

A. Some degree of azotemia is usually prerenal.

1) Dehydration

2) Vasoconstrictive preglomerular effect of calcium

B. Intrarenal lesions can be due to hypercalcemia.

1) Acute intrinsic renal failure—occasional

2) Chronic renal failure—more common

C. No specific therapy is available to alter lesions of already existing primary renal disease. Spontaneous repair and hypertrophy of function may occur in the nephron if the patient can be kept alive for a sufficient time (see Chapter 12, Renal Failure).

D. Correct dehydration and maintain hydration to decrease prerenal factors contributing to azotemia.

Disorders of Phosphorus

1. Over 80% of the phosphorus is within bone, with the rest in soft tissues such as muscle.

2. Phosphorus is predominantly located within cells as organic compounds important for cellular energy production and maintenance of cell membranes.

3. Phosphorus in the ECF is mostly inorganic and is measured in mg/dL since blood pH changes the balance, and hence the mEq/L that would otherwise be reported.

4. Normal serum phosphorus = 2.5 to 6.0 mg/dL

5. Lipemia and hemolysis will artificially increase serum phosphorus concentration.

6. Postprandial (effects can alter serum phosphorus concentration.

A. Carbohydrates decrease serum phosphorus.

B. Protein-rich foods increase serum phosphorus.

7. Serum phosphorus concentration is regulated by the dietary phosphorus intake, factors promoting or inhibiting transcellular movement of phosphorus, renal excretion, and regulatory hormone (vitamin D and PTH) interactions.

Hypophosphatemia

1. <2.5 mg/dL

2. Mild hypophosphatemia (2.0 to 2.5 mg/dL) is common and often transient.

3. Clinically important hypophospatemia is usually related to diabetes mellitus.

4. Severe hypophosphatemia (<1.5 mg/dL) is uncommon, but can be life-threatening particularly when less than 1.0 mg/dL.

5. Develops as a consequence of

A. Decreased intestinal absorption

B. Low-phosphate diet

C. Transcellular shifts (maldistribution)

D. Increased loss

1) Urinary

2) GI

3) Lactation

Conditions Associated with Hypophosphatemia

Translocation to intracellular space
    Postprandial (alkaline tide and insulin secretion)
    Glucose
    Aminoacids
    Insulin
    Respiratory alkalosis
    Steroid administration
    Diuretics
    Epinephrine
    Sodium bicarbonate
    Nutritional recovery syndrome (tissue repair)
Diabetes mellitus
Eclampsia
Hyperparathyroidism (primary/pseudo)
Starvation
Intestinal binding agents
Malabsorption
Hypovitaminosis D
Renal tubular loss
Hyperalimentation
Severe environmental hypothermia
Dialysis
Laboratory error

Consequences of Severe Hypophosphatemia

1. Decreased cellular energy production
2. Deranged carbohydrate, protein, and lipid metabolism
3. Decreased O_2 delivery to tissues (decreased 2,3-DPG)
4. Hemolysis
5. Decreased leukocyte chemotaxis, phagocytosis, and bacterial killing
    A. Decreased survival
6. Muscle pain
    A. Rhabdomyolysis
7. Anorexia/vomiting
    A. Ileus
8. Encephalopathy
9. Decreased muscle membrane potentials
10. Reduced cardiac contractility
11. Death

Treatment of Hypophosphatemia

1. Treat only if severe and persistent.
2. Oversupplementation can cause
    A. Hyperphosphatemia
    B. Hypocalcemia
    C. Tetany/seizures
    D. Soft-tissue mineralization
    E. Hyperkalemia if from K^+ phosphate
    F. Hypernatremia if from Na phosphate
3. Supplement only until phosphorus is >2.0 mg/dL.
4. Intravenous dosage
    A. .01 to .03 mmol phosphate/kg/h for three to six hours (Willard)
    B. 2.5 mg/kg phosphate over six hours also suggested as starting point
    C. Most commonly used preparations provide 3.0 mmol phosphate/ml
        1) Sodium phosphate 3.0 mmol/mL (93.0 mg/mL phosphorus)
            a) 4.0 mEq/mL Na^+
        2) Potassium phosphate 3.0 mmol/mL (99.0 mg/mL phosphorus)
            a) 4.36 mEq/mL K^+
    D. Add phosphorous supplementation to replacement and maintenance fluids.
    E. Add phosphorous supplementation to calcium-free fluids.

5. Oral dosage
    A. Phospho-soda (Fleet Co.)
        1) 4.15 mmol/mL phosphate
        2) 0.5 to 2 mmol/kg/day
    B. cow milk (whole)
        1) .029 mmol/mL phosphate
        2) 0.5 to 2 mmol/kg/day
6. Measure serum phosphate frequently and adjust or discontinue supplementation.

Hyperphosphatemia

1. >6.0 mg/dL
2. Serum phosphorus can be physiologically normal at 8.0 to 9.0 mg/dL in large-breed and small-breed puppies.
    A. Kittens also may have serum phosphorus values in excess of adult cats, but not as high as seen in dogs.
3. Hyperphosphatemia develops most commonly as a consequence of reduced renal excretion.
    A. Increased intake is the cause occasionally.
    B. Translocation of intracellular phosphate into ECF is the cause uncommonly.

Conditions Associated with Hyperphosphatemia

Lipemia
Young growing animal
Intrinsic renal failure (acute/chronic)
Obstructive nephropathy (postrenal)
Uroperitoneum
Hyperthyroid cats
Rapid cell destruction
    Hemolysis
    Rhabdomyolysis
    Tumor lysis syndrome (after treatment)
    Major tissue trauma/necrosis
Metabolic acidosis (translocation)
Radiator fluid ingestion (preservative)
Vitamin D intoxication
Hypoparathyroidism
Phosphate enema
Phosphate-supplemented IV fluids
Acromegaly
Detergent contamination of glassware
Laboratory error

Consequences of Hyperphosphatemia

1. Hypocalcemia
2. Tetany seizures
3. Stimulation of secondary hyperparathyroidism
    A. Mass-law interactions that lower ionized calcium
    B. Decreased l-alpha hydroxylase conversion to calcitriol
4. Soft-tissue mineralization
5. Enhanced progression of chronic renal failure?
6. Enhanced maintenance phase of acute intrinsic renal failure?

Treatment of Hyperphosphatemia

1. Discontinue supplementation of fluids with phosphates.
2. Discontinue vitamin D compounds if hypercalcemia also is present.
3. Maximize renal function with IV fluids.
4. Treat metabolic acidosis if severe.
5. Consider use of dextrose-containing fluid to promote transcellular lowering of serum phosphorus.
6. Correct underlying obstructions or tears in the urinary tract as needed.
7. Treat specific causes of acute or chronic intrinsic renal failure if possible (see Chapter 12, Renal Failure).
8. Provide a low phosphorus diet, usually associated with low-protein feedings.
9. Provide intestinal phosphate binders in conjunction with feeding.
10. No treatment is necessary if increased serum phosphorus is due to growth, or is an artifact from lipemia.
11. Provide vitamin D compounds to hypoparathyroid hypocalcemic patients, because the increased calcium may lower serum phosphorus by enhancing phosphaturia.

Suggested Readings

Bell FW, Osborne CA: Treatment of hypokalemia. In Kirk RW (ed): Current Veterinary Therapy IX: Small Animal Practice. Philadelphia, WB Saunders, p 101, 1986

Chew DJ: Parenteral fluid therapy. In Sherding RG (ed): The Cat. New York, Churchill Livingstone, pp 35–80, 1989

Chew DJ, Carothers M: Hypercalcemia. Vet Clin North Am [Small Anim Pract] 19: 265–287, 1989

Chew DJ, Meuten DJ: Disorders of calcium and phosphorus metabolism. Vet Clin North Am [Small Anim Pract] 12: 411–438, 1982

Cornelius LM: Abnormalities of the standard biochemical profile. In Lorenz MD, Cornelius CM (eds): Small Animal Medical Diagnosis. Philadelphia, JB Lippincott, pp 539–591, 1987

DiBartola SP: Hyponatremia. Vet Clin North Am [Small Anim Pract] 19: 215–230, 1989

Fettman MJ: Feline kaliopenic polymyopathy/nephropathy/syndrome. Vet Clin North Am [Small Anim Pract] 19: 415–432, 1989

Forrester SD, Moreland KJ: Hypophosphatemia: Causes and clinical consequences. J Vet Inter Med 3: 149–159, 1989

Hardy RM: Hypernatremia. Vet Clin North Am [Small Anim Pract] 19: 231–240, 1989

Hardy RM, Adams LG: Hypophosphatemia. In Kirk RW (ed): Current Veterinary Therapy X: Small Animal Practice. Philadelphia, WB Saunders, pp 43–47, 1989

Peterson ME: Hypoparathyroidism. In Kirk RW (ed): Current Veterinary Therapy IX: Small Animal Practice. Philadelphia, WB Saunders, pp 1039–1045, 1986

Russo EA, Lees GE: Treatment of hypocalcemia. In Kirk RW (ed): Current Veterinary Therapy IX: Small Animal Practice. Philadelphia, WB Saunders, pp 91–94, 1986

Schaer M: Disorders of potassium metabolism. Vet Clin North Am [Small Anim Pract] 12: 399–409, 1982

Scott RC: Disorders of sodium metabolism. Vet Clin North Am [Small Anim Pract] 12: 375–397, 1982

Willard MD: Disorders of potassium homeostasis. Vet Clin North Am [Small Anim Pract] 19: 241–263, 1989

CHAPTER TWENTY-SIX

Disorders in Acid–Base Balance

Dennis J. Chew and Catherine W. Kohn

Acid–Base Balance

1. In healthy animals, the quantities of acid or base taken into the body or generated by metabolic processes within the body equal the quantities lost from the body (i.e., at steady-state equilibrium there is no net loss or gain of acid or base in the body).

2. The body protects itself against abnormal H^+ concentration by a number of buffering mechanisms in the blood, interstitial fluid, and intracellular fluid. Three fourths of chemical buffering capacity is attributable to intracellular proteins. Chemical buffers consist of a weak acid and its salt (base) that resist changes in pH when either acid or base is added to the system. The carbonic acid–bicarbonate $\frac{(HCO_3^-)}{H_2CO_3}$, phosphate $\frac{(HPO_4^=)}{H_2PO_4}$, and protein $\frac{(protein^-)}{H \, protein}$ buffers are acid–base pairs operating in physiologic fluids. Knowledge of hydrogen ion status of any buffer is all that is required to determine the acid–base balance, as only one hydrogen ion concentration can exist in a physiologic solution. We customarily choose the bicarbonate–carbonic acid pair when studying the acid–base status, both because the components are readily measured and because it is the only buffer whose components may be varied independently by physiologic-control mechanisms. Chemical buffering occurs quickly within extracellular fluid following the law of mass action.

A. Hydration equation for CO_2

$$PaCO_2 \rightarrow CO_2 + H_2O \underset{\substack{\text{carbonic} \\ \text{anhydrase}}}{\rightleftarrows} H_2CO_3 \rightleftarrows H^+ + HCO_3^-$$

B. Any addition to the left side (e.g., $\uparrow$ PCO_2) or subtraction from the right side (e.g., $\downarrow$ HCO_3 from diarrhea) results in a shift of the equation to the right. Any addition to the right side ($\uparrow$ H^+ from acidosis or $\uparrow$ HCO_3 in alkalosis) or a decrease on the left (e.g., $\downarrow$ PCO_2) drives the equation to the left.

3. Sources for contributions to both ends of the hydration equation (losses or gains) (see equation at bottom of page)

$$PaCO_2 \rightarrow CO_2 + H_2O \underset{\substack{\text{carbonic} \\ \text{anhydrase}}}{\overset{\text{dissolved}}{\rightleftarrows}} H_2CO_3 \rightleftarrows H^+ + HCO_3^-$$

ventilation	dietary metabolism	dietary metabolism
hypo ($\uparrow$ PCO_2)	catabolism	$\uparrow$ intestinal loss
hyper ($\downarrow$ PCO_2)	anaerobic metabolism	$\uparrow$ or $\downarrow$ renal
metabolic by-product	$\downarrow$ renal excretion	excretion
	$\uparrow$ gastric loss	

4. Analysis of the Henderson–Hasselbalch* equation reveals that $[H^+]$ or pH is a function of the HCO_3^- concentration and of the PCO_2. Changes in plasma acidity can be adjusted only by altering the HCO_3^- (mEq/L) or the PCO_2 (mmHg). The ratio of HCO_3^- to H_2CO_3 is normally 20 to 1. Ratios less than 20 to 1 are indicative of acidemia and ratios greater than 20 to 1 are indicative of alkalemia. Hydrogen-ion concentration is increased ($\downarrow$ pH) by either an elevated PCO_2 or decreased HCO_3^- values. Hydrogen ion concentration is decreased ($\uparrow$ pH) by a decreased PCO_2 or increased HCO_3^- value.

Analysis of Blood for Acid–Base Abnormality

1. Blood-gas determinations are useful both in defining the nature of any acid–base abnormality that exists and in following the response to treatment.

2. Arterial blood is sometimes preferred over venous blood for analysis of acid–base disturbances because local factors are less likely to contribute to the laboratory values. Arterial blood is required for meaningful interpretation of PO_2.

3. Venous blood gases may be more valuable than arterial samples in assessment of an animal after cardiac arrest or during CPR.

4. Arterial blood is most often obtained from the femoral artery in dogs and cats. You may use the lingual artery in anesthetized animals, particularly when the femoral artery is not accessible owing to patient positioning or draping.

5. Perform arterial puncture with a 25-gauge needle. Approximately 1 mL of blood in a heparinized syringe is an adequate volume to analyze. Other anticoagulants are not satisfactory.

6. Quickly remove all dead space and air bubbles within the syringe and stop the needle tip with a cork. Brief exposure of the

blood to room air or air pockets within the syringe may allow significant changes in the acid–base values.

7. Determine measurements on this blood immediately (within five to ten minutes). If longer delays are unavoidable, place the blood sample into a container of crushed ice to thwart the effects of in vitro cellular metabolism and consequent erroneous laboratory values. Cooled samples remain valuable for analysis for one to two hours.

8. Enhance the value of either arterial or venous blood-gas acid–base determinations by making serial determinations.

9. Normal values for venous samples are slightly different from arterial values. In venous samples the PO_2 results are not valid for use.

Normal Blood-Gas Values

1. Measure O_2, CO_2, pH, HCO_3, and base deficit parameters or calculate them in reported blood-gas values.

2. O_2
    A. 30 to 50 mmHg venous
    B. 90 to 110 mmHg arterial

3. CO_2
    A. 40 to 48 mmHg venous (average 45)
    B. 35 to 45 mmHg arterial (average 40)

4. pH
    A. 7.35 to 7.45 (average 7.40)
    B. Venous samples tend to lie within lower limits of the above range.

5. HCO_3—Values usually approximate 20 to 25 mEq/L, with slightly higher limit values in venous versus arterial samples owing to the contribution of higher PCO_2 in venous blood.

6. Base deficit
    A. Base deficit (excess) is the number of mEq of acid or base required to titrate 1 L of blood to a pH of 7.4 under standard condition of 40 mmHg PCO_2 and temperature of 37°C. This may be determined by titration in the laboratory but is usually calculated from nomograms using the variables pH, PCO_2, and hematocrit.
    B. Normal value for base deficit is usually 1 to 8 mEq/L.
    C. Base excess or base deficit is a derived-finding index consisting of bicarbonate concentration that is corrected for PCO_2 and

$$^*pH = 6.1 + \log \frac{[HCO_3^-] \quad \text{metabolic component}}{.0301 \times PaCO_2 \quad \text{respiratory component}}$$

$$[H^+] = 24 \times \frac{PaCO_2 \quad \text{respiratory component}}{[HCO_3^-] \quad \text{metabolic component}}$$

the buffering effects of hemoglobin, phosphate, and blood protein.

D. Base deficit is not the same as the mere difference between actual and normal HCO_3 values.

E. The value in assessing base deficits or excess is that it represents the magnitude of acid–base abnormality contributed by metabolic components (nonrespiratory contribution).

7. Blood-gas machines directly measure the pH, PCO_2, and PO_2, with nomographic calculation from standard curves of HCO_3^- and base deficit. Blood-gas machines are expensive and unlikely to be found in most veterinary hospitals.

8. A less expensive alternative to a blood-gas machine is the Harleco CO_2 apparatus, which measures total plasma CO_2 after acidification of the sample. Acidification converts HCO_3^- to CO_2, which then accumulates and depresses a plunger corresponding essentially to the HCO_3 content in that sample. This technique is simple, rapid, accurate, and inexpensive. Abnormal HCO_3^- values so measured may reflect primary metabolic disturbances or primary respiratory disturbances with secondary compensatory changes in $[HCO_3^-]$ mediated by renal excretion. Integration of the HCO_3^- value with the clinical history may allow differentiation between a primary metabolic and a primary respiratory problem. (e.g., a low HCO_3^- in a dog with severe diarrhea probably represents metabolic acidosis; a low HCO_3 in a dog with a chronic respiratory condition may well represent respiratory alkalosis with a compensatory metabolic acidosis.)

9. The HCO_3^- value also may be accurately estimated from the total CO_2 (TCO_2) value reported on many automated biochemical profiles. The TCO_2 represents HCO_3^- within 1 to 2 mEq/L and may be used as discussed in the previous paragraph.

Interpretation of Acid–Base Abnormalities

1. Identify the direction in which the pH is changing. Any pH values greater than 7.45 are indicative of alkalemia, and values less than 7.35 are indicative of acidemia. Extremes in pH (values less than 6.8 or greater than 7.6) are not compatible with life.

2. Evaluate the HCO_3 and PCO_2 values to determine both what is causing the alkalemia or acidemia, and to what degree compensatory changes in either value may be taking place (Figure 26-1).

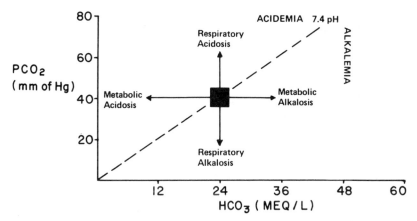

Figure 26-1. *"Pure" deviations from normal in primary acid–base disorders. Compensated states will have points lying within one of the quadrants. Normal pH of 7.4 is dependent on maintaining a fixed ratio of HCO_3^- to $H_2CO_3^-$ (.03 × PaCO₂). Rectangular area represents area of normal pH, HCO₃, and PCO₂.*

A. In acidemia, first evaluate the HCO_3. If the acidemia is of metabolic origin, the HCO_3 is lowered. If respiratory compensation to minimize the pH change has occurred, the PCO_2 also is lowered. If the acidemia is of respiratory origin, the PCO_2 is raised; if metabolic compensation for the pH change is taking place, there is also an elevation of HCO_3 (see Figure 26-1).

B. Metabolic acidosis (acidemia) is the most common acid–base abnormality found in small animals. Consequently, most of our discussion centers on this disorder.

C. In alkalemia of metabolic origin the HCO_3^- is increased; expect an increased PCO_2 if appropriate respiratory compensation has occurred. If the alkalemia is of respiratory origin, the PCO_2 is low; if metabolic compensation has occurred, the HCO_3 is low (Table 26-1).

D. Even though compensatory changes occur to minimize pH deviations, these changes are rarely adequate to return the pH completely to normal. The pH still deviates toward the side of the primary acid–base disturbance (acidemia or alkalemia).

3. Evaluate the base deficit or excess for more adequate determination of the need for supplemental buffer in treatment.

Metabolic Acidosis (Acidemia)

1. Metabolic acidosis exists when acidemia (increased $[H^+]$) occurs as a result of reduced plasma HCO_3^-.

2. Reduction in HCO_3^- may occur by

A. Excessive loss of HCO_3^- from the body (e.g., diarrhea)

B. Consumption of HCO_3^- in buffering by addition of a strong acid (e.g., ketoacidosis)

C. Consumption of HCO_3^- in buffering when decreased acid excretion occurs (e.g., renal failure)

3. Respiratory compensation to minimize pH changes occurs within minutes or hours. Reduced bicarbonate and increased hydrogen ion concentration have a direct effect on the

Table 26-1. **Acid–base imbalances**

Primary Acid–Base Abnormality	**pH**	**HCO₃⁻**	**PCO₂**
Acidemia (acidosis)			
Metabolic	↓	↓↓*	↓
Respiratory	↓	↑	↑↑
Alkalemia (alkalosis)			
Metabolic	↑	↑↑	↑
Respiratory	↑	↓	↓↓

*Double arrows indicate the initiating event in acid–base disturbance. Dashed arrows indicate compensatory changes following the primary abnormality. These compensatory changes allow a more near-normal ratio of HCO_3^- to H_2CO_3 ($.03 \times PaCO_2$) and, consequently, a less severe change in pH.

medullary centers of respiration; they result in increased alveolar ventilation and decreased $PaCO_2$.

4. In steady-state compensation the anticipated level of PCO_2 in metabolic acidosis is roughly proportional to the level of decrement in HCO_3^-.

A. $\Delta PaCO_2 = 1.2 \times (\Delta HCO_3)$
  1) Example

$$HCO_3^- \text{ normal} = 24 \text{ mEq/L}$$
$$HCO_3^- \text{ present} = 14 \text{ mEq/L}$$
$$\Delta HCO_3^- = 10$$

  2) What is the expected $PaCO_2$ after adequate respiratory compensation has occurred?

$$\Delta PaCO_2 = 1.2 \times (10)$$
$$\Delta PaCO_2 = 12$$

If normal $PaCO_2 = 40$ mmHg, the $PaCO_2$ will fall to 28 mmHg if full respiratory compensation occurs.

B. $PCO_2 = 1.54 \times (HCO_3^-) + 8.4 \pm 1$
  1) Example

$$HCO_3^- \text{ normal} = 24 \text{ mEq/L}$$
$$HCO_3^- \text{ present} = 14 \text{ mEq/L}$$

  2) What should the PCO_2 value be if respiratory compensation has occurred adequately?

$$PCO_2 = 1.54 (14) + 8.4 \pm 1$$
$$= 21.6 + 8.4 \pm 1$$
$$PCO_2 = 29 \text{ to } 31 \text{ mmHg}$$

C. The above two formulas provide a rough means to determine if the PCO_2 value is appropriate for the degree of metabolic acidosis present.

    1) Example

$$HCO_3^- \text{ normal } = 24 \text{ mEq/L}$$
$$HCO_3^- \text{ present } = 14 \text{ mEq/L}$$
$$\text{actual } PCO_2 = 38 \text{ mmHg}$$

    2) Given that this case is acidemic, is the level of PCO_2 appropriate compensation for the level of acidemia? Based on either previous formula, the PCO_2 should be approximately 28 to 31 mmHg if adequate respiratory compensation is occurring. In this instance, adequate compensation has not occurred and you must suspect an element of simultaneous respiratory acidosis. Another interpretation is that the acidemia developed very rapidly and that time for full respiratory compensation has not yet been given.

5. Patients with metabolic acidosis may be grouped further into those with a normal anion gap or those with an increased anion gap. Anion gap is a derived value reported on many automated biochemical profiles.

    A. The number of cations in the extracellular fluid (ECF) must equal the number of anions in the ECF according to the law of electroneutrality.

    B. [cations] = [anions]

$$Na + K + UC = Cl + HCO_3 + UA*$$

    C. Na + K − (Cl + HCO₃)

                     commonly measured

      = UA − UC = anion gap*

                   uncommonly measured

    D. Anion gap is a poor term to describe this equation, because electroneutrality must still exist. The gap arises because there are more unmeasured anions than measured cations reported from the laboratory. If all cations and anions could be measured, the anionic gap would be zero. Analysis of the above equation reveals that the anion gap is determined by the difference in unmeasured ions.

E. Use of the anionic gap concept is useful in providing clues to metabolic acid–base and electrolyte abnormalities.

    F. The normal anion gap for dogs is 15 to 25. Values above and below this range may provide useful diagnostic and, at times, prognostic information.

    G. Possible interpretation of abnormal anion gaps

        1) ↑ anion gap due to ↑ undetermined anions

            a) Organic acid accumulation in metabolic acidosis†

                i. Ketoacidosis†

                ii. Lactic acidosis

                iii. Renal failure (advanced)†

                iv. Hyperosmolar hyperglycemic nonketotic coma

                v. Poisonings

                    A. Ethylene glycol†

                    B. Methanol

                    C. Salicylate

                    D. Paraldehyde

                    E. Phenol

            b) Organic anion accumulation—administration of potential base therapy when metabolic conversion is limited

                i. Lactated Ringer's, lactate

                ii. Sodium acetate, acetate

                iii. Carbenicillin or penicillin, high dose not associated with acidosis, just increased gap

            c) Inorganic anion accumulation—renal failure—PO₄, SO₄

            d) Hemoconcentration

            e) Alkalosis, metabolic and respiratory

        2) ↑ anion gap due to ↓ undetermined cations

            a) ↓ calcium

            b) ↓ magnesium

        3) ↑ anion gap due to laboratory error (↑Na, ↑K, ↓Cl, ↓HCO₃)

        4) ↓ anion gap due to ↓ undetermined anions

            a) Hypoalbuminemia‡

---

*UC = undetermined cations = Ca, Mg
UA = undetermined anions = PO₄, SO₄, proteinate, organic acids

†Most important veterinary considerations.
‡Most important veterinary considerations.

b) Dilution with water or bicarbonate-poor solutions

5) ↓ anion gap due to ↑ undetermined cations

    a) ↑ calcium

    b) ↑ Mg

    c) Paraproteinemias (myeloma)

    d) Polymyxin-B use

    e) Lithium use

6) ↓ anion gap due to laboratory error (↓Na, ↓K, ↑Cl, ↑HCO_3)

6. Metabolic acidosis associated with a normal anion gap is seen when HCO_3^- is actually lost from the body, or when acid is added to the body with chloride as its anion.

    A. Loss of HCO_3^-

    1) Diarrhea*

    2) Dilutional acidosis (rapid ECF volume expansion)*

    3) Renal loss

        a) Renal tubular acidosis

        b) Obstructive nephropathy (assuming only moderate ↓ glomerular filtration rate [GFR])

        c) Carbonic anhydrase-inhibitor diuretics

    B. Addition of HCl

    1) NH_4Cl → HCL

    2) Lysine → HCl after metabolism

    3) Arginine → HCl after metabolism

7. Metabolic acidosis associated with an increased anion gap results from over-production of organic acids or from retention of anions.

    A. Overproduction of organic acids

    1) Ketoacidosis*

    2) Prolonged starvation

    3) Lactic acidosis

    4) Poisonings

        a) Methanol

        b) Ethylene glycol*

        c) Paraldehyde

        d) Salicylate

        e) Phenol

    B. Retention of anions—renal failure—PO_4, SO_4

8. Lactic acidosis

    A. Results from disordered lactate–pyruvate metabolism

*Most important veterinary considerations.

B. Not commonly measured in small animals

C. Prognostic value in small animals with metabolic acidosis is undetermined.

D. Anaerobic glycolysis due to insufficient oxygenation of tissues (hypoxia) results in overproduction of lactic acid in most instances.

E. Overproduction of lactic acid may occur transiently during severe exercise and prolonged convulsions (status epilepticus). Increased lactic-acid production also occurs during shock, cardiac arrest, severe hypoxemia, and severe anemia.

F. Spontaneous lactic acidosis may occur in disorders not characterized by tissue hypoxia, such as diabetes mellitus, pancreatitis, leukemia, and severe bacterial infections. The appearance of lactic acidosis in seriously ill patients is often regarded as a terminal occurrence.

G. The onset of lactic acidosis is usually sudden, with a precipitous decline in *p*H that may require an enormous quantity of alkali (HCO_3^-) to restore the *p*H adequately.

H. Definitive diagnosis of lactic acidosis requires measurement of serum lactate concentration.

Clinical Signs Related to Metabolic Acidosis

1. Altered activity of intracellular enzymes may ultimately account for many of the deleterious effects of acidemia.

2. You may see hyperventilation as the respiratory system attempts to increase ventilation, decrease the PCO_2, and minimize changes in *p*H.

3. Cardiovascular effects

    A. Cardiac contractility may be depressed and peripheral vessels may be dilated in response to the acidosis, resulting in hypotension.

    B. Ventricular fibrillation may occur more readily in metabolic acidosis.

4. Gastrointestinal manifestations include anorexia and vomiting.

5. Hyperkalemia and its attendant problems (see Chapter 25) may result from severe metabolic acidosis as translocation of intracellular to extracellular K^+ occurs in a buffering exchange for H^+.

Treatment of Metabolic Acidosis

1. Remove the underlying cause if possible. This alone often is adequate to allow renal excretion of H^+ and a return of pH toward normal without administration of exogenous alkali.

2. Treat the patient with parenteral alkali if the pH is 7.2 or less, even if the underlying cause can be corrected relatively rapidly.

3. With metabolic acidosis of moderate severity (pH 7.2 to 7.39), treatment with alkali may or may not be necessary depending on the severity of any clinical signs. It is not wise to treat a pH or HCO_3^- value alone.

4. Complications of alkalai ($NaHCO_3$) therapy result from too much alkali or too rapid a rate of administration.

    A. Volume overload, edema (pulmonary)*

    B. Hyperosmolality/hypernatremia

    C. Tetany from shifts of ionized calcium

    D. Paradoxic CSF acidosis*

    E. Over-correction metabolic alkalosis

    F. Hypokalemia*

5. The amount of alkali required to maintain near-normal HCO_3^- and pH values depends on the existing deficit of base and the magnitude of continuing H^+ addition to the body. Exact needs of alkali administration are difficult to formulate.

6. Estimates from formulas of HCO_3^- requirements serve only as rough guidelines to patient management. Administered alkali achieves full equilibration with ECF within 30 minutes. Consequently serial evaluations of blood-gas analysis help to determine the adequacy of HCO_3^- supplementation.

7. Complete equilibration of administered HCO_3^- with the intracellular space takes several (as long as 18) hours.

8. No. of mEq HCO_3^- needed = 0.3 kg body weight × HCO_3^- deficit† (ECF volume of distribution for HCO_3^- of 30%)

or

No. of mEq HCO_3^- needed

$$= \frac{\text{lbs body weight}}{7} \times HCO_3^- \text{ deficit}$$

    A. *Note:* give one fourth to one half of this calculated value as a slow IV-bolus injection; give the rest more slowly in the IV fluids.

    B. This formula provides treatment as if the deficit of base exists only within the ECF. This makes it most useful when multiple determinations of blood gases are evaluated serially during alkali supplementation.

        1) Example: 10 kg

Actual HCO_3^- = 15 mEq/L
Desired HCO_3^- = 25 mEq/L
HCO_3^- deficit = 10 mEq/L

        2) How many mEq of HCO_3^- should be infused to correct alkali deficit?

No. of mEq HCO_3^- needed
    = 0.3 × 10 kg × 10 mEq/L = 30 mEq

9. No. of mEq HCO_3^- needed
    = 0.6 × kg body weight × HCO_3^- deficit

This formula provides treatment regarding both intracellular and extracellular deficits of alkali. Give up to one fourth of this calculated dose as a slow bolus and place the remaining alkali in the IV fluids for slower administration.

10. Assess adequacy of alkali treatment by repeated blood-gas determinations during and following therapy. Make appropriate adjustments in dose and rate of HCO_3^- administration as correction occurs.

11. Treatment of metabolic acidosis without use of blood gases or HCO_3^- values

    A. In crisis situations in which metabolic acidosis is likely to be severe, administer 1 to 2 mEq/kg IV of HCO_3^- acutely as a bolus and reevaluate.

    B. Finco's guidelines of estimated HCO_3^- needs are intended for gradual replacement over many hours.

---

*Of most importance in small animals.

†HCO_3^- deficit = desired HCO_3^- − actual HCO_3^- (Base deficit, if available, may be substituted for HCO_3^- deficit.)

Estimated Clinical Severity of Metabolic Acidosis	*mEq HCO$_3$⁻/kg Body Weight*
Mild	3
Moderate	6
Severe	9

Respiratory Acidosis (Acidemia)

1. Primary respiratory acidosis exists when acidemia is due to elevation of PCO_2. Increased PCO_2 results from alveolar ventilation disorders encountered in the respiratory center, respiratory muscles, thoracic cage, pleural space, lung parenchyma, and airways.
2. Causes
   A. Generalized severe pulmonary disease (e.g., pulmonary edema, pneumonia)†
   B. Pleural effusion, pneumothorax, flail chest
   C. Airway obstruction
   D. Depression of ventilation by drugs†
      1) General anesthesia
      2) Tranquilizers
      3) Narcotics
      4) Barbiturates
   E. CNS lesions affecting medullary center of respiration
   F. Diseases of muscles of respiration (e.g., tick paralysis, coonhound paralysis)
   G. Cardiac arrest*
   H. Improperly adjusted mechanical ventilator

Clinical Signs

1. If increased PCO_2 occurs acutely, clinical signs tend to be more severe.
   A. Anxiety
   B. Decreased mentation
   C. Stupor or coma
2. In chronic, increased PCO_2, absence of obvious clinical signs may occur. Lethargy may be the only apparent sign.

† Of most importance in small animals

3. Papilledema may be seen in cases with severely elevated PCO_2, possibly because of increased intracranial pressure from vasodilatation.
4. Hypoxia to some degree accompanies severe hypercapnia and contributes to clinical signs.

Physiologic Compensation

1. As the hydration equation is driven to the right by the increased PCO_2, increased HCO_3⁻ is immediately generated by the law of mass action. The H⁺ generated at the same time is buffered by nonbicarbonate buffers.
   A. *Note:* for each increase in PCO_2 of 10 mmHg above 40 mmHg, the "extra" HCO_3⁻ value generated equals 1 mEq/L.
   B. Example of acute hypercapnia

$$PCO_2 = 80 \text{ mmHg}$$

$$\text{Normal } HCO_3 = 24 \text{ mEq/L}$$

   C. What will the HCO_3⁻ be as the increase in PCO_2 generates additional HCO_3⁻?

$$\Delta PCO_2 = 40 \text{ mmHg or}$$
$$4 \text{ U of 10-mmHg change}$$

$$4 \text{ U of change} \times 1 \frac{mEq/L}{U}$$

$$= 4 \frac{mEq}{L} \text{ additional}$$

$$HCO_3\text{⁻ generated}$$

   D. The expected HCO_3⁻ value is 24 mEq/L (normal) + 4 mEq/L = 28 mEq/L.
2. Adaptive renal responses begin hours after onset of the hypercapnia and may take days to reach maximal operation.
   A. Increased H⁺ secretion by renal tubules is stimulated by increased PCO_2.
   B. Increased Na⁺/H⁺ exchange promotes increased acid excretion and generation of "new" bicarbonate that is returned to the body. This process is accomplished largely by the increased excretion of ammonia.
3. Increased HCO_3⁻ levels tend to blunt the change in *p*H (acidemia) initiated by the higher PCO_2, as it is the ratio of HCO_3⁻ to .03 × PCO_2 that ultimately determines *p*H.

*Most importance in small animals.

Treatment

1. Treat or remove the underlying cause
(e.g., drain pleural fluid, administer antimicrobials for pneumonia).
2. Provide support ventilation (tracheal
intubation, mechanical ventilation).
3. Supply O_2. Be careful if the hypercapnia
is chronic, because the lower O_2 levels may
be responsible for driving respirations; sudden increases in PO_2 then would remove the
only stimulus to ventilation.
4. Sudden correction of the increased PCO_2
may lead to posthypercapnic alkalosis, because the renal adaptive mechanisms responsible for HCO_3^- generation do not instantaneously cease.

Metabolic Alkalosis

1. Primary metabolic alkalosis exists when
alkalemia ($\uparrow$ pH) is due to increased HCO_3^-.
2. To maintain electrical neutrality when
plasma bicarbonate concentration is elevated,
plasma concentration of the remaining anions
must decrease. Because chloride constitutes
the major remaining anion, hypochloremia
must exist also.

Production of Alkalosis

1. Alkali administration
  A. Bicarbonate
  B. Citrate, lactate, acetate; bicarbonate
precursors
  C. Rapid rate of administration or poor
renal function required
2. H^+ ion loss
  A. Gastric loss, vomiting
  B. Renal loss promoted by diuretics
  C. Renal loss associated with hyperaldosteronism
  D. H^+ translocation into cells in cellular
K^+ deficiency
3. Major loss of chloride and other ions in
fluid not containing HCO_3^- results in "contraction" alkalosis as HCO_3^- remains behind
in a smaller volume of fluid and its concentration consequently increases.

  A. Gastric loss of Cl^- is high.
  B. Renal loss of Cl^- without HCO_3^- loss
is high with use of potent diuretics.

Maintaining Metabolic Alkalosis

1. Alkali administration
  A. Alkali administration is associated
with volume expansion as Na is simultaneously supplied. Hypochloremia results from
the volume expansion.
  B. Volume expansion results in rapid
renal excretion of Na^+, HCO_3^-, and water
from normal kidneys.
  C. Alkalosis can be maintained only if
kidney function is impaired or if the rate of
continuing alkali administration is very high.
2. Losses of H^+ or of Cl^-
  A. Situations resulting in loss of H^+ or
Cl^- are associated with volume contraction.
  B. Volume contraction results in increased sodium reabsorption by the proximal
tubules.
  C. Sodium reabsorption must be accompanied by parallel increased anion (Cl^-) reabsorption. To maintain electroneutrality in the
absence of resorbable anion, sodium may be
reabsorbed in exchange for a cation (H^+ or
K^+).
  D. To accommodate increased sodium
reabsorption, accelerated sodium-cation exchange (Na^+–K^+, or Na^+–H^+) occurs.
  E. Na^+–H^+ exchange results in reclamation of filtered HCO_3^- to the body, rather than
in the elimination of $NaHCO_3^-$ in urine,
which would have occurred if appropriate
resorbable anion had been available (i.e., if
Cl^- had been available for reabsorption along
with Na).

Potassium Depletion

K^+ depletion is usually associated with metabolic alkalosis. In acute conditions, K^+ depletion is a more likely result and not the cause
of alkalosis.

1. K^+ loss may occur within the same fluid
losses containing H^+ or Cl^-.
2. Accelerated sodium-cation exchange may
result in increased Na–K^+ exchange.

3. Hyperaldosteronism secondary to volume depletion may occur.

4. Chronic metabolic acidosis may result in "paradoxic" K^+ depletion due to enhanced renal potassium excretion.

Causes of Metabolic Alkalosis

1. Vomiting*
2. Diuretics (furosemide, thiazides)*
3. Alkali administration
4. Hyperaldosteronism
5. Post-chronic hypercapnia
6. Severe K^+ depletion

Signs of Metabolic Alkalosis

Signs of metabolic alkalosis are nonspecific but include possible seizures or tetany from neuromuscular effects. Signs of accompanying hypokalemia (see Chapter 25) are more likely to be detected.

Treatment

Most cases of metabolic alkalosis can be corrected rapidly to a normal pH by renal clearance of excess HCO_3^-, if adequate amounts of resorbable anion in the form of Cl^- can be supplied. This is usually achieved by administering .9% NaCl IV. Often Cl^- replacement alone allows correction of pH and restoration of K^+ stores in the body.

Because K^+ often is depleted in states of metabolic alkalosis, K^+ supplementation usually is administered in the .9% NaCl solution. There are some cases in which the alkalosis and hypochloremia are not corrected until adequate K^+ replacement has been accomplished (e.g., severe K^+ deficiency and states of hyperaldosteronism).

Respiratory Alkalosis

Primary respiratory alkalosis (alkalemia) exists when alkalemia is due to decreased PCO_2. Decreased PCO_2 can occur only through hyperventilation.

*Most importance in small animals.

Causes of Hyperventilation

1. Fear, anxiety; cortical stimulation
2. Intrathoracic disease, neural reflexes
3. CNS diseases, respiratory centers
4. Hypoxia, chemoreceptor stimulation
5. Fever, respiratory-center stimulation
6. Severe liver failure, mechanism unknown
7. Septicemia (gram-negative), mechanism unknown
8. Improper mechanical ventilation

Compensatory Physiologic Changes

1. Decreased PCO_2 immediately gives rise to some decrease in HCO_3^- generation by virtue of the hydration equation and mass law.
2. Decreased PCO_2 causes decreased HCO_3^- to be reclaimed to the body by renal mechanisms. This change takes several days to be maximally effective.
3. Compensatory mechanisms are more complete at minimizing pH changes in respiratory alkalosis than in respiratory acidosis.
4. Compensatory changes resulting in decreased HCO_3^- tend to maintain a more normal ratio of HCO_3^- to $\alpha \times PaCO_2$ and hence maintain a more normal pH.

Signs

No specific signs are likely to be detected in animals with respiratory alkalosis. Increases in respiratory effort, depth, or rate may not be detected clinically even though severe decreases in PCO_2 exist.

Treatment

Treatment consists solely of removing the underlying cause.

Suggested Readings

Cohen JJ, Kassierer JP: Acid–base metabolism. In Maxwell MH, Kleeman CR (eds): Clinical Disorders of Fluid and Electrolyte Metabolism. New York, McGraw-Hill, 1980

PART V

PHYSICAL AND CHEMICAL INJURIES

CHAPTER TWENTY-SEVEN

Physical Injuries

William R. Fenner, John S. Cave, and Roy Fenner

Smoke Inhalation

Smoke inhalation occurs as a result of injury to the respiratory system produced by inhalation of hot gasses. The injury may be clinically related to the effects of the heat, toxic effects of gasses, or both.

1. Hot smoke creates mucosal damage, leading to edema, ulcers, and abnormal secretion.
2. Thermal injury may cause laryngal spasm.
3. Carbon monoxide intoxication may occur, producing tissue hypoxia.
4. Sulfate, nitrate, and very hot particles (char) inflamme mucosa, causing excessive mucus production.
5. Alveolar flooding with edema fluid may occur as an acute or a delayed process.
6. Fatal chemical pneumonitis may occur as late as 48 hours after smoke inhalation.

Clinical Picture

1. The usual history is of an animal trapped in a building during a fire. On initial presentation, the patient may appear healthy except for conjunctivitis, corneal edema, an intense odor of smoke, and evidence of charred hair.
2. A severe, persistent moist cough from irritation of the tracheal bronchial tree and excess mucous production is the earliest sign.

3. In 48 to 72 hours, the full effects of the injury to the respiratory tree may be seen. Cyanosis and dyspnea develop as the lung loses its compliance and edema develops. Remember that carbon monoxide poisoning causes a bright pink color in the blood that will mask the presence of hypoxia, normally seen as cyanosis.
4. In advanced cases the patient may be in a coma from CNS hypoxia.

Management

1. Animals that develop severe pulmonary involvement 48 to 72 hours after the fire are usually difficult to save.
2. Give IV fluids to maintain hydration and prevent drying of the mucosa of the respiratory tree. IV fluids also help in maintaining a productive cough. Do not overhydrate, because this may cause pulmonary edema.
3. Give corticosteroids for the first two to three days; prednisolone; 4 mg/kg divided three times daily is used routinely.
4. Administer humidified oxygen to prevent mucosal drying. The oxygen is especially important if you suspect CO poisoning.
5. You also may use bronchodilators and expectorants.
6. The therapy for smoke inhalation is essentially the same as for any severe chemical pneumonitis.
7. The role of prophylactic antibiotics is not

as clear. At present there is no conclusive evidence they are beneficial.

Electric-Cord Bite

1. Electric-cord bite is believed to represent a form of acute left heart failure or cardiogenic shock (see Chapter 1, Shock). It may cause neurogenic pulmonary edema.

2. There are indications that electrical current may cause damage to pulmonary capillaries, with secondary transudation of fluid into alveoli.

Clinical Picture

1. Usually young animals (i.e., puppies or kittens) presented with acute dyspnea.

2. Oral examination often shows a blanched, seared area across the tongue or lips.

3. History may disclose that the animal has a habit of playing with electric cords.

4. The animal may appear normal soon after the injury and develop pulmonary edema one to two hours after the injury.

5. Chest roentgenograms show a distribution of pulmonary edema in the caudal dorsal lung fields.

6. ECG changes are uncommon but cardiac arrhythmias may be seen in some patients.

Management

1. Observe early cases two to three hours before releasing as uncomplicated.

2. Take immediate chest roentgenograms in dyspneic cases to assess the cause of the dyspnea.

3. Adminster oxygen therapy with a face mask, as needed, and administer furosemide (Lasix) 2 mg/kg as an immediate IV dose. Continue oxygen therapy until respiration has improved. The Lasix may need to be repeated.

4. If the animal has evidence of supraventricular cardiac arrhythmias, some clinicians recommend rapid digitalization. This therapy is controversial.

5. Treat the burn in the oral cavity based on the extent of the injury (see section on burns on pages 627–628).

Snake Bite

1. If it is known that poisonous reptiles are in the area, consider the possibility of snake bite whenever a pet is presented with unexplained swelling, bleeding, or severe pain. Animals may be in shock within minutes of a poisonous bite or have only slight swelling. Not all animals develop signs from the venom.

2. For the most part, venomous snakes in the continental United States inject toxins that cause tissue necrosis. Massive tissue necrosis is the hallmark of bites by these venomous snakes.

3. Wound infection is the hallmark of non-venomous snake bites. These bite wounds are usually less painful in the acute stages, with less pronounced swelling.

4. The severity of the injury from venomous snake bites is determined by the dose of venom injected and the location of the bite. The dose of venom depends on the length of time since the snake's last feeding and the size of the snake. The size of the animal bitten also will play role in the severity of the injury.

5. Bites around the head may cause severe swelling of the area, resulting in venous obstruction or respiratory distress. Clinically, bites on the body or legs are fatal more often than head and neck bites.

Clinical Picture

1. As a rule, the first signs of snake bite are swelling and pain in the area of the bite. Usually two small fang marks can be found, although careful examination and trimming of the hair around the site may be necessary to locate them; occasionally only one fang mark is present.

2. If much venom has been injected, the area around the fang marks begins to turn black and necrotic within a short time (as quickly as 30 minutes), and the blood becomes watery and dark. The hair and the first layer of epidermis may be lifted off easily; the tissue underneath is hemorrhagic. Swelling continues to develop proximally and distally from the wound for many hours and may extend to the lower chest and abdominal region in head and leg bites.

3. Some animals present in severe pain if a large amount of venom was injected; these animals may go into shock (see Chapter 1, Shock).

Treatment

1. If the bite is recent, excise the fang marks in a pluglike incision about .5 inches deep. This is said to remove most of the venom if done within 1 hour of the bite. Although this technique is performed often in human medicine, it is seldom possible in animals, except in wounds of the head, shoulder, or thigh. Open the fang marks to allow the venom and hemolyzed blood to escape. If the bite is on a limb, a light tourniquet may be applied above the swelling.

2. The single most effective treatment is polyvalent antivenin IV and lactated Ringer's solution. The dose of fluids is determined by the animal's size and clinical condition (see Chapter 24, Fluid Therapy). Institute broad spectrum antibiotics at that time and continue until the wound has healed. Some advocate the use of adrenocorticosteroids. Steroids (dexamethasone 2 mg/kg) are used if the animal is in shock or if there is severe tissue inflammation. If the swelling continues and the animal becomes depressed, repeat the antivenin administration. Clinically, it appears to be effective even if given 24 to 48 hours after the bite has occurred. A marked improvement may be seen within a few hours of antivenin administration. The local hospital emergency room may prove to be the best source of suitable antivenin in a crisis.

3. For economic reasons, it is advisable to discuss the use of antivenin with the client before its administration. Although antivenin's effects are life-saving and dramatic, some clients prefer not to incur the expense involved in its use.

4. If several hours have elapsed and the animal seems to have only minor symptoms

(e.g., the animal is lively, apparently feeling well, and has only minor swelling around the site of the bite after several hours), it may require only antibiotics, wound cleaning, and possibly steroids. It usually is safe to send the animal home with instructions to the owner to observe it for further problems. If it seems systemically ill or has severe swelling, however, it should be hospitalized and given supportive medication.

5. Frequently, tissue around the bite sloughs in several days. If the bite is on the head, the hemolyzed blood and local tissue edema may collect in the dependent tissues under the chin and neck and cause severe swelling. This area may slough, leaving open wounds. If this occurs, treat the animal by periodically trimming away the necrotic tissue, keeping the area clean, and using topical therapy until the wound has closed. This process may require several weeks, but generally the hair grows back and little scarring is visible.

Burns

Classification

1. First-degree—injury limited to epithelium. These injuries heal rapidly (usually in ten days or less). They are not serious and are rarely detected in the animal. They will not be covered in this section.

2. Second-degree—injury to the epidermis and superficial dermis. In these injuries, there is exuding of serum and blister formation, but the skin heals within two weeks.

3. Third-degree—In third-degree burns, the full thickness of the skin is destroyed.

Basic Principles

1. Burns may be caused by a variety of thermal agents, chemical agents, or both. Regardless of cause, the pathology to the tissues and the treatment are essentially the same.

2. It may be difficult initially to define the depth of a burn, so treat a significant area of the body around the burn aggressively and observe for the first 48 hours after presentation.

3. Thermal burns are often associated with smoke inhalation, so observe for signs of respiratory distress. Caustic burns are usually associated with ingestion of caustic substances, and the primary pathology is pharyngoesophageal injury.

4. The major complications of burns involving a significant amount of the body surface are fluid loss, protein loss, overwhelming septicemia, and oliguric renal failure.

5. Extensive burns of the trunk, burns of the esophagus, and burns of the respiratory tree (smoke inhalation) are frequently fatal.

Management

1. Assess the extent of the burn and provide the owner with information about the cost and extent of therapy required to treat the animal; treatment of burn patients is expensive.

2. Sedate the animal with a narcotic analgesic agent (or ketamine hydrochloride in the cat), gently clean and debride the area. Avoid hexacloraphene-based surgical soaps because they are readily absorbed through the burned skin and may cause nervous-system injury.

3. Dress wounds with mafenide (Sulfamylon) or silver sulfadiazine cream under loose gauze; change the bandages twice daily for the first three days.

4. Weigh extensively burned animals daily and monitor urine output. Make a conscientious effort to replace all fluid lost and maintain electrolyte balance. Treat the animal intravenously with balanced electrolyte solution until it is able to maintain hydration *per os*.

5. Periodically check white cell counts and differentials, BUN, serum electrolytes, and serum albumins to detect infection, hypoproteinemia, and renal failure. Plasma transfusion and oral high-protein alimentation are the most reliable sources of protein replacement. The alimentation is the most cost effective.

6. Administer broad-spectrum antibiotics such as cephalosporins or ampicillin–aminoglycocide combinations to help avoid septicemia. Systemic antibiotic therapy is no substitute for proper wound management; keep the wound clean and treated.

7. Esophageal injury is characterized by increased salivation and immediate regurgitation of anything that is ingested. Esophageal injuries are difficult to manage; corticosteroids are the mainstay of treatment, reducing inflammation and preventing scar-tissue formation. Administer prednisolone at 2 mg/kg bid for the first ten days, given by injection. Place a feeding-tube gastrostomy and feed the animal gruel until oral test feeding is successful. Use periodic esophagrams and esophagoscopy to assess the progress of the patient. In addition, you may use pharyngostomy tubes during the healing process.

8. In burn patients with smoke inhalation, treat the smoke inhalation as well as the cutaneous burns.

9. Assess electrical burns and treat for possible cardiopulmonary injury.

10. Remove burned pieces of skin that persist longer than one week to prevent abscesses under the devitalized skin. The contracture of the devitalized skin may cause decreased excursion of the rib cage and respiratory distress; if this occurs, remove the skin.

11. The use of homografts, allografts, or xenografts is beyond the scope of most veterinarians. If necessary, refer the animal to an institution that is familiar with the techniques for skin grafting. Fortunately, most defects close, even if they take many weeks to do so. During the healing process, maintain communication with the owner and have the animal return frequently for bandage changes.

Heat Stroke

1. Heat load exceeds heat dissipation. Because of their inferior capacity to exchange heat, this problem is more common in dogs and cats than in humans.

2. As heat increases, vasodilation leads to poor organ perfusion. Build-up of heat in excess of 107°F leads to tissue damage, secondary to the poor perfusion.

A. Cerebral congestion leads to intracranial hemorrhage, neuronal death, and necrosis.

B. Necrosis of the GI mucosa occurs.

C. Disseminated intravascular coagulation (DIC) results from the release of thromboplastin from necrotic tissue and of factor XII from endothelial injury.

D. There may be both hepatic and renal injury secondary to heat prostration.

Clinical Picture

1. Signs are generally seen during hot months, especially in animals that are confined in hot, poorly ventilated areas.

2. Signs include rapid respiration, tachycardia, depression, diarrhea, vomiting, dehydration, seizures, and collapse.

3. Temperature is generally in excess of 109°F.

4. DIC is a frequent complication. Animals with petechiae of mucous membranes generally have a grave prognosis.

5. Death usually follows the development of brain-stem signs (e.g., decrease in level of consciousness, opisthotonos, abnormal eye movement).

Management

1. Immediately sedate with acepromazine (Ayerst) .5 mg/kg IV.

2. Bathe animal in cold water or rubbing alcohol and place in front of a fan to speed evaporation.

3. Stop the fan and dry the animal after the temperature has dropped to 104°F. Check the animal's temperature every hour until stable. The thermal regulatory center often is deranged after heat prostration. If this occurs, the animal may be unable to maintain adequate body temperatures. If the animal becomes hypothermic, it may need to be kept warm with heating pads or blankets.

4. Place an indwelling IV catheter, and treat the animal for hypovolemic shock (see Chapter 1, Shock).

5. Monitor urine output; if oliguric renal failure develops, treat it vigorously. Renal failure generally develops within the first 24 hours of heat prostration.

6. Some clinicians provide prophylactic treatment of animals with temperatures greater than 110°F with sodium heparin, 200 U/kg SQ every four hours to prevent the development of DIC. This therapy is controversial.

Frostbite

1. In frostbite there is freezing of tissue with ice-crystal formation.

2. The most common location of frostbite seen in veterinary medicine is on the tips of the ear. This usually demarcates and sloughs with no complications.

3. The assessment of frostbite injuries is similar to the assessment of burns (see above). The extent of the injury may not be evident for the first 24 to 48 hours.

Management

1. Warm the frostbitten area in tepid water (104° to 105°F); keep the water tepid.

2. Do not rub the area because this may cause maceration of the tissues.

3. Bandage the area under cotton if possible.

4. Demarcation may take days to occur. Once the necrotic area sloughs or is excised, manage the wound either open or closed, depending on the size of the defect. If the frostbite involves an extremity, amputation is often necessary.

5. Do not allow a previously thawed area to refreeze.

CHAPTER TWENTY-EIGHT

Intoxications

Diane F. Gerken

General Considerations

1. Intoxication in an animal results from the accidental exposure to an agent in sufficient amounts to produce clinical illness. Many of the agents that cause problems in small animals are pharmacologic or abuse substances intended for their owners.

2. Signs of intoxication are usually rapid in onset and are frequently severe. Since most toxicants potentially can cause death, intoxications should be considered true emergencies.

3. The initial clinical signs frequently involve the GI tract, the nervous system, or both.

4. Since most of the clinical signs are nonspecific, a complete history is necessary to help determine the most likely cause of the toxicosis.

5. Many intoxications result in legal proceedings so every attempt should be made to confirm the diagnosis analytically and to document the history, presenting clinical signs, therapeutic measures, and response to therapy.

6. A partial differential diagnosis list is provided in this chapter along with information about frequently encountered toxins which cause severe clinical signs.

General Clinical Management

1. If a patient has no clinical signs, try to determine the likelihood of the exposure. With or without presenting clinical signs, there is a tendency to employ heroic measures that often are unnecessary. Many emergency treatments and pharmacologic agents are not without risk to the patient.

2. Treatment of toxicosis requires a calm, rational approach.

A. Maintain vital functions just as in any emergency.

B. Remove the toxicant to decrease adsorption.

  1) Oral exposure

  a) Induce vomiting if presentation is within four to six hours after exposure.

    i. Apomorphine

      A. May be given subcutaneously or placed in the conjunctival cul-de-sac.

      B. Acts centrally

      C. May cause respiratory depression and may be contraindicated in patients with CNS depression.

      D. Vomiting may not occur

if the stomach is empty. Giving fluids orally before inducing vomiting improves the effectiveness of the emetic.

E. A narcotic antagonist may be given for apomorphine-induced depression or protracted vomiting.

ii. Syrup of ipecac

A. Can be used by the owner before arrival at veterinary clinic

b) If vomiting is contraindicated (such as in unconscious seizuring or depressed patients, or patients that may have ingested petroleum distillates, strong acids or bases, and other antiemetics), begin gastric lavage if within four to six hours after exposure.

i. Always have an endotracheal tube with an inflated cuff in place before lavage.

ii. Use a large-bore stomach tube.

iii. Wash out stomach with large volumes of warm water or with isotonic fluids.

iv. Removal of large volumes of gastric contents can cause both electrolyte and acid–base abnormalities that may require correction. For this reason, periodic evaluation of systemic electrolytes is indicated.

c) Oral activated charcoal

i. Given to prevent initial absorption of toxin or prevent enterohepatic cycling of the toxin; may be given any time during toxicosis.

ii. Do not administer any other oral agents concurrently.

iii. Commercial formulations are readily available.

d) Sodium sulfate, magnesium sulfate cathartic, or mineral oil

i. Can be given alone or after activated charcoal to increase removal of toxin from the GI tract.

ii. Should not be given if toxin caused severe inflammation of the GI tract.

iii. Mineral oil but not vegetable oils may be effective if toxin is lipid-soluble.

2) Dermal exposure

a) Thorough bathing with mild soap and large volumes of water

C. Identify toxin if possible and treat accordingly.

1) Toxic ingredients in many household products, medications, pesticides, and automotive products can be identified by the local poison control center.

2) If antidote exists, give the antidote; if the antidote is not in your clinic, contact a local hospital or pharmacy. Few antidotes are approved for animal use, therefore most will be labeled for human use or will be available as chemicals.

D. Supportive therapy

1) Fluids to promote a mild to moderate diuresis

2) Correction of acid–base and electrolyte disturbances

3) Management of target tissue toxicity such as renal failure, hepatic failure, convulsions, coma, and body temperature

E. Remove toxin from environment to prevent reexposure.

Partial Differential Diagnosis List

Nervous System Signs

Depression

Chemicals

Ethylene glycol
Anticoagulant rodenticides

Petroleum distillates
Organophosphates (OP)/carbamates
Ethanol, methanol, isopropanol
Glue, adhesives
DEET
Naphthalene
Bromethalin
Cholecalciferol

Drugs

THC
Acetaminophen, salicylates, ibuprofen
Barbiturates
Ivermectin
Benzodiazepines
5-fluorouracil

Blindness

Antidandruff shampoos
Methanol
Lead
Mercury

Seizures/Excitement

Chemicals

OP/carbamates
Chlorinated hydrocarbons
Strychnine
Camphor
Carbon monoxide
Lead
Phenol
Cyanide
Chocolate
4-aminopyridine
DEET
Pyrethrins/pyrethroids
Bromethalin
Methaldehyde
1080

Drugs

Antidepressants
Antipsychotics
β blockers (propranolol)
Hypoglycemic agents
Methylxanthines
Narcotic analgesics
Amphetamine

Phenylpropanolamine
Antihistamines
Atropine
Cocaine
Bronchodilators (terbutaline)
PCP

Tremors (from Fasciculations to Rigidity)

Chemicals

OP/carbamates
2,4-D
Metaldehyde
Strychnine
Pyrethrins/pyrethroids
4-aminopyridine
Chlorinated hydrocarbons
DEET
Naphthalene
Bromethalin
Phenols
Snake bite (pit vipers)

Drugs

Ivermectin
Cocaine

Gastrointestinal Signs

Vomiting

Chemicals

Ethylene glycol
Detergents, bleach
Lead
Chocolate
Chlorinated hydrocarbons
Naphthalene
Arsenic
Bromethalin
Cholecalciferol
Phenols
Isopropanol
Borates
Pine oil
Metaldehyde
Petroleum distillates
Poinsettia
Philodendron

Drugs

Ibuprofen
Zinc oxide
Acetaminophen
Aspirin
5-fluorouracil

Diarrhea

Detergents
OP/carbamate
Arsenic
Borates

Salivation

Chemicals

Drain cleaners
Oxalate containing plants
Chlorinated hydrocarbons
Pyrethrins/pyrethroids
DEET
OP/carbamates
Arsenic
Phenols
Borates
Pine oil
Snake bite (pit vipers)
Limonene

Drugs

Ivermectin
PCP
5-fluorouracil

Lead

1. General
   A. Sources—paint, linoleum, plaster, caulking compounds, plumbing materials, batteries, golf balls, solder, certain roof coverings, improperly glazed water bowls, fishing sinkers, drapery weights, and toys
   B. Presentation often similar to canine distemper
   C. Often occurs in young dogs because of chewing habits
2. Clinical presentation
   A. GI signs (may slightly precede neurologic signs)
      1) Abdominal pain
      2) Vomiting
      3) Anorexia
      4) Intermittent diarrhea
   B. Neurologic signs
      1) Seizures
      2) Hysteria
      3) Behavioral changes
      4) Blindness
3. Laboratory diagnosis
   A. Nucleated RBC without severe anemia
   B. RBC may have basophilic stippling or have other abnormal morphology.
   C. Blood lead concentration
      1) Inquire from laboratory whether a EDTA or heparin anticoagulant is necessary. Do not submit only serum or plasma since 90% of the circulating lead is found in the RBC. Severe anemia may affect interpretation of this parameter.
      2) Laboratory result above 60 μg/dL is considered diagnostic of lead intoxication.
      3) If laboratory result is between 25 and 60 μg/dL and patient is showing clinical signs, lead poisoning must be considered in the differential diagnosis.
   D. Abdominal radiographs may show radiopaque material—should be performed since chelation therapy can promote adsorption from the GI tract.
4. Therapy
   A. Prevent further absorption before beginning chelation therapy.
      1) Remove lead from GI tract using a cathartic or an emetic.
      2) Chelate absorbed lead with calcium disodium EDTA 100 mg/kg per day for two to five days diluted with 5% dextrose (final concentration, 10 mg EDTA/mL) for subcutaneous administration.
      3) Some dogs may require a repeat treatment after five days but this second treatment should not be started until after a short rest period.
      4) As an alternative therapy or a follow-up treatment, a patient may be given oral penicillamine at a dosage of 100 mg/kg daily for one to four weeks.
      5) If neurologic signs continue after starting EDTA therapy, steroids may be given to treat the cerebral edema.

6) If seizures persist, a short-acting anticonvulsant should be given.

Prognosis

Prognosis is good if the neurologic signs diminish with treatment.

Organophosphate and Carbamate

General Considerations

1. Compounds are effective insecticides and can be found in many commercial formulations including external parasiticides.
2. Usually the label will indicate if the one ingredient is an organophosphate/carbamate by identifying atropine as a treatment.
3. Clinical signs are indicative of central and peripheral cholinesterase inhibition.
4. Cats may be more susceptible to some compounds.
5. There may be a drug interaction with these insecticides and phenothiazine tranquilizers.

Clinical Presentation

1. Vomiting, diarrhea, salivation, urination
2. Muscle tremors progressing to paralysis
3. Miosis
4. Dyspnea due to excessive secretions
5. Usually CNS depression; occasionally CNS stimulation
6. Either bradycardia or tachycardia

Laboratory Diagnosis

1. RBC, whole blood, or plasma cholinesterase
   A. Pseudo or nonspecific cholinesterase is found in the plasma and liver.
   B. True cholinesterase is found in the RBC and in target tissues.
   C. >50% depression of plasma or RBC activity may result in cholinergic signs.
   D. The results of this test may be difficult to interpret for exposures to carbamates since carbamates are reversible inhibitors of cholinesterase.

Therapy

1. Administer atropine sulfate until signs of atropinization are seen; usually sufficient atropine has been given when a tachycardia is observed.
   A. Atropine sulfate should be given every four to six hours to maintain atropinization throughout the course of toxicosis.
   B. Atropine will alleviate the parasympathetic signs but not the muscle tremors.
2. Pralidoxime or 2-PAM—most effective if used within the first 24 hours after exposure
   A. 20 to 50 mg/kg given intravenously or intramuscularly
   B. Do not administer alone but in conjunction with atropine.
   C. Do not administer for carbamate toxicities.

Prognosis

If treatment is early in the toxicosis and treatment is maintained over a sufficient period of time, prognosis is good.

Ethylene Glycol

General Considerations

1. Sources—automobile antifreeze coolant, rust remover
2. A lethal dose in dogs can be as low as 4 mL/kg and in cats as low as 1.5 mL/kg.
3. Early clinical signs are the result of ethylene glycol toxicity but the later, more severe clinical signs are the result of ethylene glycol metabolism. Therapy is aimed at blocking the metabolism of ethylene glycol while promoting excretion of ethylene glycol and metabolites.
4. Animals may die from this poisoning from 12 hours to 7 days after ingestion.

Clinical Presentation

1. Vomiting
2. Disorientation, ataxia
3. Tachypnea
4. Animal may appear to recover within the first 12 hours after exposure.

5. Decreased awareness
6. Initial polydipsia and polyuria progressing to oliguria
7. Renal pain
8. Seizures, coma

Laboratory Diagnosis

1. Blood—clinical chemistry
  A. Early in poisoning, hyperosmolality
  B. Electrolyte abnormalities
    1) Increased potassium
    2) Decreased calcium
    3) Severe acidosis
    4) Large anion gap—>40 to 50 mEq/L
    5) Increased BUN
    6) Increased creatinine
2. Urinalysis
  A. Decreased specific gravity
  B. Hematuria
  C. Proteinuria
  D. Ca^{++} oxalate crystals

Therapy

1. Give activated charcoal.
2. Correct acid–base abnormalities.
3. Correct electrolyte abnormalities.
4. Promote excretion of unmetabolized ethylene glycol by blocking ethylene glycol metabolism with intravenous ethanol.
  A. Dose for dog—5.5 mL/kg of 20% ethanol every four hours for five treatments, then every six hours for four treatments
  B. Dose for cats—5 mL/kg of 20% ethanol intraperitoneally every six hours for five treatments, then every eight hours for four treatments
  C. Although ethanol therapy may add to CNS depression and promote pulmonary edema because of the increased fluids, ethanol is indicated in a patient present within 24 hours of exposure or before renal failure.
5. Treat renal disease
  A. Diuresis—Use either intravenous mannitol or furosemide and maintain until oxalate crystals in urine are gone.
  B. Dialysis—either peritoneal or hemodialysis if available

Prognosis

Prognosis is grave in all cases unless all recommended treatments are instituted within hours of exposure.

Strychnine

General Considerations

1. Strychnine is a plant alkaloid used as a rodenticide and previously as a gastric stimulant in large-animal practice.
2. Strychnine interfers with the spinal inhibitory neurons; therefore, the clinical signs are a result of the continual firing of the spinal excitatory neurons.
3. Clinical signs may be observed within 30 minutes after ingestion and death may occur in less than one hour.

Clinical Presentation

1. Apprehension
2. Muscular rigidity
3. Violent seizures, often induced by noise or stimulation
4. Extreme extensor rigidity
5. Hyperthermia secondary to muscular exertion

Laboratory Diagnosis

Perform a strychnine chemical analysis of vomitus or stomach contents.

Therapy

1. Prevent further absorption
  A. If patient is conscious and not showing clinical signs, induce vomiting and give activated charcoal.
  B. If patient is showing clinical signs, do not try to induce vomiting since any procedure may initiate seizures.
  C. If patient shows clinical signs, anesthetize patient and perform gastric lavage.
2. Treat seizures and muscle spasms
  A. Intravenous Valium (0.25 to 0.5 mg/kg as needed to effect) or sufficient pentobarbi-

tal intravenously to maintain muscle relaxation

B. Inhalation anesthesia may be required.

C. Intravenous glyceryl guaiacolate (110 mg/kg) may be given if the above do not produce adequate relaxation.

D. Intravenous methocarbamol (150 mg/kg) has been used to control seizures.

3. Supportive treatment

A. A respirator may be required to maintain respiration.

B. Lower body temperature if hyperthermic.

C. Institute fluid therapy to enhance diuresis.

Prognosis

1. If therapy is instituted rapidly, most animals will recover uneventfully.

2. If the animal survives the first 24 hours after exposure, there is a good chance of recovery, although the animal may need to be treated for up to three days.

Amphetamine and Amphetaminelike Compounds

General Considerations

1. Usually from exposure to owners medication—includes amphetamine, methamphetamine, and dextroamphetamine. They are commonly prescribed to humans for weight reduction, fatigue, depression, and hyperactive children.

2. These drugs are potent stimulators of the sympathetic nervous system and cardiovascular system.

Clinical Presentation

1. Cardiovascular

A. Accelerated heart rate

B. Increased blood pressure

2. CNS

A. Pupil dilation

B. Excitement

C. Agitation

D. Confusion

E. Delerium

F. Convulsions

3. Systemic

A. Hyperthermia

B. Increased metabolic rate

Laboratory Diagnosis

Perform an amphetamine chemical analysis of urine.

Therapy

1. Acepromazine maleate at a dose of 0.2 mg/kg intramuscular or thorazine 0.5 to 1.0 mg/kg intramuscular.

2. Treatment with intravenous Valium may be necessary to eliminate convulsive activity. If a barbiturate is used in conjunction with tranquilizers, be careful to avoid excessive depression of the CNS.

3. Hyperthermia—Temperatures up to 106°F are not uncommon. Give ice-water baths as necessary to get the temperature down. Check temperature frequently.

Metaldehyde

General Considerations

1. Methaldehyde has recently become popular as a snail, slug, and rat bait, usually spread on gardens and yards during spring and early summer for killing snails and slugs. The toxic dose is 400 mg/kg of body weight.

2. Clinical syndrome may be due to extreme acidosis.

Clinical Presentation

1. Lack of coordination and slight muscle tremor

2. Anxiety or agitation

3. The muscle tremors may become continuous and severe, but they are not increased with auditory or tactile stimulation, as happens with strychnine.

4. Hyperthermia, again secondary to muscle tremor

5. Polypnea and tachycardia

Laboratory Diagnosis

1. Acidosis
2. Acetaldehyde chemical analysis of the stomach contents

Therapy

1. Remove unabsorbed material either by gastric lavage or induced vomiting.
2. Treat muscle tremors; give methocarbamol (Robaxin) IM 150 mg/kg; xylazine (Rompun) slowly to effect; or Valium intravenously to effect.
3. In severe cases, general anesthesia may be required.
4. Give fluid therapy to maintain hydration and to correct acidosis.

Chlorinated Hydrocarbon

General Considerations

1. Used mainly as insecticides
2. Long biologic half-life
3. Known hepatic enzyme inducers

Clinical Presentation

1. Muscle tremors
2. Exaggerated response to stimuli
3. Generalized seizures
4. May become comatose

Laboratory Diagnosis

None

Therapy

1. Control seizures with light anesthesia.
2. Sedatives for excitability; do not use phenothiazines because they lower seizure threshold.
3. Activated charcoal to promote excretion

Prognosis

Guarded; there is no antidote.

Marijuana

General Considerations

Source of intoxication is accidental ingestion of owner's marijuana or hashish. Sometimes owners will give their dogs marijuana to "share their experience."

Clinical Presentation

1. Excitability or depression
2. Disorientation
3. Ataxia
4. Weakness
5. The most characteristic feature of marijuana intoxication is the rapidly changing nature of the clinical signs.

Laboratory Diagnosis

1. Perform a chemical analysis of urine.

Therapy

1. Give an emetic if presentation within four to six hours.
2. Keep the animal quiet.
3. Supportive care

Prognosis

Good, but complete recovery may require two to three days.

Xanthine

General Considerations

1. Substances included in the xanthine group are caffeine, theobromine, and theophylline. These compounds may be found in chocolate, over-the-counter human medications, and veterinary medications.
2. Theobromine has a long plasma half-life in the dog (17 hours).

Clinical Presentation

1. Excitability
2. Restlessness

3. Tremors
4. Cardiac arrhythmias
5. Seizures
6. Marked increase in urine volume
7. Vomiting and diarrhea
8. Coma

Laboratory Diagnosis

Perform a chemical analysis of these compounds in urine and blood.

Therapy

1. Give emetic if presentation within four to six hours after exposure.
2. Give activated charcoal to promote elimination.
3. Treat cardiac arrhythmias according to the cardiac abnormality.
4. Control seizures and muscle tremors.
5. Supportive therapy

Prognosis

Prognosis is good if treated aggressively and early after exposure.

Corrosives and Coal-Tar Derivatives

General Considerations

1. Substances found in this group of compounds are strong acids, and bases such as phenol, creosote, creosol, naphthol, tannic acid, wood tar, and others.
2. These compounds primarily cause corrosion of the skin and mucous membranes.
3. Cats are especially sensitive to the phenolic compounds because of species metabolism differences.

Clinical Presentation

1. Corrosive
   A. Edematous and hemorrhagic skin or mucous membranes depending on route of exposure
   B. Vomiting if oral exposure
2. If mildly or noncorrosive
   A. Depression, weakness

   B. Muscle fasciculations
   C. Dyspnea and perhaps seizures
   D. Icterus

Laboratory Diagnosis

1. Intravascular hemolysis of red blood cells; anemia
2. Increased bilirubin
3. Increased BUN and creatinine
4. Positive urine test for phenolic compounds
   A. Add 1 mL of ferric chloride to 10 mL urine.
   B. A violet or blue color is positive.

Therapy

1. Neutralize strong acids and bases.
   A. Acids—Give 5% sodium bicarbonate for dermal exposure only.
   B. Bases—Give vinegar.
2. Do not induce vomiting with exposure to strong acids or bases since there is a risk of more esophageal damage.
3. Gastric lavage to remove the substance
4. Bathe animal if exposure was dermal.
5. Supportive therapy

Prognosis

Prognosis is guarded in animals with clinical signs.

Salicylate (Aspirin)

General Considerations

1. Aspirin is in the process of being approved by the FDA for use in dogs.
2. Conditions for acute poisoning are accidental ingestion of owner's medication or overdosing of medication by owner.

Clinical Presentation

1. Depression
2. Vomiting and dehydration
3. Tachypnea
4. Elevated temperature

5. Progressing to possible seizures, weakness, and shock

6. Adverse effects from chronic exposure may be anemia, hepatitis, and bleeding disorders.

Laboratory Diagnosis

1. Severe acid–base dysfunction
   A. Initial respiratory alkalosis
   B. Metabolic acidosis
2. Chemical screening test for urine
   A. Add 2 drops of 10% ferric chloride to 2 mL urine.
   B. Urine turns dark red if salicylates are present.

Therapy

1. Give an emetic if within hours of ingestion.
2. Treat shock.
3. Correct acid–base status.
4. Treat seizures.
5. Give activated charcoal.
6. Excretion can be increased by alkalinization of urine with intravenous sodium bicarbonate.
7. Platelet replacement for bleeding disorder

Prognosis

Prognosis is good if treated early.

Acetaminophen

General Considerations

1. This product should not be used therapeutically in dogs or cats because of its toxicity and the availability of therapeutic alternatives.
2. Cats are intoxicated at lower doses than dogs. One 500-mg capsule can produce toxic signs in a cat.

Clinical Presentation

1. Depression
2. Anorexia
3. Cyanosis, tachypnea

4. Facial edema
5. Vomiting and abdominal pain
6. Chocolate colored urine/hematuria

Laboratory Diagnosis

1. Elevated liver enzymes and methemoglobinemia in dogs
2. Methemoglobinemia and Heinz body anemia in cats

Therapy

1. Induce vomiting if within hours of ingestion.
2. Activated charcoal
3. N-acetylcysteine (Mucomyst) administration orally or intravenously
4. Vitamin C to treat the methemoglobinemia
5. Supportive therapy

Prognosis

Prognosis is poor if severe anemia, methemoglobinemia, or hepatic necrosis are present.

Tranquilizer (Phenothiazine Class)

General Considerations

Animals may get access to opened bottles of medication and ingest them. The primary effect of these drugs are depression and hypotension.

Clinical Presentation

1. Marked depression, perhaps coma
2. Hypotensive shock

Laboratory Diagnosis

None

Therapy

1. Supportive care
2. Time to metabolize the drug
3. Induction of vomiting (only if the animal is alert)

Table 28-1. Plants commonly involved in poisoning

Name	Poisonous Part of Plant Active Principle if Known	Clinical Findings	Treatment
Arum family; calla lily, elephant ear (Dieffenbachia, Caladium, Alocasia, Colocasia, Philodendron)	All parts	Severe irritation of mucous membranes, nausea and vomiting, diarrhea, salivation; no direct systemic effects	Give demulcents (milk, oil) per os.
Oleander (Nerium oleander)	All parts (oleandrin)	Same as for digitalis	Treat as for digitalis.
Yew (Taxus)	Wood, bark, leaves, seeds	Nausea, vomiting, diarrhea, abdominal pain, dyspnea, dilated pupils, weakness, convulsions, shock, coma	*
Bird of Paradise (Caesalpinia gilliesii)	Seed pod	Nausea, vomiting, diarrhea	*Give milk, beaten eggs, liquid petrolatum; replace fluid.
Buckeye (Aesculus species)	Seed (a glycoside)	Nausea, vomiting, diarrhea, weakness and paralysis	*
Cherry (Prunus species)	Seed (amygdalin)	Stupor, vocal-cord paralysis, twitching, convulsions, and coma from chewing seeds	*Treat cyanide poisoning.
Chrysanthemum	All parts (a resin)	Exudative dermatitis from sensitivity	Wash skin.
Crowfoot family	All parts	Nausea, vomiting, diarrhea, restlessness, weak pulse, and convulsions	*Artificial resuscitation; maintain blood pressure.
Finger cherry (Rhodomyrtus macrocarpa)	Fruit	Complete and permanent blindness within 24 hours	*
Holly (Ilex species)	Berries	Vomiting, diarrhea, narcosis	*
Hydrangea	All parts (cyanogenetic)	Dizziness, respiratory stimulation, tachycardia, convulsions	*Treat cyanide poisoning.
Indian tobacco (Lobelia inflata)	All parts (α-lobeline)	Progressive vomiting, weakness, stupor, tremors, pinpoint pupils, and unconsciousness	*Give artificial respiration. Give atropine, 2 mg SQ.
Iris (Iridaceae)	Root	Nausea, violent diarrhea	*
Jessamine (Gelsemium sempervirens)	All parts (gelsemine and related alkaloids)	Muscular weakness, convulsions, and respiratory failure	*Give atropine, 2 mg (1/30 gr) SQ every 4 hr. Perform artificial respiration.

Plant	Toxic parts (toxin)	Symptoms	Treatment
Laurel (Kalmia species)	All parts (andromedotoxin)	Salivation, increased tear formation, nasal discharge, vomiting, convulsions, slow pulse, and paralysis	*
Lupin, lupine (Lupinus species)	All parts, especially berries (lupinine and related alkaloids)	Paralysis, weak pulse, depressed breathing, and convulsions	*Give artificial respiration; treat convulsions.
Machineel (Hippomane mancinella)	Sap	Severe irritation, blistering, peeling of skin from contact with the sap	Wash with soap and water or alcohol.
Mistletoe (Phoradendron flavescens)	All parts but especially in berries	Vomiting, diarrhea, and slowed pulse similar to digitalis	Treat as for digitalis.
Poinsettia (Euphorbia plucherrima)	Leaves, stems, sap	Irritation, vesication, gastroenteritis	*Wash sap from skin with soap and water.
Primrose (Primula species)	Stems and leaves	Skin reddening and irritation, itching, swelling, and blistering on contact with the plant	Wash skin with rubbing alcohol.
Privet (Ligustrum vulgare)	Berries and leaves	Gastrointestinal irritation and renal damage	*
Rayless goldenrod (Happlopappus heterophyllus)	All parts (tremetol)	Milk from animals that have been fed on white snakeroot or rayless goldrod causes nausea, loss of appetite, weakness, severe vomiting, jaundice from liver damage, constipation, and convulsions. There may be oliguria or anuria from kidney damage.	Treat liver damage; treat anuria.
Peas (Lathyrus species)	All parts but especially seeds	Paralysis, weak pulse, depressed breathing, and convulsions	*Give artificial respiration; treat convulsions.
Wild aconite (Gloriosa superba)	All parts	Pain in the abdomen, vomiting, bloody diarrhea, ataxia, convulsions, coma, and respiratory failure	*
Wisteria	All parts	Gastric upset, vomiting	*

*Remove ingested poison by gastric lavage or emesis. Treat symptoms.
(Adapted from Dreisbach RH: Poisoning, 6th ed. Palo Alto, Lange Publications, 1969)

Prognosis

Prognosis is good with proper supportive therapy.

Anticoagulant Rodenticides

General Considerations

1. These pesticides are often formulated with a blue-green dye added to the bait. This dye will not be absorbed by the gastro-intestinal tract and result in blue-green feces or vomitus. Not all rodenticides with blue-green dye added to the bait are anticoagulants.
2. These rodenticides block the recycling of vitamin K in the liver, thereby blocking the synthesis of clotting factors. Therapy is directed to providing sufficient vitamin K while the rodenticide is being metabolized and excreted. Length of therapy is dependent on the chemical structure of each compound and may vary from seven days for warfarin to five to six weeks with diphacinone.
3. Because of the chemical nature of the newer long-acting rodenticides, clinical presentation of an animal may be delayed until 5 to 8 days after a single oral exposure.

Clinical Presentation

1. Weakness
2. Dyspnea and pale mucous membranes
3. External signs of subcutaneous hemorrhage, occasionally epistaxis, bloody stools, or hematuria are observed; abnormally prolonged bleeding from venipuncture sites
4. Animal becomes progressively weaker and has cold extremities; death occurs within 24 hours after onset of clinical signs.

Laboratory Diagnosis

1. Abnormally low PCV and red cell count: usually platelet count is normal.
2. Prolonged prothrombin time; may have prolonged partial thromboplastin time; decreased Factor II (prothrombin), VII, IX, and X blood concentrations.
3. Abnormal blood vitamin K oxide: vitamin K ratio

Therapy

1. Oral vitamin K_1 administration: only vitamin K_1 should be given
A. Give orally with some type of fat-containing material; grind up tablets in a gruel of canned dog food. Vitamin K is a fat soluble vitamin which requires bile salts for absorption. When vitamin K is administered orally, it is transported directly to the target tissue, the liver.
B. May be given subcutaneously when tissue perfusion is adequate
C. Should not be administered intravenously unless diluted in fluids because of anaphylactic shock
D. Should not be administered intramuscularly until coagulation times are normal due to the risk of life-threatening intramuscular hemorrhage
E. In severe cases, administer 5 mg/kg q12h as a loading dose and maintain animals on 3 to 5 mg/kg daily for several weeks if rodenticide is not warfarin. Re-evaluate the clotting status after a 24 hour withdrawal from vitamin K. If coagulation times are abnormal, resume therapy for at least one week. The animal may need to be treated for as long as six weeks especially if the animal ingested the rodenticide more than one time.
F. If the animal ingested warfarin, treat the animal with oral vitamin K for seven days.

Prognosis

Prognosis is excellent if treated early.

Suggested Readings

Ellenhorn and Barceloux: Medical Toxicology, New York, Elsevier, 1988
Kirk RW (ed): Current Veterinary Therapy, 10th ed. Philadelphia, WB Saunders, 1989
Lampe and McCann: AMA Handbook of Poisonous and Injurious Plants, Chicago, Chicago Review Press, 1985
Osweiler, Carson, Buck, Van Gelder: Clinical and Diagnostic Veterinary Toxicology, 3rd ed. Dubuque, Kendall/Hunt Publishing, 1985

INDEX

Page numbers in italics refer to illustrations; page numbers followed by t refer to tables.